Diagnostic Radiology

Diagnostic Radiology

Editor: Coby Hawkins

FOSTER ACADEMICS

www.fosteracademics.com

www.fosteracademics.com

FOSTER ACADEMICS

Cataloging-in-Publication Data

Diagnostic radiology / edited by Coby Hawkins.
p. cm.
Includes bibliographical references and index.
ISBN 978-1-63242-629-1
1. Diagnostic imaging. 2. Medical radiology. 3. Radiography, Medical.
4. Diagnosis, Radioscopic. I. Hawkins, Coby.
RC78.7.D53 D53 2019
616.075 4--dc23

Foster Academics,
118-35 Queens Blvd., Suite 400,
Forest Hills, NY 11375, USA

ISBN 978-1-63242-629-1 (Hardback)

Contents

Preface

The world is advancing at a fast pace like never before. Therefore, the need is to keep up with the latest developments. This book was an idea that came to fruition when the specialists in the area realized the need to coordinate together and document essential themes in the subject. That's when I was requested to be the editor. Editing this book has been an honour as it brings together diverse authors researching on different streams of the field. The book collates essential materials contributed by veterans in the area which can be utilized by students and researchers alike.

Radiology is a medical specialty, which uses imaging techniques for the treatment and diagnosis of diseases occurring in the human body. Ultrasound, x-ray radiography, computed tomography (CT), magnetic resonance imaging (MRI) and positron emission tomography (PET) are some of the techniques used. Some of the subspecialties in radiology are musculoskeletal imaging, neuroradiology, pediatric radiology, nuclear medicine, emergency radiology, etc. Various forms of arthritis, congenital skeletal anomalies, bone tumors and fractures can be diagnosed by projectional radiography. Similarly using low energy projectional radiography, such as in dual-energy X-ray absorptiometry (DXA) and mammography, osteoporosis and breast cancer may be evaluated. CT scanning is the preferred diagnostic technique for detecting cerebral hemorrhage, aortic dissection, pulmonary embolism, appendicitis, etc. The various studies that are constantly contributing towards advancing technologies and evolution of diagnostic radiology are examined in detail in this book. It attempts to understand the diagnostic techniques used in this field and how such concepts have practical applications. It is a vital tool for all researching or studying diagnostic radiology as it gives incredible insights into emerging trends and concepts.

Each chapter is a sole-standing publication that reflects each author's interpretation. Thus, the book displays a multi-facetted picture of our current understanding of application, resources and aspects of the field. I would like to thank the contributors of this book and my family for their endless support.

Editor

1

An Unusual Case of Laryngeal Paraganglioma in a Patient with Carotid Body Paraganglioma: Multimodality Imaging Findings

Serap Dogan,[1] Serkan Senol,[1] Hakan Imamoglu,[1] Ummuhan Abdulrezzak,[2] Afra Ekinci,[1] Imdat Yuce,[3] and Mustafa Ozturk[1]

[1]*Department of Radiology, Erciyes University Medical Faculty, Kayseri, Turkey*
[2]*Department of Nuclear Medicine, Erciyes University Medical Faculty, Kayseri, Turkey*
[3]*Department of Otorhinolaryngology, Erciyes University Medical Faculty, Kayseri, Turkey*

Correspondence should be addressed to Serap Dogan; drserapdogan@hotmail.com

Academic Editor: Daniel P. Link

Multiple paragangliomas of the head and neck are rare conditions. Carotid paragangliomas are most common multiple paragangliomas. Laryngeal paragangliomas are very rare neuroendocrine tumors and usually are seen as symptomatic solitary lesions. We present multimodality imaging findings of incidentally detected laryngeal paraganglioma in a woman with synchronous carotid body paraganglioma and positive family history. To the best of our knowledge, this is the first case of laryngeal and carotid body paragangliomas in a patient with positive family history. Radiologists should keep in mind that paragangliomas may occur in various locations as multiple tumors.

1. Introduction

Head and neck paragangliomas (HNP) are rare neuroendocrine neoplasms. They represent 0.03% of all neoplasms and 0.6% of head and neck neoplasms [1]. The most common locations of HNP are carotid body, jugular bulb, tympanic plexus, and vagal ganglia. Other less common sites are nose, paranasal sinus, nasopharynx, larynx, parotid gland, orbit, thyroid, and thoracic inlet. Although paragangliomas are usually solitary, multiple tumors may occur in approximately 10% of sporadic tumors and 40% of the familial variety [2]. Carotid body with jugular and/or vagal paraganglioma, tympanic with vagal paraganglioma, has been reported as most common combinations [3, 4]. To the best of our knowledge there are only two cases of laryngeal with carotid body paraganglioma as a rare combination [5, 6]. Familial relationship was not mentioned in these cases. Herein we present a case of laryngeal with carotid body paraganglioma in a patient with positive family history.

2. Case Report

A 32-year-old woman presented with swelling in the left neck for the past 1.5 years. She was a nonsmoker and nondrinker. Her past medical history was negative but her mother was operated on for carotid body paraganglioma. On physical examination, mobile, soft, 1.5 cm mass was palpated anterior to the sternocleidomastoid muscle on left side. There were no cranial nerve palsies or neck lymphadenopathy. A thorough review of other systems was negative. Laryngoscopic examination was not remarkable. Blood and urine catecholamine levels were normal.

On ultrasound (US) exam well defined, oval shaped, hypoechoic, solid, 25 × 32 mm hypervascular mass was seen at the left carotid bifurcation (Figures 1(a) and 1(b)). Splaying of the internal and external carotid arteries and hypervascularity suggested that paraganglioma and thereby fine needle aspiration biopsy were not applied. Contrast enhanced computed tomography (CT) revealed hypervascular mass in the same region (Figure 2(a)). Additionally, well defined,

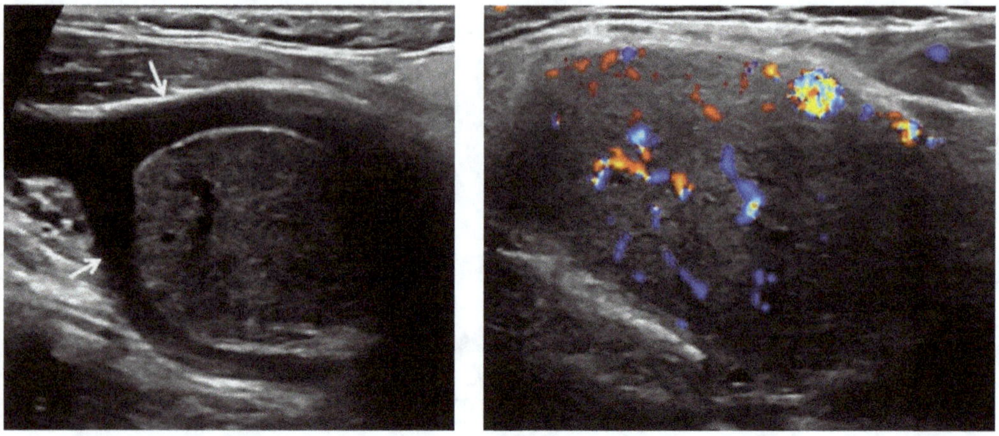

(a) (b)

FIGURE 1: Gray-scale ultrasound (a) shows well defined, solid mass that causes splaying of the internal and external carotid arteries (arrows). High vascularity of lesions is seen in Doppler ultrasound image (b).

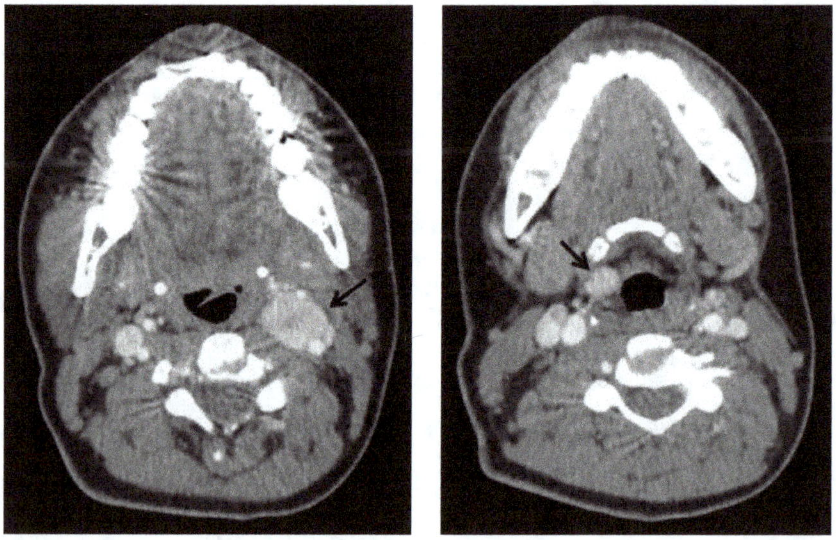

(a) (b)

FIGURE 2: Axial contrast enhanced computed tomography demonstrates vascular mass (arrow) at left carotid bifurcation (a). Right supraglottic, well defined laryngeal mass (arrow) is seen in lower level contrast enhanced computed tomography image (b).

ovoid, 10 × 12 mm hypervascular mass was seen in the right preepiglottic space (Figure 2(b)). Magnetic resonance imaging (MRI) was performed for further characterization. MRG demonstrated that both lesions had similar imaging features including isointense on T1W, hyperintense on T2W images, and homogeneous intense enhancement (Figures 3(a) and 3(b)). Imaging findings were suggestive of multicentric HNP.

Because of multicentricity and positive family history, Gallium-68 (Ga-68) DOTA-peptide positron emission tomography/computer tomography (PET/CT) was performed to verify the diagnosis and disclose whether or not another focus of paraganglioma exists anywhere in the body. 68Ga-DOTANOC PET/CT showed the laryngeal lesion with intense tracer uptake (SUV max: 35.8) and carotid body paraganglioma (SUV max: 37.5) (Figures 4(a), 4(b), 4(c), 4(d), and 4(e)). 68Ga-DOTANOC PET/CT demonstrated no additional abnormality apart from these two lesions.

Digital subtraction angiography (DSA) demonstrated right superior thyroid artery supplied laryngeal mass and left ascending pharyngeal artery supplied mass at carotid bifurcation (Figures 5(a) and 5(b)). The mass located carotid bifurcation was embolized using microcatheter with 250–350 sized polyvinyl alcohol particles (Figure 5(c)). Balloon occlusion test of the left internal carotid artery was performed and it was tolerated without any neurological deficit. Surgery was performed following embolization.

The pathologic diagnosis was paraganglioma. Microscopically, the well encapsulated tumor made characteristic clear cell nests with Zellballen pattern. Immunohistochemical analysis showed tumor cells positive for chromogranin

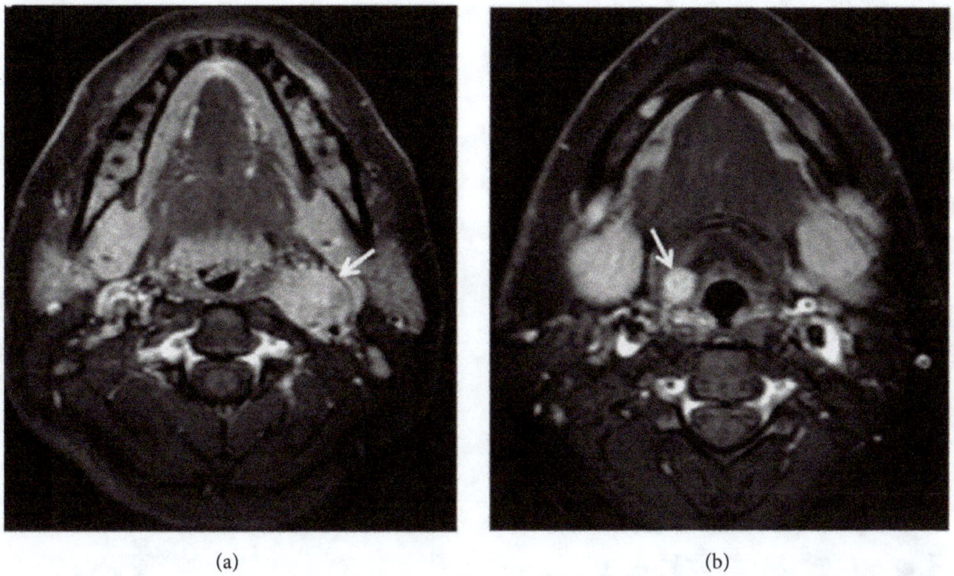

FIGURE 3: Enhanced lesions (arrows) are seen at left carotid bifurcation (a) and right supraglottic larynx (b) in axial contrast enhanced T1 weighted turbo spin echo spectral fat saturation inversion recovery image (T1 TSE SPIR).

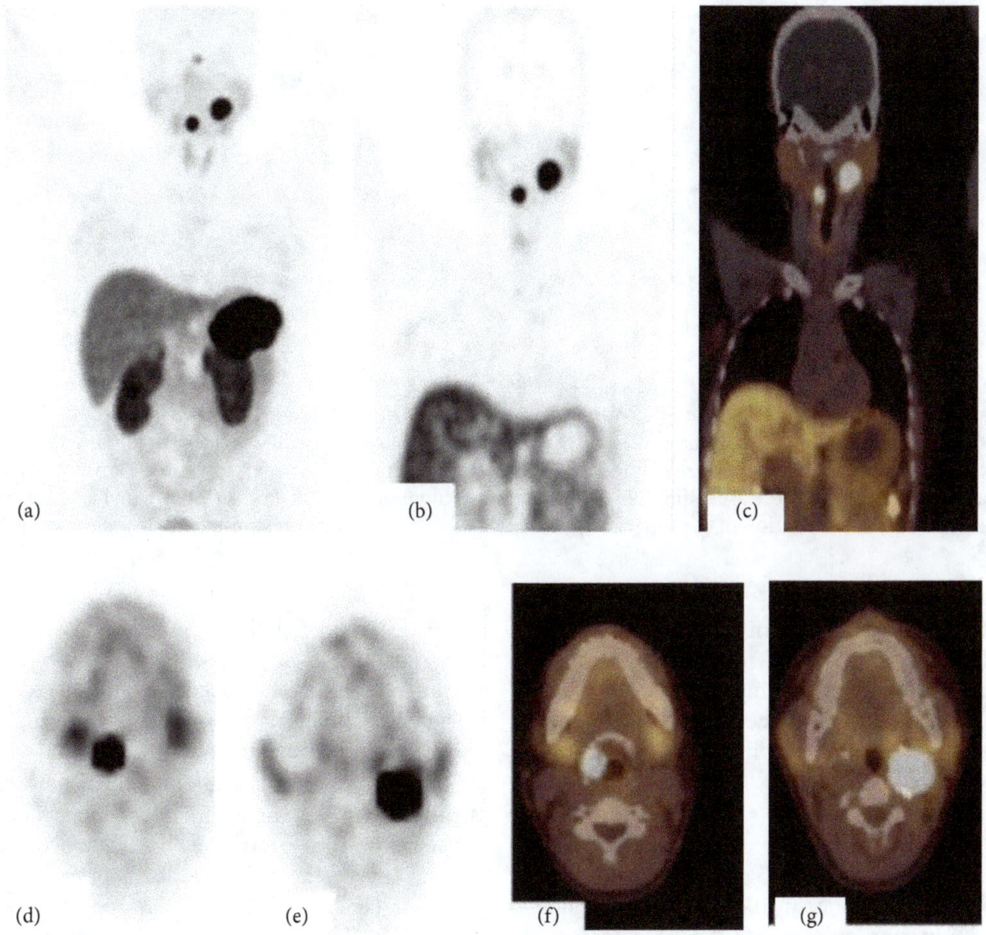

FIGURE 4: 68Ga-DOTANOC PET/CT; maximum intensity projection (MIP) image (a), coronal PET and PET/CT fusion images (b, c), and axial PET and PET/CT fusion images (d, e, f, and g) show an intense uptake by the right laryngeal paraganglioma and left carotid body paraganglioma.

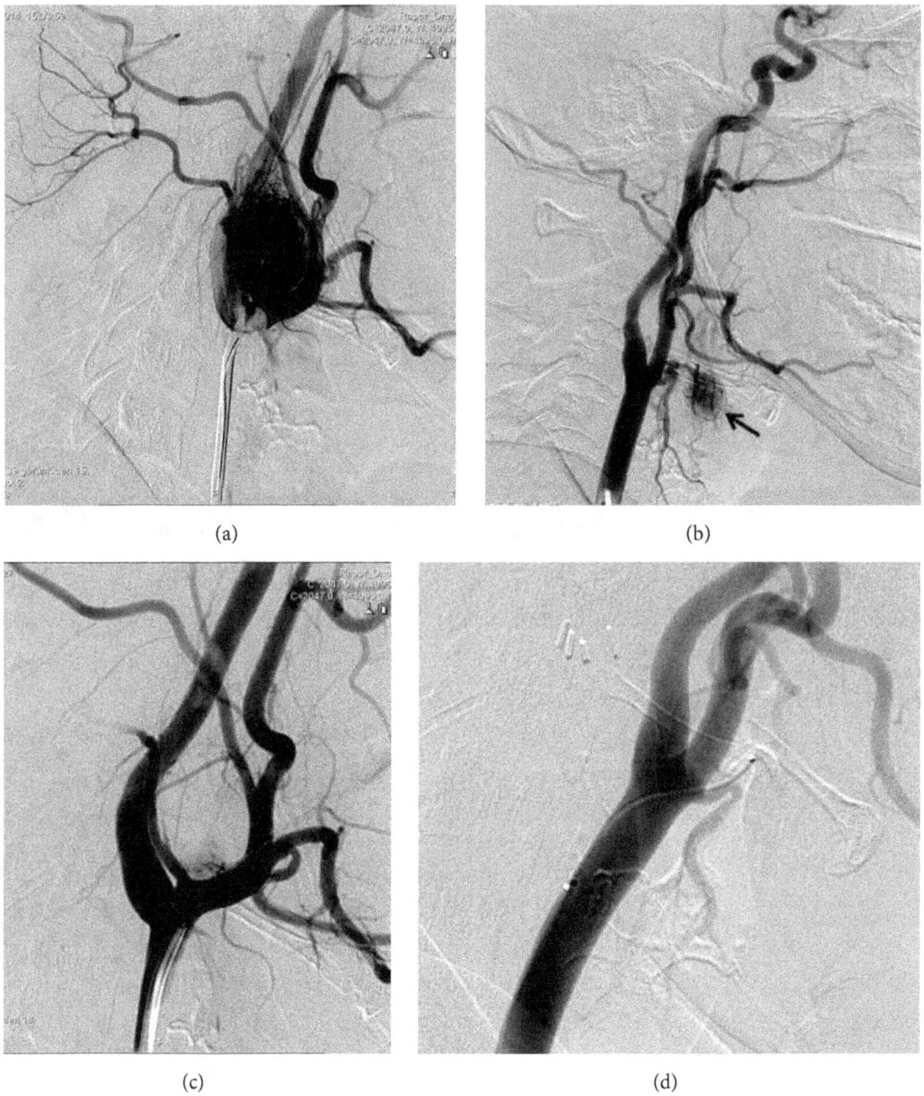

Figure 5: A lateral cervical angiogram from the left common carotid artery demonstrates the intense blush at the carotid bifurcation corresponding to the carotid body paraganglioma (a). Right common carotid artery lateral cervical angiogram shows significant tumor vascularity (arrow) at the larynx (b). Principal arterial feeder to the tumor from superior thyroid artery. Significant reduction is seen in tumor vascularity after embolization of the ascending pharyngeal and proximal occipital artery with polyvinyl alcohol particles measuring 255 to 350 (c). Superselective catheterization of the superior thyroid artery after embolization shows complete devascularization (d).

and S-100 (sustentacular cells). Staining for Ki67 showed <1% positive cells. Five months later, second operation was performed for laryngeal tumor following superior thyroideal artery embolization (Figure 5(d)). The diagnosis of laryngeal paraganglioma was confirmed on histopathology and immunohistochemistry.

3. Discussion

Multiple paragangliomas may occur in 40% of familial paragangliomas and 10% of sporadic tumors [2]. Chase described first familial paraganglioma in two sisters who both presented with bilateral carotid body tumors in 1933 [7]. Familial paragangliomas account for 10% of cases [8]. Multiple paragangliomas may arise synchronously or metachronously. Rubin et al. [5] reported that typically laryngeal paragangliomas are not found in patients with multicentric or familial paragangliomas. The case presented here is the first case of laryngeal with carotid body paraganglioma in a patient with positive family history.

Larynx is a very rare location for paragangliomas of the head and neck. The majority of laryngeal paragangliomas arise in the supraglottic larynx. They occur most commonly in the fourth to sixth decades and show a female preponderance (1 : 3), unlike other neuroendocrine tumors of the larynx [9]. Hoarseness, dysphonia, cough, and dyspnea are the commonest presenting symptoms. Its clinical features are similar to other laryngeal neoplasms. On laryngoscopy, tumors are usually seen as submucosal masses. The case presented here was asymptomatic and there were not any abnormalities on the laryngoscopic examination. There is only one asymptomatic case who presented with shortness of breath and airway compromise after intubation due to laparoscopic cholecystectomy [10].

Laryngeal paragangliomas must be differentiated from other neuroendocrine tumors of the larynx, including typical carcinoid, atypical carcinoid, small cell neuroendocrine carcinoma, and large cell neuroendocrine carcinoma [11]. Paraganglioma and other neuroendocrine tumors have different biological behavior and prognosis; thus treatment strategies are different. Because of their overlapping histological appearance, differential diagnosis is based on immunohistochemistry. Endoscopic biopsy is controversial due to the submucosal and vascular nature of the lesion. Deep biopsy may cause uncontrolled bleeding and require tracheotomy. Diagnostic imaging plays a critical role in the biopsy decision and clinical management of the patient with laryngeal submucosal mass. Differential diagnosis of laryngeal submucosal mass includes hemangioma, schwannoma, chondroma and chondrosarcoma, and minor salivary gland tumors such as adenoid cystic carcinoma [12–14].

Doppler US is a first-line imaging technique in patients with suspected carotid body paraganglioma. Well defined solid mass at the carotid bifurcation, splaying of the internal and external carotid arteries, and high vascularity are typical findings of these tumors. US cannot demonstrate jugulotympanic and most of vagal paragangliomas due to their farther cephalad localization. Contrast enhanced computed tomography is a useful technique for defining bone changes in patients with jugular paraganglioma such as irregular widening of the jugular foramen with cortical erosion and permeative bone destruction. MRI provides better tissue characterization and allows detailed evaluation of tumor localization, size, vascularity, its relationship with major arteries and surrounding structures, and presence of intracranial extension. The typical MRI finding of paragangliomas is "salt and pepper" appearance that results from slow flow or hemorrhage and signal void areas due to high velocity flow, respectively. CT and MRI may also show asymptomatic synchronous HNP especially in patients with familial paraganglioma. Imaging findings of laryngeal paraganglioma are similar to other HNP. In our case, similar imaging features of both lesions confirmed diagnosis of multiple paragangliomas.

DSA is most commonly used for preoperative vascular mapping and tumor embolization rather than diagnosis. Also, balloon occlusion test can be performed to assess collateral cerebral perfusion in patients with carotid body paragangliomas to determine the risk for ischemia and stroke following ICA ligation.

68Ga-DOTA-peptide PET/CT has higher sensitivity and advanced spatial resolution for the detection of well differentiated neuroendocrine tumors than conventional somatostatin receptor scintigraphic agents. Apart from characterizing a lesion as neuroendocrine tumor, 68Ga-DOTA-peptide PET/CT can reveal extension of disease and exclude synchronous and metastatic lesions. 68Ga-DOTA-peptide PET/CT study may further assist in choosing the right treatment and selection of patients for peptide receptor radionuclide therapy with 177 Lu or 90 Y labeled peptides in such patients with extensive disease.

In conclusion, radiologists should keep in mind that paragangliomas may arise in head and neck region as synchronous or metachronous multiple tumors. All areas within the images should be carefully evaluated to avoid missing asymptomatic lesions. Earlier detection and treatment of these tumors can reduce morbidity and mortality rates of surgery.

References

[1] L. A. B. Borba and O. Al-Mefty, "Intravagal paragangliomas: report of four cases," *Neurosurgery*, vol. 38, no. 3, pp. 569–575, 1996.

[2] P. H. Bikhazi, E. Roeder, A. Attaie, and A. K. Lalwani, "Familial paragangliomas: the emerging impact of molecular genetics on evaluation and management," *American Journal of Otology*, vol. 20, no. 5, pp. 639–643, 1999.

[3] A. Szymańska, M. Szymański, E. Czekajska-Chehab, W. Gołabek, and M. Szczerbo-Trojanowska, "Diagnosis and management of multiple paragangliomas of the head and neck," *European Archives of Oto-Rhino-Laryngology*, vol. 272, no. 8, pp. 1991–1999, 2015.

[4] M. S. Persky, A. Setton, Y. Niimi, J. Hartman, D. Frank, and A. Berenstein, "Combined endovascular and surgical treatment of head and neck paragangliomas—a team approach," *Head & Neck*, vol. 24, no. 5, pp. 423–431, 2002.

[5] A. D. Rubin, S. S. Cheng, and C. R. Bradford, "Laryngeal paraganglioma in a patient with multiple head and neck paragangliomas," *Otolaryngology—Head and Neck Surgery*, vol. 132, no. 3, pp. 520–522, 2005.

[6] K. W. Sanders, F. Abreo, E. Rivera, F. J. Stucker, and C.-A. O. Nathan, "A diagnostic and therapeutic approach to paragangliomas of the larynx," *Archives of Otolaryngology—Head and Neck Surgery*, vol. 127, no. 5, pp. 565–569, 2001.

[7] W. H. Chase, "Familial and bilateral tumors of the carotid body," *Journal of Pathology & Bacteriology*, vol. 36, pp. 1–12, 1933.

[8] K. Y. Lee, Y.-W. Oh, H. J. Noh et al., "Extraadrenal paragangliomas of the body: imaging features," *American Journal of Roentgenology*, vol. 187, no. 2, pp. 492–504, 2006.

[9] A. Ferlito, K. O. Devaney, and A. Rinaldo, "Neuroendocrine neoplasms of the larynx: advances in identification, understanding, and management," *Oral Oncology*, vol. 42, no. 8, pp. 770–788, 2006.

[10] J. R. Smolarz, E. Y. Hanna, M. D. Williams, and M. E. Kupferman, "Paraganglioma of the endolarynx: a rare tumor in an uncommon location," *Head and Neck Oncology*, vol. 2, article 2, 2010.

[11] A. Ferlito, C. E. Silver, C. R. Bradford, and A. Rinaldo, "Neuroendocrine neoplasms of the larynx: an overview," *Head and Neck*, vol. 31, no. 12, pp. 1634–1646, 2009.

[12] L. Plisson, V. Patron, B. Luna Azoulay, E. Babin, and M. Hitier, "Laryngeal paraganglioma mimicking a laryngeal haemangioma," *Revue de Laryngologie Otologie Rhinologie*, vol. 134, no. 2, pp. 109–112, 2013.

2

New Method of Parent Catheter Advancement in the Balloon Anchor Technique during Balloon-Occluded Transarterial Chemoembolization for Hepatic Tumors

**Kei Shibuya,[1] Hiroki Tahara,[2] Suguru Takeuchi,[2]
Yoshinori Koyama,[1] and Yoshito Tsushima[1]**

[1]*Department of Diagnostic and Interventional Radiology, Gunma University Hospital, 3-39-22 Showa-machi, Maebashi, Gunma 371-8511, Japan*
[2]*Department of Gastroenterology, Saiseikai Maebashi Hospital, 564-1 Kamishinden-machi, Maebashi, Gunma 371-0821, Japan*

Correspondence should be addressed to Kei Shibuya; shibukei@gunma-u.ac.jp

Academic Editor: Dimitrios Tsetis

Balloon-occluded transarterial chemoembolization (B-TACE) using a microballoon catheter is a promising method for improvement of lipiodol emulsion accumulation and local control relative to conventional transarterial chemoembolization. This method has been referred to as the balloon anchor technique in previous reports. We report a new technique for successful parent catheter advancement for achievement of stable backup for the selective insertion of a microballoon catheter during B-TACE using the microballoon as an anchor, even in patients with tortuous anatomy of the hepatic and celiac arteries. Deep cannulation of parent catheters was accomplished in all three cases and complications such as vascular injury were not observed in the postprocedure angiograms.

1. Introduction

Balloon-occluded transarterial chemoembolization (B-TACE) using a microballoon catheter improves lipiodol emulsion accumulation in cancer nodules and, thus, local control compared with conventional transarterial chemoembolization [1–4]. Selective microballoon catheter cannulation into the feeding artery is important in reducing hepatobiliary complications related to B-TACE; however, unstable backup of the parent catheter prevents the advance of the microballoon catheter. This is caused by certain characteristics of the celiac artery. We report a new technique for successful parent catheter advancement for achievement of stable backup for the selective insertion of a microballoon catheter during B-TACE using the microballoon as an anchor, even in patients with tortuous anatomy of the hepatic and celiac artery. We call this method the balloon anchor technique. In this report, we describe our experience using the balloon anchor technique in three cases with primary hepatic malignancies.

2. Technique

The balloon anchor technique was only adapted to cases that required selective cannulation that could not be accomplished by conventional methods. The schematic of this technique is shown in Figure 1. Transfemoral access was achieved using a 5 Fr sheath, and a 5 Fr catheter was used as the parent catheter for the microballoon catheter. An over-the-wire microballoon was inserted and inflated in a peripheral branch of the hepatic artery that was not a feeding artery for the target tumors. Following inflation and fixation of the microballoon catheter, the parent catheter was advanced to the proper or common hepatic artery by gentle retraction of the microballoon catheter as a guide wire. Based on stable backup of the parent catheter, selective B-TACE was

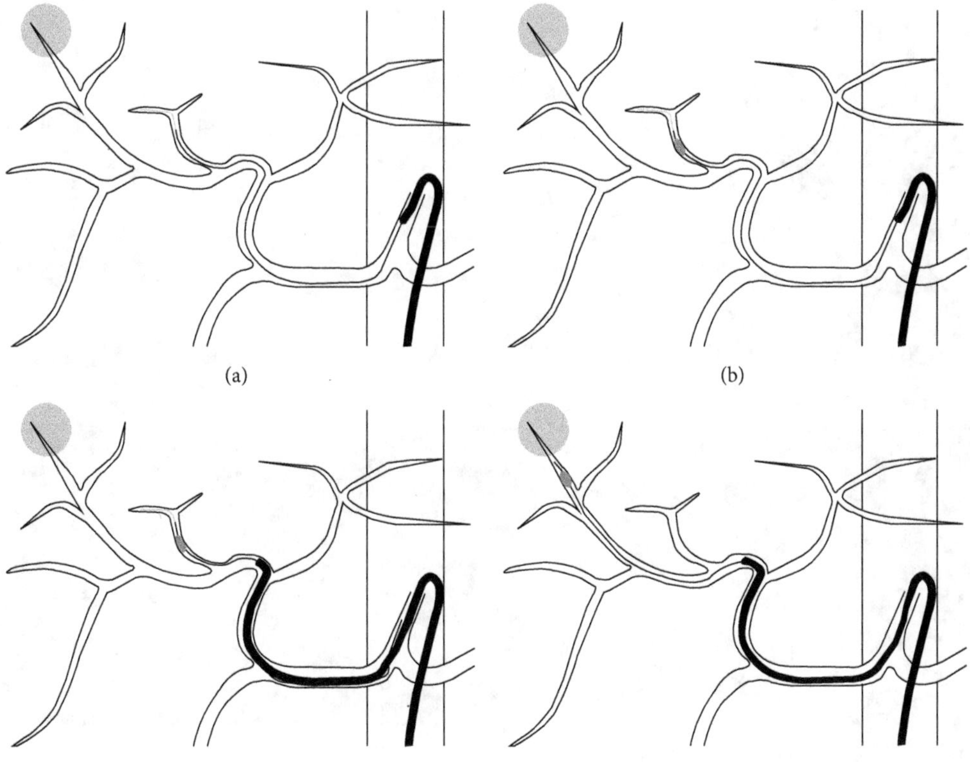

Figure 1: Schematic of the balloon anchor technique. (a) When selective cannulation of the feeding artery of the tumor was not possible using conventional methods, a microballoon catheter was inserted into a nontarget branch. (b) The balloon was inflated and fixed in the vessel. (c) The parent catheter was advanced along the fixed microballoon catheter. (d) The microballoon catheter was advanced into the feeding artery and selective balloon-occluded transarterial chemoembolization was performed.

then achieved in all cases. Postprocedure diagnostic angiography was performed to confirm the absence of vascular complications related to this technique. Written informed consent was obtained from all individual participants before the procedure. For this type of study, formal consent is not required.

3. Case Presentation

3.1. Case 1. A 70-year-old woman with liver cirrhosis caused by the hepatitis C virus was admitted for the treatment of a hepatocellular carcinoma (HCC). Although the liver tumor was solitary, surgical resection was avoided because of poor liver function and transarterial chemoembolization (TACE) was planned as the initial treatment. Diagnostic angiography was performed using a 5 Fr shepherd-hook catheter (FANSAC: Terumo Clinical Supply, Gifu, Japan). Digital subtraction angiography, computed tomography (CT) during arterial portography and CT hepatic arteriography demonstrated a hypervascular tumor in segment eight. Because the size and location of the tumor was not suitable for local ablation therapy, B-TACE was planned for better local control than could be achieved using conventional TACE. We exchanged the 5 Fr shepherd-hook catheter for a 5 Fr Cobra-shaped catheter (Selecon SNCC: Terumo Clinical Supply) for deep cannulation into the hepatic artery. Although we tried to advance the catheter to the proper hepatic artery, it would not cross because of the vessel's tortuous anatomy. A 1.8 Fr tip coaxial microballoon catheter (Logos: PIOLAX, Kanagawa, Japan) was inserted into the right hepatic artery via the parent catheter. However, selective cannulation into the tumor feeders was not possible because of the tortuous arterial anatomy and unstable backup of the parent catheter. Deep cannulation and stable backup of the parent catheter were essential in this situation, but the parent catheter could not be advanced using a 0.035-inch hydrophilic coated guide wire (Radifocus, Terumo, Tokyo, Japan). Therefore, we selected the balloon anchor technique for the advancement of the parent catheter (Figure 2). A microballoon catheter with a 0.014-inch guide wire (Transend EX: Boston Scientific, Marlborough, MA, USA) was inserted into an intrahepatic branch that was unrelated to the feeding artery, via the parent catheter. The microballoon was then inflated and fixed in the vessel. Using the microballoon catheter as a guide wire, we advanced the parent catheter into the right hepatic artery through the tortuous proper hepatic artery. Finally, we performed super-selective B-TACE into the feeding arteries of the tumor with stable support of the parent catheter.

3.2. Case 2. The second case was a 60-year-old man with hypovascular hepatic tumors diagnosed as poorly differentiated adenocarcinoma of unknown origin. Surgical resection

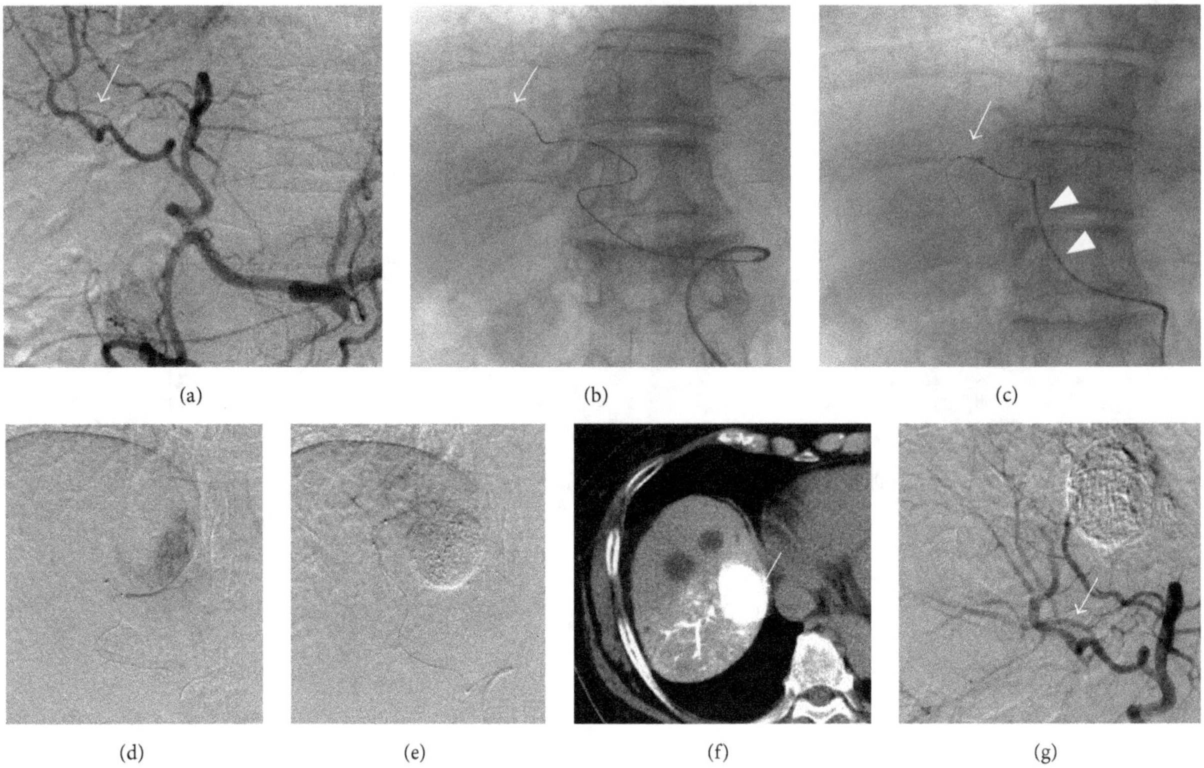

FIGURE 2: ((a) and (b)) A 1.8 Fr tip coaxial microballoon catheter was inserted into a branch in segment five (arrow) that was unrelated to the feeding arteries of the tumor in segment eight. (c) The microballoon was inflated in the vessel (arrow) and the parent catheter was advanced into the right hepatic artery (arrowheads). ((d), (e), and (f)) Selective transarterial chemoembolization using miriplatin was performed and dense lipiodol deposition in the tumor was visible in the postprocedure computed tomography images. (g) Including the vessel in which the microballoon was inflated (arrow), no vascular complications were confirmed in the postprocedure angiogram.

was not indicated and cisplatin-based transarterial infusion chemotherapy, followed by TACE under feeder occlusion using a microballoon catheter, was planned for the treatment of the main tumor in the right liver lobe. Diagnostic angiography performed using a 5 Fr modified spiral-shaped catheter (Gridecath, Terumo, Tokyo, Japan) revealed stenosis at the origin of the celiac artery, and collateral blood flow from the superior mesenteric artery to the proper hepatic artery via dilated arterial arcades around the pancreas head. Deep cannulation of the 5 Fr catheter using a 0.035-inch guide wire was impossible; consequently, we selected the balloon anchor technique. As in Case 1, a 1.8 Fr tip microballoon catheter was inserted into the left hepatic artery via the parent catheter and the 5 Fr catheter was then successfully advanced into the common hepatic artery (Figure 3). Subsegmental B-TACE was then performed and good drug distribution was achieved.

3.3. Case 3. An 80-year-old woman presented with a large recurrent HCC in the medial segment after conventional TACE. We planned B-TACE for the recurrent tumor to achieve superior drug distribution to that of the previously used TACE technique. Celiac angiography was carried out using a 5 Fr Cobra-shaped catheter. However, as a result of severe arteriosclerosis, backup of the 5 Fr catheter was unstable and deep cannulation by means of guide wires was impossible. Similar to Cases 1 and 2, a 1.8 Fr tip microballoon catheter was inserted into a branch in segment six and fixed by inflation of the balloon. The 5 Fr catheter was then successfully advanced into the proper hepatic artery using the balloon anchor technique and the recurrent HCC was treated by means of selective B-TACE. Obvious vascular injury was not observed in the postprocedure angiogram in all three cases.

4. Discussion

In the present case report, we describe the balloon anchor technique, a new technique that assists the advancement of parent catheters through regions of tissue with difficult anatomy, to achieve reliable support of catheters during B-TACE for hepatic tumors. Deep cannulation of the parent catheter facilitated clear angiograms as a result of high-flow injection of contrast medium, and selective TACE was supported by stable backup. Techniques to stabilize the guiding catheter using a balloon as the anchor or guide wire have been reported previously in the fields of coronary intervention, neurointervention, and endoscopic intervention [5–8]. Our new technique was developed based on the results reported in these previous studies.

Reduction of mean arterial stump pressure by means of balloon occlusion is important in obtaining dense lipiodol

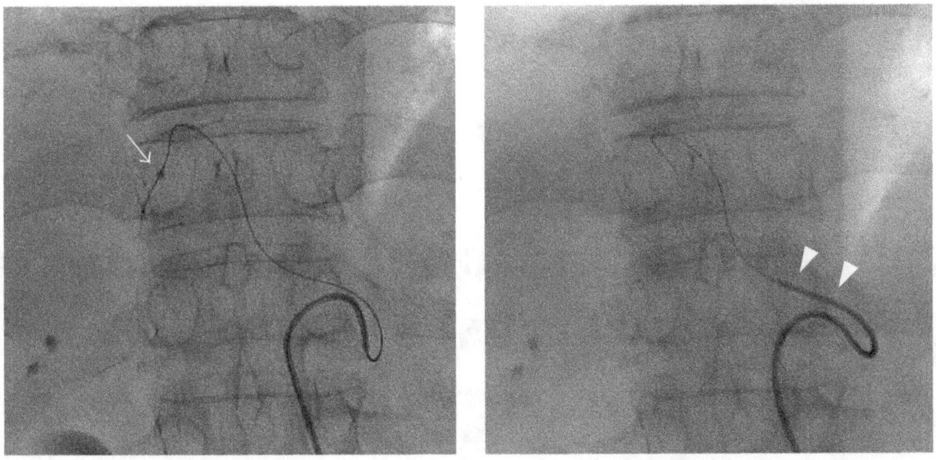

(a) (b)

FIGURE 3: (a) A microballoon catheter was inserted into a branch of the left medial segment and inflated (arrow). (b) The 5 Fr catheter was advanced into the common hepatic artery (arrowheads). In this figure, the microballoon had already been deflated.

accumulation during B-TACE [2]; consequently, selective insertion of a microballoon is required to prevent inflow from the collateral arteries. However, the flexibility and selectivity of microballoon catheters are lower than conventional microcatheters; in addition, it is sometimes difficult to advance a microballoon catheter because of kick-back movement in the parent catheter. All three of our patients had difficult anatomy regarding reliable support of the parent catheters during B-TACE. Also, 3 Fr or thinner microballoon catheters are required for the performance of B-TACE using a standard coaxial system. As a result of this structural limitation, angiograms from the proper or left/right hepatic artery via a microballoon catheter are insufficient in most cases; this is because of the lower injection rate of the contrast medium. Although these problems can usually be resolved by advancing the parent catheter into the hepatic artery, this is occasionally impossible because of tortuous anatomy or angulation of the celiac artery. The balloon anchor technique is useful in these situations. We consider that the balloon anchor technique could also be used to improve catheter backup in embolization for aneurysms or other abdominal vascular interventions, and further investigation is proceeding.

Additional study will be required to confirm the safety of the balloon anchor technique; however, technique-related complications such as vascular injuries were not observed in the postprocedure angiograms in our three cases. In addition, we inserted the anchor balloon into a nontarget artery and inflated it gently to avoid vascular injury to the feeding artery.

In conclusion, the balloon anchor technique can be applied to TACE for hepatic malignancies. It is a promising choice when selective catheter insertion is not readily achievable by other methods and more stable backup is required.

References

[1] H. Arai, T. Abe, H. Takayama et al., "Safety and efficacy of balloon-occluded transcatheter arterial chemoembolization using miriplatin for hepatocellular carcinoma," *Hepatology Research*, vol. 45, no. 6, pp. 663–666, 2015.

[2] T. Irie, M. Kuramochi, and N. Takahashi, "Dense accumulation of lipiodol emulsion in hepatocellular carcinoma nodule during selective balloon-occluded transarterial chemoembolization: measurement of balloon-occluded arterial stump pressure," *CardioVascular and Interventional Radiology*, vol. 36, no. 3, pp. 706–713, 2013.

[3] T. Matsumoto, J. Endo, K. Hashida et al., "Balloon-occluded transarterial chemoembolization using a 1.8-French tip Coaxial microballoon catheter for hepatocellular carcinoma: technical and safety considerations," *Minimally Invasive Therapy and Allied Technologies*, vol. 24, no. 2, pp. 94–100, 2015.

[4] T. Ishikawa, S. Abe, R. Inoue et al., "Predictive factor of local recurrence after balloon-occluded TACE with miriplatin (MPT) in hepatocellular carcinoma," *PLoS ONE*, vol. 9, no. 7, Article ID e103009, 2014.

[5] S. Fujita, H. Tamai, E. Kyo et al., "New technique for superior guiding catheter support during advancement of a balloon in coronary angioplasty: the anchor technique," *Catheterization and Cardiovascular Interventions*, vol. 59, no. 4, pp. 482–488, 2003.

[6] T. Itoi, A. Sofuni, and F. Itokawa, "Large dilating balloon to allow endoscope insertion for successful endoscopic retrograde cholangiopancreatography in patients with surgically altered anatomy (with video)," *Journal of Hepato-Biliary-Pancreatic Sciences*, vol. 17, no. 5, pp. 725–728, 2010.

[7] K. V. Snyder, S. K. Natarajan, F. F. Hauck et al., "The balloon anchor technique: a novel technique for distal access through a giant aneurysm," *Journal of Neurointervention Surgery*, vol. 2, no. 4, pp. 363–367, 2010.

[8] K. Wagatsuma, "Anchor balloon technique for very tortuous lesions by transradial coronary intervention," *Indian Heart Journal*, vol. 60, no. 1, pp. A42–A44, 2008.

3

Ileocaecal Intussusception with a Lead Point: Unusual MDCT Findings of Active Crohn's Disease Involving the Appendix

Ebru Ozan,[1] Gokce Kaan Atac,[1] Egemen Akincioglu,[2] Mete Keskin,[3] and Kamil Gulpinar[3]

[1]*Department of Radiology, Ufuk University School of Medicine, 06520 Ankara, Turkey*
[2]*Department of Pathology, Ufuk University School of Medicine, 06520 Ankara, Turkey*
[3]*Department of General Surgery, Ufuk University School of Medicine, 06520 Ankara, Turkey*

Correspondence should be addressed to Ebru Ozan; ebrusanhal@yahoo.com

Academic Editor: Stefania Rizzo

Adult intussusception is a rare entity accounting for 1% of all bowel obstructions. Unlike intussusceptions in children, which are idiopathic in 90% of cases, adult intussusceptions have an identifiable cause (lead point) in the majority of cases. Crohn's disease (CD) may affect any part of the gastrointestinal tract, including the appendix. It was shown to be a predisposing factor for intussusception. Here, we report a rare case of adult intussusception with a lead point, emphasizing diagnostic input of multidetector computed tomography (MDCT) in a patient with active CD that involves the appendix.

1. Introduction

Crohn's disease (CD) is a chronic granulomatous inflammatory disease of the gastrointestinal tract, which can involve almost any segment from the mouth to the anus [1]. CD can involve the appendix extending from the terminal ileum or the cecum. Appendiceal involvement is seen in about 25% of patients with ileal CD [2].

Intussusception is the invagination of a bowel loop with its mesenteric fold (intussusceptum) into the lumen of a contiguous portion of bowel (intussuscipiens) as a result of peristalsis. A few cases of small bowel or colonic intussusceptions in patients with Crohn's disease have been reported; hence CD is considered as a predisposing factor for intussusception [3]. In adults, intestinal obstruction due to intussusception is a relatively rare phenomenon and it accounts for minority of intestinal obstructions [4].

Different imaging techniques have been proposed for the diagnosis of intussusception. Although ultrasound is the modality of choice in children, computed tomography (CT) is mandatory in adults to make the diagnosis, to determine the underlying cause, to find the lead point, and to evaluate the complications [5].

We describe an unusual case of acute intestinal obstruction due to ileocaecal intussusception in a patient with CD. The case also presents multidetector CT (MDCT) findings of active CD with appendiceal involvement. To our knowledge, this report is the first that illustrates MDCT findings of intussusception with a lead point and appendiceal involvement in an adult patient with active CD.

2. Case Presentation

A 25-year-old male, known to have CD for 5 years, presented to the emergency room with abdominal pain and vomiting. He had no history of previous surgery. A moderate amount of free fluid in the peritoneal cavity with distended bowel loops was described on ultrasound in another institution a few hours before. Physical examination revealed a tenderness in the lower quadrants. Bowel sounds were hypoactive and the rectum showed no feces on digital rectal examination. Routine laboratory investigation of blood sample showed an elevated white blood cell count (15,200/mL).

MDCT of the abdomen with oral (1.5 liters of water mixed with 50 mL sodium and meglumine diatrizoate, Urografin 50 mL, Schering) and IV (ioversol, Optiray 300/100, Mallinckrodt) nonionic iodinated contrast material administration revealed small bowel obstruction due to long segment ileocolic intussusception with invaginated mesenteric fat and

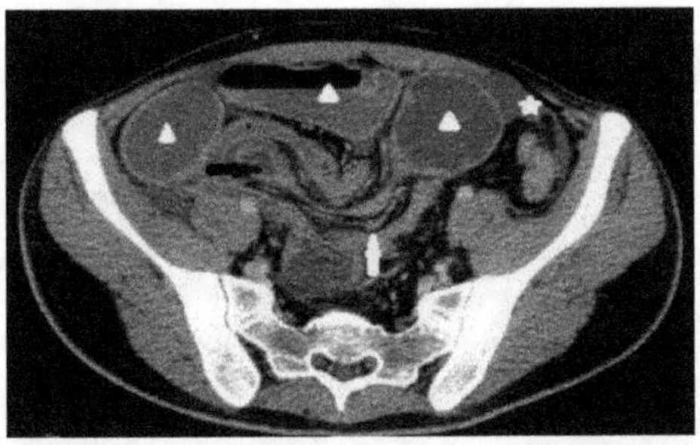

FIGURE 1: Contrast enhanced axial MDCT image demonstrates the presence of intussusception (black arrow) with an accompanying complex of mesenteric fat and blood vessels (white arrow). Dilated small bowel loops due to obstruction (arrowheads) and a moderate amount of free fluid (five-pointed star) are seen.

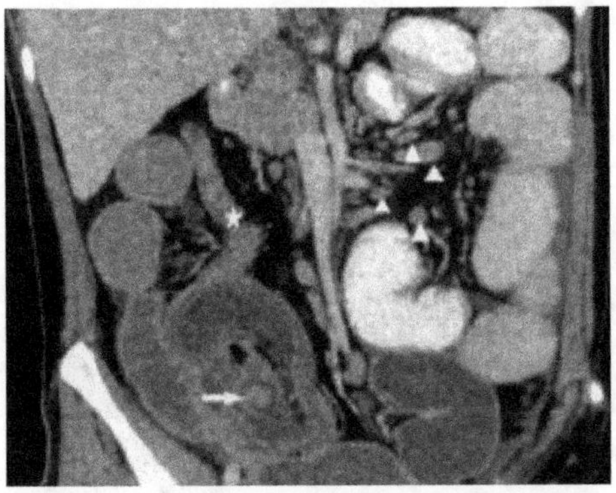

FIGURE 2: Coronal multiplanar reformatted (MPR) image demonstrates the entire intussusception with a round soft-tissue mass serving as a lead point (white arrow), collapsed colon distal to the intussusception (five-pointed star), and multiple enlarged lymph nodes (arrowheads).

vessels, dilated small bowel loops, and moderate amount of free peritoneal fluid (Figure 1). Coronal multiplanar reformatted (MPR) images clearly demonstrated the lead point. Collapsed colonic segment distal to the intussusception and multiple enlarged lymph nodes were also seen (Figure 2). Sagittal MPR images showed enlarged appendix with enhancing wall indicating appendiceal involvement in this patient with CD. "Comb" sign representing engorgement of vasa recta in the mesentery was also nicely demonstrated on sagittal MPR images (Figure 3).

Preoperative diagnosis of ileocaecal intussusception with a lead point was made based on MDCT findings, and also enlarged appendix with wall enhancement was found to be highly suspicious for appendiceal involvement in this case of active CD.

An open surgical laparotomy showed a long segment of ileocaecal intussusception (Figure 4). Appendix was enlarged and inflamed as preoperatively illustrated on MDCT. Surgical resection of the affected bowel segments including terminal ileum, ileocaecal valve, and appendix was performed.

On gross examination the 25 cm long specimen composing terminal ileum, ileocaecal valve, and appendix was evaluated in the pathology department. Terminal ileum was invaginated through the ileocaecal valve and appendix was enlarged. A polypoid lesion, measuring 1,5 cm in diameter corresponding to the lead point, was on the mucosal surface of the invaginated terminal ileum (Figure 5).

Microscopic examination revealed that the polypoid lesion (lead point) was an inflammatory polyp. Mucosal glands and lamina propria of the intussusceptum and the intussuscipiens had ischemic changes. There were lymphoid follicles, vasodilatation, and edema in the mucosa of the colonic wall covering the invaginated part. The wall of the appendix was thick (Figure 6). There were lymphoid aggregates and chronic inflammatory cells on the whole section of the appendix and periappendiceal fat tissue. A final diagnosis of inflammatory Crohn's disease affecting the terminal ileum, ileocaecal valve, and appendix was made.

3. Discussion

Intussusception occurs when a proximal segment of bowel and its associated mesentery invaginate into the lumen of the adjacent distal segment. It is a rare entity in adults and it accounts for only 1% of all cases of intestinal obstructions and 5% of all intussusceptions [6].

Cases of intestinal obstruction secondary to small bowel intussusception by a segment of active Crohn's ileitis have been rarely reported. There have been reports of intussusception in adult patients with Crohn's disease and history of previous surgery [7]. Transient nonobstructive intussusception in two patients with Crohn's disease was also described and repeated abdominal CT showed spontaneous resolution of intussusceptions in both patients [8]. In the presented case the patient had no history of previous surgery and presented with a persistent intussusception leading to small bowel obstruction.

The current case clearly demonstrates that intussusception should be considered in the differential diagnosis of an adult patient with CD presenting with signs of small bowel obstruction. Hence it is critical to keep intussusception in mind and perform abdominal CT, which is considered as a useful tool for making an accurate diagnosis in this group of patients.

It is stated that identifying the presence or absence of a lead point when dealing with intussusception is crucial. Thus, the former is a serious condition likely to persist and require surgery, while the latter is more likely to resolve spontaneously [9]. When a mass is demonstrated at CT separately from edematous bowel, it can be regarded as a reliable predictor of an intussusception with a lead point and surgery should be recommended. As in the presented case, use of MDCT with multiplanar reformations can be helpful to characterize an intussusception, determine an underlying lead point, and demonstrate evidence of obstruction.

CD can affect any part of the gastrointestinal tract. Appendix is involved in approximately 25% of patients with CD of the terminal ileum and in more than 50% of patients with colonic CD [2]. Inappreciable attention has been given to the CT appearance of the appendix in patients with this condition. Increased appendiceal wall enhancement is

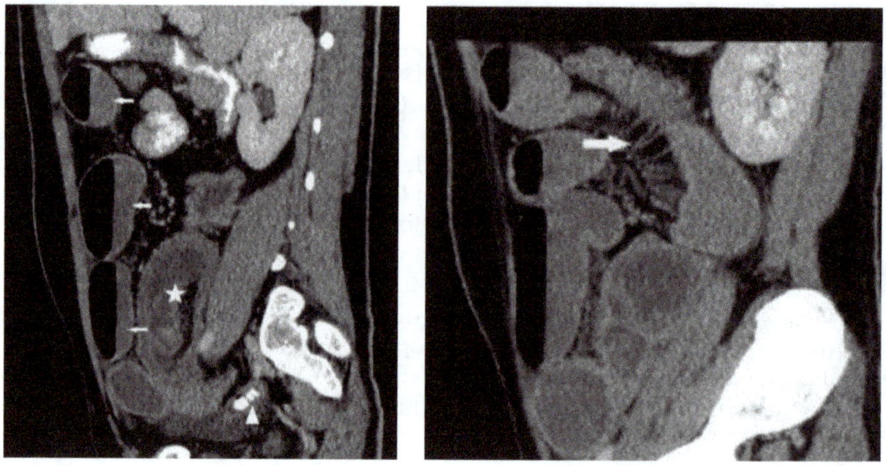

FIGURE 3: (a) Sagittal MPR images show intussusception (five-pointed star) and dilated loops (arrows). Enlarged appendix showing wall enhancement (arrowhead) is seen. (b) Engorgement of vasa recta, "comb" sign, is nicely demonstrated (arrow).

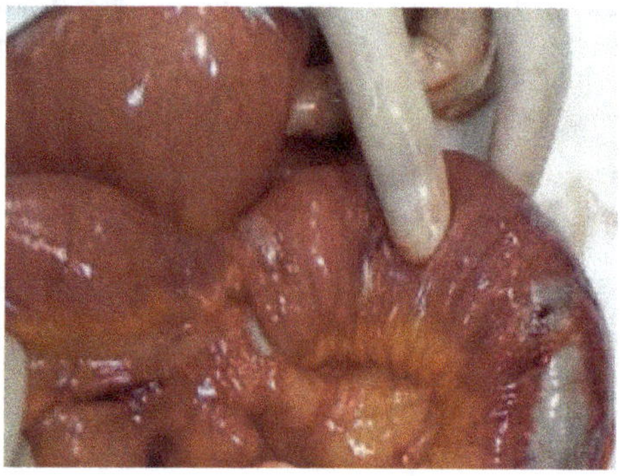

FIGURE 4: Intraoperative view of the intussusception.

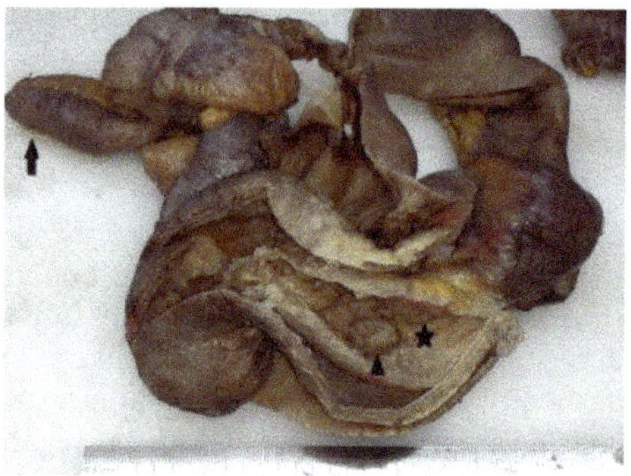

FIGURE 5: Gross appearance of the resected material composing the invaginated terminal ileum (five-pointed star), polypoid lesion (arrowhead), and enlarged appendix (arrow).

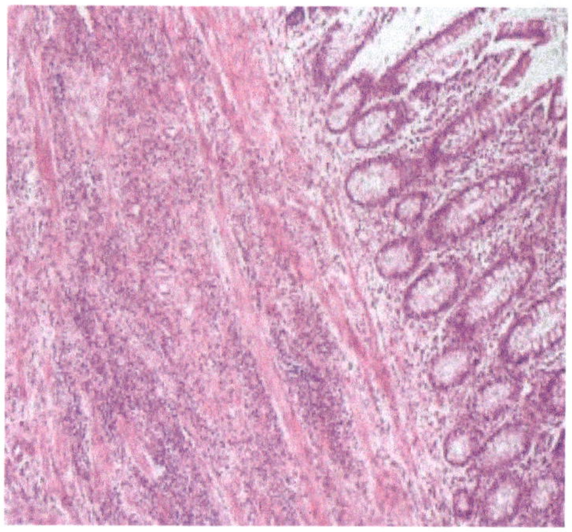

FIGURE 6: Microscopic examination demonstrates lymphoid aggregates and chronic inflammatory cells on the thick appendiceal wall, H&E stain, ×100.

more frequently observed in patients with active disease by comparison with patients who have inactive CD [10]. In this case, appendiceal involvement which was shown to be an activity sign in CD was clearly demonstrated. Another sign of activity, the "comb" sign, representing engorgement of the vasa recta was also shown.

This case illustrates an unusual cause of small bowel obstruction in an adult patient with CD. It also demonstrates MDCT findings of appendiceal involvement and signs of active disease.

References

[1] G. Gatta, G. Di Grezia, V. Di Mizio et al., "Crohn's disease imaging: a review," *Gastroenterology Research and Practice*, vol. 2012, Article ID 816920, 15 pages, 2012.

[2] R. Shaoul, Y. Rimar, A. Toubi, J. Mogilner, R. Polak, and M. Jaffe, "Crohn's disease and recurrent appendicitis: a case report," *World Journal of Gastroenterology*, vol. 11, no. 43, pp. 6891–6893, 2005.

[3] A. Shah, J. Roberts, H. Lipsky, Y. Twersky, M. Hirth, and K. Chawla, "Enteroenteric intussusception: an unusual presentation of Crohn's disease in an adult patient," *The American Journal of Gastroenterology*, vol. 90, no. 12, pp. 2231–2232, 1995.

[4] K. Shaheen, N. Eisa, A. H. Alraiyes, M. C. Alraies, and S. Merugu, "Telescoping intestine in an adult," *Case Reports in Medicine*, vol. 2013, Article ID 292961, 4 pages, 2013.

[5] S. Baleato-González, J. C. Vilanova, R. García-Figueiras, I. B. Juez, and A. M. de Alegría, "Intussusception in adults: what radiologists should know," *Emergency Radiology*, vol. 19, no. 2, pp. 89–101, 2012.

[6] M. Barussaud, N. Regenet, X. Briennon et al., "Clinical spectrum and surgical approach of adult intussusceptions: a multicentric study," *International Journal of Colorectal Disease*, vol. 21, no. 8, pp. 834–839, 2006.

[7] A. J. Greenstein, M. Wertkin, G. Doughlin, and A. Sicular, "Enteroenteric intussusception in Crohn's disease," *The Mount Sinai Journal of Medicine*, vol. 46, no. 1, pp. 69–73, 1979.

[8] M. C. Knowles, E. K. Fishman, J. E. Kuhlman, and T. M. Bayless, "Transient intussusception in Crohn disease: CT evaluation," *Radiology*, vol. 170, no. 3, p. 814, 1989.

[9] S. Tresoldi, Y. H. Kim, M. A. Blake et al., "Adult intestinal intussusception: can abdominal MDCT distinguish an intussusception caused by a lead point?" *Abdominal Imaging*, vol. 33, no. 5, pp. 582–588, 2008.

[10] P. Soyer, M. Boudiaf, X. Dray et al., "Crohn's disease: multidetector row CT-enteroclysis appearance of the appendix," *Abdominal Imaging*, vol. 35, no. 6, pp. 654–660, 2010.

4

Successful Localization of the Source of Hemorrhage in Patient with Post-Whipple Surgery by ^{99m}Tc-Labelled Red Blood Cell Scintigraphy

Ahmed Fathala, Alaa Alduraibi, and Moheieldin M. Abouzied

Department of Radiology, Division Nuclear Medicine Division & Cardiothoracic Radiology Division, King Faisal Specialist Hospital & Research Centre, P.O. Box 3354, MBC 28, Riyadh 11211, Saudi Arabia

Correspondence should be addressed to Ahmed Fathala; ahm35799@hotmail.com

Academic Editor: Samer Ezziddin

Gastrointestinal Bleeding Scintigraphy (GIBS) of ^{99m}Tc-labelled red blood cells is a relatively simple examination to perform, with high diagnostic accuracy and a relatively lower radiation dose. A positive scan can either suggest surgery without further investigation or can indicate angiography, a more targeted procedure. Whipple pancreatoduodenectomy is most often performed for tumors of the head of the pancreas. Pancreatoduodenectomy has 30%–40% morbidity and mortality, and while post-pancreatoduodenectomy hemorrhage is seen in less than 10% of patients, it accounts for 11%–38% mortality. The role of imaging in patients to detect relative hemodynamic stability is essential. Computed tomography angiography (CTA) shows the cause, site, and nature of bleeding, while digital subtraction angiography (DSA) has a diagnostic as well as a therapeutic role. We present a patient who presented with active gastrointestinal bleeding (GI) bleeding after undergoing a Whipple procedure, to highlight the role of GIBS in the successful localization of a bleeding site and the guidance of digital DSA in the embolization and control of the active bleeding.

1. Introduction

Gastrointestinal Bleeding Scintigraphy (GIBS) of ^{99m}Tc-labelled red blood cells blood cells is a relatively simple examination, where the scan is useful for diagnosing active gastrointestinal bleeding (GI bleeding) and for guiding therapeutic angiography. The technique is very sensitive and can detect bleeding rates of 0.05– 0.1 cc/min, while conventional angiography allows the detection of bleeding at rates of only 0.5–1.0 mi/min and above [1], and computed tomography angiography (CTA) can detect bleeding rates of 0.3–1 ml [2]. A positive scan can either indicate surgery without further investigation or can suggest a more targeted angiography procedure. Whipple pancreatoduodenectomy is most often performed for tumors of the head of the pancreas. Pancreatoduodenectomy has 30%–40% morbidity and mortality, while post-pancreatoduodenectomy hemorrhage accounts for 11%–38% mortality even though it is seen less than 10% of patients [3]. Several vascular lesions and sources have been discerned using this method. But it is essential to use imaging in patients to detect relative hemodynamic stability; CTA shows the cause, site, and nature of bleeding [4], while digital subtraction angiography (DSA) has a diagnostic as well as a therapeutic role [5].

There has been very little emphasis on the role and utilization of GIBS with a ^{99}Tc-labelled red blood cell scan in the following clinical situation. We present a patient who presented with active GI bleeding after undergoing a Whipple procedure in order to highlight the role of GIBS in the successful localization of the bleeding site and the guidance of digital DSA in the embolization and control of the active bleeding.

2. Case Presentation

A 53-year-old patient was recently diagnosed with pancreatic cancer with obstructive jaundice, for which he underwent a Whipple procedure. Unfortunately, the procedure

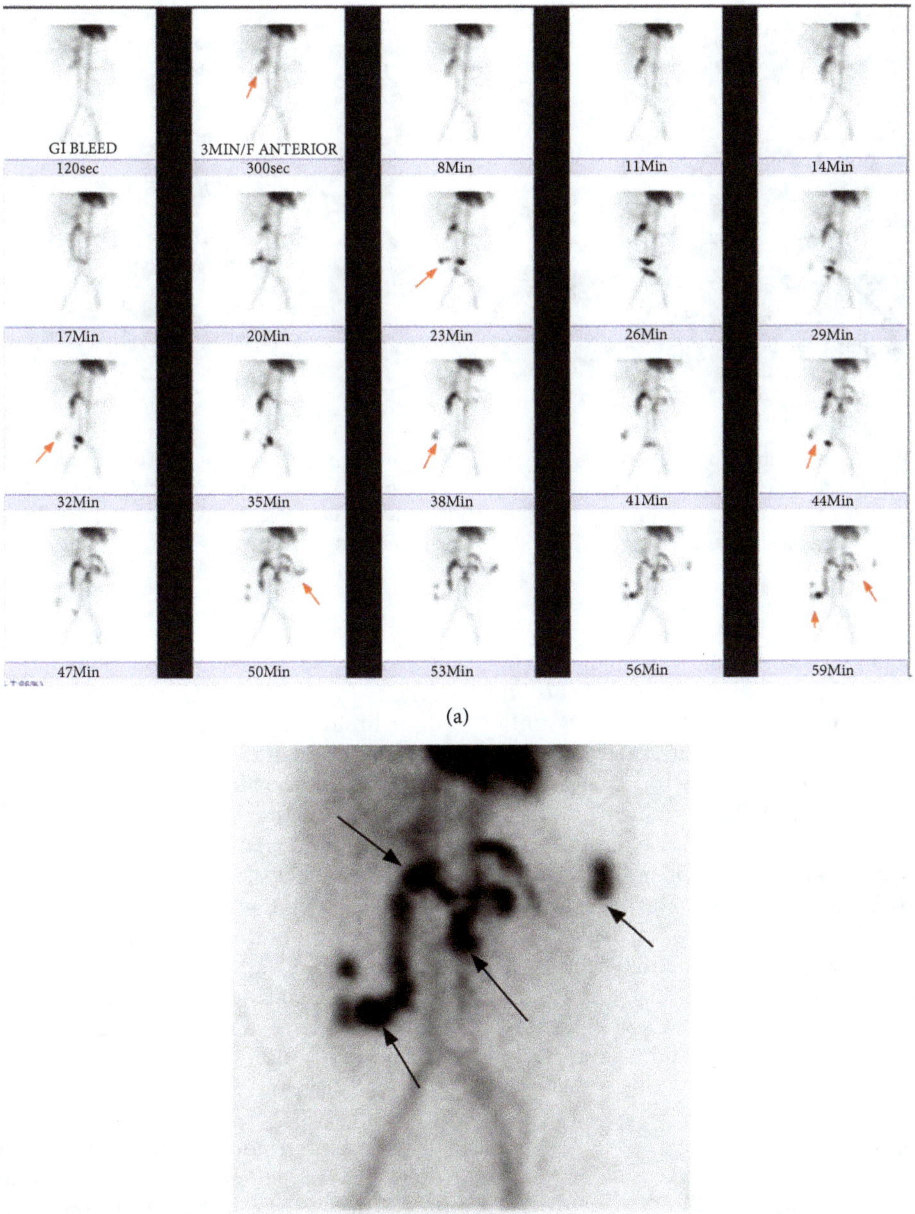

(a)

(b)

FIGURE 1: (a) Dynamic imaging sequence of a ^{99}Tc-labelled erythrocyte scan. The initial image (2 min image) demonstrates normal biodistribution of the radiotracer. A focus of increasing intensity is noted in the right upper abdomen at the 3 min image (red arrow). This focus of abnormal accumulation of the radiotracer shows antegrade and retrograde movement, confirming the bowel lumen appearance, and it crosses the midline several times (on cine images). This pattern is compatible with small bowel bleeding. (b) This selected late image from the ^{99}Tc-labelled erythrocyte bleeding scan (59 min image) shows the typical pattern of small bowel bleeding (multiple red arrows).

was complicated with a pancreatojejunostomy anastomosis leak, deep vein thrombosis deep vein thrombosis (DVT), and postoperative-bleeding. He was taken for exploratory laparotomy and a revision of gastrojejunostomy anastomosis without the successful localization of the source of the bleeding; later the same day, the patient underwent diagnostic DSA, which also failed to localize the source of the bleeding. GIBS was requested for better localization of the GI bleeding source.

The study was positive for active bleeding, which had started primarily high in the right upper abdomen, supposedly from the region of the hepaticojejunostomy (Figures 1(a) and 1(b)). Therefore, the patient was transferred to the angiography suite for another diagnostic and therapeutic DSA. Selective catheterization of the superior mesenteric artery was performed followed by an angiogram, which showed no active contrast extravasation and identified no abnormality. Then selective catheterization of the celiac trunk

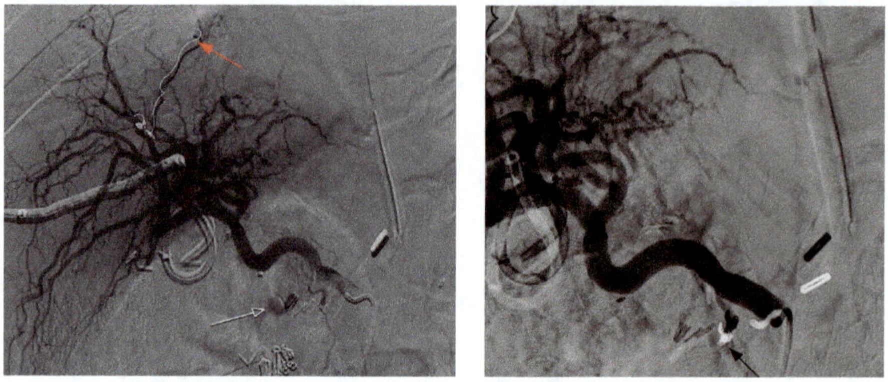

(a) (b)

FIGURE 2: (a) Digital subtraction angiogram (DSA) with selective injection through the common hepatic artery shows active extravasation from a small artery arising from the gastroduodenal artery stump. The red arrow indicates previous coil embolization in the right hepatic artery branch, due to previous hepatic trauma from the prior insertion of a percutaneous transhepatic biliary drain. (b) DSA shows the embolization coil placed in the gastroduodenal artery stump with excellent hemostasis (arrow).

was followed by an angiogram, which showed small contrast extravasation originating from the proximal common hepatic artery, most likely from the gastroduodenal artery stump (Figure 2(a)). Using a coaxial microcatheter/microwire utilizing an Echelon catheter and synchro-wire, contrast was injected for the selective catheterization of the small arterial branches originating from the proximal main common hepatic artery. A small extravasation was confirmed, and while the catheter remained in the same position, coil embolization was performed utilizing three coils measuring 2 mm. After that, an angiogram was performed that showed no extravasation and no abnormality (Figure 2(b)). And upper abdominal angiogram was also performed, again demonstrating no abnormalities. No immediate complications were encountered.

3. Discussion

GIBS contributed very significantly to the management of this postoperative high-risk patient; this procedure accurately confirmed that the patient was actively bleeding, it found the location of the bleed, and it provided guidance for radiologic intervention. The main advantage of GIBS compared to CTA is its ability to detect GI bleeding at a very low threshold, at a rate of 0.05–0.2ml/min [6]. The sensitivity and specificity of GIBS have been reported to be 93% and 95%, respectively [7, 8]. There are certain predictors of GIBS that correlate with the positivity of DSA, its prompt performance, and the higher intensity of the radiotracer accumulation at the site of the bleeding [9]. GIBS may be considered the initial test in the management of a post-Whipple patient presenting with hemorrhage, as it provides greater diagnostic accuracy, is relatively simple to perform, and uses a lower radiation dose than those of other methods.

An alternative diagnostic test for lower GI bleeding in post-Whipple patients is CTA, which is widely available, provides a faster diagnosis, particularly in patients who cannot be tested in other ways, and delineates other possible etiologies, such as vascular anomalies. But the drawbacks of CTA include higher relative costs, a higher radiation dose, limited time for evaluation, lower sensitivity compared to GIBS, and iodine contrast IV administration. GIBS is preferred, especially in the pediatric population, because of its lower radiation dose compared to CTA [10].

Several previous studies have suggested that GIBS can be effective as the sole tool in surgical planning [11], but others have suggested that it is useful only as a screening tool before angiography and intervention [12]. The value of SPECT/CT GIBS for localization, sensitivity, and specificity has yet to be investigated. Bleeding in the small bowel may be more difficult to detect and localize compared to colonic bleeding, since the location of the small bowel is more variable and more central, and it is more prone to overlap with vascular structures [13].

Post-pancreatoduodenectomy hemorrhage is seen in less than 10% of patients, but as mentioned, it accounts for 11%–38% of mortality [3]. Intramural hemorrhage may present as hematemesis, bleeding from the nasogastric tube, or melena. The possible sources of bleeding in post-pancreatoduodenectomy include the gastroduodenal artery stump, common and proper hepatic artery erosion, or splenic and inferior pancreaticoduodenal artery erosions or aneurysm, besides other etiologies [14].

4. Conclusion

Post-Whipple pancreatoduodenectomy hemorrhage is a common but important complication with high mortality. GIBS may be viewed as an initial diagnostic test in stable patients; it is simple and easy to perform, with the highest diagnostic accuracy and a relatively lower radiation dose, and it may guide therapeutic percutaneous radiologic intervention. CTA is an alternative diagnostic test resulting in faster diagnosis, it delineates other possible causes of bleeding such as vascular anomalies, and it can guide endovascular therapy. But CTA is more expensive, it has a higher radiation dose, and it needs iodinated contrast IV administration. DSA has a role in both diagnosis and intervention, but the role of DSA has changed from diagnostic to therapeutic. Radiologic intervention is preferred in the management of post-Whipple pancreatoduodenectomy hemorrhage, because of the lower resulting mortality.

References

[1] M. Chung, G. J. Dubel, R. B. Noto et al., "Acute lower gastrointestinal bleeding: Temporal factors associated with positive findings on catheter angiography after 99mTc-labeled RBC scanning," *American Journal of Roentgenology*, vol. 207, no. 1, pp. 170–176, 2016.

[2] E. Grady, "Gastrointestinal bleeDing scintigraphy in the early 21st century," *Journal of Nuclear Medicine*, vol. 57, no. 2, pp. 252–259, 2016.

[3] R. B. Jagad, M. Koshariya, J. Kawamoto, G. S. Chude, R. V. Neeraj, and N. J. Lygidakis, "Postoperative hemorrhage after major pancreatobiliary surgery: an update," *Hepato-Gastroenterology*, vol. 55, no. 82-83, pp. 729–737, 2008.

[4] L. Lepanto, D. Gianfelice, R. Dery, M. Dagenais, R. Lapointe, and A. Roy, "Postoperative changes, complications, and recurrent disease after Whipple's operation: CT features," *American Journal of Roentgenology*, vol. 163, no. 4, pp. 841–846, 1994.

[5] F. Makowiec, H. Riediger, W. Euringer, M. Uhl, U. T. Hopt, and U. Adam, "Management of delayed visceral arterial bleeding after pancreatic head resection," *Journal of Gastrointestinal Surgery*, vol. 9, no. 9, pp. 1293–1299, 2005.

[6] D. A. Zuckerman, T. P. Bocchini, and E. H. Birnbaum, "Massive hemorrhage in the lower gastrointestinal tract in adults: Diagnostic imaging and intervention," *American Journal of Roentgenology*, vol. 161, no. 4, pp. 703–711, 1993.

[7] A. R. Siddiqui, D. S. Schauwecker, H. N. Wellman, and B. H. Mock, "Comparison of technetium-99m sulfur colloid and in vitro labeled technetium-99m RBCs in the detection of gastrointestinal bleeding," *Clinical Nuclear Medicine*, vol. 10, no. 8, pp. 546–549, 1985.

[8] S. R. Bunker, R. J. Lull, D. E. Tanasescu et al., "Scintigraphy of gastrointestinal hemorrhage: Superiority of 99mTc red blood cells over 99mTc sulfur colloid," *American Journal of Roentgenology*, vol. 143, no. 3, pp. 543–548, 1984.

[9] D. A. Ng, F. G. Opelka, D. E. Beck et al., "Predictive value of technetium Tc 99m-labeled red blood cell scintigraphy for positive angiogram in massive lower gastrointestinal hemorrhage," *Diseases of the Colon & Rectum*, vol. 40, no. 4, pp. 471–477, 1997.

[10] F. H. Fahey, S. T. Treves, and S. J. Adelstein, "Minimizing and communicating radiation risk in pediatric nuclear medicine," *Journal of Nuclear Medicine Technology*, vol. 40, no. 1, pp. 13–24, 2012.

[11] R. Dusold, K. Burke, W. Carpentier, and W. P. Dyck, "The Accuracy of Technetium-99m-Labeled Red Cell Scintigraphy in Localizing Gastrointestinal Bleeding," *American Journal of Gastroenterology*, vol. 89, no. 3, pp. 345–348, 1994.

[12] J. M. Hunter and M. E. Pezim, "Limited value of technetium 99m-labeled red cell scintigraphy in localization of lower gastrointestinal bleeding," *The American Journal of Surgery*, vol. 159, no. 5, pp. 504–506, 1990.

[13] D. M. Howarth, K. Tang, and W. Lees, "The clinical utility of nuclear medicine imaging for the detection of occult gastrointestinal haemorrhage," *Nuclear Medicine Communications*, vol. 23, no. 6, pp. 591–594, 2002.

[14] S. Puppala, J. Patel, S. McPherson, A. Nicholson, and D. Kessel, "Hemorrhagic complications after whipple surgery: Imaging and radiologic intervention," *American Journal of Roentgenology*, vol. 196, no. 1, pp. 192–197, 2011.

Spontaneous Rupture of Pyometra Causing Peritonitis in Elderly Female Diagnosed on Dynamic Transvaginal Ultrasound

Sharad M. Malvadkar, Madhuri S. Malvadkar, Shilpa V. Domkundwar, and Shariq Mohd

Department of Radiodiagnosis, Grant Medical College and Sir JJ Group of Hospitals, Byculla, Mumbai 400008, India

Correspondence should be addressed to Sharad M. Malvadkar; drsharadmed@gmail.com

Academic Editor: Yoshito Tsushima

Pyometra is collection of pus within the uterine cavity and is usually associated with underlying gynaecological malignancy or other benign causes. Spontaneous rupture of pyometra is a rare complication. We report a case of a 65-year-old female who presented with acute abdomen and was diagnosed with a ruptured uterus secondary to pyometra and consequent peritonitis on dynamic transvaginal sonography (TVS) which was later confirmed on contrast enhanced computed tomography (CECT). An emergency laparotomy was performed and about 800 cc of pus was drained from the peritoneal cavity. A rent was found in the anterior uterine wall and hence hysterectomy was performed. Histopathology revealed mixed inflammatory cell infiltrate with no evidence of malignancy. There are only 31 cases of ruptured pyometra reported till date, most of which were definitively diagnosed only on laparotomy. In only two of these cases the preoperative diagnosis was made on CECT. We report this case, as the correct and definitive diagnosis was made preoperatively on dynamic TVS. To our knowledge, *this is the first case report revealing spontaneous ruptured pyometra being diagnosed preoperatively on dynamic TVS*. This report is aimed at giving emphasis on the use of simple dynamic TVS for accurate diagnosis of rare spontaneous ruptured pyometra causing peritonitis.

1. Introduction

Pyometra is collection of pus in the uterine cavity with several aetiologies like malignancy of genital tract more commonly and sometimes benign lesions and other benign conditions. Clinical presentation of pyometra is a whitish discharge per vaginum and sometimes lower abdominal pain and bleeding per vaginum also. Spontaneous rupture of pyometra is a rare complication. Usually a definite diagnosis of spontaneous rupture pyometra was made only by laparotomy. This report is aimed at giving emphasis on the use of simple dynamic TVS for accurate diagnosis of rare spontaneous ruptured pyometra causing peritonitis.

2. Case History

A 65-year-old postmenopausal diabetic female presented to the emergency department with complaints of abdominal pain, fever, and distension along with white discharge per vaginum for seven days. Her vital parameters were stable except for mild tachycardia (pulse rate being 110 beats/min). Blood pressure was 110/70 mm Hg. Temperature was 100 degree F. Diffuse guarding, rigidity, and tenderness were present on abdominal palpation. On per speculum cervix was stenosed with minimal white discharge through external os. Per vaginal examination revealed retroverted normal sized uterus with free fornices.

Laboratory investigations revealed neutrophilic leukocytosis (white cell count of 14,800/cc with 66% neutrophils), elevated ESR of 32 mm/hour, and a low haemoglobin 10.7 gm/dL.

First, a transabdominal ultrasound (USG) was performed which revealed moderate free fluid with thick echoes within the peritoneal cavity and mild collection within endometrial cavity. TVS was performed to look for a cause of endometrial collection, which revealed a collection with thick echoes within the uterine cavity suggestive of pyometra and a defect of size 2.0 × 2.0 cm in the anterior wall near fundus (Figure 1). Using a transvaginal probe gentle pressure was exerted over the cervix and uterus, which showed the real

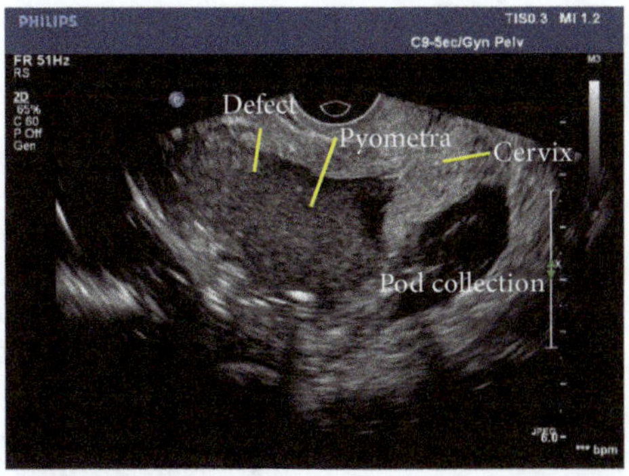

FIGURE 1: B mode TVS reveals large pyometra distending endometrial cavity with defect in anterior wall near fundus and collection in pouch of Douglas.

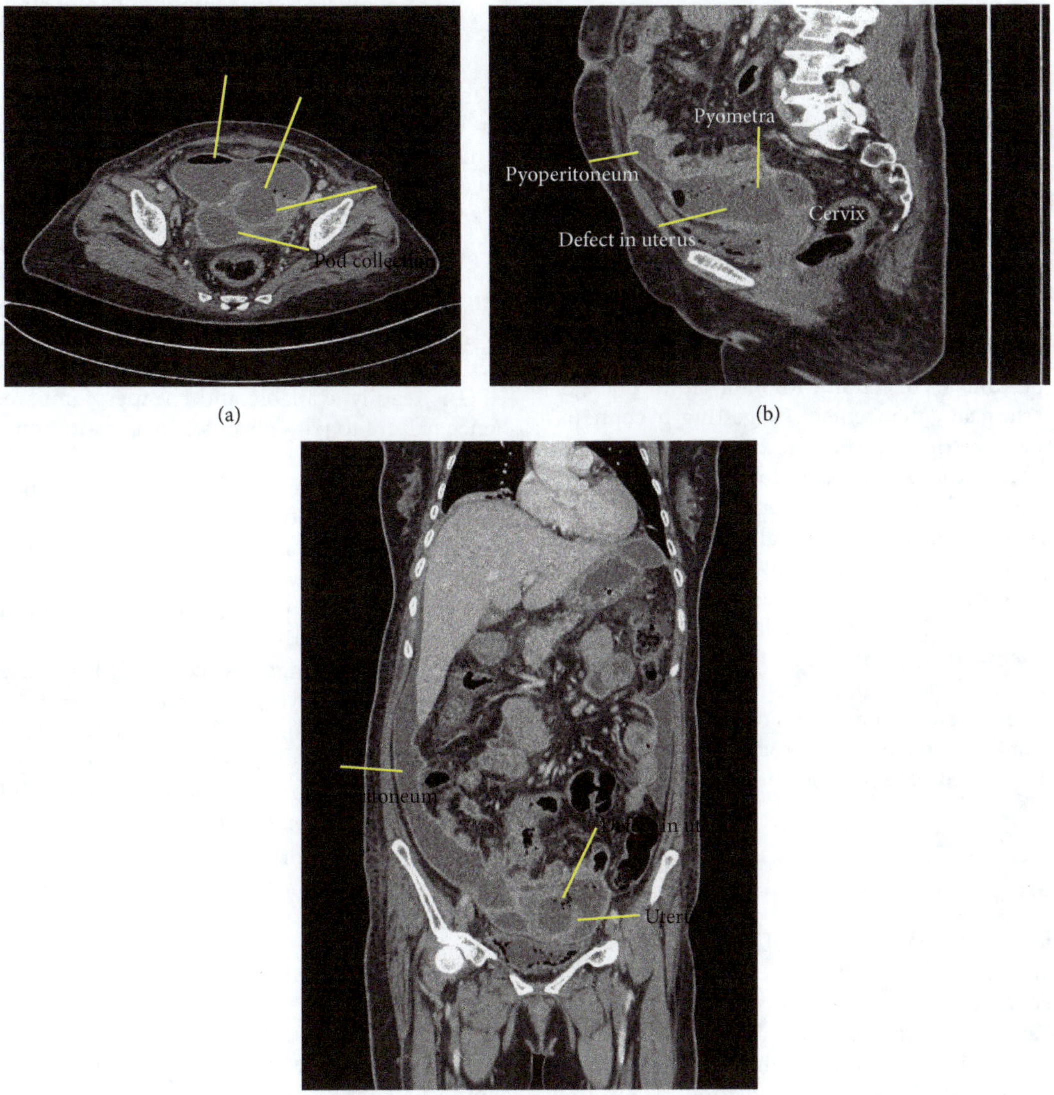

(a) (b) (c)

FIGURE 2: (a) Axial contrast enhanced CT in venous phase reveals pyometra communicating with peritoneal collection through defect in anterior wall of the uterus near fundus. Free nondependant air with smooth peritoneal enhancement suggesting pyopneumoperitoneum. (b) Sagittal contrast enhanced CT in venous phase reveals pyometra communicating with peritoneal collection through defect in anterior wall of the uterus near fundus. (c) Coronal contrast enhanced CT abdomen in venous phase reveals pyometra communicating with peritoneal collection through defect in the uterus near fundus.

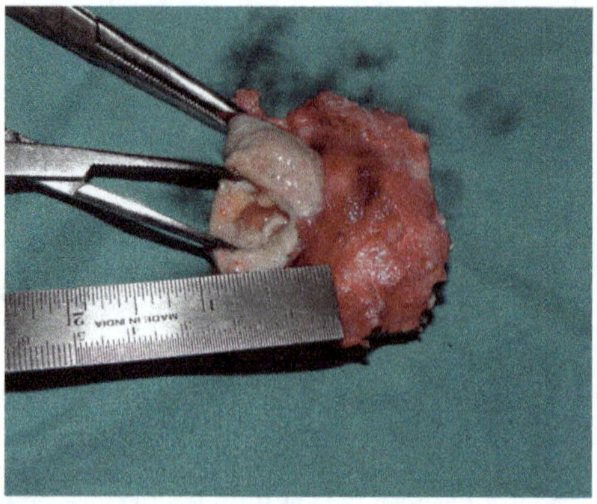

FIGURE 3: Postoperative surgical specimen showing 2 × 2 cm defect in the anterior wall near fundus of the uterus.

time movement of the endometrial collection through the defect into peritoneal collection with near complete emptying of the cavity. On releasing pressure, movement in the reverse direction was noticed with refilling of the endometrial cavity (See video in Supplementary Material available online at http://dx.doi.org/10.1155/2016/1738521). Based on these findings a diagnosis of spontaneous rupture of pyometra into peritoneal cavity was suggested. Emergency CECT abdomen and pelvis was performed which confirmed the pyometra, defect of 2.0 × 2.0 cm in the anterior wall of the uterus, and moderate peritoneal collection with multiple air pockets and smooth peritoneal enhancement suggesting pyeopneumoperitoneum with peritonitis (Figures 2(a), 2(b), and 2(c)).

An emergency exploratory laparotomy was done. At laparotomy a defect of 2 × 2 cm was found in the anterior wall of the uterus and hence abdominal hysterectomy was performed (Figure 3). No evidence of any uterine or cervical malignancy was found. 800 cc of pus was drained from the peritoneal cavity followed by peritoneal lavage. Histopathology revealed haemorrhage along with fibrovascular tissue infiltrated with mixed inflammatory cell infiltrate comprising of polymorphs and a few lymphocytes confirming pyogenic infection. The patient was started on broad spectrum antibiotic and was discharged on 28th postoperative day without complication.

3. Discussion

Pyometra is defined as the collection of pus in the uterine cavity. The main cause of pyometra is cervical canal occlusion usually secondary to carcinoma cervix; however, other benign causes are endometrial polyp, leiomyoma, infection especially senile cervicitis, a forgotten intrauterine device, cervical occlusion after surgery, and radiation [1–3]. The usual presentation of pyometra is a whitish discharge per vaginum. Sometimes the patients may present with the clinical triad of abdominal pain, purulent vaginal discharge, and postmenopausal bleeding. However, more than 50% of all cases are asymptomatic [4].

Spontaneous rupture of pyometra is a rare complication, the incidence being 0.01–0.5% of all gynaecological patients and more common in postmenopausal females [5]. There are only 31 cases of ruptured pyometra reported till date [6–8].

Spontaneously perforated pyometra is difficult to diagnose preoperatively. Clinically it commonly mimics the symptoms of gastrointestinal tract diseases. Misdiagnoses are common and most frequent preoperative diagnosis is generalised peritonitis secondary to gastrointestinal perforation [9]. It is mentioned in prior case reports that, in most cases, a correct and definite diagnosis of spontaneous rupture pyometra was made only by laparotomy [8].

Preoperative diagnosis of perforated pyometra on CECT was made in only two cases in which CT suggested the diagnosis and surgical intervention was performed [10, 11]. Abdominal USG has high sensitivity in assessing pyometra, but it plays a limited role in the diagnosis of perforated pyometra because of its inability to demonstrate the uterine breach and the limited sonographic window available due to pneumoperitoneum [10]. However, this limitation can be overcome by TVS using a window of cervix and pyometra for detecting uterine defect and using dynamic TVS for demonstrating the real time movement of the endometrial collection through the defect into peritoneal collection. *There is no case report suggesting perforated pyometra being diagnosed preoperatively on dynamic TVS till date.* This report is aimed at giving emphasis on the use of simple dynamic TVS for accurate diagnosis of rare spontaneous ruptured pyometra causing peritonitis. *The advantage of USG over CT is accessibility, affordability, and no risk of radiation.* USG is readily available and cheaper compared to CT and hence helpful to patients of smaller institutions especially in developing countries.

In our case, the patient presented with symptoms of generalised peritonitis and TVS demonstrated the pyometra and a defect in the anterior wall of the uterus near fundus. Dynamic TVS showed real time movement of endometrial collection and peritoneal collection through defect in either direction further confirming diagnosis of perforated pyometra. The findings were confirmed on subsequent CECT abdomen, which revealed pyometra, uterine perforation in anterior wall near fundus, and pyeopneumoperitoneum. *To our knowledge this is the first such case report revealing spontaneous ruptured pyometra causing peritonitis being diagnosed preoperatively on dynamic TVS.*

The treatment of spontaneously ruptured pyometra is emergency laparotomy, peritoneal lavage and drainage, and hysterectomy.

4. Conclusion

Although spontaneous rupture of pyometra is rare, it should be kept in mind as a differential diagnosis in postmenopausal women presenting with acute abdomen and dynamic transvaginal sonography should be advised prior to laparotomy for definitive diagnosis. USG is more accessible and cheaper compared to CT and hence helpful in diagnosis of ruptured pyometra in patients from smaller institutions especially in developing countries. A carefully performed dynamic transvaginal sonography will give the accurate diagnosis so as to help with early intervention and proper treatment to reduce the associated morbidity and mortality.

References

[1] S. Vyas, A. Kumar, M. Prakash, R. Kapoor, P. Kumar, and N. Khandelwal, "Spontaneous perforation of pyometra in a cervical cancer patient: a case report and literature review," *Cancer Imaging*, vol. 9, no. 1, pp. 12–14, 2009.

[2] S.-L. Lee, L.-W. Huang, K.-M. Seow, and J.-L. Hwang, "Spontaneous perforation of a pyometra in a postmenopausal woman with untreated cervical cancer and 'forgotten' intrauterine device," *Taiwanese Journal of Obstetrics and Gynecology*, vol. 46, no. 4, pp. 439–441, 2007.

[3] P.-H. Chen, Hsien-Liu, S.-L. Lee, C.-Y. Chang, and C.-C. Chang, "Pneumoperitoneum caused by perforation of pyometra associated with a lost intrauterine device and perforated malignancy of the sigmoid colon," *Taiwanese Journal of Obstetrics & Gynecology*, vol. 50, no. 1, pp. 124–125, 2011.

[4] N. M. Nuamah, E. Hamaloglu, and A. Konan, "Spontaneous uterine perforation due to pyometra presenting as acute abdomen," *International Journal of Gynecology and Obstetrics*, vol. 92, no. 2, pp. 145–146, 2006.

[5] L. Geranpayeh, M. Fadaei-Araghi, and B. Shakiba, "Spontaneous uterine perforation due to pyometra presenting as acute abdomen," *Infectious Diseases in Obstetrics and Gynecology*, vol. 2006, Article ID 60276, 2 pages, 2006.

[6] Z. Yousefi, N. Sharifi, and M. Morshedy, "Spontaneous uterine perforation caused by pyometra: a case report," *Iranian Red Crescent Medical Journal*, vol. 16, no. 9, Article ID e14491, 2014.

[7] S. F. Lim, S. L. Lee, A. K. H. Chiow, C. S. Foo, A. S. Y. Wong, and S.-M. Tan, "Rare cause of acute surgical abdomen with free intraperitoneal air: spontaneous perforated pyometra. A report of 2 cases," *American Journal of Case Reports*, vol. 13, pp. 55–57, 2012.

[8] F. Mallah, T. Eftekhar, and M. Naghavi-Behzad, "Spontaneous rupture of pyometra," *Case Reports in Obstetrics and Gynecology*, vol. 2013, Article ID 298383, 2 pages, 2013.

[9] B. Yildizhan, E. Uyar, A. Sişmanoğlu, G. Güllüoğlu, and Z. N. Kavak, "Spontaneous perforation of pyometra," *Infectious Diseases in Obstetrics and Gynecology*, vol. 2006, Article ID 26786, 2006.

[10] H.-S. Jeon, H.-J. Shin, I.-H. Kim, H. Chung, and D.-Y. Chung, "Spontaneous uterine perforation of pyometra presented as an acute abdomen: a case report," *Korean Journal of Obstetrics & Gynecology*, vol. 55, no. 6, pp. 437–440, 2012.

[11] K.-S. Chan, C.-K. Tan, C.-W. Mak, C.-C. Chia, C.-Y. Kuo, and W.-L. Yu, "Computed tomography features of spontaneously perforated pyometra: a case report," *Acta Radiologica*, vol. 47, no. 2, pp. 226–227, 2006.

6

Unusual Presentations of Focal Periphyseal Edema Zones: A Report of Bilateral Symmetric Presentation and Partial Physeal Closure

Nicholas Beckmann and Susanna Spence

Department of Diagnostic and Interventional Imaging, Memorial Hermann, University of Texas Health Science Center, 6431 Fannin Street, No. 2.130B, Houston, TX 77030, USA

Correspondence should be addressed to Nicholas Beckmann; nicholas.m.beckmann@uth.tmc.edu

Academic Editor: Maria Raissaki

Focal periphyseal edema (FOPE) zones are areas of periphyseal edema seen near the time of physeal closure which are believed to be a physiologic phenomenon related to changes in distribution of forces around the physis as it closes. Since the original case series describing these areas of periphyseal edema, there has been little published in regard to FOPE zone outside of review articles. We present a set of three patients identified with focal periphyseal edema zones around the knee and compare our findings with the initial case series. We include a patient presenting with bilateral, nearly symmetric, focal periphyseal edema zones of the proximal tibia physis and a patient with partial closure of the physis at time of presentation, which were not reported in the original case series.

1. Introduction

In 2011, Zbojniewicz and Laor described areas of bone marrow edema centered on physes of the knee nearing closure in adolescent patients [1]. They coined these areas of marrow edema focal periphyseal edema, or FOPE, zones. Since their original case series in 2011, FOPE zones have been referred to in a few other review publications [2–4], but, to the best of our knowledge, there have not been any additional published case studies describing the imaging and clinical features of FOPE zones. The three adolescent patients presented in this series have areas of periphyseal edema around the knee consistent with FOPE zones previously described by Zbojniewicz and Laor. However, two of the patients had an imaging appearance of FOPE zones not previously described in their paper. One of the patients had bilateral nearly symmetric FOPE zones while another patient had partial closure of her physis associated with the FOPE zone.

2. Materials & Methods

2.1. Case 1. An adolescent female softball player presented with gradually worsening right anterior knee pain and knee stiffness of several months duration. She had focal tenderness in the right infrapatellar region on palpation and mild pain during knee flexion. Initial radiographs of the right knee (Figure 1) were interpreted as normal. The patient was treated with a presumed diagnosis of patellar tendinitis and instructed to undergo a brief period of rest followed by physical therapy with gradual return to normal activity.

She returned 9 months later with persistent anterior right knee pain and mild knee pain with deep knee flexion. At this time, mild medial joint line tenderness was also elicited on palpation. Due to the medial joint line tenderness, a right knee MRI was performed to assess for medial meniscal pathology. A 1.6 × 1.4 cm osteochondral lesion of the medial femoral condyle was identified on MRI with mild marrow edema and cystic change at the interface between the osteochondral lesion and femoral condyle (Figure 2). There was no defect in the overlying cartilage or fluid-like signal at the interface of the osteochondral lesion and femoral condyle. The remainder of the MRI exam was normal.

The patient's medial joint line pain improved, but she continued to have mild anterior knee pain. A repeated MRI of the right knee was performed 6 months after the initial

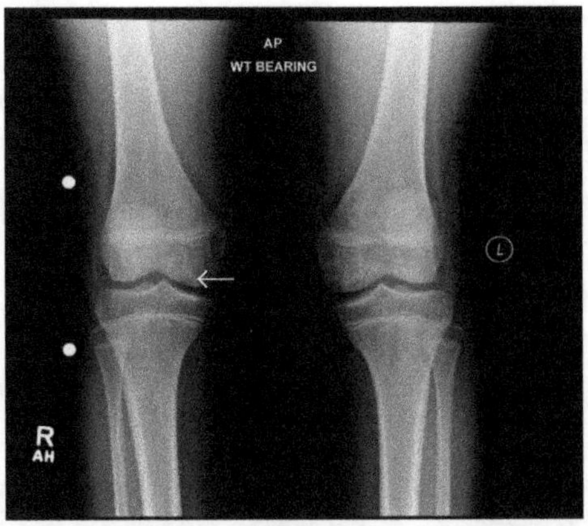

FIGURE 1: A 13-year-3-month-old female with FOPE zones at both proximal tibiae. Findings: AP radiograph of the bilateral knees at time of initial presentation shows a subtle lytic lesion abutting the articular surface of the right medial femoral condyle (arrow). The radiographs were initially interpreted as normal. Technique: AP radiograph kVp = 77, mAs = 4.

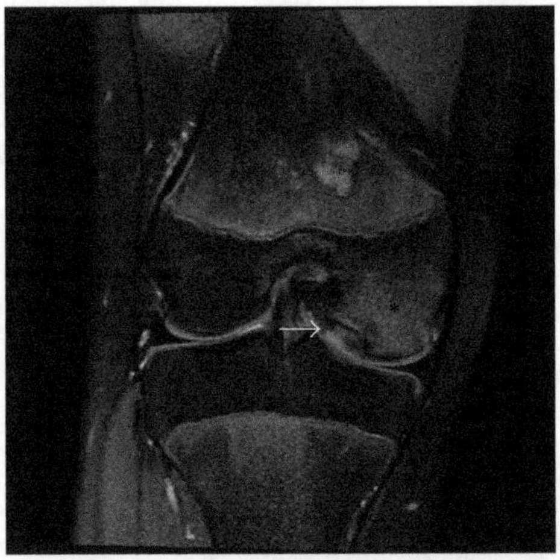

FIGURE 2: A 13-year-3-month-old female with FOPE zones at both proximal tibiae. Findings: coronal proton density fat-saturated image from right knee MRI obtained 9 months after initial presentation shows an osteochondral lesion (arrow) with mild surrounding marrow edema (asterisk) of the medial femoral condyle corresponding to subtle lytic lesion present on initial radiographs. Technique: coronal PD fat-saturated MRI (TR = 2,825.7, TE = 30), ST = 2.5 mm, spacing = 3.264 mm, FOV = 14 cm, and matrix = 312 × 244.

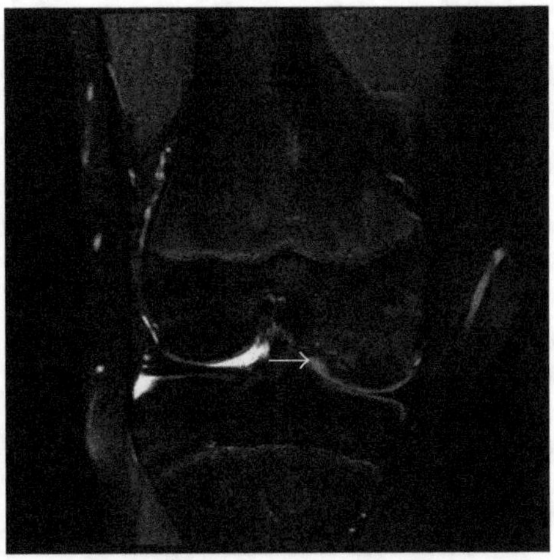

FIGURE 3: A 13-year-3-month-old female with FOPE zones at both proximal tibiae. Findings: coronal proton density fat-saturated image from follow-up of right knee MRI obtained 6 months after initial MRI shows decrease in the marrow edema surrounding the osteochondral lesion of the medial femoral condyle. The osteochondral lesion (arrow) is otherwise unchanged in appearance. Technique: coronal PD fat-saturated MRI (TR = 2,472.4, TE = 30), ST = 2.5 mm, spacing = 3.3 mm, FOV = 14 cm, and matrix = 312 × 244.

MRI to assess for changes in the osteochondral lesion. MRI of the left knee was performed at the same time due to the patient complaining of vague anterior left knee pain similar to the presenting right knee pain, which raised clinical concern for an occult osteochondral lesion of the left knee. She was at chronologic age of 13 years and 3 months at the time of the bilateral knee MRI. The osteochondral lesion of the right medial femoral condyle was unchanged in appearance between the two MRI exams (Figure 3). However, in the interim, a 9 mm focal periphyseal edema (FOPE) zone developed in the anterolateral aspect of the central proximal right tibia (Figure 4). A similar appearing 13 mm FOPE zone was present in the anterior aspect of the central proximal left tibia on the left knee MRI (Figures 5 and 6). While the distribution of FOPE zone periphyseal edema was equal on the epiphyseal and metaphyseal sides of the proximal right tibia, the periphyseal edema was more exuberant on the epiphyseal side of the proximal left tibia. The remainder of the left knee MRI was normal. The proximal tibial physis was narrowed, but open, bilaterally.

It was uncertain whether the patient's bilateral anterior knee pain was due to the FOPE zones or another etiology not elucidated on the MRI. However, the patient pain resolved after a several-week period of rest. She was released to continue activity as tolerated with instruction to return if pain increased. She did not return for follow-up.

2.2. Case 2. An adolescent female dancer and cheerleader at chronological age of 14 years and 2 months presented with right knee pain beginning after twisting her knee one month prior to presentation. The knee pain was initially medial but had migrated to the anterior knee by the time of presentation. The patient was focally tender to palpation in the infrapatellar region on physical exam and had patella crepitus. She had diminished flexion due to pain.

There was no abnormality on presenting knee radiographs, which showed bilateral symmetric partial closure of the central portion of the proximal tibial physis (Figure 7). Right knee MRI was performed to assess for possible patellofemoral chondromalacia. A 14 mm FOPE zone was present in the anteromedial aspect of the central proximal tibia physis on MRI (Figure 8). The right knee MRI was otherwise unremarkable. The proximal tibia physis was partially closed centrally on the knee MRI (Figure 9).

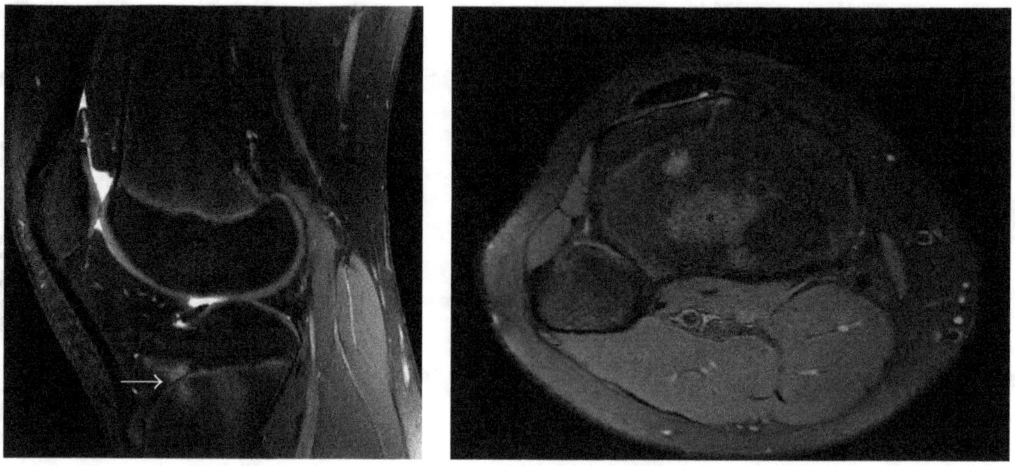

(a) (b)

Figure 4: A 13-year-3-month-old female with FOPE zones at both proximal tibiae. Findings: (a) sagittal proton density fat-saturated image on the 6-month follow-up MRI of the right knee shows interval development of 9 mm in diameter area of periphyseal edema on both the epiphyseal and metaphyseal sides of the proximal tibia physis (arrow). The proximal tibia physis is narrowed but remains open. (b) Axial proton density fat-saturated image at the level of the proximal tibia physis shows the periphyseal edema located at the anterolateral aspect of the central physis (asterisk). Technique: (a) sagittal PD fat-saturated MRI (TR = 2,958.3, TE = 30), ST = 3 mm, spacing = 3.3 mm, FOV = 14 cm, and matrix = 364 × 261; (b) axial PD fat-saturated MRI (TR = 2,843.3, TE = 30), ST = 3 mm, spacing = 3.3 mm, FOV = 15 cm, and matrix = 376 × 297.

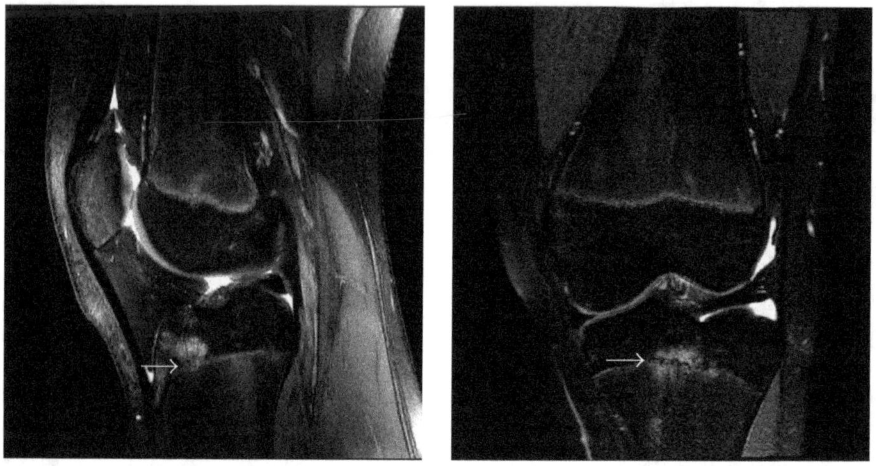

(a) (b)

Figure 5: A 13-year-3-month-old female with FOPE zones at both proximal tibiae. Findings: (a) sagittal proton density fat-saturated image of the left knee shows 13 mm in diameter area of periphyseal edema at the metaphyseal side of the proximal tibia physis (arrow). The proximal tibia physis is narrowed but remains open. (b) Coronal proton density fat-saturated image shows the periphyseal edema to be on both sides of the proximal tibia physis. The coronal image better demonstrates the periphyseal edema involvement of both the epiphyseal and metaphyseal sides of the physis (arrow). Technique: (a) sagittal PD fat-saturated MRI (TR = 2,959.1, TE = 30), ST = 3 mm, spacing = 3.3 mm, FOV = 14 cm, and matrix = 364 × 261; (b) coronal PD fat-saturated MRI (TR = 2,504.2, TE = 30), ST = 2.5 mm, spacing = 3.3 mm, FOV = 15 cm, and matrix = 312 × 244.

The patient underwent a short period of rest followed by physical therapy with gradual return to activity. She reported significant improvement in knee pain 2 months after initial presentation and has not returned for follow-up.

2.3. Case 3. An adolescent female at chronological age of 13 years and 10 months presented with acute right knee pain after hyperextending her knee while playing basketball. She felt a "pop" during the hyperextension and had been unable to bear weight after injury. On physical examination, she had lateral joint line pain without ligamentous laxity. There was limited knee range of motion, and a moderate joint effusion was present.

Presenting radiographs of the right knee were normal (Figure 10). MRI of the right knee showed pivot-shift bone marrow contusion pattern in the lateral compartment and

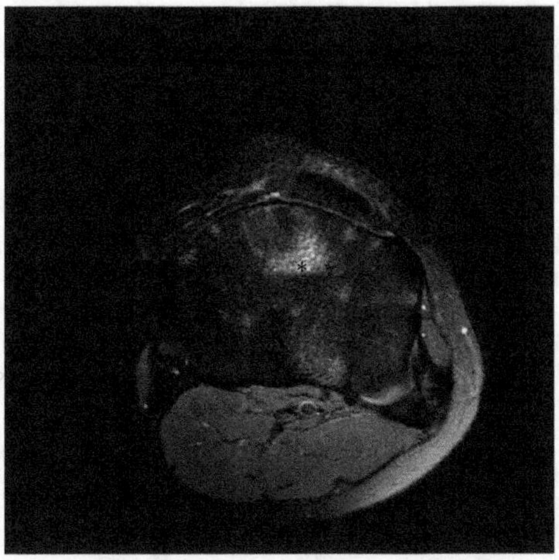

FIGURE 6: A 13-year-3-month-old female with FOPE zones at both proximal tibiae. Findings: axial proton density fat-saturated image at the level of the proximal tibia physis shows the periphyseal edema located at the anterocentral aspect of the central physis (asterisks). Technique: axial PD fat-saturated MRI (TR = 2,843.2, TE = 30), ST = 3 mm, spacing = 3.3 mm, FOV = 15 cm, and matrix = 376 × 297.

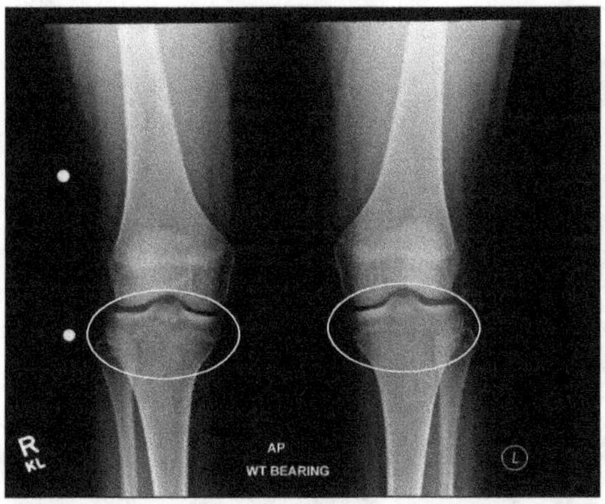

FIGURE 7: A 14-year-2-month-old female with FOPE zone of the proximal tibia. Findings: AP radiograph of both knees shows bilateral symmetric partial closure of the central portion of the proximal tibial physis (ovals). Technique: AP radiograph kVp = 70, mAs = 7.

root ligament avulsion of the lateral meniscus posterior horn (Figure 11). A 5 mm FOPE zone was also present in the central portion of the distal femur physis (Figure 12). The distal femur physis was still open.

She underwent 2 months of conservative management without relief in symptoms. The patient subsequently had knee arthroscopy for repair of the lateral meniscus posterior horn root ligament. The right knee pain and joint effusion resolved after surgery with return of normal range of motion by 3 months after meniscal repair. The patient has not returned for additional follow-up.

3. Discussion

The etiology of FOPE zones is uncertain; however, it is postulated that these areas of edema may be physiologic and related to normal physeal closure [1]. Physeal closure starts centrally and proceeds peripherally. The central portion of the physis has increased susceptibility to trauma, which is believed to be due to decreased elasticity of the central physis relative to the periphery during the early closure of the central physis [2]. This decreased elasticity could also potentially predispose the central physis to increased stress during physeal closure. Bone marrow edema on MRI has been shown to be a manifestation of increased stress placed on the bone [5], which could explain the appearance of marrow edema around the narrowed central physis typically seen in FOPE zones. While some FOPE zones may be physiologic, two of the three patients we reported had knee pain in the region of the FOPE zones without other explanations for pain on their knee MRIs, suggesting that the FOPE zones may represent a painful phenomenon related to mechanical strain placed on the physis during physeal closure.

In Zbojniewicz and Laor's paper, all 12 patients with FOPE zones were between 12 and 16 years of age. This age range coincides with the expected age of physeal closure at the knee, which supports the theory that FOPE zones are related to physeal closure. The physes of the knee typically close between 12 and 15 years of age with 5% of patients having closed physes by 12 years of age and 94% of patients having closed physes at 15 years of age [6]. All three of our patients were between the ages of 13 and 15 at time of presentation.

No gender or racial predilection has been described for FOPE zones. However, seven of the 12 patients in the case series by Zbojniewicz and Laor were female, and all three of the patients in our series were female. This suggests that there could be a higher incidence of FOPE zones in females.

It is uncertain whether FOPE zones can present with clinical symptoms. Five of the twelve patients in Zbojniewicz and Laor's study had no MRI finding beyond the FOPE zone to explain their pain, suggesting that FOPE zones may be a source of pain. However, a little more than half of the patients in the study did have other explanations for their pain, and bone marrow edema has been shown to be an incidental finding in asymptomatic, active adolescents [7]. In our series, patient #3 had a clear source for her pain other than the FOPE zone, patient #2 had no clear source of her pain, and patient #1 had a potential source of knee pain on the right and no clear source of pain on the left one. It should be noted that the anterior right knee pain in patient #1 was not clearly referable to the right medial femoral condyle osteochondral lesion.

FOPE zones appear as areas of T1 hypointense and T2 hyperintense marrow edema on both the epiphyseal and metaphyseal sides of the physis with the areas of edema demonstrating contrast enhancement [2]. The edema is typically slightly eccentrically centered in the central portion of the physis with a great deal of variability in the extent of edema present. The physis has previously been described as being narrowed but open in the region of periphyseal edema [1, 2]. However, in one of our cases, the central portion of the physis was closed with surrounding periphyseal edema, which has not been previously described. Multiple physes can be involved at the same time [1, 2].

A FOPE zone is a self-limited process that requires no imaging follow-up or diagnostic intervention. FOPE zones

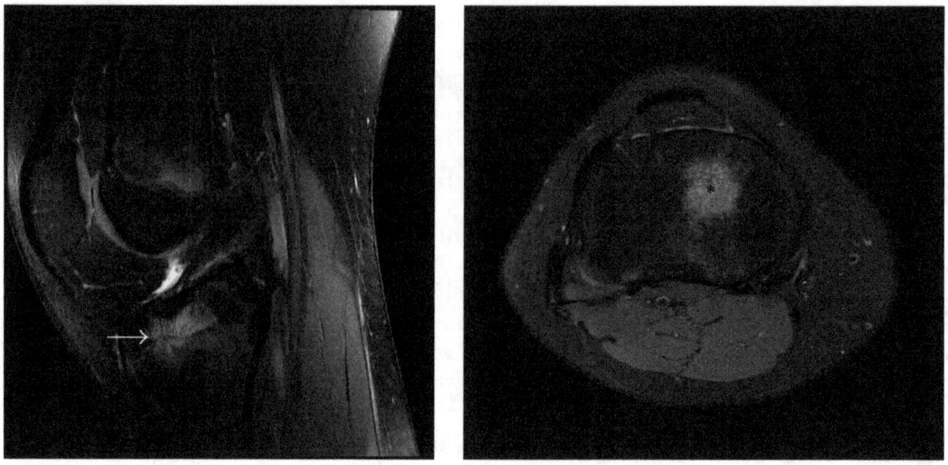

(a) (b)

Figure 8: A 14-year-2-month-old female with FOPE zone of the proximal tibia. Findings: (a) sagittal proton density image shows 14 mm in diameter area of periphyseal edema involving both sides of the proximal tibia physis (arrow). Edema is greater along the epiphyseal side of the physis. (b) Axial proton density image at the level of the proximal tibia physis shows the area of periphyseal edema within the anteromedial aspect of the central proximal tibia (asterisk). Technique: (a) sagittal PD fat-saturated MRI (TR = 2,922.8, TE = 30), ST = 3 mm, spacing = 3.3 mm, FOV = 14 cm, and matrix = 364 × 261; (b) axial PD fat-saturated MRI (TR = 2,803.1, TE = 30), ST = 3 mm, spacing = 3.3 mm, FOV = 15 cm, matrix = 376 × 297.

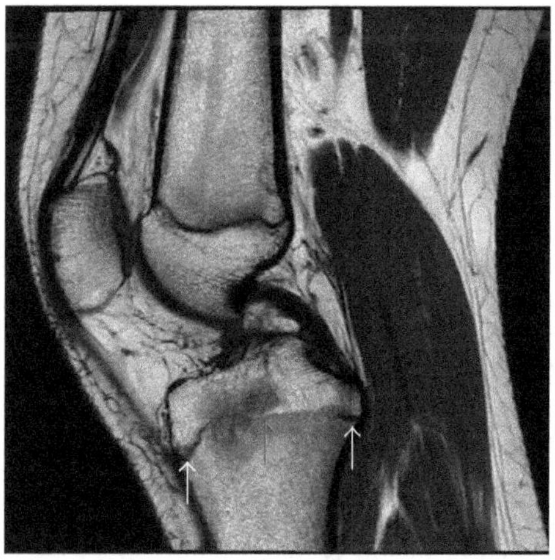

Figure 9: A 14-year-2-month-old female with FOPE zone of the proximal tibia. Findings: Sagittal T1 weighted image shows partial closure of the proximal tibia physis centrally (red arrow) with the physis still open along the periphery of the tibia (yellow arrows). The distal femur physis is narrowed but still open by comparison. Low T1 signal intensity corresponding to the periphyseal edema is again seen spanning the proximal tibia physis. Technique: sagittal T1 MRI (TR = 621.991, TE = 15), ST = 3 mm, spacing = 3.3 mm, FOV = 14 cm, and matrix = 340 × 277.

likely resolve quickly once physeal closure occurs, although our patient with partial closure of her physis demonstrates that FOPE zones can persist during physeal closure. While there is no standard treatment for FOPE zones, symptomatic FOPE zones can generally be treated with periods of rest and activity cessation similar to the treatment for stress reaction of the bone. A clinical summary of FOPE zones is included at the end of the paper (Table 1).

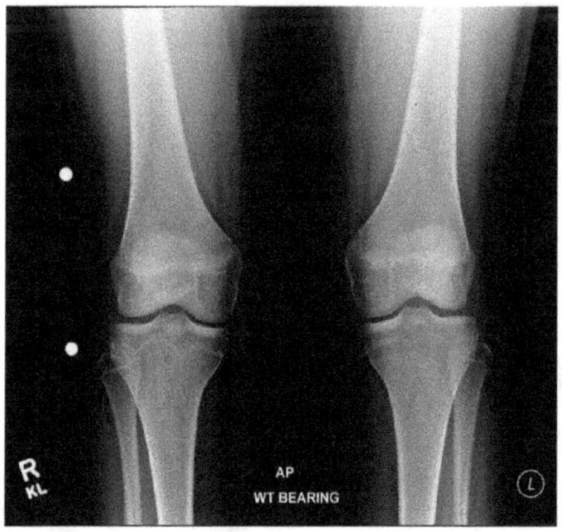

Figure 10: A 13-year-10-month-old female with FOPE zone of the distal right femur. Findings: presenting radiographs of the knees were normal. There is partial closure centrally of the bilateral proximal tibia physes. The bilateral distal femur physes are narrowed but remain open. Technique: AP radiograph kVp = 70, mAs = 8.

The physis acts as a relative barrier, preventing the spread of most tumors from the metaphysis to the epiphysis [8], although aggressive pediatric tumors such as Ewing's or osteosarcoma can cross the physis [9] and could be considered in the differential for FOPE zones. However, the typical presenting age and location, symmetric uniform appearance of marrow edema on both sides of the physis, and lack of aggressive features should allow for the distinction between FOPE zones and malignancy without much difficulty. Malignancy will often demonstrate heterogenous enhancement while the enhancement of edema in FOPE zones tends to be relatively uniform.

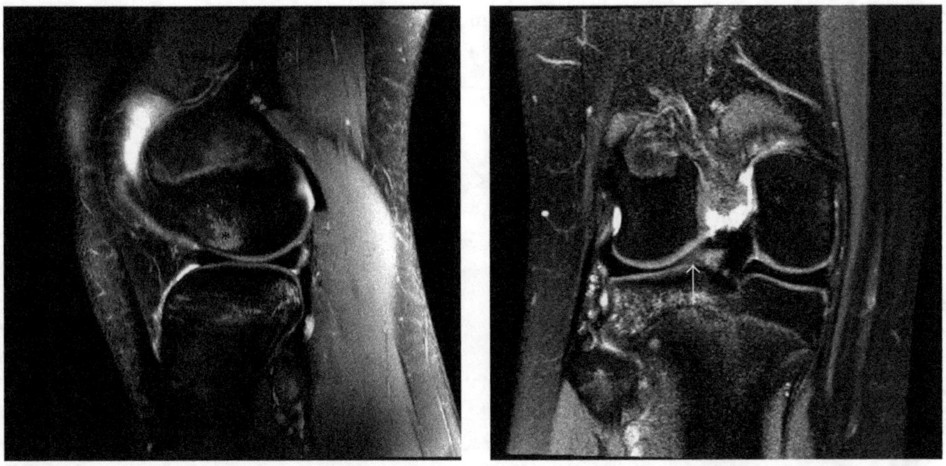

(a) (b)

FIGURE 11: A 13-year-10-month-old female with FOPE zone of the distal right femur. Findings: (a) sagittal proton density fat-saturated image shows pivot-shift pattern of bone marrow edema at the weight-bearing aspect of the lateral femoral condyle and posterior aspect of the lateral tibial plateau (asterisks). (b) Coronal proton density fat-saturated image shows increased signal in the lateral meniscus posterior horn root ligament (arrow) consistent with tearing of the ligament. Tear of the root ligament was confirmed on arthroscopy. Technique: (a) sagittal PD fat-saturated MRI (TR = 2,557, TE = 30), ST = 3 mm, spacing = 3.3 mm, FOV = 14 cm, and matrix = 364 × 261; (b) coronal PD fat-saturated MRI (TR = 2,826.1, TE = 30), ST = 2.5 mm, spacing = 3.3 mm, FOV = 15 cm, and matrix = 312 × 244.

TABLE 1: FOPE zone clinical summary.

Etiology	Unknown. Likely due to mechanical stress placed on the physis during early physeal closure.
Incidence	Rare. Only a small case series reported in the literature.
Gender ratio	Unknown. There may be a higher incidence in females.
Age of predilection	12–16 years old.
Risk factors	No known risk factors.
Treatment	No treatment for asymptomatic lesions. Symptomatic lesions treated conservatively with protected weight bearing.
Prognosis	Excellent. Self-limited process that likely resolves shortly after physeal closure.
Imaging findings	Focal enhancing bone marrow edema on both sides of a central portion of a narrowed or partially closed physis.

Infection is more likely to present with enhancing periphyseal edema that could mimic a FOPE zone. FOPE zones will lack the exuberant marrow edema and intraosseous fluid collections frequently seen with infection, and the clinical presentation as well as elevated inflammatory markers typically makes differentiating between infection and FOPE zone possible. A table summarizing the MRI characteristics of FOPE zones and the major differential considerations is included (Table 2).

Chronic physeal stress injury could present with chronic knee pain and physeal signal changes similar to a FOPE zone. On MRI, though, FOPE zones demonstrate periphyseal edema around a narrowed physis, while chronic physeal stress injuries appear as physeal widening, typically without periphyseal edema [10].

4. Conclusion

FOPE zones are a phenomenon seen at time of physeal closure, typically in the knee. While some FOPE zones may be physiologic, our cases would suggest that FOPE zones may be a possible source of pain potentially from alterations in mechanical stress across the physis as it closes. FOPE zones typically are seen as a unilateral process prior to physeal closure; as our cases show, FOPE zones can occur both after the physis begins to close and as a bilateral symmetric process. FOPE zones should be recognized as a benign self-limited entity and not mistaken for an aggressive process crossing the physis.

Abbreviations

cm: Centimeter
FOPE: Focal periphyseal edema
FOV: Field of view
kVp: Peak kilovoltage
mAs: Milliampere-second
mm: Millimeter
MRI: Magnetic resonance imaging
PD: Proton density
ST: Slice thickness
TR: Relaxation time
TE: Echo time.

TABLE 2: Differential diagnosis MRI characteristics.

Pathology	MRI, T1	MRI, T2	MRI enhancement
FOPE zone	Relatively symmetric focal decreases signal intensity on both sides of central portion of narrowed or partially closed physis.	Relatively symmetric focal increased signal intensity on both sides of central portion of narrowed or partially closed physis.	Avid, uniform enhancement of areas of bone marrow edema.
Infiltrative bone tumor	Low signal typically on one side of the physis. Low signal distribution will be asymmetric if tumor does cross physis.	High signal typically on one side of the physis. High signal distribution will be asymmetric if tumor does cross physis.	Typically avid enhancement of areas of increased T2 signal. Enhancement is often heterogeneous.
Osteomyelitis	Low signal that may cross the physis. Distribution of low signal across physis is typically asymmetric. Other findings of infection such as cortical disruption, fluid collections, and periosteal reaction are often present.	High signal that may cross the physis. Distribution of high signal across physis is typically asymmetric. Other findings of infection such as cortical disruption, fluid collections, and periosteal reaction are often present.	Typically avid, heterogenous enhancement. Nonenhancing fluid collections may be present.
Chronic physeal stress injury	Widening of the physis typically without periphyseal low signal.	Widening of the physis typically without periphyseal high signal.	Typically no increased periphyseal enhancement.

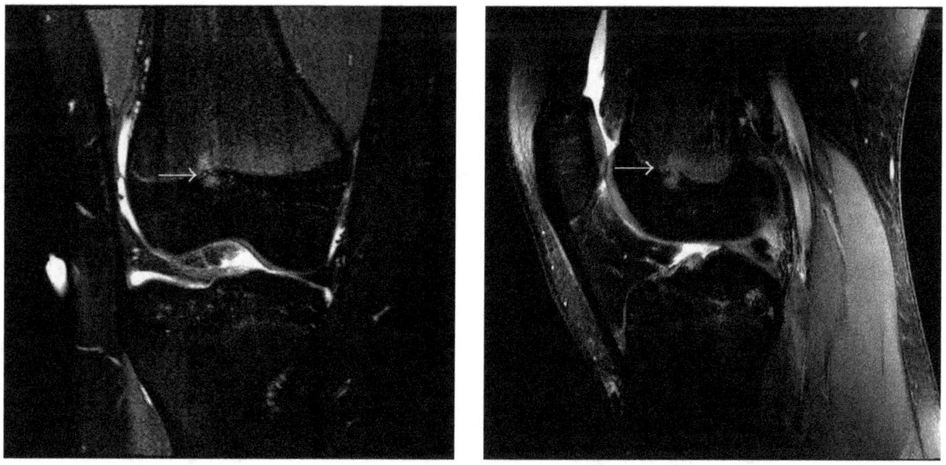

(a) (b)

FIGURE 12: A 13-year-10-month-old female with FOPE zone of the distal right femur. Findings: (a) coronal proton density fat-saturated image shows a 5 mm area of periphyseal edema slightly eccentrically located on both sides of the distal femur physis (arrow). The edema is slightly more prominent on the epiphyseal side of the physis. (b) Sagittal proton density fat-saturated image again shows the eccentrically located area of periphyseal edema in the distal femur physis (arrow) with the edema again slightly more prominent on the epiphyseal side. The distal femur physis is narrowed but remains open. Technique: (a) coronal PD fat-saturated MRI (TR = 2,826.1, TE = 30), ST = 2.5 mm, spacing = 3.3 mm, FOV = 15 cm, and matrix = 312 × 244; (b) coronal PD fat-saturated MRI (TR = 2,826.1, TE = 30), ST = 2.5 mm, spacing = 3.3 mm, FOV = 15 cm, and matrix = 312 × 244.

Authors' Contribution

Nicholas Beckmann is the primary author and contributed to case contributions. Susanna Spence helped with paper editing and case contributions.

References

[1] A. M. Zbojniewicz and T. Laor, "Focal periphyseal edema (FOPE) zone on mri of the adolescent knee: a potentially painful manifestation of physiologic physeal fusion?" *American Journal of Roentgenology*, vol. 197, no. 4, pp. 998–1004, 2011.

[2] S. L. Viana, M. C. Machado-Ribeiro, and B. Beber-Machado, "Peculiar aspects of the anatomy and development of the growing skeleton," in *Joint Imaging in Childhood and Adolescence*, pp. 23–36, Springer, Berlin, Germany, 2013.

[3] K. G. Gill, B. A. Nemeth, and K. W. Davis, "Magnetic resonance imaging of the pediatric knee," *Magnetic Resonance Imaging Clinics of North America*, vol. 22, no. 4, pp. 743–763, 2014.

[4] C. Bateni, J. Bindra, and B. Haus, "MRI of sports injuries in children and adolescents: what's different from adults," *Current Radiology Reports*, vol. 2, article 45, 2014.

[5] N. M. Major, "Role of MRI in prevention of metatarsal stress fractures in collegiate basketball players," *American Journal of Roentgenology*, vol. 186, no. 1, pp. 255–258, 2006.

[6] T. Sasaki, Y. Ishibashi, Y. Okamura, S. Toh, and T. Sasaki, "MRI evaluation of growth plate closure rate and pattern in the normal knee joint," *Journal of Knee Surgery*, vol. 15, no. 2, pp. 72–76, 2002.

[7] R. B. Soder, J. D. Simoes, J. B. Soder, and M. Baldisserotto, "MRI of the knee joint in asymptomatic adolescent soccer players: a controlled study," *American Journal of Roentgenology*, vol. 196, no. 1, pp. W61–W65, 2011.

[8] L. T. Staheli, "Features of the immature skeleton," in *Fundamentals of Pediatric Orthopedics*, Lippincott Williams & Wilkins, 2008.

[9] M. Panuel, J. C. Gentet, C. Scheiner et al., "Physeal and epiphyseal extent of primary malignant bone tumors in childhood. Correlation of preoperative MRI and the pathologic examination," *Pediatric Radiology*, vol. 23, no. 6, pp. 421–424, 1993.

[10] T. Laor, E. J. Wall, and L. P. Vu, "Physeal widening in the knee due to stress injury in child athletes," *American Journal of Roentgenology*, vol. 186, no. 5, pp. 1260–1264, 2006.

7

Skeletal Muscle Involvement in B-Cell Lymphoma: Two Cases Illustrating the Contribution of Imaging to a Clinically Unsuspected Diagnosis

Elijah Burton,[1] Kristian Schafernak,[2,3] Elaine Morgan,[4] and Jonathan Samet[4]

[1]*David Grant USAF Medical Center, Fairfield, CA, USA*
[2]*University of Arizona College of Medicine, Phoenix, AZ, USA*
[3]*Mayo Clinic College of Medicine, Phoenix, AZ, USA*
[4]*Northwestern University Feinberg School of Medicine, Chicago, IL, USA*

Correspondence should be addressed to Elijah Burton; elburto8@gmail.com

Academic Editor: Atsushi Komemushi

Skeletal muscle lymphoma is rare, comprising only a very small subset of lymphoma cases. There are characteristic imaging features which, if recognized, can prevent delay in diagnosis and treatment, particularly when not suspected clinically. Herein, we report two cases of skeletal muscle lymphoma with nearly identical imaging features; the first is an example of primary muscle lymphoma in a 17-year-old boy with back and thigh pain, and the second represents lymphoma recurrence in a 55-year-old man with HIV. Characteristic features seen on MRI were key in raising suspicion for the disease and helped prevent a delay in pathologic diagnosis.

1. Introduction

Extranodal involvement is relatively common in NHL (non-Hodgkin Lymphoma), present in up to 30% of cases [1]. Involvement of the muscle, however, is much less frequent, representing 1.5–5% of extranodal lymphoma cases [2, 3]. Most of these cases showed contiguous spread from adjacent bone or other tissues, indicating that the musculature was not the primary origin of disease. In a study of 7000 patients with malignant lymphoma, primary muscle lymphoma was seen in only 8 patients [4]. By comparison, lymphoma of bone represents 5% of extranodal lymphomas and 7% of bone malignancies [4].

We report two cases of lymphoma presenting in muscle with progressive swelling and pain, one in a 17-year-old boy, and the other in a 55-year-old man with HIV. We aim to highlight the characteristic imaging findings of muscle lymphoma and to emphasize the importance of suggesting lymphoma as pathologic evaluation requires specific biopsy considerations.

2. Case Reports

2.1. Case 1. This patient is a 17-year-old boy who presented with a four-week history of intermittent back and thigh pain refractory to conservative therapy. The pain had progressively worsened, awakening him at night, and there was swelling in the thigh and buttocks. He denied fevers, night sweats, or weight loss at presentation. His past medical history was otherwise unremarkable and he had no history of trauma to the involved area. His exam and labs revealed that he was HIV-negative and afebrile without leukocytosis. Neurologic exam of the lower extremities showed no weakness or sensory deficit. After failing initial therapy with anti-inflammatory medications, his pediatrician sent him for an outpatient MRI. However, the pain was so severe that he was referred to the emergency department for adequate pain control prior to imaging.

MRI demonstrated diffuse unilateral expansion of the right-sided paraspinal and gluteal musculature without a focal measurable mass. There was striking effacement of the normally identified fatty striations within the affected

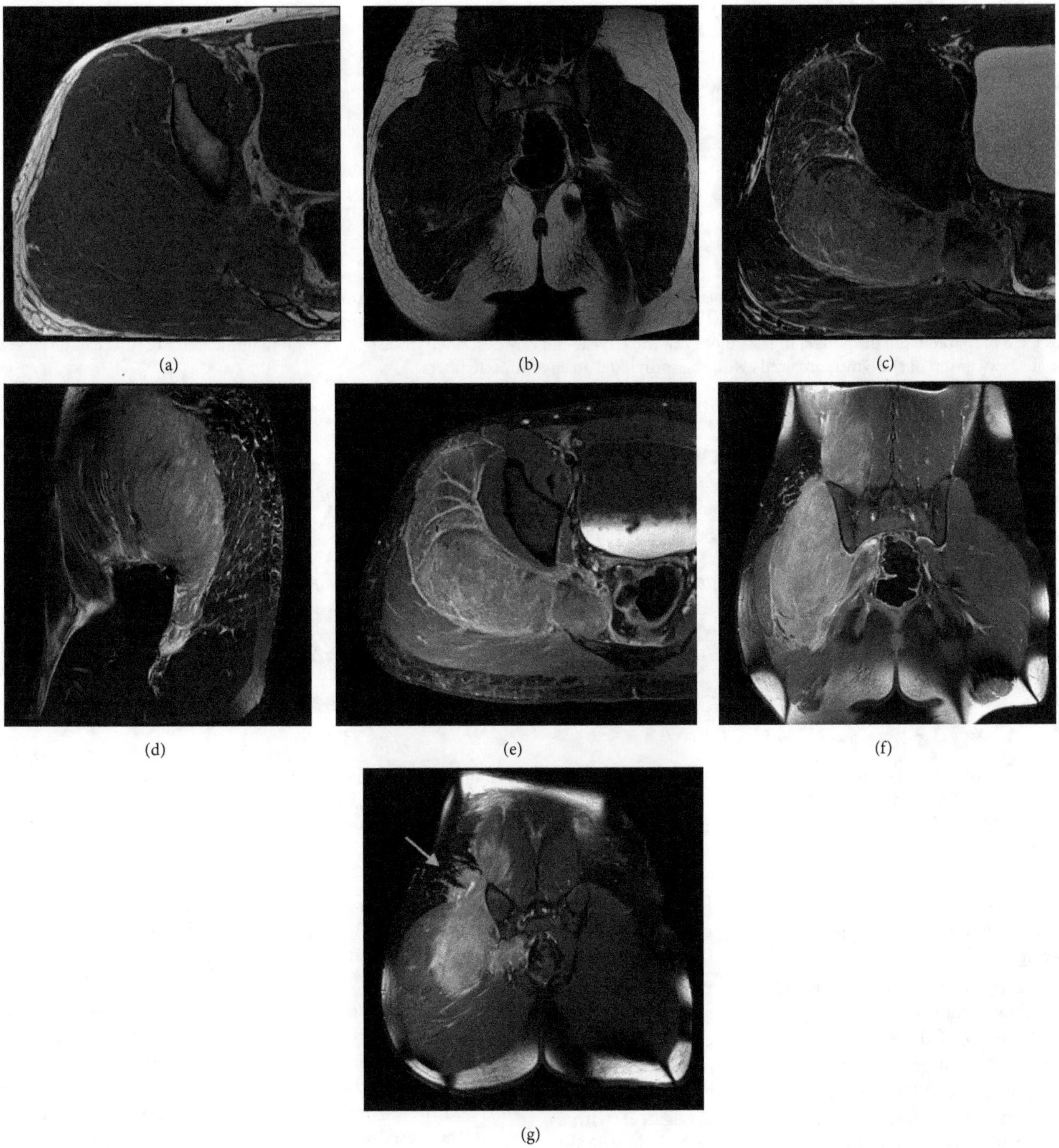

FIGURE 1: Axial T1 (a), coronal T1 (b), axial T2 (c), sagittal T2 (d), axial T1 FS postcontrast (e), coronal T1 FS postcontrast (f), and coronal T1 FS postcontrast (g) images of the involved lumbar spine and pelvis in the 17-year-old boy from case 1. There is unilateral marked expansion of the right gluteal, piriformis, and paraspinal muscles, exhibiting T1 isointensity and T2 hyperintensity. The muscle enlargement results in effacement of intramuscular fat. The postcontrast images demonstrate diffuse striated enhancement, giving an infiltrative appearance. Enhancing nodules are seen in the adjacent subcutaneous tissues. There is also subcutaneous fat stranding (indicated by the arrow, image (g)). Aside for the enlargement, note the overall preservation of muscle morphology and lack of a focal mass.

muscles. Relative to other muscles, the signal was isointense on T1. The muscle was diffusely mildly T2 hyperintense, with more dominant linear T2 hyperintense signal in a striated pattern along the muscle fibers. Following administration of gadolinium, the involved muscles exhibited diffuse enhancement with additional linear hyperenhancement in a striated pattern. Additionally, small enhancing soft tissue nodules adjacent to the affected muscles were seen in the overlying subcutaneous tissues (Figures 1(a)–1(g)). Although small, the presence of soft tissue masses was a clue pointing toward a neoplastic process and would be atypical for inflammatory or infectious myositis. These nodules were located over the

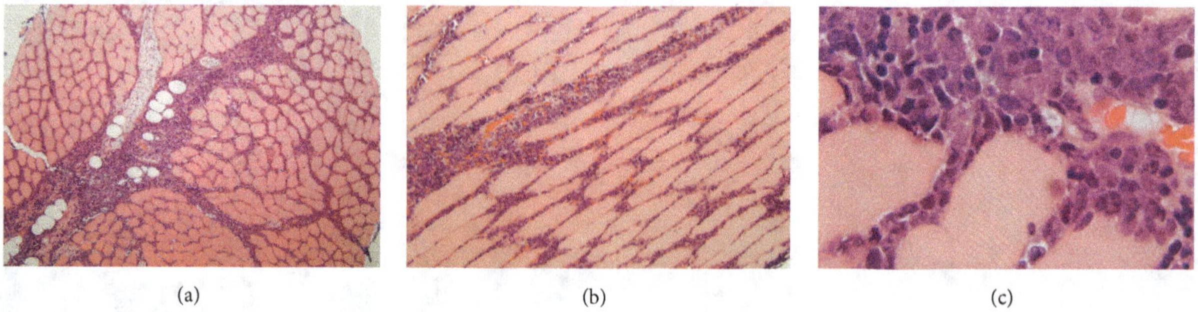

Figure 2: Transverse (a) and longitudinal (b) hematoxylin and eosin-stained histologic sections showing an infiltrate of intermediate-sized to large lymphoid cells in the endomysium between muscle fibers and the perimysium investing the fascicles or bundles of these fibers; these slides were prepared from the gluteal muscle biopsy of the 17-year-old boy described in case 1. On high magnification (c) one can observe the intimate association of the lymphoma cells with the individual striated muscle fibers.

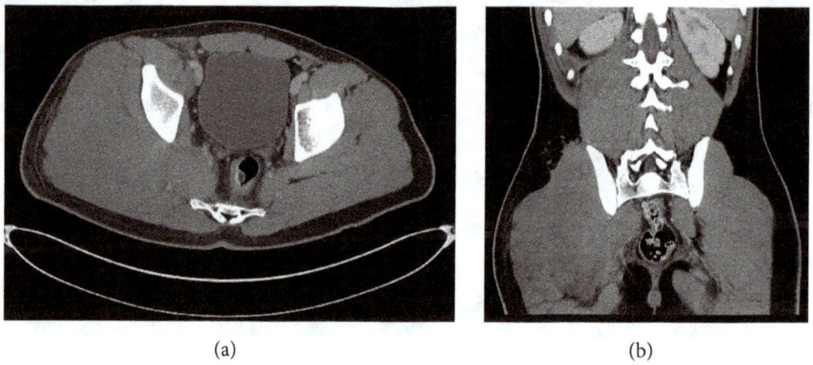

Figure 3: Axial (a) and coronal contrast enhanced CT (b) images of the abdomen and pelvis from the 17-year-old boy in case 1. There is striking asymmetric enlargement of the right gluteal and paraspinal muscles, isodense to adjacent muscle.

buttocks, an unusual site for lymph nodes. Regardless, infectious myositis was also considered highly on the radiologic differential.

This appearance was suspicious for an infiltrative process, specifically lymphoma, which promptly led to ultrasound-guided biopsy of the involved gluteal musculature. A high-grade CD10 positive B-cell lymphoma was diagnosed (it was CD45 positive, CD19 positive, CD20 negative, CD10 positive, surface immunoglobulin negative, and BCL2 negative, with a Ki67 proliferation index approaching 100% based on limited phenotyping by combined flow cytometry and immunohistochemistry), but additional fresh tissue via open biopsy was requested for additional studies to attempt to refine the diagnosis. Ultimately, the lymphoma is perhaps best classified as a high-grade B-cell lymphoma, not otherwise specified, following the 2016 revision of the World Health Organization classification of lymphoid neoplasms (histopathology depicted in Figures 2(a)–2(c)). CT scan of the chest, abdomen, and pelvis was obtained for staging purposes and similar to the MRI, there was diffuse unilateral enlargement of the gluteal and paraspinal muscles (Figures 3(a) and 3(b)). There were a few suspicious local subcentimeter lymph nodes adjacent to the right psoas muscle enlargement. No other sites of involvement or additional lymph node enlargement were seen on the CT. Bone marrow biopsy and lumbar puncture were negative for involvement by lymphoma.

2.2. Case 2. This patient is a 55-year-old HIV-positive man who presented with several weeks of worsening pain and swelling in the lower leg. His past medical history was significant for CD10 positive diffuse large B-cell lymphoma of the kidney without bone marrow involvement, 15 months prior to presentation. He went into initial remission with chemotherapy. On exam, the patient was afebrile but his calf was exquisitely tender and enlarged. There was no neurologic deficit. After these symptoms progressed despite conservative therapy, MRI was ordered.

Similar to case 1, MRI demonstrated diffuse enlargement of multiple posterior calf muscles, with effacement of intramuscular fat (Figures 4(a)–4(f)). Postcontrast images showed diffuse enhancement of the affected muscles, but no focal mass (Figures 4(d)–4(f)).

Myositis was favored over recurrent lymphoma clinically and radiologically. However, due to persistent symptoms, an open biopsy was performed, which revealed diffuse large B-cell lymphoma of the gastrocnemius muscle; histology is demonstrated in Figures 5(a) and 5(b). CT was subsequently

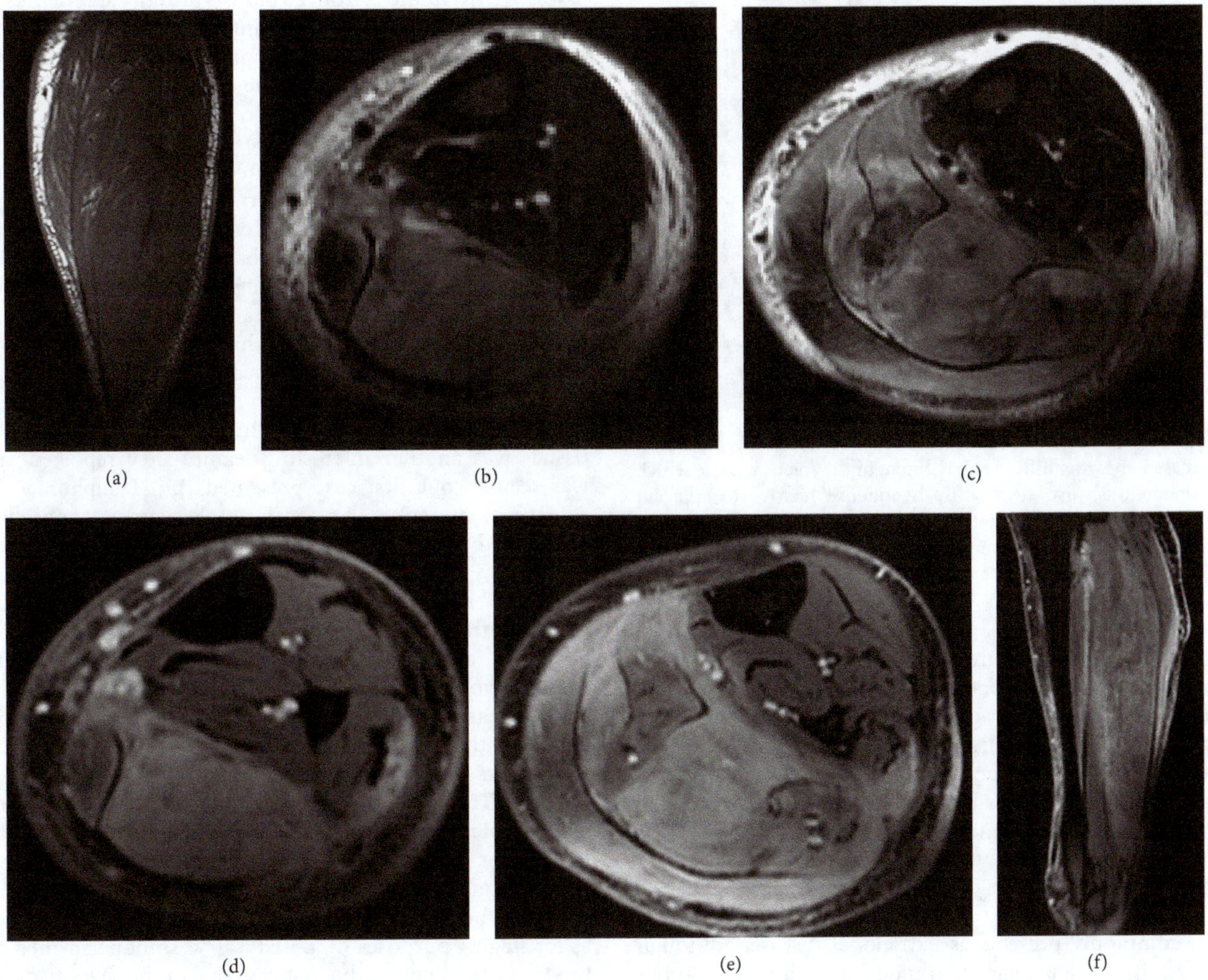

FIGURE 4: Sagittal T1 (a), axial STIR (b, c), axial T1 fat saturated postcontrast (d, e), and sagittal T1 fat saturated postcontrast (f) images of the involved lower leg in the 55-year-old man with HIV described in case 2. There is marked enlargement of the posterior calf muscles with effacement of the intramuscular fat. The affected muscle demonstrates T2 hyperintense signal and diffuse enhancement on postcontrast sequences. The overall findings should raise the suspicion for an infiltrative process such as lymphoma.

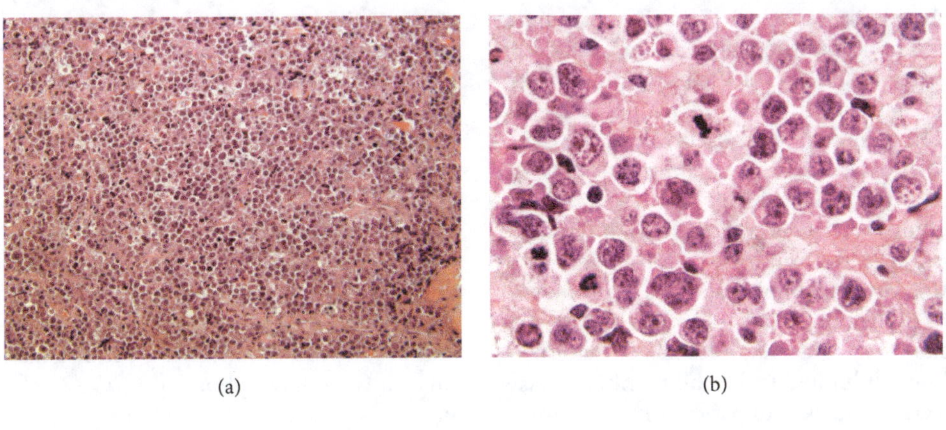

FIGURE 5: The 55-year-old patient's lymphoma from case 2 showed microscopically a more diffuse infiltrate of large cells with abundant mitotic figures (a, b).

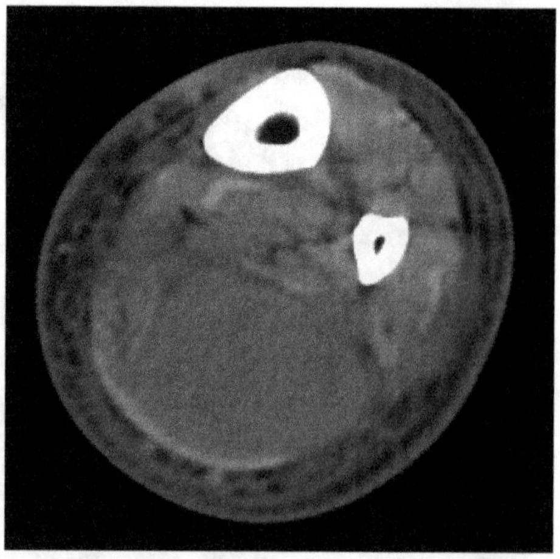

FIGURE 6: Axial contrast enhanced CT image of the 55-year-old man from case 2 showing diffuse enlargement of the soleus muscle which is homogenously iso- to slightly hypodense relative to adjacent muscle. Note the skin thickening and subcutaneous fat stranding, which can also be seen in lymphoma.

ordered to assess for progression of disease, which redemonstrated diffuse enlargement of the posterior calf musculature and subcutaneous fat stranding of the leg (Figure 6). There was no lymph node enlargement in the chest, abdomen or pelvis, indicating that the muscle was the primary site of recurrence. Bone marrow biopsy and lumbar puncture were also negative for malignancy.

3. Discussion

NHL commonly presents as extranodal disease. Although the definition of primary extranodal lymphoma is somewhat controversial, the commonly accepted definition is involvement of an organ with no or minor local lymph node enlargement [5]. Infiltration of the muscle is a very uncommon manifestation of lymphoma and most commonly occurs in the gluteal and pelvic musculature as a result of hematogenous dissemination or direct spread from adjacent lymph nodes or bone; primary involvement of the muscle is exceedingly rare [6]. By 1997, fewer than 50 cases of primary muscle lymphoma had been described [7]. Primary muscle lymphoma was found to account for just 0.1% of over 7,000 cases of lymphoma diagnosed over a 10-year period at the Mayo Clinic [8]. By comparison, in a study of 1168 patients with NHL, <1% involved the ovary and 3% involved bone [5].

Primary skeletal muscle NHL most commonly has an aggressive B-cell immunophenotype, but aggressive mature T-cell lymphoma has also been rarely reported [9]. It typically presents with a mass, swelling, and pain [10]. As imaging is often part of the initial workup, radiologists have the opportunity to direct further evaluation by suggesting the diagnosis.

Knowledge of the imaging findings associated with primary muscle lymphoma is limited to a small number of case reports and retrospective studies. Our patients' imaging findings correspond well with those described in the literature [7, 8, 10–13]. In a recent retrospective study, Chun et al. [14] assessed MRI findings from 20 biopsy-proven cases of muscle lymphoma. All patients had diffuse enlargement of the muscle. Nine of these were primary muscle lymphoma and 11 represented recurrence in the muscle. On T1-weighted images, all patients had equal to or slightly higher signal than normal surrounding muscle. All lesions demonstrated intermediate signal on T2-weighted imaging. In cases using contrast, the most common pattern was diffuse enhancement (seen in 13 of 19 cases); peripheral enhancement and marginal septal enhancement were the enhancement patterns seen in the remaining cases. A majority of patients showed stranding in the subcutaneous fat, with a minority demonstrating overlying skin thickening. Suresh et al. found that muscle lymphoma had a propensity to involve multiple muscle compartments, distinguishing it from most soft tissue sarcomas. Extension of muscle lymphoma into adjacent subcutaneous tissues was another interesting feature they reported and was seen in our first case presented [15]. Lymphoma can sometimes present with a focal muscle mass as opposed to an infiltrative ill-defined abnormality, but this is less common [16].

On CT, nearly all reports describe diffuse expansion of the muscle with iso- to hypodensity of the involved areas [2, 17–20]. There are two reported cases of NHL with extranodal muscle involvement which showed hyperdensity on CT. Both of these cases occurred in HIV-positive patients [21]. Our patient with HIV demonstrated iso- to hypodense muscle infiltration.

PET/CT was not performed in either of these cases and is not typically performed in the initial workup of muscle lymphoma. PET/CT is, however, often performed after a tissue diagnosis is made to obtain a baseline for which future scans can be compared to gauge response to therapy as well as for staging purposes [22]. PET/CT was not performed on the 17-year-old boy in the first case due to the severity of his disease at presentation and desire to initiate prompt therapy.

The differential diagnosis includes denervation muscle edema, infectious and inflammatory myositis, sarcoidosis, rhabdomyolysis, sarcoma, and metastatic disease, among other etiologies. Denervation edema of skeletal muscle can result in T2 hyperintensity and muscle expansion but may also present with weakness and evidence of nerve compression on imaging [23]. Inflammatory myositis such as polymyositis and juvenile dermatomyositis can display T2 hyperintensity in skeletal muscle but is rarely unilateral and can typically be excluded on the basis of normal laboratory values [24]. Muscle involvement of sarcoidosis on MRI shows multiple elongated nodules with a characteristic low signal center, producing a striped appearance. In addition, patients will typically have other manifestations of this systemic disease [25]. Rhabdomyolysis shows diffuse T2 hyperintense signal in a muscle and can be unilateral or bilateral. Postcontrast imaging can show diffuse enhancement or rim enhancement depending on the severity and time course. Laboratory tests and predisposing underlying conditions would differentiate this entity from lymphoma [26]. On MRI, primary soft tissue sarcomas typically present with a distinct rounded mass [27]. Intramuscular metastases appear as enhancing masses with central necrosis and peritumoral edema [28]. The absence of clinical and laboratory parameters of the aforementioned differential diagnoses should allow one to suggest lymphoma as the leading diagnosis.

Patients with HIV have a 60-fold greater risk of developing NHL compared to the general population. This risk is mainly present in individuals with CD4+ counts less than 200/mm^3. There is a propensity for the development of extranodal disease in these patients as well, including primary or metastatic muscular involvement [29, 30]. When considering muscle lymphoma in an HIV-positive patient, infectious myositis should also be kept in mind. With this type of infection, most patients present with severe pain, fever, and muscle swelling. In its early stages, MRI will show muscle enlargement and T2 hyperintensity. In more progressed cases, MRI demonstrates intramuscular fluid collections which can represent abscesses or myonecrosis [31]. Nonbacterial myositis can have a wide spectrum of imaging findings depending on the organism. Viral infection, for example, in the setting of inclusion body myositis, will have MRI features similar to polymyositis and does not form abscesses [32].

While imaging cannot definitively establish the diagnosis of primary muscle lymphoma, the imaging characteristics described above can strongly suggest this diagnosis. Lymphoma is important to suspect because it can guide the workup, limit unnecessary testing, and avoid delay in diagnosis. When intramuscular lymphoma is suspected, more generous sampling than normal of fresh tissue is often needed for pathological analysis, which may influence the strategy for obtaining biopsy [33]. Proper treatment is predicated on precise diagnosis; the current World Health Organization approach to lymphoma diagnosis is multiparametric but has become increasingly complex and typically relies on the convergence of clinical, morphologic, immunophenotypic, and genetic data. Techniques such as flow cytometry, immunophenotyping, and conventional cytogenetic analysis can only be performed on fresh [not formalin-fixed] tissue. Therefore to facilitate these studies, additional tissue may be required, which needs to be placed in sterile saline or a nutrient medium such as RPMI (Roswell Park Memorial Institute) medium to keep the cells viable.

In summary, primary and secondary muscle lymphomas are rare but present with characteristic findings on MRI and CT. The radiologist can be the first provider to suggest this diagnosis and anticipate the special biopsy preparation needed for definitive diagnosis.

Disclosure

One of the cases in this manuscript was presented previously in a poster format at the Society of Pediatric Radiology's annual conference in April 2015.

References

[1] C. Freeman, J. W. Berg, and S. J. Cutler, "Occurrence and prognosis of extranodal lymphomas," *Cancer*, vol. 29, no. 1, pp. 252–260, 1972.

[2] H. S. Glazer, J. K. T. Lee, D. M. Balfe, M. A. Mauro, R. Griffith, and S. S. Sagel, "Non-Hodgkin lymphoma: Computed tomographic demonstration of unusual extranodal involvement," *Radiology*, vol. 149, no. 1, pp. 211–217, 1983.

[3] G. Carroll, W. Breidahl, and P. Robbins, "Musculoskeletal lymphoma: MRI of bone or soft tissue presentations," *Journal of Medical Imaging and Radiation Oncology*, vol. 57, no. 6, pp. 663–673, 2013.

[4] C. Y. Lim and K. O. Ong, "Imaging of musculoskeletal lymphoma," *Cancer Imaging*, vol. 13, no. 4, pp. 448–457, 2013.

[5] A. D. G. Krol, S. le Cessie, S. Snijder, J. C. Kluin-Nelemans, P. M. Kluin, and E. M. Noordijk, "Primary extranodal non-Hodgkin's lymphoma (NHL): the impact of alternative definitions tested in the Comprehensive Cancer Centre West population-based NHL registry," *Annals of Oncology*, vol. 14, no. 1, pp. 131–139, 2003.

[6] M. Komatsuda, T. Nagao, and S. Arimori, "An autopsy case of malignant lymphoma associated with remarkable infiltration in skeletal muscles (author's transl)," *(Rinsho ketsueki) The Japanese Journal of Clinical Hematology*, vol. 22, no. 6, pp. 891–895, 1981.

[7] I. Beggs, "Primary muscle lymphoma," *Clinical Radiology*, vol. 52, no. 3, pp. 203–212, 1997.

[8] W. D. Travis, P. M. Banks, and H. M. Reiman, "Primary extranodal soft tissue lymphoma of the extremities," *The American Journal of Surgical Pathology*, vol. 11, no. 5, pp. 359–366, 1987.

[9] T. J. Alekshun, D. Rezania, E. Ayala, H. Cualing, and L. Sokol, "Skeletal muscle peripheral T-cell lymphoma," *Journal of Clinical Oncology*, vol. 26, no. 3, pp. 501–503, 2008.

[10] K. Hongsakul, T. Laohawiriyakamol, and K. Kayasut, "A rare case of primary muscular non-Hodgkin's lymphoma and a review of how imaging can assist in its diagnosis," *Singapore Medical Journal*, vol. 54, no. 9, pp. e179–e182, 2013.

[11] A. Ueno, K. Kuribayashi, S. Iyama et al., "Two cases of primary skeletal muscle lymphoma, and a review of the literature," *(Rinsho ketsueki) The Japanese Journal of Clinical Hematology*, vol. 46, no. 10, pp. 1141–1145, 2005.

[12] V. S. Lee, S. Martinez, and R. E. Coleman, "Primary muscle lymphoma: clinical and imaging findings," *Radiology*, vol. 203, no. 1, pp. 237–244, 1997.

[13] J. Chong, P. M. Som, A. R. Silvers, and J. F. Dalton, "Extranodal non-Hodgkin lymphoma involving the muscles of mastication," *American Journal of Neuroradiology (AJNR)*, vol. 19, no. 10, pp. 1849–1851, 1998.

[14] C. W. Chun, W.-H. Jee, H. J. Park et al., "MRI features of skeletal muscle lymphoma," *American Journal of Roentgenology*, vol. 195, no. 6, pp. 1355–1360, 2010.

[15] S. Suresh, A. Saifuddin, and P. O'Donnell, "Lymphoma presenting as a musculoskeletal soft tissue mass: MRI findings in 24 cases," *European Radiology*, vol. 18, no. 11, pp. 2628–2634, 2008.

[16] A. Surov, "Imaging findings of skeletal muscle lymphoma," *Clinical Imaging*, vol. 38, no. 5, pp. 594–598, 2014.

[17] N. D. Grunshaw and A. G. Chalmers, "Skeletal muscle lymphoma," *Clinical Radiology*, vol. 45, no. 6, pp. 399–400, 1992.

[18] M. Hosono, H. Kobayashi, Y. Kotoura, T. Tsuboyama, K. Tsutsui, and J. Konishi, "Involvement of muscle by malignant

lymphoma: MR and CT appearances," *Journal of Computer Assisted Tomography*, vol. 19, no. 3, pp. 455–459, 1995.

[19] P. C. Malloy, E. K. Fishman, and D. Magid, "Lymphoma of bone, muscle, and skin: CT findings," *American Journal of Roentgenology*, vol. 159, no. 4, pp. 805–809, 1992.

[20] M. V. Pilepich and B. L. Carter, "Muscle enlargement in lymphoma patients," *Radiology*, vol. 134, no. 2, pp. 521–523, 1980.

[21] D. R. Radin, J. A. Esplin, A. M. Levine, and P. W. Ralls, "AIDS-related non-Hodgkin's lymphoma: abdominal CT findings in 112 patients," *American Journal of Roentgenology*, vol. 160, no. 5, pp. 1133–1139, 1993.

[22] M. Hutchings and S. F. Barrington, "PET/CT for Therapy response assessment in lymphoma," *Journal of Nuclear Medicine*, vol. 50, supplement 1, pp. 21S–30S, 2009.

[23] N. J. Fischbein, M. J. Kaplan, R. K. Jackler, and W. P. Dillon, "MR imaging in two cases of subacute denervation change in the muscles of facial expression," *American Journal of Neuroradiology*, vol. 22, no. 5, pp. 880–884, 2001.

[24] E. Dion, P. Cherin, C. Payan et al., "Magnetic resonance imaging criteria for distinguishing between inclusion body myositis and polymyositis," *Journal of Rheumatology*, vol. 29, no. 9, pp. 1897–1906, 2002.

[25] S. Otake, "Sarcoidosis involving skeletal muscle: imaging findings and relative value of imaging procedures," *American Journal of Roentgenology*, vol. 162, no. 2, pp. 369–375, 1994.

[26] C.-H. Lu, Y.-M. Tsang, C.-W. Yu, M.-Z. Wu, C.-Y. Hsu, and T. T.-F. Shih, "Rhabdomyolysis: magnetic resonance imaging and computed tomography findings," *Journal of Computer Assisted Tomography*, vol. 31, no. 3, pp. 368–374, 2007.

[27] E. Robinson, R. R. Bleakney, P. C. Ferguson, and B. O'Sullivan, "Multidisciplinary management of soft-tissue sarcoma," *Radiographics*, vol. 28, no. 7, pp. 2069–2086, 2008.

[28] T. Arpaci, G. Ugurluer, T. Akbas, R. B. Arpaci, and M. Serin, "Imaging of the skeletal muscle metastases," *European Review for Medical and Pharmacological Sciences*, vol. 16, no. 15, pp. 2057–2063, 2012.

[29] A. C. Jung and D. S. Paauw, "Diagnosing HIV-related disease: using the CD4 count as a guide," *Journal of General Internal Medicine*, vol. 13, no. 2, pp. 131–136, 1998.

[30] L. M. Baddour, K. H. Haden, and J. W. Allen, "Primary skeletal muscle lymphoma presenting as refractory cellulitis," *Cutis*, vol. 68, no. 3, pp. 223–226, 2001.

[31] S. J. Theodorou, D. J. Theodorou, and D. Resnick, "MR imaging findings of pyogenic bacterial myositis (pyomyositis) in patients with local muscle trauma: illustrative cases," *Emergency Radiology*, vol. 14, no. 2, pp. 89–96, 2007.

[32] D. A. May, D. G. Disler, E. A. Jones, A. A. Balkissoon, and B. J. Manaster, "Abnormal signal intensity in skeletal muscle at MR imaging: patterns, pearls, and pitfalls," *Radiographics*, vol. 20, pp. S295–S315, 2000.

[33] P. L. Farmer, D. J. Bailey, B. F. Burns, A. Day, and D. P. LeBrun, "The reliability of lymphoma diagnosis in small tissue samples is heavily influenced by lymphoma subtype," *American Journal of Clinical Pathology*, vol. 128, no. 3, pp. 474–480, 2007.

8

Focal Xanthogranulomatous Pyelonephritis with Pulmonary Lesions on the Background of Type Two Diabetes Mellitus

Ahmad Enshaei,[1] Arash A. Boora,[2] Diana Taheri,[3] Zahra Changizi,[4] and Nahid Bahmani[5]

[1]*Isfahan University of Medical Science, Kashani Hospital, Kashani Ave, Isfahan, Iran*
[2]*University of Queensland, St. Lucia, QLD, Australia*
[3]*Department of Pathology, Isfahan Kidney Diseases Research Centre, Isfahan University of Medical Sciences, Isfahan, Iran*
[4]*Department of Internal Medicine, Saadi Hospital, Isfahan, Iran*
[5]*Department of Radiology, Saadi Hospital, Isfahan, Iran*

Correspondence should be addressed to Arash A. Boora; arash.boora@gmail.com

Academic Editor: Vincent Low

Focal Xanthogranulomatous pyelonephritis is a rare chronic inflammatory condition of kidneys which usually is associated with postrenal obstruction or renal stone leading to chronic bacterial infection and eventually chronic glomerular inflammation. About 90% of cases are of the diffuse type and associated with staghorn renal calculi. The case presented in this paper is of the focal type in a 58-year-old diabetic female. Interestingly she did not have symptoms or laboratory presentation of chronic renal bacterial infection except for elevated ESR. She sought medical attention due to severe pulmonary infection of the background of morbid obesity. Imaging studies revealed several pulmonary lesions and a large mass of the right kidney which was indistinguishable from renal malignancy. After surgical resection of the right kidney, the lesion is pathologically diagnosed to be a focal Xanthogranulomatous pyelonephritis. The pulmonary lesions were spontaneously resolved about three months following right nephrectomy.

1. Introduction

Xanthogranulomatous pyelonephritis (XGP) is a chronic inflammatory renal condition [1]. It is manifested in three types: diffuse (83%–90%), segmental, and focal (together 10%–17%) [2]. The pathogenesis of the disease constitutes lipid-laden macrophages replacing the renal parenchyma [3, 4]. The focal form has a reputation for imitating more serious pathologies [5]. Symptomatically XGP presents with urinary tract infection resistant to antibiotics, fever, haematuria, dysuria, abdominal pain, a palpable mass, anorexia, and weight loss [6]. The aetiology is uncertain. However, association with *E. coli* and Proteus Mirabilis urinary infection has been shown [7, 8]. Also, XGP has been linked to obstruction of the renal tract by infected calculi [9–12]. XGP has been presented as a complication of renal transplant [13]. In addition, XGP has been correlated with metabolic syndrome and diabetes mellitus.

2. Case Report

A 58-year-old female presented to infectious disease department of the hospital with a severe pulmonary infection on the background of morbid obesity (BMI 43) and type 2 diabetes mellitus for the last 17 years which was under treatment with insulin in addition to hypertension and hyperlipidaemia. She has past surgical history of cholecystectomy. Recently she has lost 25 kg using Liraglutide (Victoza) injections. She weighed 110 kg at the time of admission.

She has no urological symptoms; no flank pain, dysuria, or frequency or gross haematuria, and neither had she reported experiencing any of these symptoms in the past. She had an elevated ESR for a long time with unknown cause. Urine analysis revealed microscopic haematuria. Besides treatment for pulmonary infection, work-up has been initiated to find the cause of elevated ESR and microscopic haematuria.

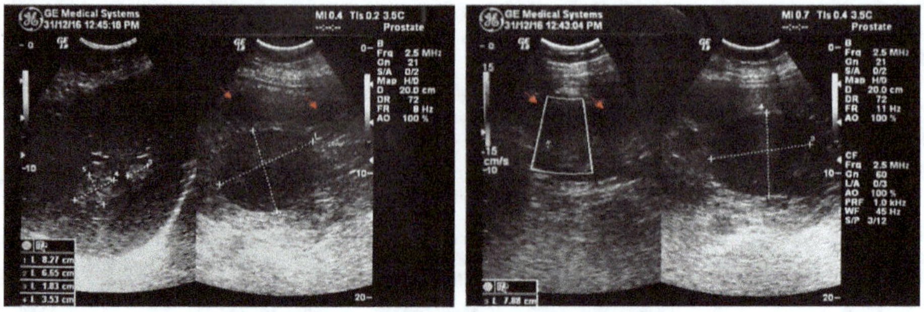

FIGURE 1: The right kidney masses probably are liver hematomas (red arrows).

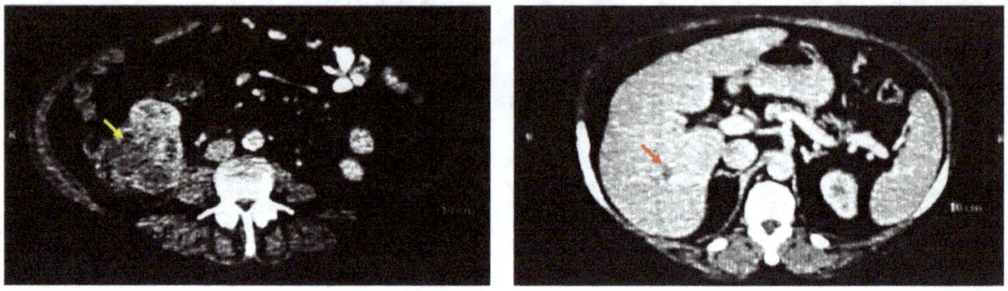

FIGURE 2: CT of Abdomen. Yellow arrow: mass attached to the right kidney (yellow arrow) on CT scan with bear paw sign. Red arrows: probably liver hemangiomas.

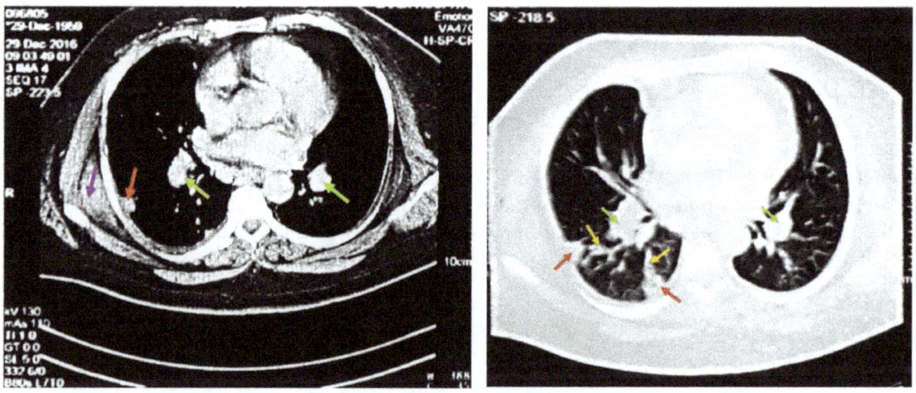

FIGURE 3: CT of Chest. Lung lesions. Hilar adenopathies (green arrows), probable septic embolization (red arrows), feeding vessels (yellow arrow), and serratus anterior muscle (purple arrow).

An ultrasonography of abdomen and pelvis was performed which revealed a large round hypoechoic solid appearing mass at the lower pole of the right kidney. The mass is virtually indistinguishable from a renal malignancy. The ultrasonography of her abdomen and pelvis was otherwise unremarkable except for evidence of previous cholecystectomy and two small lesions in the liver suspected to be hemangiomas. Then abdominal Computed Tomography with and without administration of contrast medium injection was performed to further investigate the lesion visualized by ultrasonography (Figure 1). A 10 cm × 8 cm heterogeneous soft tissue mass in the lower pole of the right kidney was reported. The mass had faint enhancement and adjacent fatty stranding and pararenal facial thickening.

Also, bear's paw sign was observed due to dilation of the renal calyces on CT of the abdomen (Figure 2). Complex cystic renal mass or renal malignancy and cystic degeneration were mentioned as a probable diagnosis.

In addition, chest X-ray revealed mild pleural effusion and a soft tissue density pleural based lesion in right hemithorax. A thoracic CT scan with and without contrast medium injection was advised to investigate the latter findings further (Figure 3).

Thoracic CT revealed bilateral smaller than 2 cm irregular bordered nodules in both lung fields. Also, a 3.5 cm × 2.5 cm cavitating lesion in the right upper lobe, a wedge-shaped consolidation in the right lower lobe, right pleural effusion, and right hilar adenopathy were seen in thoracic CT scan. Thoracic metastasis was suggested.

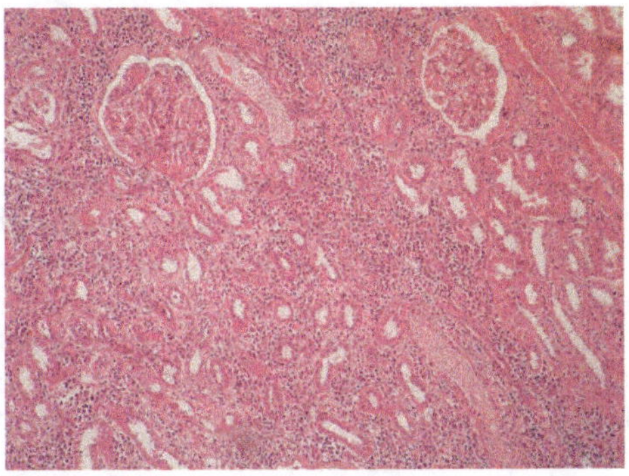

FIGURE 4: There is marked mixed inflammation in renal parenchyma in the background of diabetic nephropathy (nodular sclerosis). H&E 100x.

On laboratory investigations before treatment, other than elevated ESR (99 in 1 hour), urinalysis shows protein, glucose, and blood in a turbid sample. Urine culture was negative; therefore antibiotics were not administered. Biochemistry shows low sodium (130 normal range: 136–145). Complete blood count shows normocytic anaemia (Hb: 10.3 normal range: 12–17) and slightly elevated white cell count (10.1 normal range 4–10). Tumour markers, CEA, CA19-9, CA125, and CA15-3, were not elevated.

With regard to the imaging findings, renal malignancy (Figure 2) with pulmonary metastasis (Figure 3) was suggested. After consultation with the urologist, the patient was scheduled for right radical nephrectomy. In semiflank position (mild elevated patient right flank), with transperitoneal subcostal incision, classic right radical nephrectomy was performed. Nephrectomy is recommended in patients with an irretrievably impaired kidney due to symptomatic, chronic infection, calculus disease, or severe traumatic injury [14]. The mass had severe adhesions to adjacent organs which were released during operation. The entire mass was sent for pathologic examination.

After operation (right nephrectomy) the patient is in good condition without fever and pulmonary symptoms. Also, ESR is reduced to 65 mm/hr. White cell count was reduced to 7.1 and is within the normal range. It seems that her pulmonary nodules had been septic pulmonary embolisms. There is a similar case presentation in the literature which reports XGP complicated with pulmonary embolism [6]. Our case is the second presenting with this complication.

On pathological examination, Xanthogranulomatous pyelonephritis (XGP) was diagnosed. On microscopic examination, there is the focal replacement of renal parenchyma by severe mixed inflammatory cells infiltration including lymphoplasma cells, neutrophils and foamy histiocytes infiltration, and fibrosis with extension to perirenal soft tissue. Diabetic nephropathy including nodular sclerosis and arteriolar hyalinosis is seen in the background (Figure 4).

Prophylactic antibiotics were administered at surgery. About three months following right nephrectomy, the pulmonary nodules were found to have spontaneously resolved on chest CT scan.

3. Discussion

XGP is a renal chronic granulomatous inflammatory process commonly associated with *E. coli* and *Proteus mirabilis* infection; other likely organisms include *Pseudomonas*, *Enterococcus faecalis*, and *Klebsiella* [8]. XGP usually affects middle-aged females and children [9]. Most instances of diffuse XGP develop in the setting of obstruction due to infected renal calculi [9]. One study showed about 34% of the affected individuals have a staghorn calculus [12]. Usually, there is massive destruction of renal parenchyma by the time of diagnosis [12]. Rarely XGP may present as a complication of renal transplant [13].

XGP appears in three forms: diffuse (typical and common form, 83–90%), segmental, and focal forms (rare 10–17%) [2]. In focal form, the disease is located in renal cortex without renal pelvic communication and, in this form, the renal stone may not be seen. The focal XGP is an imitator of renal neoplasm and is a pseudotumour of the kidney and simply may be mistaken as a renal tumour [15].

Symptomatically, XGP usually presents with stigmata of chronic pyelonephritis including flank pain, fever, malaise, reduced appetite, and weight loss [13]. XGP in children may present differently with fever, abdominal and flank pain, and growth and weight retardation [16].

However, large focal XGP can be symptomless and silent. Sometimes it is found as an incidental finding in an abdominal sonogram that is recommended for other reasons [17]. Interestingly, our patient has not had any symptom related to urinary infection in contrast to almost all these patients as already mentioned in literature who have either symptomatic urinary infection or pyuria (60%) and positive urinary culture (90%) in case of a silent urinary infection [18].

CT scan has been substituted by renal angiography as the diagnostic tool of choice [19]. It has several advantages including the demonstration of the extension of the lesion into pararenal tissue and renal stones as the usual original cause [20]. Also in cases with no renal stone visible on CT, obstruction due to malignancy should be considered as the initiating aetiology of obstruction and the following chronic infection and inflammation [21, 22]. Furthermore, there is no imaging modality that can definitely distinguish between focal XGP and renal malignancy.

On pathological examination, macroscopically, the kidney is enlarged which is unilateral in the majority of cases. Renal stones are enclosed by the mass. If a tumour has infiltrated the perirenal tissue adherence to the adjacent structures may be observed, although uncommon fistula formation may be seen in case the tumour invades gastrointestinal tract [23]. Microscopically, the lesion is composed of three layers around a calyx. The inner zone is composed of necrosis, lymphocytes, leukocytes, plasma cells, and macrophages. The middle zone includes vascularized granulation tissue scattered with haemorrhage. The inflammatory cells are mostly lipid-laden macrophages, hence the yellow colour. The outer section of the lesion is recognized by giant cells and cholesterol clefts [24]. The pathophysiology of XGP involves defected processing of infective bacteria by macrophages which present as giant cells. The pathologic cause of accumulation of lipid in macrophages is not fully understood [10].

The main differential diagnosis of XGP is renal malignancy which cannot be differentiated confidently using CT scan alone. But evidence of chronic renal infection increases the likelihood of XGP. Other renal inflammatory conditions including renal parenchymal malakoplakia and megalocytic interstitial nephritis need to be differentiated from XGP based on their histologic characteristics [25].

Due to a high incidence of the destruction of the kidney parenchyma and the majority of unilateral incidence of XGP, the treatment is almost always surgical en bloc nephrectomy which involves removal of all involved tissues and closure of fistulas if developed. However, an interval of antibiotic is necessary to control the local infection prior to surgery [26]. There is a report of nonsurgical management of XGP [27]. Also, an alternative invasive treatment involving surgical drainage and renal artery embolization is introduced [28]. In case the lesion is focal and has not invaded adjacent structures, a partial nephrectomy may be performed [29]. Laparoscopic nephrectomy may be possible depending on the extension of the lesion and involvement of other structures [26].

4. Conclusion

A case of Xanthogranulomatous pyelonephritis (XGP) complicated with pulmonary lesions is presented. Considering that there is no imaging modality which can differentiate focal XGP form renal malignancy, it is important to include the diffuse form of XGP as a differential diagnosis particularly on the background of chronic urinary tract infection and obstruction of the urinary tract by renal calculi. Alternatively, diabetes mellitus has been shown to be associated with focal XGP which has no association with renal calculi.

References

[1] S. Butticè, A. Inferrera, G. Ascenti et al., "Xanthogranulomatous pyelonephritis can simulate a complex cyst: Case description and review of literature," *Urology Case Reports*, vol. 2, no. 3, pp. 113–115, 2014.

[2] D. G. Bostwick and L. Cheng, *Urologic surgical pathology*, Elsevier Health Sciences, 2008.

[3] C.-C. Kuo, C.-F. Wu, C.-C. Huang et al., "Xanthogranulomatous pyelonephritis: Critical analysis of 30 patients," *International Urology and Nephrology*, vol. 43, no. 1, pp. 15–22, 2011.

[4] A. E. Hartley and T. Page, "Renal and retroperitoneal abscess," *Oxford Textbook of Urological Surgery*, 2017.

[5] N. Arrighi, A. Antonelli, D. Zani et al., "Renal mass with caval thrombus as atypical presentation of xantogranulomatous pyelonephritis. A case report and literature review.," *Urologia*, vol. 80, pp. 44–47, 2013.

[6] A. Yousof, A. Aldhilan, A. Alamer, and A. Fahad, "Renal squamous cell carcinoma presented with bone metastasis and coexistence with xanthogranulomatous pyelonephritis: A case report," *Urology Case Reports*, vol. 2, no. 2, pp. 35–37, 2014.

[7] S. Hori, Y. Toyoshima, S. Takada et al., "A case of xanthogranulomatous pyelonephritis complicated by simultaneous septic pulmonary embolism," *Acta Urologica Japonica*, vol. 61, no. 1, pp. 13–18, 2015.

[8] M. Goodman, T. Curry, and T. Russell, "Xanthogranulomatous pyelonephritis (XGP): a local disease with systemic manifestations. Report of 23 patients and review of the literature," *Medicine*, vol. 58, no. 2, pp. 171–181, 1979.

[9] C. K. Chuang, M. K. Lai, P. L. Chang et al., "Xanthogranulomatous pyelonephritis: experience in 36 cases," *The Journal of Urology*, vol. 147, no. 2, pp. 333–336, 1992.

[10] M. A. Parsons, S. C. Harris, A. J. Longstaff, and R. G. Grainger, "Xanthogranulomatous pyelonephritis: a pathological, clinical and aetiological analysis of 87 cases," *Diagnostic Histopathology*, vol. 6, no. 3-4, pp. 203–219, 1983.

[11] K. S. Bourm, C. O. Menias, K. Ali, K. Alhalabi, and K. M. Elsayes, "Spectrum of Xanthogranulomatous processes in the abdomen and pelvis: A pictorial review of infectious, inflammatory, and proliferative responses," *American Journal of Roentgenology*, vol. 208, no. 3, pp. 475–484, 2017.

[12] F. Korkes, R. L. Favoretto, M. Bróglio, C. A. Silva, M. G. Castro, and M. D. C. Perez, "Xanthogranulomatous pyelonephritis: clinical experience with 41 cases," *Urology*, vol. 71, no. 2, pp. 178–180, 2008.

[13] E. A. Elkhammas, K. H. Mutabagani, D. D. Sedmak, R. J. Tesi, M. L. Henry, and R. M. Ferguson, "Xanthogranulomatous pyelonephritis in renal allografts: Report of 2 cases," *The Journal of Urology*, vol. 151, no. 1, pp. 127-128, 1994.

[14] S. Falahatkar, A. Enshaei, A. A. Allahkhah, M. M. Asli, Z. Panahandeh, and N. Okhovatpoor, "Comparison of open vs laparoscopic nephrectomy: Outcomes and complications," *UroToday International Journal*, vol. 3, no. 1, 2010.

[15] R. Loffroy, B. Guiu, J. Watfa, F. Michel, J. P. Cercueil, and D. Krausé, "Xanthogranulomatous pyelonephritis in adults: clinical and radiological findings in diffuse and focal forms," *Clinical Radiology*, vol. 62, no. 9, pp. 884–890, 2007.

[16] L. Li and A. Parwani, "Xanthogranulomatous pyelonephritis," *Archives of Pathology & Laboratory Medicine*, vol. 135, no. 5, pp. 671–674, 2011.

[17] T. K. Huisman and J. P. Sands, "Focal xanthogranulomatous pyelonephritis associated with renal cell carcinoma," *Urology*, vol. 39, no. 3, pp. 281–284, 1992.

[18] U. S. Dwivedi, N. K. Goyal, V. Saxena et al., "Xanthogranulomatous pyelonephritis: Our experience with review of published reports," *ANZ Journal of Surgery*, vol. 76, no. 11, pp. 1007–1009, 2006.

[19] I. Zorzos, V. Moutzouris, G. Korakianitis, and G. Katsou, "Analysis of 39 cases of xanthogranulomatous pyelonephritis with emphasis on CT findings," *Scandinavian Journal of Urology*, vol. 37, no. 4, pp. 342–347, 2003.

[20] S. M. Goldman, D. S. Hartman, and E. K. Fishman, "CT of Silverman xanthogranulomatous pyelonephritis: Radiologic-pathologic correlation," *American Journal of Roentgenology*, vol. 142, no. 5, pp. 963–969, 1984.

[21] F. Piscioli and L. Luciani, "Association of xanthogranulomatous pyelonephritis with small renal cell carcinoma. Case report and review of the literature," *European Urology*, vol. 10, no. 1, pp. 62–66, 1984.

[22] F. V. Ordones, K. Das, S. Prowse, P. Cohen, and N. R. Brook, "High-grade transitional cell carcinoma masquerading as a xanthogranulomatous pyelonephritis and perinephric abscess," *Radiology Case Reports*, vol. 12, no. 2, pp. 281–284, 2017.

[23] W. Hitti, C. Drachenberg, M. Cooper et al., "Xanthogranulomatous pyelonephritis in a renal allograft associated with xanthogranulomatous diverticulitis: Report of the first case and review of the literature," *Nephrology Dialysis Transplantation* , vol. 22, no. 11, pp. 3344–3347, 2007.

[24] G. S. Hill, Renal infection. In: Uropathology, 1st Ed, G. S. Hill (Ed), Churchill Livingstone, New York, NY, USA, p.333, 1989.

[25] M. H. Al-Sulaiman, A. A. Al-Khader, D. H. Mousa, R. Y. Al-Swailem, J. Dhar, and A. Haleem, "Renal parenchymal malacoplakia and megalocytic interstitial nephritis: Clinical and histological features: Report of two cases and review of the literature," *American Journal of Nephrology*, vol. 13, no. 6, pp. 483–488, 1993.

[26] T. J. Guzzo, T. J. Bivalacqua, P. M. Pierorazio, J. Varkarakis, E. M. Schaeffer, and M. E. Allaf, "Xanthogranulomatous pyelonephritis: presentation and management in the Era of laparoscopy," *BJU International*, vol. 104, no. 9, pp. 1265–1268, 2009.

[27] P. S. Brown Jr., M. Dodson, and P. S. Weintrub, "Xanthogranulomatous pyelonephritis: report of nonsurgical management of a case and review of the literature," *Clinical Infectious Diseases*, vol. 22, no. 2, pp. 308–314, 1996.

[28] A. Upasani, A. Barnacle, D. Roebuck, and A. Cherian, "Combination of Surgical Drainage and Renal Artery Embolization: An Alternative Treatment for Xanthogranulomatous Pyelonephritis," *CardioVascular and Interventional Radiology*, vol. 40, no. 3, pp. 470–473, 2017.

[29] L. M. Perez, J. B. Thrasher, and E. E. Anderson, "Successful management of bilateral xanthogranulomatous pyelonephritis by bilateral partial nephrectomy," *The Journal of Urology*, vol. 149, no. 1, pp. 100–102, 1993.

9

Endovascular Repair with a Stent Graft in a Patient with Aortoduodenal Fistula after Radiation Therapy

Kazuhiko Morikawa,[1] Hirokazu Ashida,[1] Yosuke Nozawa,[1] Kenji Motohashi,[1] Takao Igarashi,[1] Hiroya Ojiri,[1] Yuji Kanaoka,[2] and Takao Ohki[2]

[1]*Department of Radiology, The Jikei University School of Medicine, Tokyo, Japan*
[2]*Department of Vascular Surgery, The Jikei University School of Medicine, Tokyo, Japan*

Correspondence should be addressed to Kazuhiko Morikawa; k.morikawa@jikei.ac.jp

Academic Editor: Dimitrios Tsetis

Primary aortoduodenal fistula (ADF) is a direct communication between the abdominal aorta and the gastrointestinal tract without any previous vascular intervention and represents a rare but critical cause of repeated and massive gastrointestinal bleeding. Primary ADF often occurs as a result of atherosclerotic aneurysm and infection, but ADF involving a normal-size aorta is rare; furthermore, ADF related to radiation therapy is extremely rare. We present the case of a 56-year-old man with a history of bowel obstruction due to radiation enteritis who was admitted with severe hematemesis and hemorrhagic shock. Gastroduodenal endoscopy and contrast-enhanced computed tomography findings were unremarkable. Aortoduodenal fistula was suspected based on the diffuse calcification of the abdominal aorta confined to the radiation field and the presence of an aortoduodenal communication on angiography. Endovascular repair with a stent graft seemed to be a safer option than open surgery and was suited to the rapid control of bleeding from ADF because of the patients' unstable hemodynamic state and the presence of intestinal adhesions. The fistula was successfully sealed by endovascular stent graft placement. Hematemesis did not recur postoperatively and anemia gradually improved. The patient died from pneumonia 33 days later.

1. Introduction

Aortoduodenal fistula (ADF) is a direct communication between the abdominal aorta and the gastrointestinal tract and represents a rare but critical cause of repeated and massive gastrointestinal bleeding. Therefore, accurate diagnosis and immediate treatment are necessary. AEF is classified into the following two types: primary and secondary. Most commonly, ADF occurs from surgical repair of a prior aortic aneurysm (secondary ADF); however, ADF can arise due to the spontaneous development of a connection between the duodenum and the abdominal aorta (primary ADF) [1]. Primary ADF often occurs as a result of atherosclerotic aneurysm and infection [1]. ADF involving a normal-size aorta is rare [2]; furthermore, ADF related to radiation therapy is extremely rare. Herein, we present a case of ADF related to radiation-induced arteriosclerosis/aortopathy and enteritis, treated with an endovascular stent graft.

2. Case Presentation

A 56-year-old man with a recent history of duodenal ulcer was admitted with severe hematemesis and hemorrhagic shock. On arrival, the patient presented with hematemesis and mild epigastric pain. There was no sign of sepsis including fever, chills, rigors, and highly elevated inflammatory markers. Laboratory findings showed low hemoglobin level (8.3 g/dL), mildly elevated leukocyte count (11600/dL), and low C-reactive protein level (0.3 mg/dL). The patient's respiration was unstable and chest radiography revealed bilateral aspiration pneumonia; immediate endotracheal intubation was performed. The patient had a history of orchiectomy for seminoma followed by radiation therapy for para-aortic lymph node metastases approximately 30 years before the events described herein. Additionally, the patient had undergone several open surgeries for small bowel obstruction related to radiation-induced enteritis and adhesions.

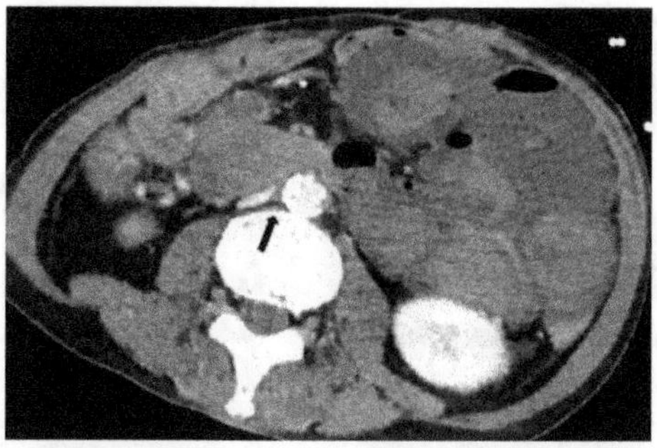

FIGURE 1: Contrast-enhanced computed tomography image on admission. A massive hematoma is visible in the small intestine, with mucosal thickening of the duodenal wall, duodenal stenosis at the level of the third and fourth portions of the duodenum, and soft-tissue density (arrow) with fat stranding between the duodenum and aorta.

Although an ulcer and stenosis of the third portion of the duodenum had been revealed one month before admission, emergency gastroduodenal endoscopy on admission failed to reveal the source of bleeding due to the massive amount of fresh blood in the stomach and duodenum. Moreover, contrast-enhanced computed tomography (CT) identified no extravasation around the duodenum, but it revealed mucosal thickening of the duodenal wall, duodenal stenosis at the level of the third and fourth portion of the duodenum, and soft-tissue density with fat stranding between the duodenum and the abdominal aorta (Figure 1). Contrast CT on admission also revealed the presence of diffuse calcification and stenosis from the left common iliac artery to the abdominal aorta, which was confined to the radiation field (Figure 2). Because these findings were suggestive of ADF, emergency aortography was performed, revealing occlusion of the origin of the celiac and superior mesenteric arteries, which were supplied via the collateral circulation. Furthermore, extravasation from the right lateral wall of the abdominal aorta and diffusion of the contrast agent along the duodenum were also observed (Figure 3), which suggested that the source of bleeding was a direct communication between the abdominal aorta and the duodenum.

A covered stent graft was deployed under fluoroscopic guidance via cannulation of the right femoral artery. The diameter of the infrarenal abdominal aorta was 12 mm, but it was only 11 mm at the narrowest site. Because it was predicted that the advancement of the aortic wall would be poor due to a high degree of arteriosclerotic change, we chose a covered stent graft (Endurant II iliac extension; width, 13 mm; length, 82 mm; Medtronic Inc., Minneapolis, MN) that was slightly bigger than the diameter of the aorta among the immediately usable devices. For adequate sealing of the stent graft, ballooning of the proximal and distal neck was performed. There were no intraoperative complications and angiography showed good positioning of the stent graft and complete exclusion of the extravasation. The ADF was completely sealed with the covered stent graft (Figure 3(d)).

After the procedure, the patient received intravenous broad-spectrum antibiotics for treatment of aspiration pneumonia and to prevent infection from ADF throughout hospital stay. Hematemesis did not recur and anemia gradually improved. Although the patient's condition temporarily recovered enough to allow rehabilitation, he died 33 days after the procedure as a result of acute exacerbation of pneumonia.

3. Discussion

AEF is a direct communication between the abdominal aorta and the gastrointestinal tract and represents a rare but critical cause of repeated and massive gastrointestinal bleeding. Since the first description of primary ADF was published by Astley Cooper in 1839, less than 200 primary aortoenteric fistula (AEF) cases have been reported in the English-language literature; 73% of primary AEF were from atherosclerotic aneurysms, 26% were from traumatic or mycotic aneurysms, and the remaining 1% were caused by radiation, metastases, pancreatic carcinoma, ulcers, gallstones, diverticulitis, appendicitis, and cystic medial necrosis [1]. As described in the Introduction, primary ADF involving a normal-size aorta is rare [2]; furthermore, ADF related to radiation therapy is extremely rare. Puccio reviewed the research on this uncommon condition and reported that radiation related AEF was not associated with aneurysm in all eight cases, including their own case [3]. ADF typically occurs between the third and fourth portions of the duodenum (70%–90%) [4]. Initial bleeding is usually minor and often intermittent in approximately two-thirds of cases, but this small amount of bleeding can lead to severe bleeding and hemorrhagic shock (herald bleeding) [5–7], resulting in significant mortality of up to 40%–70% [5]. The period from herald bleeding to massive bleeding ranges from hours to months.

Several reports have mentioned acute or chronic radiation-induced damage to tissues as a potential cause for ADF and suggested that minor, but sustained, damage to either of or both the duodenal wall and aortic wall can result in tissue necrosis and perforation of these walls [3, 8–12]. Histological changes related to radiotherapy include mucosal and submucosal damage due to obliteration of small vessels, telangiectasia, and new vessel formation, resulting in tissue damage and subsequent formation of fibrosis and chronic erosion (ulcer). Therefore, several authors have hypothesized that a chronic ulcer slowly erodes through the duodenal wall and eventually perforates a weakened aortic wall [3, 8]. Radiation-induced tissue damage also accelerates arteriosclerosis and aortopathy. Peripheral fibrosis, calcification, thrombosis, and severe stenosis or even occlusion of small blood vessels including the vasa vasorum induce fragility of large vessels, eventually resulting in perforation of the aorta [3, 8–12]. ADF can develop years or decades after radiation therapy [3]. As described above, the fragility of both the duodenum and aorta due to chronic radiation-induced histological damage is considered the cause of ADF in our patient, who had a history of severe enteritis and intestinal adhesions that occurred after radiation therapy. Moreover, the presence of duodenal stenosis at the level of the third and fourth portion

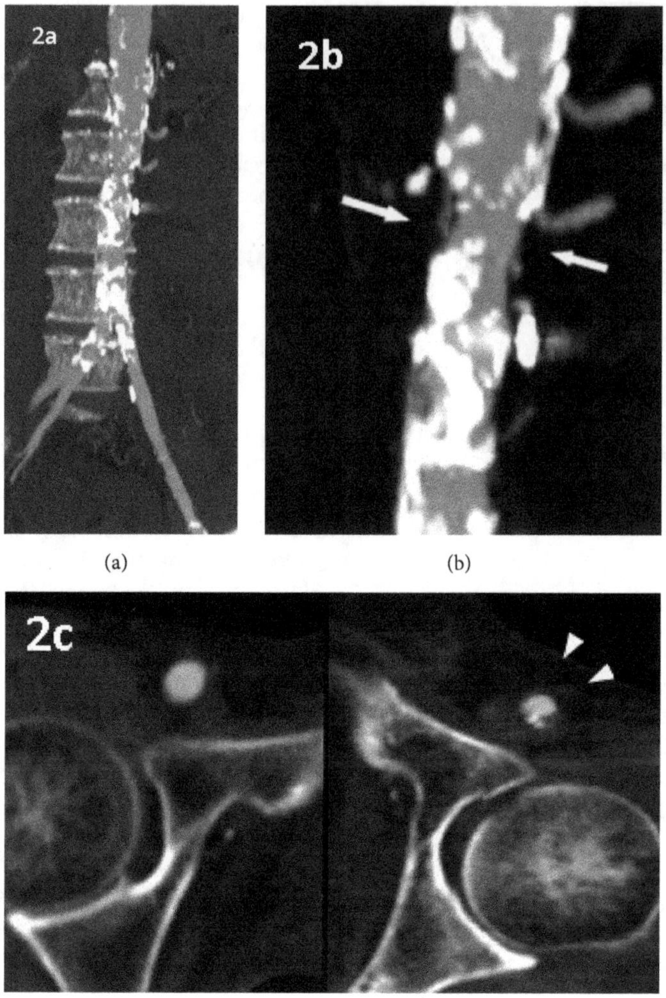

(a) (b)

(c)

FIGURE 2: Maximum intensity projection reconstruction of coronal computed tomography angiogram and transverse plane at the level of inguinal region on admission. (a) Diffuse calcification from the abdominal aorta to the left common iliac artery was observed, which was confined to the irradiation field. ((b) and (c)) Irregular stenosis of the abdominal aorta (white arrows) and left femoral artery (arrowhead).

of the duodenum, identified on contrast CT, indicated chronic inflammation and secondary fibrosis. Thus, it was estimated that the ulcer observed in the third portion of the duodenum one month before admission was also associated with radiation-induced complications. Since it is known that chronic inflammation may lead to erosion in the surrounding tissue, the CT findings of soft-tissue density with fat stranding between the duodenum and aorta suggested the presence of chronic inflammation between the duodenum and aorta. Furthermore, our patient also had diffuse calcification and stenosis confined to the radiation field, which also corresponded to findings indicative of radiation-induced arteriosclerosis or aortopathy. Hence, we believe that, in our patient, ADF was caused by radiation therapy.

Although CT typically has high diagnostic ability (sensitivity, 93%; specificity, 85.7%) for ADF formation [13], intermittent bleeding may be undetectable on contrast-enhanced CT, as it was in our patient. If ADF is suspected, angiography should be performed.

Despite prompt surgical repair, open surgeries including extra-anatomic bypass, aortic ligation, and graft replacement or open intestinal repair are associated with high mortality (27% to 50%) [13–16] and morbidity rates (66% to 80%) [13, 15, 16]. Furthermore, operative mortality rates are higher in patients with sepsis or shock [13, 15]. With respect to the optimal treatment method in the initial management of patients with severe hemorrhagic shock, endovascular aortic repair is preferred to open surgery because it is faster and less invasive, allowing rapid control of blood loss in patients with hemodynamic instability. Some researchers reported that, compared to those in laparotomy, the use of an endovascular stent graft seemed to be associated with decreased perioperative mortality and shorter hospital stay, allowing for acceptable survival given the presence of coexisting medical comorbidities [12–14, 17]; however, the mortality rate is worse

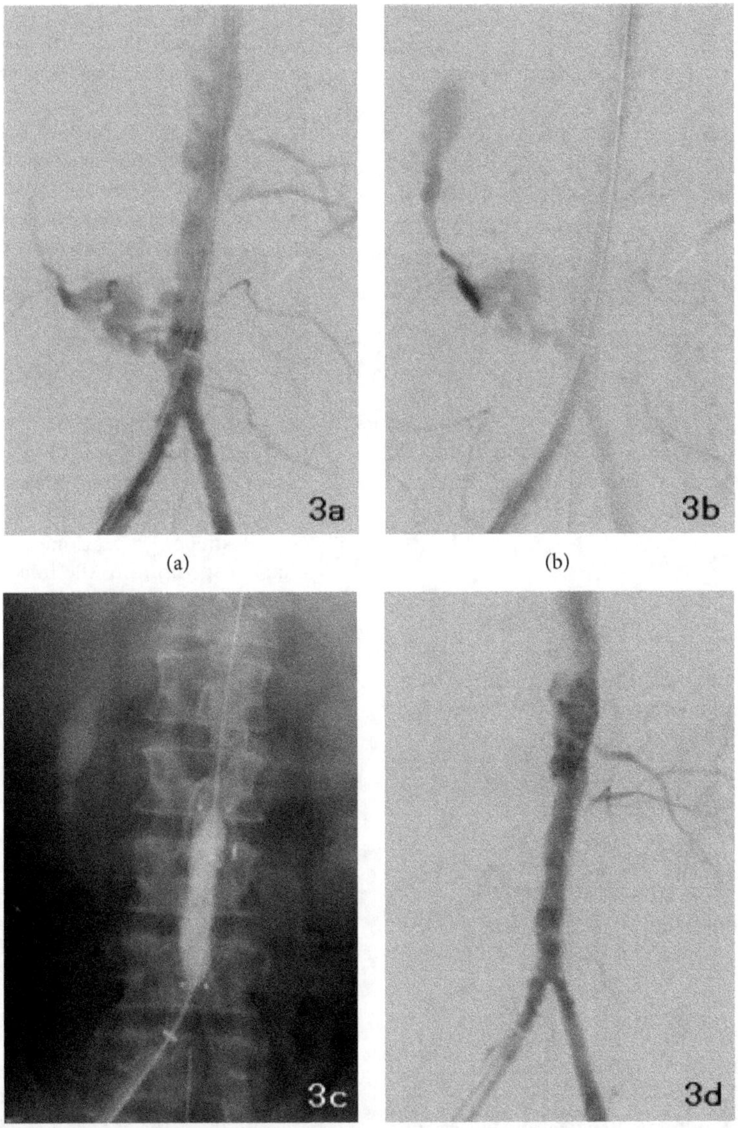

FIGURE 3: Perioperative digital subtraction angiograms. Extravasation from the right lateral wall of the abdominal aorta (a) and diffusion of the contrast agent along the duodenum (b) were observed. The celiac, superior mesenteric, and right renal arteries were occluded. A covered stent graft was successfully deployed into the abdominal aorta, and a leak at the end of the graft was treated with balloon angioplasty (c). After placement of the endovascular stent graft, aortography showed no extravasation from the right lateral wall of the abdominal aorta (d).

for patients with sepsis [13, 14]. The reported perioperative morbidity rates of endovascular repair are lower than that of open surgery and range from 25% to 60% [13–15, 17].

In our patient, mild leukocytosis was observed before the procedure, which was most likely caused by aspiration pneumonia. However, there were no signs of sepsis preoperatively. Immediate control of bleeding was necessary, and thus endovascular repair with a stent graft seemed to be a safer option than open surgery because of the patients' unstable hemodynamic state and the presence of intestinal adhesions.

The remaining aortoduodenal communication may serve as a nidus for continuing bacterial growth and lead to infection of the new implanted endovascular stent graft; therefore, long-term intravenous antibiotic therapy is necessary. Baril et al. [13] reported that all patients treated with endovascular repair were placed on lifelong suppressive oral antibiotics, which may allow for freedom from further complications related to ADF. Postoperative stent graft infection and recurrent bleeding are known as the most frequent causes of death; such an event is significantly more frequent in patients with sepsis before endovascular treatment. However, even if patients have ongoing sepsis or other infectious complications, endovascular repair may serve as a bridging therapy to open surgery [13–15, 17]. In our case, laparotomy was expected to be difficult due to severe adhesions; however, a variety of adjunctive therapies including fibrin sealant or n-butyl 2-cyanoacrylate insulation into a fistula tract might be an option [18, 19].

We reported the case of ADF related to radiation-induced arteriosclerosis/aortopathy and enteropathy that was successfully sealed with an endovascular stent graft. While ADF related to radiotherapy is extremely rare, it may be the cause of fatal gastrointestinal bleeding in patients with a history of radiotherapy. When gastroduodenal endoscopy and CT fail to detect ADF, angiography and endovascular repair with a stent graft can be employed to rapidly diagnose and repair ADF.

Ethical Approval

This report was approved by the institutional review board and complied with the provisions of Good Clinical Practice guidelines, Declaration of Helsinki, and local laws.

Disclosure

The case in this manuscript was presented previously in a poster format at the 45th Annual Conference of the Japanese Society of Interventional Radiology in May 2016.

References

[1] D. W. Lemos, J. D. Rafferto, T. C. Moore, and J. O. Menzoian, "Primary aortoduodenal fistula: A case report and review of the literature," *Journal of Vascular Surgery*, vol. 37, no. 3, pp. 686–689, 2003.

[2] C. Klonaris, G. Vourliotakis, A. Katsargyris, S. Tsiodras, and E. Bastounis, "Primary aortoduodenal fistula without abdominal aortic aneurysm in association with psoas abscess," *Annals of Vascular Surgery*, vol. 20, no. 4, pp. 541–543, 2006.

[3] F. Puccio, G. Pandolfo, S. Chiodini, F. Benzi, and M. Solazzo, "Primary Aorto-Duodenal Fistula as a Late Complication of Radiotherapy: Report of a Case and Review of the Literature," *Case Reports in Gastroenterology*, vol. 2, no. 3, pp. 415–423, 2008.

[4] T. J. Bunt, "Synthetic vascular graft infections. II. Graft-enteric erosions and graft-enteric fistulas," *Surgery*, vol. 94, no. 1, pp. 1–9, 1983.

[5] S. J. Busuttil and J. Goldstone, "Diagnosis and management of aortoenteric fistulas," *Seminars in Vascular Surgery*, vol. 14, no. 4, pp. 302–311, 2001.

[6] G. R. Capaldo and R. M. Amin, "Aortoduodenal fistula. Two case reports and review of literature," *The Journal of Cardiovascular Surgery*, vol. 37, no. 6, pp. 567–570, 1996.

[7] D. E. Szilagyi, R. F. Smith, F. J. DeRusso, J. P. Elliott, and F. W. Sherrin, "Contribution of abdominal aortic aneurysmectomy to prolongation of life.," *Annals of Surgery*, vol. 164, no. 4, pp. 678–699, 1966.

[8] D. R. Kalman, G. F. Barnard, G. J. Massimi, and R. S. Swanson, "Primary Aortoduodenal Fistula after Radiotherapy," *American Journal of Gastroenterology*, vol. 90, no. 7, pp. 1148–1150, 1995.

[9] T. P. Poon, J. Kanshepolsky, and V. Tchertkoff, "Rupture of the Aorta Due to Radiation Injury: Report of a Case and Electron Microscopic Study," *Journal of the American Medical Association*, vol. 205, no. 12, pp. 875–878, 1968.

[10] M. J. Butler, R. H. S. Lane, and J. H. H. Webster, "Irradiation injury to large arteries," *British Journal of Surgery*, vol. 67, no. 5, pp. 341–343, 1980.

[11] M. P. Parikh, M. Sherid, S. Panginikkod, H. A. Rawal, and V. Gopalakrishnan, "Radiation therapy-induced aortoesophageal fistula: a case report and review of literature," *Gastroenterology Report*, vol. 4, no. 2, pp. 165–167, 2016.

[12] C. S. Restrepo, D. Ocazionez, R. Suri, and D. Vargas, "Aortitis: imaging spectrum of the infectious and inflammatory conditions of the aorta," *RadioGraphics*, vol. 31, no. 2, pp. 435–451, 2011.

[13] D. T. Baril, A. Carroccio, S. H. Ellozy et al., "Evolving strategies for the treatment of aortoenteric fistulas," *Journal of Vascular Surgery*, vol. 44, no. 2, pp. 250–257, 2006.

[14] G. A. Antoniou, S. Koutsias, S. A. Antoniou, A. Georgiakakis, M. K. Lazarides, and A. D. Giannoukas, "Outcome after endovascular stent graft repair of aortoenteric fistula: a systematic review," *Journal of Vascular Surgery*, vol. 49, no. 3, pp. 782–789, 2009.

[15] S. K. Kakkos, P. N. Antoniadis, C. N. Klonaris et al., "Open or endovascular repair of aortoenteric fistulas? A multicentre comparative study," *European Journal of Vascular and Endovascular Surgery*, vol. 41, no. 5, pp. 625–634, 2011.

[16] R. J. Valentine, C. H. Timaran, G. J. Modrall, S. T. Smith, F. R. Arko, and G. P. Clagett, "Secondary Aortoenteric Fistulas Versus Paraprosthetic Erosions: Is Bleeding Associated with a Worse Outcome?" *Journal of the American College of Surgeons*, vol. 207, no. 6, pp. 922–927, 2008.

[17] T. Kotsis, C. Lioupis, A. Tzanis et al., "Endovascular repair of a bleeding secondary aortoenteric fistula with acute leg ischemia: A case report and review of the literature," *Journal of Vascular and Interventional Radiology*, vol. 17, no. 3, pp. 563–567, 2006.

[18] V. W. K. Mok, A. C. W. Ting, S. Law, K. H. Wong, S. W. K. Cheng, and J. Wong, "Combined endovascular stent grafting and endoscopic injection of fibrin sealant for aortoenteric fistula complicating esophagectomy," *Journal of Vascular Surgery*, vol. 40, no. 6, pp. 1234–1237, 2004.

[19] L. Finch, R. B. Heathcock, T. Quigley, G. Jiranek, and D. Robinson, "Emergent treatment of a primary aortoenteric fistula with N-butyl 2-cyanoacrylate and endovascular stent," *Journal of Vascular and Interventional Radiology*, vol. 13, no. 8, pp. 841–843, 2002.

10

Pseudoaneurysm of the Common Carotid Artery in an Infant due to Swallowed Fish Bone

Moulion Tapouh Jean Roger,[1] Fokou Marcus,[2] Fongang Emmanuel,[3] Moifo Boniface,[4,5] and Juimo Alain Georges[3,4]

[1] *Yaounde University Hospital Center, Yaounde, Cameroon*
[2] *Department of Surgery, Yaounde General Hospital, Yaounde, Cameroon*
[3] *Radiology Department, Yaounde General Hospital, Yaounde, Cameroon*
[4] *Faculty of Medicine and Biomedical Sciences (FMBS), Yaounde, Cameroon*
[5] *Radiology Department, Yaounde Gynaeco-Obstetric and Paediatric Hospital, Yaounde, Cameroon*

Correspondence should be addressed to Moulion Tapouh Jean Roger; tapouh@yahoo.fr

Academic Editor: Atsushi Komemushi

Carotid artery pseudoaneurysm is a rare condition, particularly in the paediatric population. Only about 30 cases of carotid artery aneurysms in infants have been published until now. This paper reports the case of a giant pseudoaneurysm of the left common carotid artery due to swallowed fish bone by an 8-year-old boy. This pseudoaneurysm was 5.5 cm transverse-diameter and resulted in severe respiratory distress. It was treated by resection and end-to-end anastomosis with satisfactory outcome after one-year follow-up. To the best of our knowledge, this is the largest carotid artery pseudoaneurysm ever described in children.

1. Introduction

Cervical masses in infants are frequent during routine clinical practice. They are usually congenital or of infectious origin and are often due to benign adenitis [1–3]. Vascular abnormalities, such as extracranial carotid aneurysms, are very uncommon. These aneurysms could be true aneurysms involving all the layers of the arterial wall or pseudoaneurysms in which there is no organic wall [4–6]. To our knowledge just about 30 cases of carotid artery aneurysms in infants have been published, a third of which were posttraumatic pseudoaneurysms which were either due to an accident or iatrogenic [5, 7, 8]. We report the case of an 8-year-old boy with no particular past history who underwent imaging for a suspected giant pseudoaneurysm of the left common carotid artery. This case is peculiar because of the exceptional aetiology which was the ingestion of an unnoticed fish bone.

2. Observation

An 8-year-old boy was investigated in the radiology department for a left-sided neck swelling which was observed 3 weeks earlier and was gradually increased in size. Physical examination revealed a painless pulsatile left-lateral cervical mass with a smooth outline, mild edema of the left hemiface, and a normal temperature. The infant looked generally well. A systolic murmur was present and suggestive of aneurysm. A contrast-enhanced computed tomography (CT) scan of the neck was performed (Figure 1) and showed a 42 mm × 55 mm × 28 mm ($H \times W \times$ AP) saccular dilatation of the left common carotid artery situated 20 mm proximally to the bifurcation. There was mass effect on adjacent structures notably the oesophagus and the trachea without significant stenosis. On reformatted images, a 45 mm long linear hyperdensity was depicted inside the aneurysm.

The infant was admitted in the surgery department for a comprehensive preoperative work-up. A severe inspiratory dyspnea ensued which led to patient transfer to the intensive care unit where endotracheal intubation was performed. Heparin was administered and an emergency surgical operation was performed through a left posterior cleidomastoid incision, followed by clamping of the ipsilateral common, internal, and external carotid arteries. The aneurysmal sac

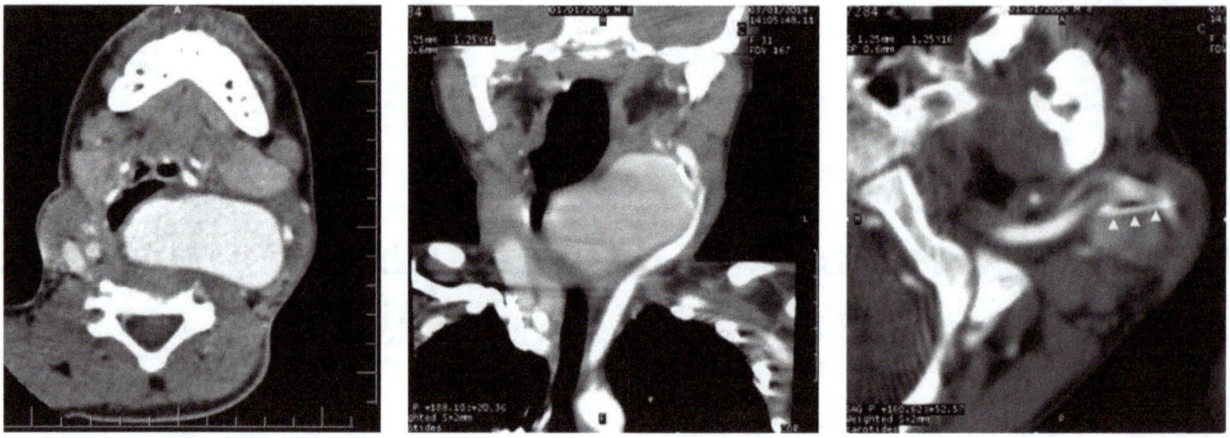

(a) (b) (c)

FIGURE 1: Axial (a) and coronal reformatted (b) contrast-enhanced CT scan images of the neck showing a saccular dilatation of the left common carotid artery with mass effect on the trachea and adjacent vascular structures. Axial bone window image (c) along the upper portion of the aneurysm shows a linear hyperdensity denoted with arrow-heads (later confirmed to be a fish bone).

was resected and a fish bone was found inside which had perforated the common carotid wall. An end-to-end anastomosis was carried out using Prolene 5/0 and cerebral blood-flow was reestablished. On day 2 after surgery there was complete regression of the dyspnea and one year later the patient was completely asymptomatic (Figure 2).

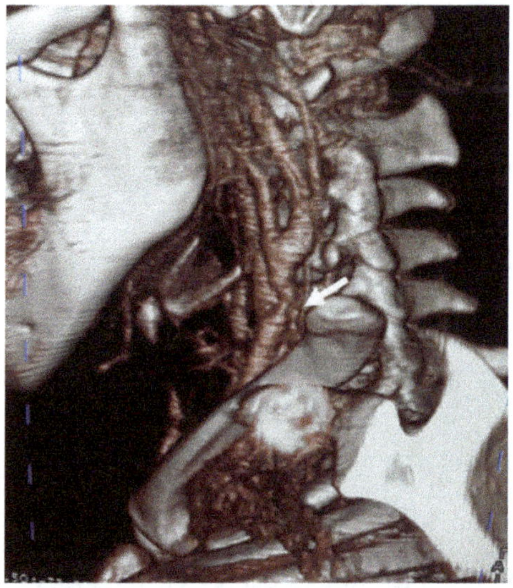

FIGURE 2: VRT CT picture at one-year follow-up. The common carotid is permeable without any residual dilation, with some mild scar narrowing at the anastomotic site (white arrow).

3. Discussion

Pseudoaneurysm is a hematoma that forms as the result of a leaking hole in an artery. It arises when a tear occurs in the arterial wall allowing blood to leak into the surrounding tissue, with persistent communication between the arterial lumen and the blood-filled cavity [9]. The main difference between true aneurysm and pseudoaneurysm is the lack of adventitia in pseudoaneurysm, where the whole wall is lacerated [8].

Pseudoaneurysms are particularly uncommon in the paediatric population. In a study of 57 659 infants with blunt trauma, Lew et al. reported only 15 cases (0.03%) of blunt carotid trauma [10] which are known to be potentially causative of pseudoaneurysms [11].

They generally are caused by direct arterial injury, which may result from trauma, vascular diagnostic or interventional procedures, adenotonsillectomy, and, in a lesser extent, deep infections [12]. Posttraumatic pseudoaneurysms of the carotid arteries are secondary to penetrating wounds or neck contusions. In these cases the tunica intima or media or the entire arterial wall is affected, resulting in extravasation into surrounding tissues [4, 7]. Iatrogenic pseudoaneurysms occur when the arterial wall is accidentally injured by a suture running too deeply [13] or a needle inserted for lymph node aspiration, for instance [9].

In our case, the child swallowed a fish bone two months before the cervical mass appeared. The fish bone perforated the wall of the oropharynx and injured the common carotid artery resulting in extravasation of blood into adjacent tissues. To our knowledge, this is the first report of a common carotid artery pseudoaneurysm resulting from food intake accident.

We found only 13 cases of noninfectious carotid pseudoaneurysms reported in the paediatric population from which 8 were iatrogenic (Table 1).

The most common site of extracranial carotid artery pseudoaneurysms is the external carotid artery [5, 14] while aneurysms often involve the bifurcation of the common carotid artery. In this case, the pseudoaneurysm was located 20 mm proximal to the carotid bifurcation.

Extracranial carotid arteries aneurysms (either true or false) can be asymptomatic or present as a pulsating cervical mass [15]. This mass can compress the upper airways leading

TABLE 1: Noninfectious carotid pseudoaneurysms reported in the paediatric population.

Authors and year	Sex and age	Carotid location	Mechanism	Treatment
Mahmoud et al., 2012 [8]	M, 4 years	Left common	Stabbing	Balloon trapping
Binning et al., 2010 [20]	F, 11 weeks	Right internal	Motor vehicle collision	Direct suture of the arterial defect and muslin sling wrapping
Singhal et al., 2009 [9]	M, 2 years M, 8 years	Right internal	Fine needle aspiration of cervical lymph node	Proximal and distal coiling Ligation
Beena et al., 2007 [7]	M, 3 years	Right internal	Needle aspiration of a parotid abscess	Not reported
DeFatta et al., 2005 [17]	F, 8 years	Left internal	Unclear : infection or transoral parapharyngeal abscess drainage	Ligation after coiling failure
Cuff and Thomas, 2005 [11]	M, 12 years	Left common	Elbow-strike during a basketball match	Resection and saphenous graft interposition
Hoff et al., 2005 [21]	M, 7 year	External	Tonsillectomy	Ligation
Chambers et al., 2002 [19]	F, 11 months	Right internal	Fall with a spoon inside the mouth	Coiling
Windfuhr, 2001 [15]	F, 5 years	Left internal	Fall with blunt trauma of head and neck	Ligation
Henriksen et al., 2000 [4]	F, 7 years	Right lateral aberrant internal	Myringotomy	Balloon embolization
Karas et al., 1997 [22]	M, 6 years	Right external	Tonsillectomy	Surgical trapping
Tovi et al., 1987 [13]	F, 14 years	Right internal	Tonsillectomy	Ligation of the sac with proximal and distal coiling

M: male. F: female.

to dyspnoea [16] as in this case. Rarely, it can lead to a recurrent laryngeal nerve palsy [14], dysphagia, Horner syndrome, neck pain, or thromboembolic conditions (cerebral ischemia). Less frequent presentations include a mass mimicking a peritonsillar abscess, epistaxis, nasopharyngeal mass, paranasal sinus mass, and a pharyngeal mass [17]. The onset of neck pain should prompt the clinician to search for complications such as rupture, mural thrombosis, or dissection [5, 7].

The diagnosis of pseudoaneurysms may be made with Doppler ultrasonography, CT Angiography (CTA), magnetic resonance imaging (MRI), and angiography [5]. Conventional radiographs may show nonspecific findings like a homogeneous cervical opacity of water density with smooth outline that may be calcified. Doppler ultrasonography would confirm this to be of vascular origin and permit blood-flow assessment but it does not give sufficient information to plan management decision [18]. On CTA, pseudoaneurysm is a mass that is enhanced homogeneously in continuity with a blood vessel. This study will permit an assessment of surrounding structures. If thrombosis is present, there is a peripheral hypodense rim surrounding the blood that is flowing [14]. CTA is the preferred modality since it provides information about the feeding artery to the pseudoaneurysm, status of surrounding vessels and structures, and intracranial circulation. MRI, which is not necessary for the diagnosis, can enable visualisation of the pseudoaneurysm and thrombus if present and moreover permit a 3D rendering of the other arteries. Catheter angiography remains the gold standard for the diagnosis despite the fact that it is invasive. It is essential in determining the extent of a thrombus and the presence of arteriovenous fistulas and permits an assessment of collateral circulation [7, 15]. Usually, It is used when therapeutic procedures are being contemplated [9]. It has been recommended that duplex ultrasound could be used for neurologically asymptomatic patients and invasive angiography be reserved for those with deficits, evidence of vessel disruption, or abnormality on duplex scanning [11]. In our setting (low income country), only Doppler ultrasound and CTA are feasible, with the latter being less affordable because of its cost (at least 240 US $).

As stated by Singhal et al., the treatment of pseudoaneurysms depends on its morphology, the segment involved, the age of the patient, and most importantly the status of collateral circulation to brain [9]. However, the economic environment and the technical platform can seriously influence therapeutic choices. The primary goals of treatment are to isolate the pseudoaneurysm from circulation in order to prevent its rupture, to permit distal thromboembolism, and to relieve compression on adjacent vital structures [9].

Three therapeutic options could be considered in the treatment of carotid pseudoaneurysms: conservative management, endovascular treatment, or surgical repair. Conservative management with close long-term follow-up and anticoagulation should be reserved to very small aneurysms [15]. Endovascular treatment includes stent insertion and coiling and parent vessel occlusion. It can be efficiently used particularly when the cerebral circulation is satisfactory through the Willis circle [9, 12]. However, although several authors have already used endovascular treatment successfully [4, 8, 9, 19], it is not considered advisable on children because of insufficient data and some doubts about its long-term outcomes [5, 11]. In this case, surgical approach was chosen for two reasons. Firstly, there was a huge hematoma impairing airway that needed to be evacuated rapidly. The second reason was the level of the lesion, since common carotid artery is accessible to surgical approach without need to manipulate mandibular of other bones and nerves.

Surgical treatment includes five options summarized by Garg et al. [6]: clipping, resection and primary end-to-end anastomosis, resection with graft interposition, extracranial to intracranial bypass, and carotid artery ligation. Carotid artery ligation in children my cause stroke and possibly death if the collateral circulation is insufficient and should be reserved as last resort or in cases of aneurysm rupture. Restoring vascularization after surgical resection by direct anastomosis or bypass is the most recommended approach [5, 6, 13]. For lesions that are not accessible to surgical management, anticoagulation with or without stenting and close follow-up are appropriate [11]. Usually, anticoagulation is considered as a temporary treatment to reduce the embolic risk prior to surgery. The technique often used is resection of the pseudoaneurysm followed by end-to-end anastomosis or insertion of a venous graft [6]. In our case the end-to-end anastomosis was performed.

Several complications can follow the operation: transient ischemic attacks, stroke, cervical or cranial nerve injuries, graft occlusion, or death [5, 6]. Despite those complications, surgical management is the most frequently used option for the treatment of carotid pseudoaneurysm in children and is considered to have the better long-term prognosis. In 2007 Pourhassan et al. described 4 cases of surgically managed pseudoaneurysms in children with favourable outcome after 25-year follow-up [5].

4. Conclusion

Carotid artery pseudoaneurysm is an uncommon pathology particularly in the paediatric population. It is mostly due to trauma but can also occur during unexpected circumstances such as food intake. For the treatment, endovascular and surgical options could be considered, each possibility having its precise indications. When possible, surgical management by resection and end-to-end anastomosis would be preferred in order to avoid the risk of compression on neighbouring organs and rupture. This approach seems to provide the most favourable long-term outcome.

References

[1] M. K. Badawy, "Pediatric neck masses," *Clinical Pediatric Emergency Medicine*, vol. 11, no. 2, pp. 73–80, 2010.

[2] M. R. Goins and M. S. Beasley, "Pediatric neck masses," *Oral and Maxillofacial Surgery Clinics of North America*, vol. 24, no. 3, pp. 457–468, 2012.

[3] E. R. Friedman and S. D. John, "Imaging of pediatric neck masses," *Radiologic Clinics of North America*, vol. 49, no. 4, pp. 617–632, 2011.

[4] S. D. Henriksen, M. W. Kindt, C. B. Pedersen, and H. J. Nepper-Rasmussen, "Pseudoaneurysm of a lateral internal carotid artery in the middle ear," *International Journal of Pediatric Otorhinolaryngology*, vol. 52, no. 2, pp. 163–167, 2000.

[5] S. Pourhassan, D. Grotemeyer, M. Fokou et al., "Extracranial carotid arteries aneurysms in children. Single-center experiences in 4 patients and review of the literature," *Journal of Pediatric Surgery*, vol. 42, no. 11, pp. 1961–1968, 2007.

[6] K. Garg, C. B. Rockman, V. Lee et al., "Presentation and management of carotid artery aneurysms and pseudoaneurysms," *Journal of Vascular Surgery*, vol. 55, no. 6, pp. 1618–1622, 2012.

[7] N. V. Beena, M. S. Kishore, A. Mahale, and V. Poornima, "Pseudoaneurysm of internal carotid artery," *Indian Journal of Pediatrics*, vol. 74, no. 3, pp. 307–309, 2007.

[8] M. Mahmoud, E. Roshdi, and D. Benderbous, "Traumatic pseudoaneurysms of the common carotid and vertebral artery in a four-year-old child," *Interventional Neuroradiology*, vol. 18, no. 3, pp. 348–352, 2012.

[9] M. Singhal, V. Gupta, P. Singh, A. Lal, A. Behra, and N. Khandelwal, "Iatrogenic life-threatening pseudoaneurysms of extracranial internal carotid artery after fine-needle aspiration of cervical Lymph nodes: report of two cases in children," *CardioVascular and Interventional Radiology*, vol. 32, no. 6, pp. 1260–1263, 2009.

[10] S. M. Lew, C. Frumiento, and S. L. Wald, "Pediatric blunt carotid injury: a review of the National Pediatric Trauma Registry," *Pediatric Neurosurgery*, vol. 30, no. 5, pp. 239–244, 1999.

[11] R. F. Cuff and J. H. Thomas, "Pediatric blunt carotid injury from low-impact trauma: a case report and review of the literature," *Journal of Trauma—Injury, Infection and Critical Care*, vol. 58, no. 3, pp. 620–623, 2005.

[12] U. Tannuri, N. Mendes De Almeida, R. Piske, and T. Matsumoto, "Giant pseudoaneurysm of the internal carotid artery causing upper airway obstruction in a 10-month-old infant treated by endovascular occlusion and surgical drainage," *Journal of Pediatric Surgery*, vol. 38, no. 9, pp. 1393–1395, 2003.

[13] F. Tovi, A. Leiberman, Y. Herizanu, and L. Golcman, "Pseudoaneurysm of the internal carotid artery secondary to tonsillectomy," *International Journal of Pediatric Otorhinolaryngology*, vol. 13, no. 1, pp. 69–75, 1987.

[14] W. Zamiati, M. I. Kably, and R. Kadiri, "A rare cause of recurrent laryngeal nerve palsy," *Journal de Radiologie*, vol. 86, no. 9, part 1, pp. 1038–1039, 2005.

[15] J. P. Windfuhr, "Aneurysm of the internal carotid artery following soft tissue penetration injury," *International Journal of Pediatric Otorhinolaryngology*, vol. 61, no. 2, pp. 155–159, 2001.

[16] N. De Luccia, E. S. da Silva, M. Aponchik, F. Appolonio, and L. A. Benvenuti, "Anévrysme congénital de l'artère carotide externe," *Annales de Chirurgie Vasculaire*, vol. 24, no. 3, pp. 457.e7–457.e10, 2010.

[17] R. J. DeFatta, D. J. Verret, and P. Bauer, "Extracranial internal carotid artery pseudoaneurysm," *International Journal of Pediatric Otorhinolaryngology*, vol. 69, no. 8, pp. 1135–1139, 2005.

[18] H. Constantinides, C. Passant, and A. N. Waddell, "Mycotic pseudoaneurysm of common carotid artery mimicking parapharyngeal abscess," *Journal of Laryngology and Otology*, vol. 114, no. 10, pp. 796–797, 2000.

[19] N. Chambers, D. Hampson-Evans, K. Patwardhan, and L. Murdoch, "Traumatic aneurysm of the internal carotid artery in an infant: a surprise diagnosis," *Paediatric Anaesthesia*, vol. 12, no. 4, pp. 356–361, 2002.

[20] M. J. Binning, R. Eskandari, and W. T. Couldwell, "Direct surgical repair of carotid pseudoaneurysm in an infant," *Child's Nervous System*, vol. 26, no. 9, pp. 1151–1153, 2010.

[21] M. Hoff, S. Graumüller, and H. W. Pau, "Arterial aneurysms as cause of gushing post-tonsillectomy hemorrhage," *Laryngo-Rhino-Otologie*, vol. 84, no. 9, pp. 680–682, 2005.

[22] D. E. Karas, R. S. Sawin, and K. C. Y. Sie, "Pseudoaneursym of the external carotid artery after tonsillectomy. A rare complication," *Archives of Otolaryngology—Head and Neck Surgery*, vol. 123, no. 3, pp. 345–347, 1997.

11

Two Unusual Aspects of Posterior Reversible Encephalopathy Syndrome Mimicking Primary and Secondary Brain Tumor Lesions

Mazamaesso Tchaou,[1,2] Nicoleta Modruz,[2] Lama K. Agoda-Koussema,[1] Anthony Michelot,[2] Samer Naffa,[2] Véronique Jeudy,[2] and Raymond Kaczmarek[2]

[1]*Department of Radiology, Lomé Teaching Hospital, University of Lomé, Lomé, Togo*
[2]*Department of Radiology, Cornouaille Intercommunal Hospital, 29000 Quimper, France*

Correspondence should be addressed to Mazamaesso Tchaou; joseph_tchaou@yahoo.fr

Academic Editor: Yoshito Tsushima

The posterior reversible encephalopathy syndrome (PRES) is a rare clinical-radiological entity well described with typical clinical and radiological manifestations. Atypical presentation, especially in imaging, exists. The authors report here two cases of posterior reversible encephalopathy in which imaging aspects were atypical, mimicking, in the first case, hemorrhagic cerebral metastasis of cholangiocarcinoma and, in the second case, a brain tumor. The diagnosis has been retrospectively rectified due to clinical and radiological outcome.

1. Introduction

Described for the first time in 1996 by Hinchey et al. [1], the posterior reversible encephalopathy syndrome (PRES) is a clinical-radiological entity combining clinical manifestations such as seizures, headache, visual disturbances, consciousness impairment, nausea/vomiting, and focal neurological signs [1–3]. In imaging, posterior reversible encephalopathy is typically characterized by partially or completely reversible bilateral and symmetrical subcortical vasogenic edema preferentially affecting the posterior regions of the brain [1]. In addition to its typical appearance, there is a great variability both in clinical manifestations and in the imaging aspects of this syndrome.

We report here two cases of posterior reversible encephalopathy in which imaging aspects were atypical, mimicking, in the first case, hemorrhagic cerebral metastasis of cholangiocarcinoma and, in the second case, a brain tumor because of its unilateral localization.

2. Cases Presentation

2.1. Case 1. A 71-year-old male patient with known hypertension and history of myocardial infarction that required a double bypass surgery 38 years ago, cardiac arrhythmias due to atrial fibrillation (AF), and an old thrombocytopenia has been urgently admitted for onset of neurological disorders manifested as visual disturbances. Clinical examination found an acute hypertensive episode with an elevated blood pressure of 180/110 mmHg.

A brain noncontrast CT-scan was performed and found bilateral occipital nodular hematomas, predominantly in the right hemisphere, surrounded by edematous hypodense white matter (Figure 1(a)). Faced with this aspect, the hypothesis of hemorrhagic brain metastases secondary to a neoplastic tumor was raised as first line. The search for a primary neoplastic lesion by performing thoracic-abdominal-pelvic CT-scan revealed dilatation of the intrahepatic bile ducts upstream of a hilar hepatic lesion—which was proved to be

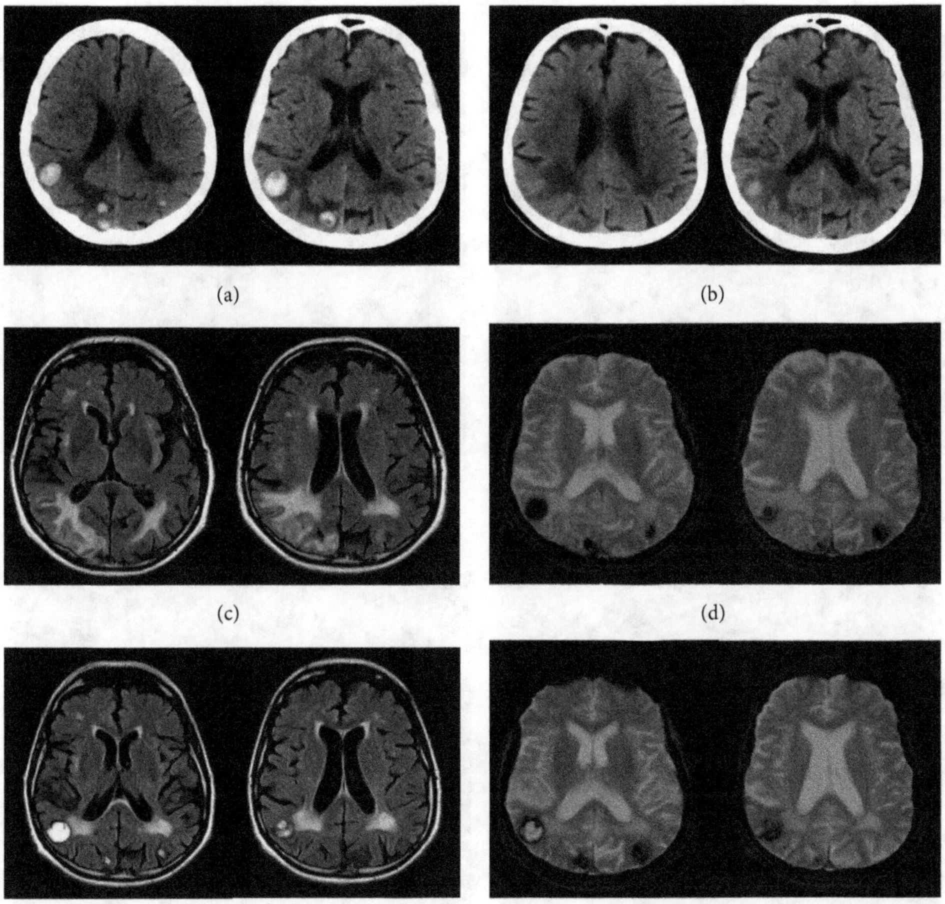

(a) (b) (c) (d) (e) (f)

Figure 1: Patient 1: noncontrast brain CT-scan showing occipital bilateral hyperdense nodules, predominantly on the right side, surrounded by edema, corresponding to brain hematomas (a). Noncontrast brain CT-scan 18 days later showing regression of the size and number of hematomas with a decrease in the degree of the surrounding edema (b). MRI-scan 6 weeks later, axial Fluid Attenuated Inversion Recovery, FLAIR (c), and Gradient Echo, GRE (d), weighted sequences showing a marked susceptibility effect confirming the haemorrhagic lesions and the presence of surrounding edema. Follow-up MRI-scan 4 months later with same sequences, showing regression of the size and number of hematomas with increase in the size of the vasogenic edema in the left occipital lobe (e and f).

a cholangiocarcinoma. A follow-up brain CT-scan performed 18 days later, following the disappearance of the visual disturbances, with the only treatment to control the hypertension, found a partial regression of the lesions (Figure 1(b)).

A brain MRI-scan performed 6 weeks later (Figures 1(c) and 1(d)) and another follow-up brain MRI-scan performed 4 months later (Figures 1(e) and 1(f)) confirmed the hemorrhagic nature and evolution of the lesions, the absence of new hemorrhagic lesions, and the increase in size of the vasogenic edema in the left occipital area. No abnormal brain enhancement was proven.

Given the evolution of radiological images and the disappearance of neurological disorders in the absence of a specific treatment except the one for controlling the hypertension and the chemotherapy for his cholangiocarcinoma, the final diagnosis was intracerebral hemorrhagic complicated form of PRES. For his hepatobiliary tumor he had initially benefited from chemotherapy by GEMOX that allowed stabilizing the lesions and in a second phase he had a right hepatectomy.

2.2. Case 2. A 77-year-old woman was admitted in emergency room for persistent headache in a context of high blood pressure at 175/115 mmHg. Noncontrast and contrast brain CT-scans were performed and showed a diffuse area of unilateral hypoattenuation in the right white matter in the parietooccipital lobes finger in glove appearance with a discrete mass effect on the occipital horn of the lateral ventricle, without contrast enhancement, in favour of a space occupying lesion of the brain (Figures 2(a) and 2(b)). The brain MRI-scan confirmed the presence of a vasogenic edema in the right white matter in the parietooccipital lobes (Figures 2(c) and 2(d)). No contrast enhancement was proved. The hypothesis of a low grade glioma was raised. A new brain follow-up MRI-scan performed a month later after the control of blood pressure and the disappearance of headache (Figures 2(e) and 2(f)) showed the disappearance of the parietooccipital hyperintense area, confirming a PRES, corresponding to a vasogenic edema. No contrast enhancement was proved. At this moment, the final diagnosis was unilateral atypical PRES.

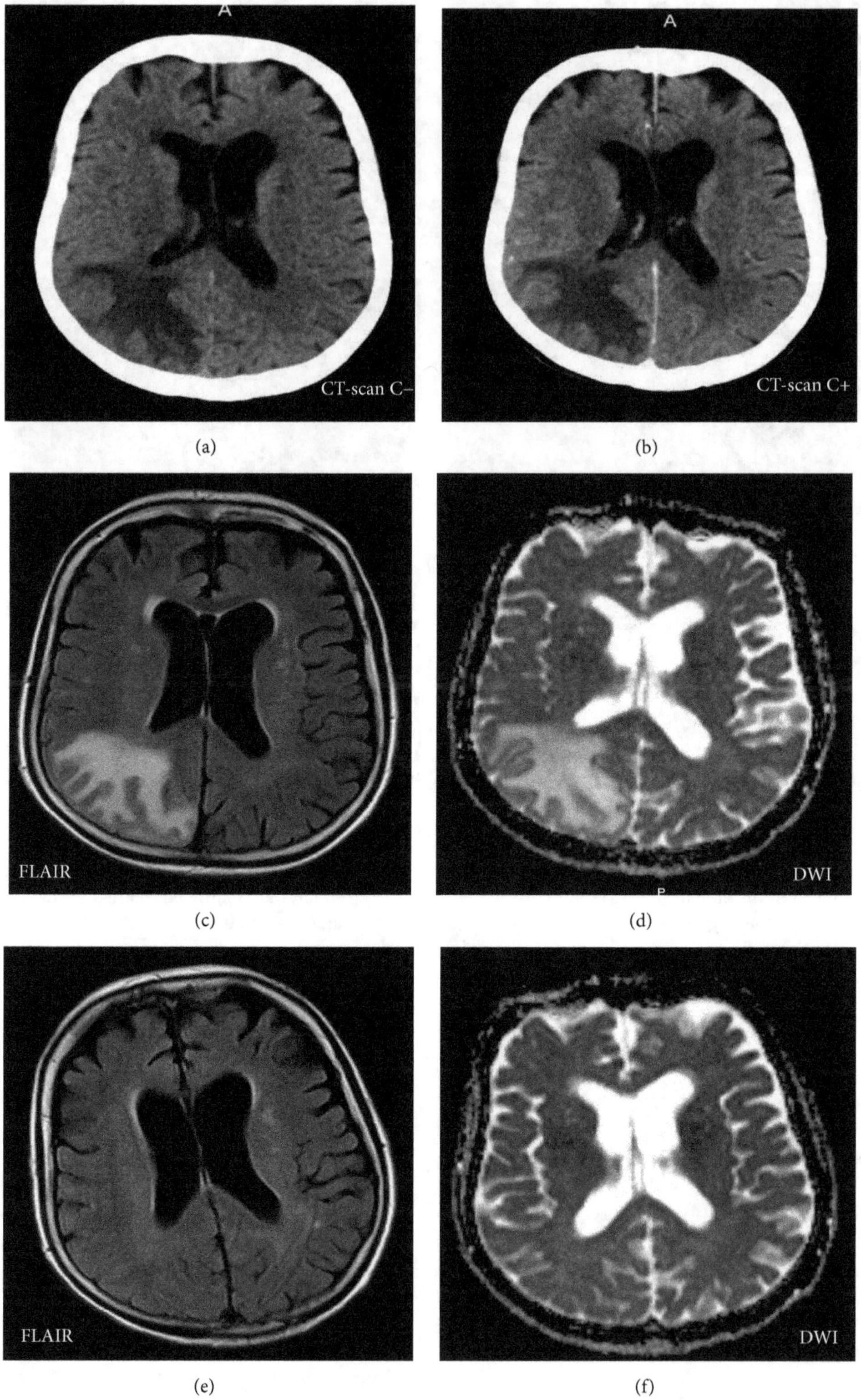

FIGURE 2: Patient 2: noncontrast brain CT-scan (a) showing a diffuse area of unilateral hypoattenuation in the right white matter in the parietooccipital lobes with a discrete mass effect on the occipital horn of the lateral ventricle, without contrast enhancement (b), in favour of a space occupying lesion of the brain. MRI-scan, axial FLAIR (c) and Diffusion Weighted Imaging, DWI (d), showing an area of FLAIR hyperintensity without diffusion restriction and without contrast enhancement with the same localization as on the CT-scan corresponding to a vasogenic cerebral edema. Follow-up MRI-scan one month later, axial FLAIR (e) and DWI (f), showing the disappearance of the parietooccipital hyperintense area corresponding to a vasogenic cerebral edema, confirming PRES.

She was followed up during one year and there were no new symptoms or sequelae.

3. Discussion

3.1. Epidemiology. Posterior reversible encephalopathy syndrome (PRES) is a clinical-radiological entity that was well described by Hinchey et al. [1] in 1996 based on 15 cases. Its global incidence is unknown [4]. But there are a lot of scientific publications about it. Of course, since 1996, there has been a range of more than 1000 publications describing its diverse etiology, variety of clinical symptoms, and typical neuroradiological features [5].

3.2. Pathophysiology. The pathophysiology of PRES remains controversial. The two main hypotheses contradict each other. One involves impaired cerebral autoregulation responsible for an increase in cerebral blood flow (CBF), whereas the other involves endothelial dysfunction with cerebral hypoperfusion [6]. This hypoperfusion hypothesis may be most relevant to cases of PRES associated with cytotoxic therapy. Under both hypotheses, the result of the cerebral blood perfusion abnormalities is blood-brain barrier dysfunction with cerebral vasogenic edema [3].

3.2.1. Typical Pattern of PRES. Typically, PRES presents as widespread, symmetrical, and bilateral, usually reversible vasogenic edema, cortical and subcortical, which backs up into the deep white matter as it becomes more severe [6, 7]. Predominant locations are the occipital and parietal lobes [1]. In large retrospective studies, this is the most common pattern of edema [6–9]. In addition to the occipital and parietal symmetric pattern of vasogenic edema, wide variations of distribution have been described in the literature.

3.3. Atypical Pattern in Our Cases

3.3.1. Atypical Distribution: Unilateral Form. Although typically symmetrical and bilateral, asymmetrical or unilateral distributions of vasogenic edema in PRES can also be seen. This is designed as "tumefactive PRES" by McKinney et al. [6]. That is the situation in our case. The problem of this situation is that confusion can exist with a space occupying lesion. Patel et al. reported the same situation in one case [10], where a plain head CT imaging revealed the presence of a space occupying lesion and surrounding vasogenic edema in the left occipital lobe. Grey matter around the edema gave the impression of a space occupying lesion. A preliminary diagnosis of a space occupying primary malignant tumor lesion was made on initial presentation following CT imaging. However, this was revised after follow-up MRI, to PRES. The main risk in this situation is an unnecessary and contraindicated biopsy.

3.3.2. Atypical Initial Presentation: Cerebral Hemorrhage, Focal Hematomas. Our first case has been diagnosed with an intracerebral haemorrhagic complicated form of PRES. The aspect was bilateral multiple focal hematomas. Cerebral hemorrhage is a potential complication that is known to occur in PRES. Hemorrhage is said to be an uncommon complication in PRES (5% [11] to 17% [6] of patients), based on older sequences such as FLAIR and T2*, but it is antiquated relative to SWI (susceptibility-weighted imaging) and other newer and postprocessed sequences. The incidence of hemorrhage (particularly microhemorrhage) is higher; its frequency is more than 50%; McKinney et al. found 58.1% at presentation and 64.7% at follow-up [12]. The pathological mechanism of bleeding in PRES is still not well understood but is thought to relate to hypertension and hyperperfusion or vasculopathy with resulting hypoperfusion. Varying patterns of hemorrhage have been identified, including large focal hematomas, subarachnoid hemorrhage, or multiple minute foci of hemorrhage [8]. The differential diagnosis in this case was with cerebral metastasis of cholangiocarcinoma. But brain metastasis secondary to cholangiocarcinoma is exceedingly rare, with only a few cases reported in the literature [13, 14]. In addition, there is no hemorrhagic brain metastasis of cholangiocarcinoma reported.

3.4. Retrospective Diagnosis of PRES. In all of our two cases, the diagnostic of PRES has been made after partial or complete regression of the initial clinical and radiological abnormalities. In some cases, the diagnosis of PRES remains in doubt. In this situation, regression of the clinical and radiological abnormalities with appropriate treatment supports the diagnosis. Thus, repeated brain imaging is helpful [4].

4. Conclusion

The posterior reversible encephalopathy syndrome is a rare radioclinical syndrome. This diagnosis is easy when the clinical and radiological presentation is typical. In atypical forms, it poses the problem of differential diagnosis, which can be confused with a primary brain tumor or brain metastasis. It is often the evolution that allows rectifying the diagnosis.

References

[1] J. Hinchey, C. Chaves, B. Appignani et al., "A reversible posterior leukoencephalopathy syndrome," *The New England Journal of Medicine*, vol. 334, no. 8, pp. 494–500, 1996.

[2] W. S. Bartynski, "Posterior reversible encephalopathy syndrome. Part 2. Controversies surrounding pathophysiology of vasogenic edema," *American Journal of Neuroradiology*, vol. 29, no. 6, pp. 1043–1049, 2008.

[3] W. S. Bartynski, "Posterior reversible encephalopathy syndrome. Part 1. Fundamental imaging and clinical features," *American Journal of Neuroradiology*, vol. 29, no. 6, pp. 1036–1042, 2008.

[4] S. Legriel, F. Pico, and E. Azoulay, "Understanding posterior reversible Encephalopathy syndrome," in *Annual Update in Intensive Care and Emergency Medicine 2011*, J.-L. Vincent, Ed., vol. 1 of *Annual Update in Intensive Care and Emergency Medicine 2011*, pp. 631–653, Springer, Berlin, Germany, 2011.

[5] D. Morina, G. Ntoulias, H. Maslehaty, M. Scholz, and A. K. Petridis, "Posterior reversible encephalopathy syndrome mimicking cerebral metastasis: contraindication for biopsy," *Clinics and Practice*, vol. 4, article 632, 2014.

[6] A. M. McKinney, J. Short, C. L. Truwit et al., "Posterior reversible encephalopathy syndrome: incidence of atypical regions of involvement and imaging findings," *American Journal of Roentgenology*, vol. 189, no. 4, pp. 904–912, 2007.

[7] W. S. Bartynski and J. F. Boardman, "Distinct imaging patterns and lesion distribution in posterior reversible encephalopathy syndrome," *American Journal of Neuroradiology*, vol. 28, no. 7, pp. 1320–1327, 2007.

[8] C. J. Stevens and M. K. S. Heran, "The many faces of posterior reversible encephalopathy syndrome," *The British Journal of Radiology*, vol. 85, no. 1020, pp. 1566–1575, 2012.

[9] J. Ni, L.-X. Zhou, H.-L. Hao et al., "The clinical and radiological spectrum of posterior reversible encephalopathy syndrome: a retrospective series of 24 patients," *Journal of Neuroimaging*, vol. 21, no. 3, pp. 219–224, 2011.

[10] K. Patel, A. Durnford, N. Owen, and R. Dardis, "Posterior reversible encephalopathy syndrome mimicking a cerebral tumour," *BMJ Case Reports*, 2012.

[11] V. H. Lee, E. F. M. Wijdicks, E. M. Manno, and A. A. Rabinstein, "Clinical spectrum of reversible posterior leukoencephalopathy syndrome," *Archives of Neurology*, vol. 65, no. 2, pp. 205–210, 2008.

[12] A. M. McKinney, B. Sarikaya, C. Gustafson, and C. L. Truwit, "Detection of microhemorrhage in posterior reversible encephalopathy syndrome using susceptibility-weighted imaging," *American Journal of Neuroradiology*, vol. 33, no. 5, pp. 896–903, 2012.

[13] Y. Okamura, A. Harada, A. Maeda et al., "Carcinomatous meningitis secondary to cholangiocarcinoma without other systemic metastasis," *Journal of Hepato-Biliary-Pancreatic Surgery*, vol. 15, no. 2, pp. 237–239, 2008.

[14] B. M. William and J. L. Grem, "Brain metastasis and leptomeningeal carcinomatosis in a patient with cholangiocarcinoma," *Gastrointestinal Cancer Research*, vol. 4, no. 4, pp. 144–145, 2011.

12

Giant Splenorenal Shunt in a Young Patient with Autoimmune Hepatitis/Primary Biliary Cholangitis Overlap Syndrome and Portal Vein Thrombosis

F. Chegai,[1] A. U. Cavallo,[1] M. Forcina,[1] V. Giuricin,[1] F. Castellani,[1] L. Greco,[1] M. Manuelli,[2] T. M. Manzia,[2] and G. Sergiacomi[1]

[1]*Department of Diagnostic and Molecular Imaging, Radiation Therapy and Interventional Radiology, University Hospital Tor Vergata, Viale Oxford 81, 00133 Rome, Italy*
[2]*Organ Transplantation Unit, University Hospital Tor Vergata, Rome, Italy*

Correspondence should be addressed to F. Chegai; fabrizio.chegai@hotmail.it

Academic Editor: Atsushi Komemushi

We present a case of giant Splenorenal Shunt (SRS) associated with portal vein thrombosis in a 37-year-old woman with a twelve-year history of autoimmune hepatitis/primary biliary cholangitis overlap syndrome. At the moment of the CT examination laboratory tests showed creatinine 1.5 mg/dl, bilirubin 1.5 mg/dl, INR 3, and Na 145 mmol/l and the Model End-Stage Liver Disease score was 24. Extensive calcified thrombosis causing complete occlusion of the portal vein lumen and partially occluding the origin of the superior mesenteric vein was present and a small calcified thrombus in the Splenic Vein lumen was also evident. SRS was located among the spleen hilum and the left kidney with a maximum diameter of 3.25 cm and was associated with dilatation of left renal vein and inferior vena cava. After a multidisciplinary evaluation the patient was put on the Regional Liver Transplant waiting list and liver transplantation was performed successfully. Although portal vein thrombosis and SRS are common occurrences in cirrhotic patients, the impact in the natural history of the disease is still unclear. Careful management and accurate imaging protocols are essential in the evaluation of those patients.

1. Introduction

Portal hypertension (PH) in patients with cirrhosis is caused by an increase in resistance to portal outflow and by a growth in splanchnic blood flow [1].

Likewise portal vein thrombosis (PVT) is frequent in these patients, particularly in the advanced stages of liver disease [2]. In a later phase of PH and cirrhosis specific changes occur, leading to a hyperkinetic circulation that raises cardiac output and reduces systemic vascular resistance as well as perfusion pressure [3]. The associated vasodilation and vasoconstriction with sinusoidal remodelling and related vascular distortion had a role in the pathophysiology of PH concurring to circulatory impairment and expansion of the collateral circulation. Frequent manifestations of PH include indeed the onset of large spontaneous shunts. As a consequence of increased vascular pressure, blood can be rerouted in the systemic circulation by collateral vessels which surround the portal vein, forming a "portal vein cavernoma" or by portosystemic shunts. Splenorenal Shunt (SRS) is defined as one of several spontaneous shunts, which may be created by reopening the embryonic venous route, in patients with portal hypertension. In patients with advanced liver disease who were candidates for liver transplantation (LT), the incidence varied from 3.8% to 60% [1]. This condition seems to be protective from variceal development by avoiding fatal bleeding but could complicate splenoliver surgery because of the difficulties of retroperitoneal dissection and preparation of the shunt. Few studies have evaluated the importance of SRS size changes after liver transplantation (LT). Recently Chikamori et al. [4] showed that the increase in the SRS/portal vein ratio is associated with reduction of liver function, hyperdynamic status, and narrowed arteriovenous oxygen content difference (C(a-v) O_2).

Imaging of the portal venous system and large spontaneous shunts has a crucial role on evaluation of this clinical situation. Usually it is performed with color Doppler ultrasonography, contrast enhanced computed tomography (ceCT), and magnetic resonance imaging (MRI). Triphasic dynamic contrast enhanced CT is a useful tool for assessing abnormalities of the portal venous system.

We report the case of a young patient with autoimmune hepatitis/primary biliary cirrhosis overlap syndrome and PVT associated with solitary giant SRS.

2. Case Report

A 37-year-old woman with autoimmune hepatitis/primary biliary cholangitis overlap syndrome in good clinical conditions underwent routine CT examination.

The patient's clinical history dates back to 2004 when she noticed yellowish discoloration of sclera and skin associated with generalized itching, with no symptoms of biliary obstruction.

She did not report alcohol abuse and laboratory tests for HBV-HCV were negative. On physical examination, she was jaundiced and pale and abdominal examination revealed hepatomegaly.

Subsequent laboratory tests showed increased level of alkaline phosphatase (AP), Anti-Mitochondrial Antibodies (AMA) and Anti-Smooth Muscle Cells Antibodies (ASMA).

Histopathological examination after liver biopsy revealed mild to moderate chronic inflammatory portal tract infiltrates consisting of lymphocytes, polymorphs, and plasma cells and significant portal fibroplasia, bile ductular proliferation, and fibrosis.

After the clinical diagnosis the patient was treated with ursodeoxycholic acid (UDCA) and corticosteroids combination therapy with normalization of liver function tests in about six months.

In order to be placed in the waiting list for LT the patient underwent multislice CT using a 64-row MDCT scanner (Lightspeed VCT; General Electric, USA) with triphasic technique (30, 65, and 180 s) after intravenous administration of 120 ml of 350 mgI/ml iodine contrast media, injected at a rate of 3 ml/s with an automatic injector and followed by 20–30 ml of saline solution. CT was obtained with the following parameters: rotation time, 0.6 s; 2.5 to 5 mm thick sections with the possibility of back-reconstructions up to 0.6 mm; automatic milliamperage (mA) (min 300 mA, max 450 mA), and 120 kV. All reconstructed datasets were transferred to a dedicated offline workstation (VitreaWorkStation; Toshiba Medical, Japan) to obtain 2-dimensional Multiplanar Reconstruction (MPR) and Maximum Intensity Projection (MIP) and 3-dimensional (volume rendering, VR, technique) reconstructions.

At the moment of the CT examination blood laboratory tests showed the following: creatinine: 1.5 mg/dl (NV: 0.6–1.2 mg/dl); bilirubin: 1.5 mg/dL (NV: 3–1 mg/dl); INR: 3 (NV: 0.8–1.2); Na: 145 mmol/l (NV: 135–145 mmol/l).

CT showed liver with reduced size and hypertrophy of caudate lobe and no evidence of intrahepatic focal lesions. Extensive calcified thrombosis causing complete occlusion of the portal vein lumen and partially occluding the proximal superior mesenteric vein (SMV) (Yerdel grade 3) [2] was present (Figures 1(a)–1(c)) and a small calcified thrombus in the Splenic Vein (SV) lumen was also evident (Figure 1(a)). Among the spleen hilum and the left kidney a massive SRS was evident: hypodense structure in basal scans, made of tortuous tubular structures detectable in the venous phase scans (Figures 1(d) and 1(e)). Multiplanar Reconstruction allowed accurately measuring the maximum axial diameter. The shunt had a maximum diameter of 3.25 cm and was associated with dilatation of left renal vein and Inferior Vena Cava (Figures 1(d) and 1(e)).

A subsequent color Doppler evaluation showed a forward flow direction in the SV.

A multidisciplinary meeting including a radiologist, a hepatologist, and a transplant surgeon evaluated risks and benefits of LT. Because of the young age and the 20% estimated survival expectancy without transplantation according to Mayo Clinic Risk score, the patient was put on the Regional Liver Transplant waiting list.

At the time of LT, the Model End-Stage Liver Disease (MELD) score was 24 and the Mayo Risk Score was 9.0. Surgeons performed the transplant procedure using a 1992-Belghiti piggyback technique. Due to the presence of calcific portal vein sclerosis extending into the proximal SMV a portal thrombectomy was excluded. Hence, after side-to-side vena cava anastomosis, SRS was sectioned at the confluence to the left renal vein and the renal side was brought behind the stomach, in order to perform a T-T anastomosis between portal vein and venous shunt.

The procedure was performed successfully and then the patient was kept in the Intensive Care Unit (ICU) 24 hours. Postoperative course was uneventful and the patient was discharged on postoperative day 7 with excellent graft function and in good clinical conditions.

3. Discussion

The portal venous system comprises the veins draining the abdominal tract of the digestive system, including the lower esophagus, except the lower anal canal. The main tributaries of the portal vein are the splenic, left gastric, right gastric, superior mesenteric, paraumbilical, and cystic veins [3]. In patients with portal hypertension blood flow is diverted in the systemic vessels by different kinds of collateral pathways, including esophageal, paraesophageal, coronary gastric, inferior phrenic, paraumbilical, abdominal wall, splenorenal, gastrorenal, retrocaval, and mesocaval collateral.

Angiography was considered the gold standard for the evaluation of varices but, with the availability of cross-sectional imaging techniques, the demonstration of collateral portal vessels can be obtained in all parts of the abdomen and thorax without the risks associated with the catheterization. Although endoscopy is considered the best modality for detection of esophageal varices, angiography and computed tomography (CT) can demonstrate more reliably varices in other locations [5]; MR imaging can ease the diagnosis and the evaluation of these conditions and in particular cases is complementary to CT evaluation [6].

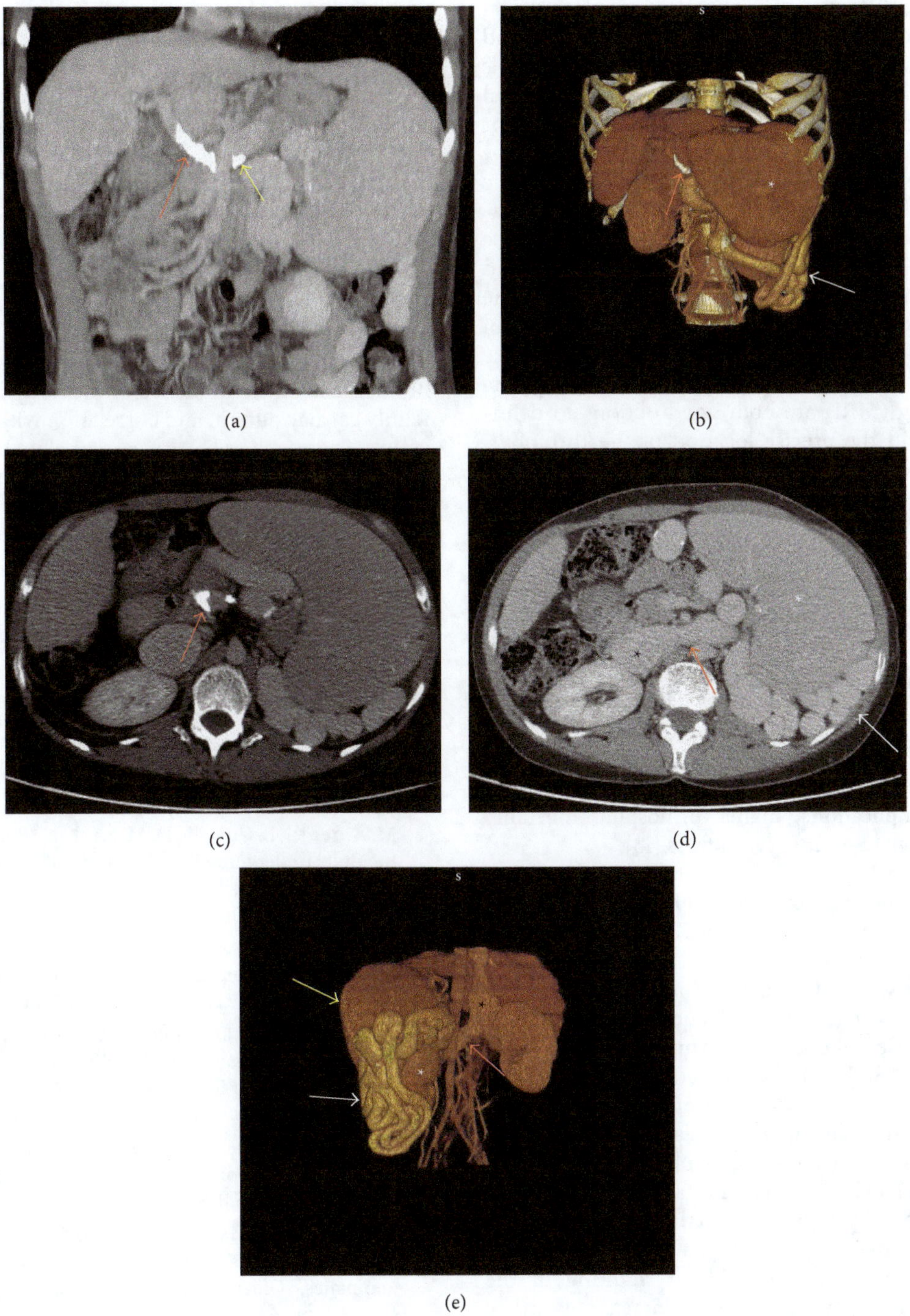

FIGURE 1: (a) MIP sagittal reconstruction showing portal vein calcified thrombosis. The thrombus appears as hyperdense structure occluding the portal vein lumen (red arrow). A little thrombus in the Splenic Vein is also evident (yellow arrow). (b) VR reformation showing portal vein calcified thrombosis (red arrow). The thrombus appears as hyperdense structure occluding the portal vein lumen (red arrow). Spleen (white star) and Splenorenal Shunt (white arrow) are also evident. (c) Axial view (portal phase) showing calcified thrombi partially occluding the superior mesenteric vein lumen (red arrow). (d) Axial view (portal phase) showing the Splenorenal Shunt (white arrow) behind the spleen (white star). Renal vein (red arrow) and Inferior Vena Cava (black star) dilatation is also evident. (e) VR reformation showing the Splenorenal Shunt (white arrow) among the spleen (yellow arrow) and the left kidney (white star). Renal vein (red arrow) and Inferior Vena Cava (black star) dilatation is also evident.

With CT imaging techniques, varices appear as smooth, well-defined structures, round, tubular, or serpentine in shape, with homogeneous attenuation, often surrounded by fat in the retroperitoneum, greater and lesser omentum, and mesentery, with a similar enhancement to the adjacent vessels after the administration of contrast medium, which is useful for distinguishing them by bowel loops, tumor masses, or adenopathy [5].

Color Doppler ultrasound is the first-line diagnostic approach for the detection of PVT; the sensitivity and specificity vary from 66% to 100%, depending on the expertise of the individual examiner and the extent of PVT, and are reduced when bowel gas and obesity are present. The main limitation is delimiting the extension of the thrombi to SV or SMV [7]. When technical conditions are adverse contrast enhanced computed tomography (CT) and magnetic resonance imaging (MRI) are both good options to delineate the extent and the precise location of the thrombus. Unenhanced CT can display fresh thrombi as hyperdense, but this condition does not often occur and contrast medium administration is often required [8]. CT and US examinations are also useful for detecting calcifications within the wall of the vessel or the thrombus, which can eventually complicate the LT procedure [8]. The impact of the development of PVT on the natural history of liver cirrhosis is unclear. Different studies did not show a real impact of PVT on the progression of the disease [9, 10]. Even if PVT does not seem to increase the wait list mortality in patient scheduled for LT [11, 12], it represents a relevant occurrence in patients undergoing LT because it is associated with more difficult surgery, more postoperative complications, higher in-hospital mortality rates [2], and reduced 5-year survival rates [13].

In this particular case PVT was associated with SRS, a quite common consequence of portal hypertension.

Due to the long course of the disease and the progressive increase of portal resistance it is likely that the development of a calcified thrombus in the portal vein can be considered as a slow and progressive event that has advanced up to determine the complete occlusion of the venous trunk.

The presence of SRS and hemodynamic changes related to it might explain the slight symptoms of the patient, as well as the modest alterations of laboratory tests.

In patients with advanced cirrhosis, in fact, the incidence of SRS is approximately 35% [13]. Portal venous flow and velocity are reduced in patients with cirrhosis and large SRS, compared with normal subjects and patients with chronic hepatitis [14] due to the venous blood shunting in the systemic circulation which determines an increase of cardiac output. The enhanced portal blood flow tends to counterpoise the hypotensive effect of the portosystemic shunt. As portal blood flow grows, collateral blood flow multiplies and is nearly totally shunted in the systemic circulation [15].

Due to these hemodynamic changes SRS prevents the formation of gastroesophageal varices but does not reduce the risk of bleeding [16, 17] and is associated with an increased risk of complications such as hepatic encephalopathy [18] and HCC [15].

Chikamori et al. [4] claimed that SRS/portal vein ratio can be an indicator of hyperdynamic status in patients with liver cirrhosis. Authors demonstrated that there is a relationship between the SRS/PV ratio and the degree of hyperdynamic circulatory status in patients with cirrhosis.

SRS management in LT remains controversial, as there is still no consensus on indications to LT and modalities of care. In our case ceCT with MPR and volume rendering reconstruction helped surgeons to properly plan the LT.

In our case ceCT with MPR and volume rendering reconstruction helped surgeons to properly plan the LT

4. Conclusions

Careful management is necessary for patients with PVT and SRS because of the influence on hemodynamic parameters, mainly cardiac output, and correlation with increased risk of complication such as hepatic encephalopathy.

Imaging plays a pivotal role in the evaluation and follow-up of cirrhotic patients, and ceCT is especially useful in the evaluation of vascular alterations such as PVT and SRS.

References

[1] M. Primignani, G. Tosetti, and V. La Mura, "Therapeutic and clinical aspects of portal vein thrombosis in patients with cirrhosis," *World Journal of Hepatology*, vol. 7, no. 29, pp. 2906–2912, 2015.

[2] M. A. Yerdel, B. Gunson, D. Mirza et al., "Portal vein thrombosis in adults undergoing liver transplantation: risk factors, screening, management, and outcome," *Transplantation*, vol. 69, no. 9, pp. 1873–1881, 2000.

[3] C. Gallego, M. Velasco, P. Marcuello, D. Tejedor, L. De Campo, and A. Friera, "Congenital and acquired anomalies of the portal venous system," *Radiographics*, vol. 22, no. 1, pp. 141–159, 2002.

[4] F. Chikamori, H. Okamoto, and N. Kuniyoshi, "Relationships between splenorenal shunt/portal vein diameter ratio and systemic hemodynamics in patients with liver cirrhosis," *Digestion*, vol. 89, no. 2, pp. 133–138, 2014.

[5] K. Cho, Y. D. Patel, R. H. Wachsberg, and J. Seef, "Varices in portal hypertension: evaluation with CT," *Radiology*, vol. 195, no. 2, pp. 553–556, 1995.

[6] I. Lupescu, N. Masala, R. Capsa, N. Câmpeanu, and Ş. A. Georgescu, "CT and MRI of acquired portal venous system anomalies," *Journal of Gastrointestinal and Liver Diseases*, vol. 15, no. 4, pp. 393–398, 2006.

[7] H. Chen, F. Turon, V. Hernández-Gea et al., "Nontumoral portal vein thrombosis in patients awaiting liver transplantation," *Liver Transplantation*, vol. 22, no. 3, pp. 352–365, 2016.

[8] A. Berzigotti, Á. García-Criado, A. Darnell, and J.-C. García-Pagán, "Imaging in clinical decision-making for portal vein thrombosis," *Nature Reviews Gastroenterology and Hepatology*, vol. 11, no. 5, pp. 308–316, 2014.

[9] F. Nery, S. Chevret, B. Condat et al., "Causes and consequences of portal vein thrombosis in 1,243 patients with cirrhosis: results of a longitudinal study," *Hepatology*, vol. 61, no. 2, pp. 660–667, 2015.

[10] A. Luca, S. Caruso, M. Milazzo et al., "Natural course of extrahepatic nonmalignant partial portal vein thrombosis in patients with cirrhosis," *Radiology*, vol. 265, no. 1, pp. 124–132, 2012.

[11] B. V. John, R. Konjeti, A. Aggarwal et al., "Impact of untreated portal vein thrombosis on pre and post liver transplant outcomes in cirrhosis," *Annals of Hepatology*, vol. 12, no. 6, pp. 952–958, 2013.

[12] M. J. Englesbe, D. E. Schaubel, S. Cai, M. K. Guidinger, and R. M. Merion, "Portal vein thrombosis and liver transplant survival benefit," *Liver Transplantation*, vol. 16, no. 8, pp. 999–1005, 2010.

[13] F. Chikamori, S. Nishida, G. Selvaggi et al., "Effect of liver transplantation on spleen size, collateral veins, and platelet counts," *World Journal of Surgery*, vol. 34, no. 2, pp. 320–326, 2010.

[14] K. Ohnishi, M. Saito, S. Sato et al., "Direction of splenic venous flow assessed by pulsed Doppler flowmetry in patients with a large splenorenal shunt. Relation to spontaneous hepatic encephalopathy," *Gastroenterology*, vol. 89, no. 1, pp. 180–185, 1985.

[15] G. Tarantino, V. Citro, P. Conca et al., "What are the implications of the spontaneous spleno-renal shunts in liver cirrhosis?" *BMC Gastroenterology*, vol. 9, article 89, 2009.

[16] H. Maruyama, T. Kondo, S. Kiyono, T. Sekimoto, M. Takahashi, and O. Yokosuka, "Influence of splenorenal shunt on long-term outcomes in cirrhosis," *Scandinavian Journal of Gastroenterology*, vol. 50, no. 5, pp. 593–600, 2015.

[17] P. Aseni, C. Beati, G. Brambilla, M. Bertini, and L. Belli, "Does large spontaneous portal systemic shunt in cirrhosis protect from the risk of gastroesophageal bleeding?" *Journal of Clinical Gastroenterology*, vol. 8, no. 3, pp. 235–238, 1986.

[18] S. Iannello, L. Libertini, R. Martini et al., "A large spontaneous splenorenal shunt in a patient with liver cirrhosis and uncomplicated portal hypertension," *Digestive Diseases*, vol. 17, no. 4, pp. 248–255, 1999.

13

Radiological Diagnosis of a Rare Premature Aging Genetic Disorder: Progeria (Hutchinson-Gilford Syndrome)

Haji Mohammed Nazir, Akshiitha Ramesh Baabhu, Yuvaraj Muralidharan, and Seena Cheppala Rajan

Saveetha Medical College and Hospital, Saveetha Nagar, Thandalam, Chennai, Tamil Nadu 602105, India

Correspondence should be addressed to Akshiitha Ramesh Baabhu; whityna27@gmail.com

Academic Editor: Daniel P. Link

Hutchinson-Gilford Progeria Syndrome (HGPS) is a rare disease with a combination of short stature, bone abnormalities, premature ageing, and skin changes. Though the physical appearance of these patients is characteristic, there is little emphasis on the characteristic radiological features. In this paper, we report a 16-year-old boy with clinical and radiological features of this rare genetic disorder. He had a characteristic facial appearance with a large head, large eyes, thin nose with beaked tip, small chin, protruding ears, prominent scalp veins, and absence of hair.

1. Introduction

Hutchinson-Gilford Progeria Syndrome is an extremely rare genetic disease, which was named after the two doctors who first described it in England, in 1886 by Dr. Hutchinson and in 1897 by Dr. Hastings Gilford [1]. The reported prevalence rate of progeria is one in eight million births and if unreported cases are taken into account, the estimated birth prevalence is one in four million [2]. According to the Progeria Research Foundation database as of January 2017, there are 144 progeric children worldwide, residing in 46 countries [3]. The average survival age is 13.5 years (life expectancy about 8–21 years) and death occurs mostly due to stroke, myocardial infarction, heart failure, or atherosclerosis [4].

2. Case Presentation

A 16-year-old boy, born to nonconsanguineous parents presented to our hospital with difficulty in walking and bilateral hip deformity, following a trivial trauma, four months before the presentation. The boy was short and had a bird-like facial appearance (Figure 6). History from the mother revealed that perinatal period was uneventful and had two siblings who were normal. On general examination, the boy had prominent eyes, prominent scalp veins, small chin, small face and large head, beaked nose, loss of subcutaneous fat, muscular atrophy, kyphosis, brown pigmentation all over the trunk, coarse thickened skin, broad stumpy fingers, and short wide toes. The boy resembled a little old person with loss of scalp hair, eyebrows, and eyelashes. He had normal intelligence. The first visible abnormality his parents noticed was excessive hair loss at three months of age. Based on the history and clinical diagnosis, a provisional diagnosis of progeria was made.

Routine biochemical tests were normal except for elevated serum cholesterol. The patient was sent to our radiology department and was subjected for the skeletal survey. Frontal chest radiograph showed cardiomegaly, sloping slender fifth, and sixth posterior ribs. The absence of lateral and medial ends of both clavicles with a tiny bone fragment was seen in the acromial ends of both clavicles (Figure 1). Skull radiograph in lateral view showed disproportionate large calvarium with hypoplastic facial bones, small mandible with small ascending ramus, and obtuse mandibular angle with the overcrowding of teeth (Figures 2(a) and 2(b)). CT head showed open anterior fontanelle, large cranial vault with thin diploic space, and no abnormality in the brain (Figure 2(c)). Radiograph of the dorsal spine in the lateral projection showed the presence of mild concavity in the anterior aspect of vertebral

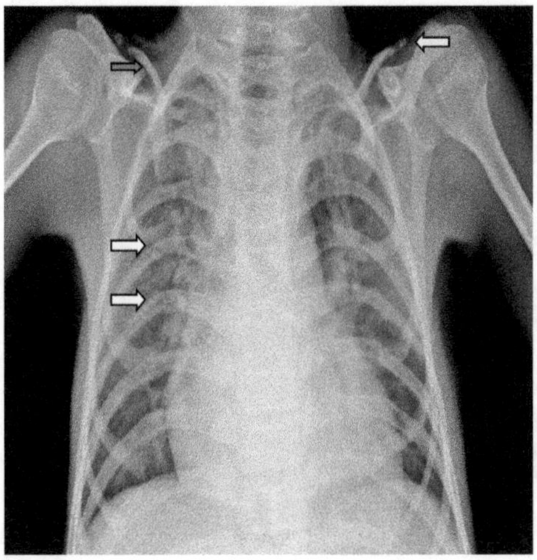

FIGURE 1: Frontal chest radiograph showing cardiomegaly, sloping slender fifth and sixth posterior ribs (white arrows). The absence of lateral and medial end of both clavicles (red arrow) with a tiny bone fragment was seen in the acromial end of both clavicles (yellow arrow).

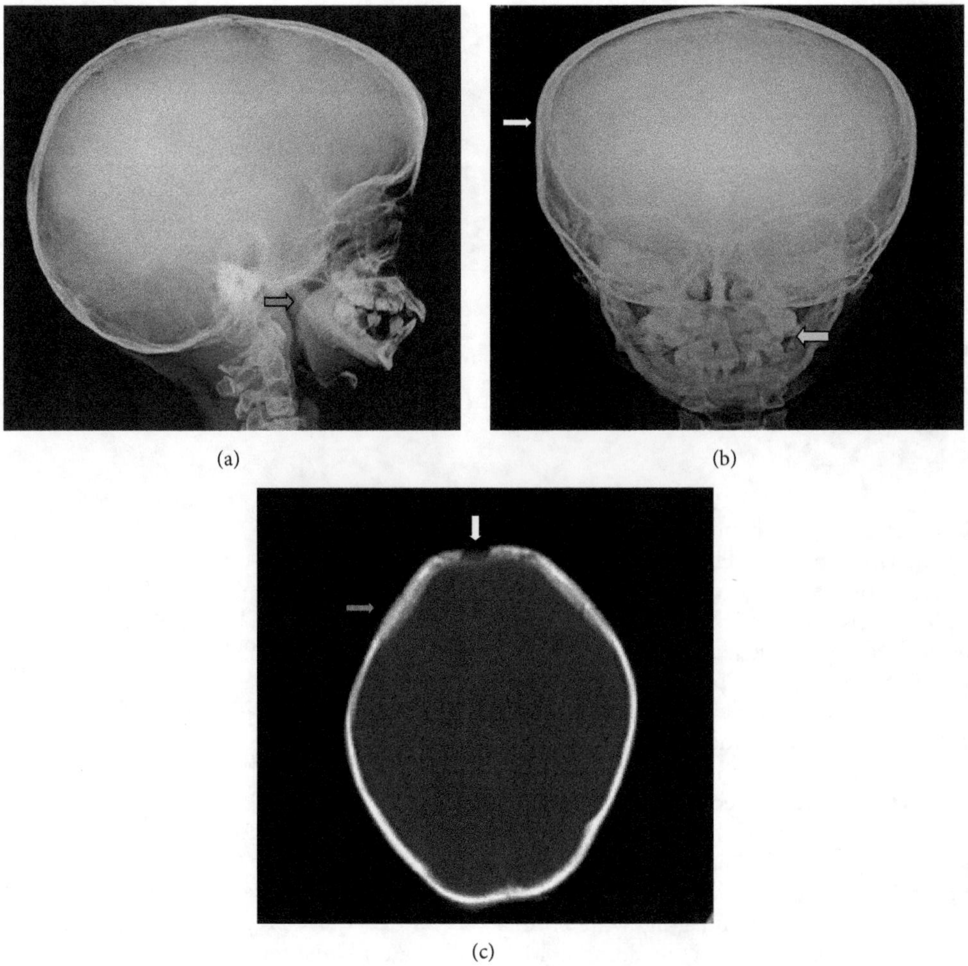

FIGURE 2: Skull radiograph lateral and anteroposterior views (a, b) showing disproportionate large calvarium with hypoplastic facial bones, small mandible with small ascending ramus, and obtuse mandibular angle (red arrow) and overcrowding of teeth (blue arrow). CT head (c) showing open anterior fontanelle (white arrow) and large cranial vault with thin diploic space (red arrow).

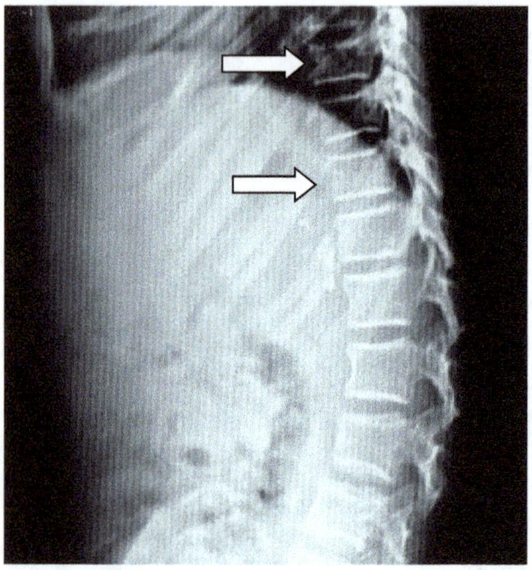

FIGURE 3: Radiograph of the dorsal spine (lateral projection) showing thoracic kyphosis and mild concavity in the anterior aspect of vertebral bodies (arrows). Prevertebral calcific foci seen adjacent to lower thoracic vertebrae.

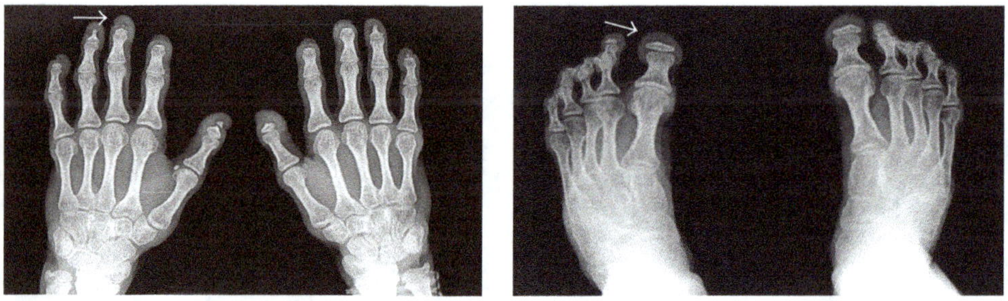

(a) (b)

FIGURE 4: Anteroposterior radiograph of both hands (a) and foot (b) showed resorption of terminal phalanges with preservation of soft tissue (white arrow).

bodies ("fish mouth" vertebra) and kyphotic curvature [5]. Prevertebral calcifications are shown in Figure 3. Radiograph of both hands' anteroposterior view showed resorption of terminal phalanges with preservation of soft tissue (Figure 4(a)). Radiograph of both feet's anteroposterior view showed resorption of terminal phalanges with preservation of soft tissue (Figure 4(b)). Radiograph of pelvis with both hip joints in anteroposterior view showed widening of pubic symphysis, bilateral shallow acetabulum, abnormal contour of bilateral femoral head with increased neck shaft angle (coxa valga deformity), enlarged and elongated bilateral greater trochanter, superolateral migration of bilateral femoral head overlying adjacent to iliac bones, and slender proximal femoral shafts (Figure 5(a)). Further imaging with computed tomography (CT) of pelvis confirmed the radiographic findings of pubic diastasis, bilateral shallow acetabulum, bilateral coxa valga deformity, bilateral hip dislocation, and pseudoarticulation of the left femoral head with iliac bone (Figure 5(b)). Bones appeared diffusely osteopenic in all the radiographs.

3. Discussion

Progeria is a genetic disease which is extremely rare and characterised by accelerated premature ageing. Gilford in 1904 coined the term progeria which is derived from the Greek word "geros" meaning old. In progeria the pattern of premature aging is segmental as cataracts, Alzheimer's disease or cancers typical of aging do not occur in progeric children. Also the typical balding pattern and bone changes of progeria do not occur with normal aging [6]. The affected individual ages seven times faster than that of normal individuals. The disease occurs due to the sporadic mutation in the LMNA gene, which provides instructions for making proteins lamins A and C. These proteins are the main components of intermediate filamentous lamina which function as a structural support [7]. This disorder is confirmed by a genetic test for the point mutation in LMNA gene [8]. Genetic analysis was not performed for this case due to lack of such facilities in and around our institution. Our case was mainly diagnosed by classical clinical and characteristic radiology features.

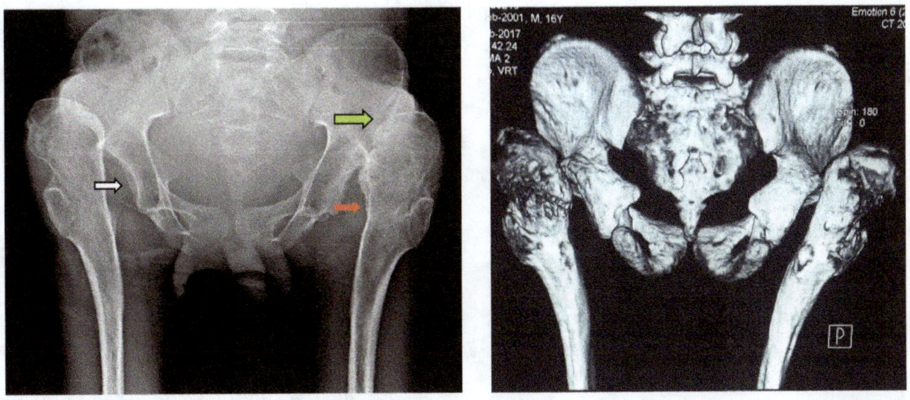

(a) (b)

FIGURE 5: Anteroposterior radiograph of pelvis with both hip joints (a) showed widening of pubic symphysis, bilateral shallow acetabulum (white arrow), abnormal contour of bilateral femoral head with increased neck shaft angle (coxa valga deformity) (red arrow), enlarged and elongated bilateral greater trochanter, superolateral migration of bilateral femoral head overlying adjacent to iliac bones (green arrow), and slender proximal femoral shafts. CT of pelvis (b) confirming pubic diastasis, bilateral shallow acetabulum, bilateral coxa valga deformity, bilateral hip dislocation, and pseudoarticulation of the left femoral head with iliac bone.

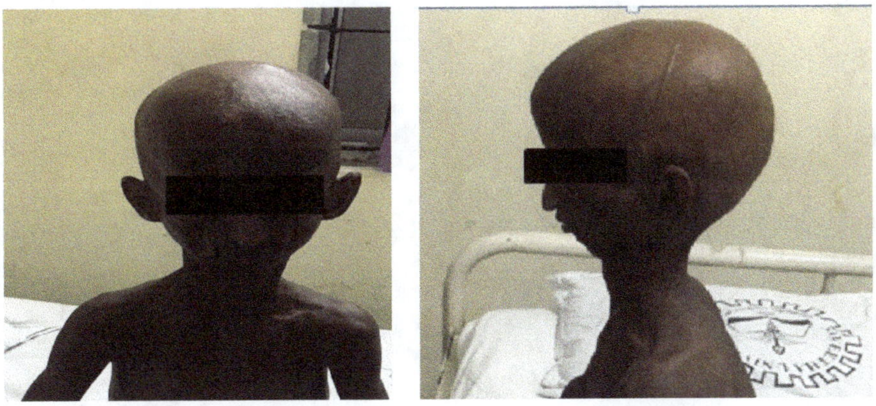

(a) (b)

FIGURE 6: Real life pictures of the 16-year-old male patient with bird-like facies: (a) en face view and (b) profile view.

Elevated levels of serum triglycerides, total cholesterol low-density lipoprotein cholesterol, and reduced levels of high-density lipoprotein cholesterol have been reported [9]. Elevated levels of hyaluronic acid excretion in the urine may be seen but are not diagnostic.

Progeric children are normal at birth and within the first year of life develop severe growth deficiency with sclerodermatous skin changes. Loss of subcutaneous fat with alopecia changes in the skin give the typical "plucked-bird" appearance at about 6–12 months of age. Simultaneously, scalp hair and eyelashes are progressively lost and finally resulting in baldness with prominent scalp veins. Abnormal dentition, beaked nose, receding chin, and exophthalmos are the typical facial features in these patients. Muscular atrophy with joint deformities is additional features. Intelligence is normal or above normal in these patients. All these physical features were seen in our patient, giving a physical appearance of "a wizened little old man." Commonest cause of death in progeria is heart disease due to genetic predisposition in the affected persons.

A review of the previously reported radiography findings in affected individuals with progeria disclosed a notable similarity of changes [10]. Diffuse osteopenia, prominent vascular markings in skull, thin and large calvarium with shallow diploic space, multiple wormian bones, small mandible with infantile obtuse angle and short ascending rami, hypoplastic facial bones, open cranial fontanelles, thin short clavicles, dwarfism, abnormally gracile ribs involving the posterior segments of the upper ribs, slender long bones, kyphosis, coxa valga, and progressive acroosteolysis of the terminal phalanges were the major roentgen findings previously reported. All the above findings were seen in our patient, except wormian bones. Bilateral coxa valga deformity with bizarre greater trochanters and shallow acetabulum with bilateral hip dislocation were seen in our patient. Coxa magna, coxa valga, acetabular dysplasia, hip subluxation, and dislocation are the common orthopaedic hip manifestations which have been previously reported [11]. Avascular necrosis of the femoral head, flared long bone metaphysis/epiphysis, enlarged capitulum of the distal humerus have also been reported.

The radiological findings of our case were consistent with those of which were present in more than fifty percent of cases of a largely appreciated study by Cleveland et al. on HGPS [12].

This discussion will be incomplete without a mention on "nonclassical" progeria in which the patients show less growth retardation, presence of scalp hair for a longer time, more slowly progressive lipodystrophy, and survival well into adulthood [13].

Differential diagnoses are other ageing syndromes like Werner's syndrome (adult progeria), Cockyane's syndrome, Acrogeria, and Rothmund-Thomson syndrome which can be differentiated by their clinical features. Progeric individuals rarely survive beyond the second decade and the cause of death is usually due to myocardial infarction or congestive heart failure.

4. Conclusion

The presented case provides important teaching points with regard to clinical and radiological findings of progeria syndrome which is an extremely rare genetic disorder with fatal outcome. Adequate knowledge on the radiological findings can aid in excluding mimics of progeria at diagnosis. The rarity of the disease and limited availability of literature prompted us to report this case.

References

[1] J. Hutchinson, "Case of congenital absence of hair, with atrophic condition of the skin and its appendages, in a boy whose mother had been almost wholly bald from alopecia areata from the age of six," *Lancet*, vol. 1, no. 923, 1886.

[2] R. L. Pollex and R. A. Hegele, "Hutchinson-Gilford progeria syndrome," *Clinical Genetics*, vol. 66, no. 5, pp. 375–381, 2004.

[3] Progeria Research Foundation (PRF) webpage, http://www.progeriaresearch.org/assets/files/pdf/PRF-By-the-Numbers_-Jan-2017-Update.pdf.

[4] S. Pereira, P. Bourgeois, C. Navarro et al., "HGPS and related premature aging disorders: From genomic identification to the first therapeutic approaches," *Mechanisms of Ageing and Development*, vol. 129, no. 7-8, pp. 449–459, 2008.

[5] R. Rastogi and S. M. Chander Mohan, "Progeria syndrome: a case report," *Indian Journal of Orthopaedics*, vol. 42, no. 1, pp. 97–99, 2008.

[6] Progeria Research Foundation (PRF) webpage, https://www.progeriaresearch.org/assets/files/pdf/info_sheets/18_Progeria-Aging_0410.pdf.

[7] D. K. Shumaker, E. R. Kuczmarski, and R. D. Goldman, "The nucleoskeleton: lamins and actin are major players in essential nuclear functions," *Current Opinion in Cell Biology*, vol. 15, no. 3, pp. 358–366, 2003.

[8] M. Eriksson, W. T. Brown, L. B. Gordon et al., "Recurrent de novo point mutations in lamin A cause Hutchinson-Gilford progeria syndrome," *Nature*, vol. 423, no. 6937, pp. 293–298, 2003.

[9] P. K. Sarkar and R. A. Shinton, "Hutchinson-Guilford progeria syndrome," *Postgraduate Medical Journal*, vol. 77, no. 907, pp. 312–317, 2001.

[10] N. J. Ullrich, V. M. Silvera, S. E. Campbell, and L. B. Gordon, "Craniofacial abnormalities in Hutchinson-Gilford Progeria syndrome," *American Journal of Neuroradiology*, vol. 33, no. 8, pp. 1512–1518, 2012.

[11] P. Akhbari, S. Jha, K. D. James, B. L. Hinves, and J. A. Buchanan, "Hip pathology in Hutchinson–Gilford progeria syndrome," *Journal of Pediatric Orthopaedics B*, vol. 21, no. 6, pp. 563–566, 2012.

[12] R. H. Cleveland, L. B. Gordon, M. E. Kleinman et al., "A prospective study of radiographic manifestations in Hutchinson-Gilford progeria syndrome," *Pediatric Radiology*, vol. 42, no. 9, pp. 1089–1098, 2012.

[13] R. C. M. Hennekam, "Hutchinson-Gilford progeria syndrome: review of the phenotype," *American Journal of Medical Genetics*, vol. 140, no. 23, pp. 2603–2624, 2006.

14

Imaging of Posterior Interosseous Neuropathy following Distal Biceps Repair: A Report of 3 Cases

Darren Fitzpatrick,[1] Catherine Petchprapa,[2] and Leon Rybak[2]

[1]*Department of Radiology, Mount Sinai Medical Center, 1 Gustave Levy Place, New York, NY 10029, USA*
[2]*Department of Radiology, NYU School of Medicine, 660 1st Avenue, 1st Floor, New York, NY 10016, USA*

Correspondence should be addressed to Darren Fitzpatrick; darren.fitzpatrick.md@gmail.com

Academic Editor: Yoshito Tsushima

Three cases of PIN palsy following biceps repair are presented with clinical and imaging correlation. The imaging findings in these cases will be discussed and the orthopedic literature, as regards possible surgical approaches and technical factors believed to predispose to or prevent this complication, will be reviewed. It is important for radiologists to serve as consultants in these uncommon but sometimes devastating complications, helping to quickly and accurately recognize the imaging findings corresponding to the clinical symptoms and aiding the surgeon in diagnosis and treatment by identifying the possible causes and sites of nerve compression.

1. Introduction

The elbow is a complex anatomical region, with multiple fine structures in close proximity working in concert to result in efficient function of the upper extremity. Radiologists interpreting MRI of this joint must be well versed with these relationships. Injury to the posterior interosseous nerve (PIN) and its branches is a well-known complication of surgical repair of the distal biceps tendon. Though much has been published in the radiology literature as regards the posterior interosseous nerve syndrome as well as the imaging diagnosis of distal biceps tear, there is lack of literature on imaging of iatrogenic injury to the PIN.

2. Cases

2.1. Case 1. A healthy, right hand dominant, 51-year-old male sustained a complete rupture of the biceps tendon while shoveling dirt. Within one week of the injury, the patient underwent single incision anterior repair. At the time of surgery, 90% of the biceps tendon was avulsed from the radial tuberosity. The biceps was repaired utilizing a cortical fixation button to secure it to the posterior aspect of the radius.

Immediately following the procedure, the patient complained of increased paresthesia and numbness along the lateral volar aspect of his forearm as well as an inability to extend his wrist (2/5) and fingers (1/5). These findings were attributed to neuropraxia of both the lateral antebrachial cutaneous nerve (LACN) and PIN secondary to operative retraction.

The patient was placed in an extension splint and was started on active range of motion exercises. When the symptoms failed to resolve in 4-week time, electromyographic (EMG) testing was performed which revealed the expected motor and sensory deficits in the radial nerve and LACN distribution. A magnetic resonance imaging study (MRI) (Figure 1) demonstrated a denervation related edema-like pattern of homogenous high signal on fluid sensitive sequences in the extensor compartment, involving the extensor carpi ulnaris (ECU), extensor digitorum communis (EDC), extensor digiti minimi (EDM), and supinator muscles. No muscle atrophy or fatty infiltration was noted on the T1 weighted images. A surgical scar was noted in the antecubital region with no evidence of a posterior incision. The surgical tunnel within the proximal radius was clearly identified and appeared to be oriented slightly in a proximal to distal direction.

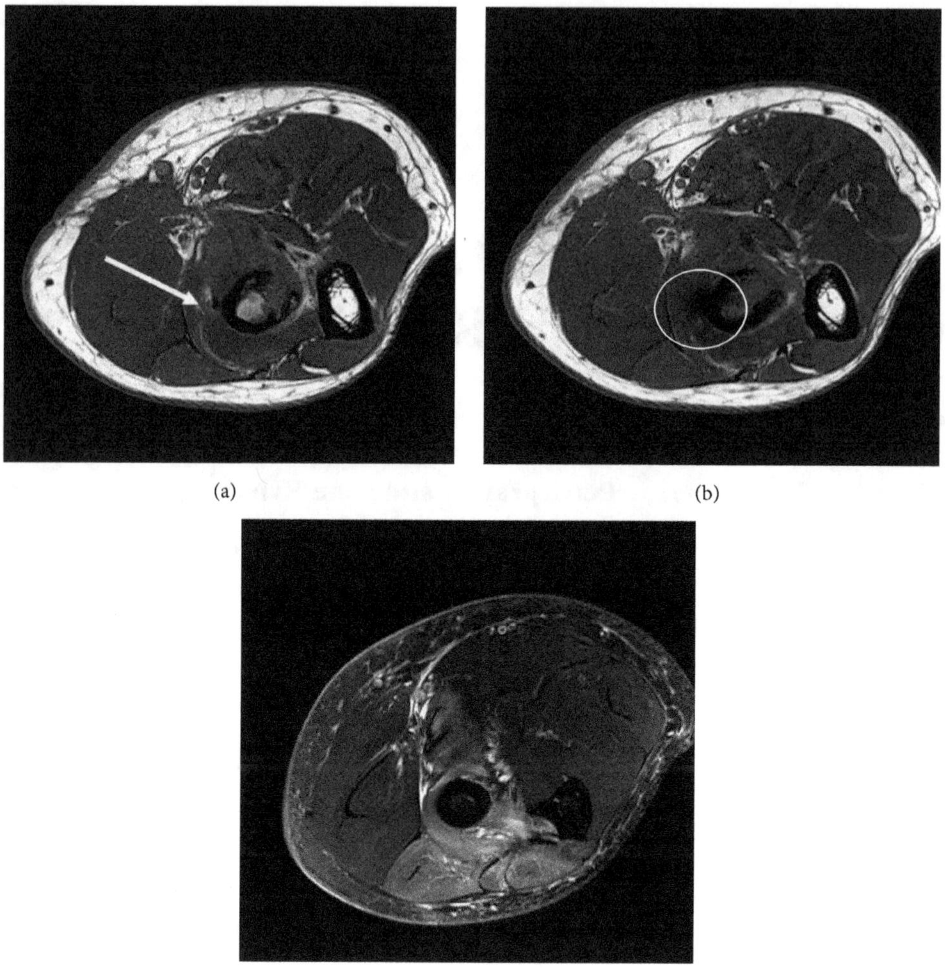

(a) (b) (c)

FIGURE 1: Axial T1 ((a), (b)) and T2 fat saturated images (c) from patient 1. (a) demonstrates the PIN in the supinator tunnel just proximal to the exit point of the radial tunnel posterolaterally where it is clearly identified (white arrow). Slightly more distally, (b), artifact from the cortical fixation button obscures the plane of the PIN (circle). A pattern of muscle edema involving the ECU, EDC, EDM, and supinator muscles is consistent with injury to the PIN in (c).

In the area of cortical button deployment, along the posteromedial radial cortex, the PIN and corresponding fat plane within the supinator tunnel were focally obscured by small susceptibility artifact. The biceps tendon was not clearly visualized at its insertion prompting the interpreting radiologist to suggest rerupture. However, clinical examination demonstrated intact biceps function and the findings at imaging were attributed to edema and hemorrhage related to the recent postoperative state.

A decision was made to pursue a course of conservative, nonoperative therapy with aggressive physical and occupational therapy. The patient began to recover PIN function by 6 months. At one year, motor function throughout the arm returned to 5/5 with persistent loss of sensation in the LACN distribution.

2.2. Case 2. A 44-year-old male presented to the surgeons office with an approximately two-month history of pain along the anterior aspect of the elbow. An MRI was ordered which demonstrated a near-full thickness tear of the distal biceps tendon. Surgery was performed 1 month after presentation and approximately 3 months after the onset of symptoms. At the time of surgery, there was high grade, near-full thickness tear of the tendon just proximal to the insertion site. The torn tendon fibers were retracted to the level of the elbow crease. Repair was performed via a single incision anterior approach with fixation achieved using both cortical fixation button and a biotenodesis screw.

Beginning on postoperative day 4, the patient was noted to have numbness along the dorsal aspect of his thumb, index, and middle digits as well as mild weakness of wrist extension. The patient complained predominantly of loss of function of his thumb. When symptoms failed to resolve with conservative therapy, an EMG was performed which showed evidence of conduction loss in the distribution of both the deep and superficial radial branches.

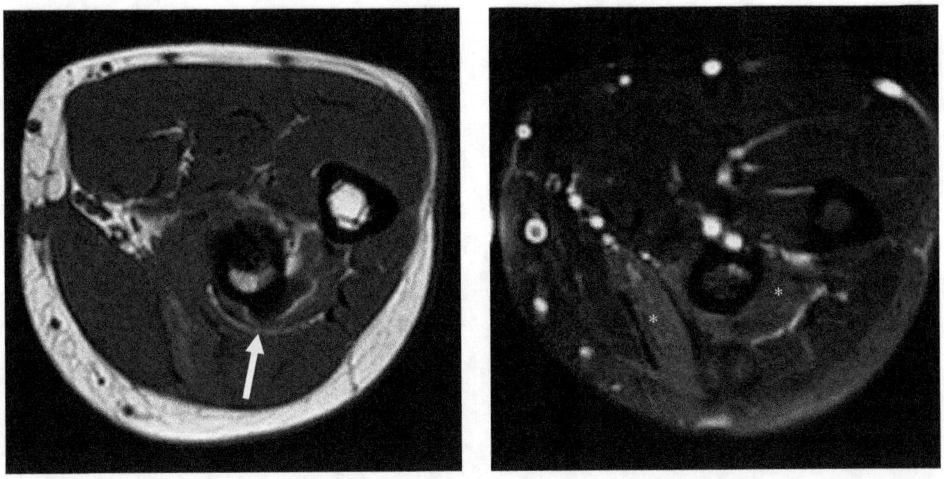

(a) (b)

FIGURE 2: Axial T1 (a) and T2 (b) fat saturated images from patient 2. In (a), surgical artifact along the posterolateral margin of the radius can be seen approaching but not definitively compressing or obscuring the deep radial nerve or proximal PIN (white arrow). Neurogenic edema is noted in the ECRB and supinator muscles in (b) (asterisks).

Approximately 4 months after the surgery and 7 months after the initial injury, a second MRI was performed (Figure 2) which demonstrated an edema-like pattern within the supinator and extensor carpi radialis brevis muscles consistent with denervation. No muscle atrophy was noted. As with the first case, a single anterior scar was identified with no evidence of a posterior incision. Artifact from the area of the cortical fixation button was noted in proximity to the plane of the traversing PIN, but without effacement of the nerve or surrounding fat plane. The biceps repair was intact.

The patient was treated conservatively with physical therapy without resolution of his symptoms. One year later, he opted for nerve exploration and repair at another institution, the details of which are not available. At last contact, he has shown no significant improvement.

2.3. Case 3. A 54-year-old, right hand dominant, male sustained a complete rupture of the left distal biceps tendon while playing baseball. The patient underwent surgical repair of the tendon approximately 2 weeks later using a 2-incision approach with suture fixation.

In the immediate postoperative period, the patient reported a burning type pain along the dorsal aspect of his forearm and an inability to extend his fingers. On examination, he had extensor carpi radialis longus function with complete lack of function of the ECU, EPL, and EDC. The consistency of the biceps repair site was noted to be spongy on palpation. A subsequent EMG confirmed the lack of response in the distribution of the PIN. An MRI was performed approximately 1 month after surgery (Figure 3) which demonstrated scattered susceptibility artifact posteriorly along the expected course of the PIN and denervation-like edema signal on fluid sensitive images in all of the muscles of the posterior extensor compartment (supinator, ECU, EDC, and EDM). Mild atrophy and fatty infiltration of the muscles were also noted. Retear of the biceps tendon was identified with proximal tendon retraction of approximately 6 cm. There were surgically created defects in the area of the bicipital tuberosity and adjacent posterolateral radial cortex with no discrete transosseous tunnel. Scarring and susceptibility artifact in the planes between the ECU and EDM muscles posteriorly were consistent with a second posterolateral incision.

Surgical therapies including reexploration and tendon transfer were discussed with the patient who opted instead for conservative treatment consisting of physical therapy and medications. At last visit, the patient has made partial recovery of PIN function but continues to have a significant deficit.

3. Discussion

Tears of the distal biceps tendon are relatively uncommon injuries, with most affecting the dominant arm of males in their 40s and 50s. Because conservative treatment may result in a loss of both flexion and supination strength in up to 30% and 40% of cases, respectively, most of these injuries are surgically repaired [1, 2]. The vast majority of patients will return to function; however, complications may occur. Perhaps the most dreaded of these is injury to the posterior interosseous nerve, which can take the form of limited, self-resolving neuropraxia or have devastating implications for function of the hand, requiring tendon transfers or nerve grafting procedures [3]. Though PIN injury can be recognized by classic symptomatology and is treated successfully with conservative therapy, MRI imaging is occasionally necessary to confirm the findings and to elucidate the cause of nerve injury.

Current MRI techniques, with multichannel coils and higher gradients, can accurately image around the surgical artifact produced by distal biceps tendon repair. Metal susceptibility artifact from radial tunnel drilling is usually

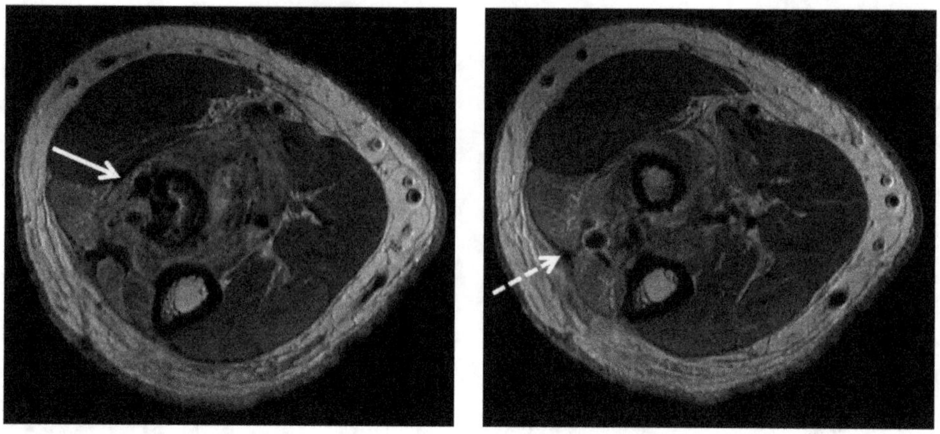

(a) (b)

Figure 3: Two sequential axial proton density images ((a), (b)) in patient 3. Susceptibility artifact is noted in the expected location of the PIN along the posterolateral margin of the proximal radius (solid arrow, (a)). Note the scarring posteriorly indicating a two-incision approach (dashed arrow, (b)).

minimal and does not affect image resolution or obscure the fat planes around the PIN. Bioabsorbable suture anchors in the radial tuberosity also produce minimal artifact. When metallic suture anchors or cortical fixation buttons are placed, the protocol of the MRI exam may be altered to utilize a higher bandwidth, increased echo train length, increased matrix, and increased field of view to maximize visualization of the metallic surgical components and tissue planes adjacent to the PIN.

We have presented three illustrative cases with postoperative imaging of PIN injury sustained at the time of surgical repair of the biceps. In all three cases, a pattern of edema-like signal abnormality was noted within muscles supplied by the PIN, with early atrophy and fatty replacement in one case. This pattern of signal change, which is well defined and confluent and conforms to the boundaries of the specific muscles supplied by a nerve, has a well-documented association with denervation injury. Furthermore, it allows the radiologist to distinguish this injury from other forms of muscle signal abnormality such as the patchy edema seen in postoperative cases such as what is discussed in this report. To further understand the specific imaging findings in these cases, however, it is necessary to be familiar both with the anatomy of the nerve at the elbow and with the different surgical techniques and attendant risks involved in biceps repair.

4. Anatomic Considerations

The posterior interosseous nerve is the motor branch of the radial nerve that arises at the level of the elbow and innervates the posterior musculature of the forearm. The nerve gives off small branches to the supinator muscle proximally and has two main terminal branches. The medial or recurrent branch supplies the superficial musculature of the forearm consisting of the extensor digitorum communis (EDC), extensor digiti minimi (EDM), and extensor carpi ulnaris (ECU) while the lateral or descending branch innervates the deep extensors consisting of the abductor pollicis longus (APL), extensor pollicis brevis (EPB), extensor pollicis longus (EPL), and extensor indicis proprius (EIP) [4]. The extensor carpi radialis brevis (ERCB) can be innervated by the PIN as well. The PIN is, thus, responsible for wrist and finger extension and integral to coordinated use of the hand. Depending on the site of injury to the PIN, the patient can present with failure of extension at all metacarpophalangeal (MCP) joints, weakness of thumb abduction and weakness of extension of the wrist with a radial drift (due to the unopposed pull by the unaffected ECRB and extensor carpi radialis longus (ECRL)), loss of extension of the little and ring fingers alone (recurrent branch injury), or loss of extension of the index and thumb and loss of abduction of the thumb alone (descending branch injury) [5].

The PIN originates on average 3-4 cm proximal to the leading edge of the supinator and travels through a space, approximately 3-4 fingerbreadths long, known as the radial tunnel. This tunnel lies along the anterior aspect of the proximal radius with the floor consisting of the radiocapitellar joint capsule proximally and the deep head of the supinator distally. The nerve quickly travels into the posterior forearm, diving deep to the superficial head of the supinator muscle. PIN syndrome, the name given to compression of the nerve with loss of motor function, can be the result of any number of pathologies in this area. Entrapment of the nerve is usually said to occur at 5 common locations: compression by the leading edge of the ECRB, prominent recurrent radial vessels (Leash of Henry), a fibrous leading edge of the supinator tunnel (Arcade of Frohse), within the supinator muscle tunnel itself, or exiting the tunnel. Other etiologies include trauma to the proximal radius, with either acute injury to the nerve or entrapment by subsequent fibrous scarring and compressive masses such as a ganglion cyst, radiobicipital bursa, or distended annular recess of the elbow joint, as can occur with rheumatoid arthritis [4, 5]. Other iatrogenic etiologies include injury during fixation of proximal radial fractures or, as illustrated in these cases, at the time of surgical repair of the biceps tendon.

Knowledge of the course of the radial nerve and PIN and patterns of innervation may suggest the site of compression and branches involved. Based on the distribution of muscle denervation in our cases, involvement of the medial branch of the PIN in case 1 (ECU, EDC, and EDM) and medial (ECU and EDM) and recurrent (EPL) branches in case 3 could be implied. On the other hand, inclusion of the extensor carpi radialis brevis muscle may indicate a more proximal lesion at the level of the radial nerve or variant innervation of the ECRB by the PIN [6].

5. Factors Related to Surgical Technique

Surgical techniques of biceps tendon repair have been adapted in part to avoid PIN injury while achieving the strongest and most anatomic repair possible. All techniques require an anterior incision in the antecubital crease to retrieve the biceps tendon. The difference lies in whether an additional posterolateral incision is also utilized. Early reports of biceps repair, involving the classic anterolateral incision first used by Henry, noted a high incidence of injury to the radial, posterior interosseous, and antebrachial nerves. To address this issue, Boyd and Anderson in 1961 suggested use of an anterior incision to retrieve the tendon and a second posterolateral incision to reattach the tendon [7]. This second incision would allow visualization and protection of the radial nerve and PIN during exposure of the radial tuberosity. The 2-incision approach, while decreasing the incidence of PIN injury, has led in some cases to heterotopic ossification (HO) and radioulnar synostosis. More recently, with new available techniques of fixation, including cortical fixation button devices, the single anterior incision approach has experienced resurgence [8].

Further mention of the specific technique of cortical fixation button repair is merited, as this procedure has gained popularity and was performed in the first two cases reported here. With this single anterior incision technique, the tendon edge, attached to a cortical fixation button, can be passed through a tunnel in the radial tuberosity. The cortical fixation button is subsequently deployed on the back side of the tunnel, securing the biceps in place. This repair has been touted as resulting in rapid restoration of strength of the biceps tendon and, thus, early physical therapy and return to activity. It has been criticized, however, for limited exposure to the medially positioned radial tuberosity, thereby preventing accurate reconstruction of the original biceps footprint and resulting in decreased supination strength [9]. It is possible, furthermore, when deploying the cortical fixation button on the posterior tuberosity to trap the PIN between the button and the radius, resulting in nerve damage [10]. Double intramedullary cortical button fixation technique has been shown to be an alternative to the cortical fixation button technique as it has the highest load to failure with theoretical decreased risk of potential PIN injury and more anatomic repair of the biceps footprint because of dual fixation [11].

If information about the surgical technique is not readily available, the radiologist might be able to glean this information by assessing signs of a posterolateral incision. It is likely in these patients that the injury was due to posterior dissection and careful inspection for signs of hemorrhage, scarring, nerve discontinuity, or susceptibility obscuring the PIN, as was seen in case 3, is warranted. Conversely, if a single anterior incision was used, the site of nerve injury is likely at the posterior aspect of the surgically created radial tunnel and may have been sustained at time of tunnel creation or deployment of the fixation devices used (i.e., cortical fixation button). Thus, inspection of the fixation device and its relationship to the PIN should be attempted. In case 2, the PIN was noted in close proximity to the cortical fixation button, whereas in case 1, the nerve was completely obscured by susceptibility artifact in proximity to the device.

The trajectory of the tunnel has been pointed out as critical when performing cortical button fixation. Several groups have demonstrated that creation of the tunnel in 30 degrees of ulnar deviation results in greater distance between the posterior exit site of the tunnel and the PIN [10, 12]. Lo et al. found that tunnel drilling from proximal to distal placed the PIN at the greatest risk [13]. These authors further noted that a small transverse anterior antebrachial incision advocated by some authors may in fact force the surgeon to angle distally and suggested a slightly larger longitudinal incision to allow the surgeon more latitude in tunnel trajectory. The slightly proximal to distal orientation of the tunnel in case 1 may have increased the risk of nerve injury.

6. Future Role for Imaging

Most cases of PIN palsy following distal biceps surgery are believed to be temporary in nature and, in many cases, related to stretch of the nerve, pressure due to the pronated position, or inadvertent placement of a retractor in proximity to the nerve. Most of these are treated conservatively and, even in those cases with no resolution, the surgeon may opt to confirm the findings with an EMG and proceed directly to surgical exploration without imaging.

Is there a role for imaging in the prevention, diagnosis, and treatment of this complication? In the preoperative scenario, is it possible that high resolution MRI can help identify normal anatomic variants, which might predispose the patient to this complication. It has been noted that when using a two-incision technique, up to 20% of patients will fail to have complete restoration of supination strength, attributed to disruption of some of the smaller PIN branches to the supinator [13]. Duquin et al. studied the anatomy of the PIN and found 25% of the specimens to have at least 1 branch to the supinator, originating within 5 mm or less of the distal margin of the bicipital tuberosity, and suggested that greater care should be used when dissecting in this area [14]. Other investigators have noted that direct contact of the PIN with the periosteum of the proximal radius, with lack of interposed soft tissue, may place the nerve at greater risk during surgery [15]. With high resolution MR neurography now in use, it might be possible to alert the surgeon to these variants in advance.

Clearly, as indicated in our 3 cases, MRI can identify the pattern of muscle denervation and provide an indirect map of the nerve branches involved. Furthermore, with recent advances in metal artifact reduction MRI techniques, the radiologist can guide therapy by identifying cases where the nerve is transected or entrapped by surgical devices and nothing short of surgical intervention will suffice. Thus, MRI guidance can prevent unnecessary delays, with prolonged periods of conservative therapy, which may doom the patient to permanent deficit [16].

7. Conclusion

In conclusion, injury to the radial nerve and its branches, particularly the PIN, is a well recognized complication of surgical repair of the distal biceps tendon that has been described extensively in the orthopedic literature but, to the best of the authors' knowledge, has not been discussed in the radiology literature. Multiple technical factors as well as normal anatomic variations have been identified which increase injury to the PIN during biceps tendon repair. The authors describe 3 cases in which MRI revealed a pattern of marrow edema consistent with neurogenic injury and suggested the site of injury along the course of the PIN. With advancing MRI techniques, including MR neurography and metal suppression, imaging may play an even greater role in the presurgical identification of patients with anatomic variations, which may place them at greater risk for surgical nerve injury as well as identifying the cause of postsurgical nerve damage.

References

[1] B. E. Baker and D. Bierwagen, "Rupture of the distal tendon of the biceps brachii. Operative versus non-operative treatment," *Journal of Bone and Joint Surgery A*, vol. 67, no. 3, pp. 414–417, 1985.

[2] B. F. Morrey, L. J. Askew, K. N. An, and J. H. Dobyns, "Rupture of the distal tendon of the biceps brachii. a biomechanical study," *The Journal of Bone and Joint Surgery—American Volume*, vol. 67, no. 3, pp. 418–421, 1985.

[3] D. B. Mokhtee, J. M. Brown, S. E. Mackinnon, and T. H. Tung, "Reconstruction of posterior interosseous nerve injury following biceps tendon repair: case report and cadaveric study," *Hand*, vol. 4, no. 2, pp. 134–139, 2009.

[4] A. C. Dang and C. M. Rodner, "Unusual compression neuropathies of the forearm, part I: radial nerve," *The Journal of Hand Surgery*, vol. 34, no. 10, pp. 1906–1914, 2009.

[5] P. K. Givissis, S. I. Stavridis, K. T. Ditsios, and A. G. Christodoulou, "Isolated injury of the posterior interosseous nerve complicating a deep laceration of the proximal forearm dorsolateral muscles: a case report," *The Journal of Trauma*, vol. 67, no. 6, pp. E194–E196, 2009.

[6] M. M. al-Qattan, "The nerve supply to extensor carpi radialis brevis," *Journal of Anatomy*, vol. 188, part 1, pp. 249–250, 1996.

[7] H. B. Boyd and L. D. Anderson, "A method for reinsertion of the distal biceps brachii tendon," *The Journal of Bone & Joint Surgery—American Volume*, vol. 43, no. 7, pp. 1041–1043, 1961.

[8] G. I. Bain, H. Prem, R. J. Heptinstall, R. Verhellen, and D. Paix, "Repair of distal biceps tendon rupture: a new technique using the Endobutton," *Journal of Shoulder and Elbow Surgery*, vol. 9, no. 2, pp. 120–126, 2000.

[9] S. A. Hasan, C. L. Cordell, R. B. Rauls, M. S. Bailey, D. Sahu, and L. J. Suva, "Two-incision versus one-incision repair for distal biceps tendon rupture: a cadaveric study," *Journal of Shoulder and Elbow Surgery*, vol. 21, no. 7, pp. 935–941, 2012.

[10] N. Saldua, J. Carney, C. Dewing, and M. Thompson, "The effect of drilling angle on posterior interosseous nerve safety during open and endoscopic anterior single-incision repair of the distal biceps tendon," *Arthroscopy*, vol. 24, no. 3, pp. 305–310, 2008.

[11] S. Siebenlist, A. Buchholz, J. Zapf et al., "Double intramedullary cortical button versus suture anchors for distal biceps tendon repair: a biomechanical comparison," *Knee Surgery, Sports Traumatology, Arthroscopy*, vol. 23, no. 3, pp. 926–933, 2015.

[12] P. R. Chavan, T. R. Duquin, and L. J. Bisson, "Repair of the ruptured distal biceps tendon: a systematic review," *The American Journal of Sports Medicine*, vol. 36, no. 8, pp. 1618–1624, 2008.

[13] E. Y. Lo, C.-S. Li, and J. M. Van den Bogaerde, "The effect of drill trajectory on proximity to the posterior interosseous nerve during cortical button distal biceps repair," *Arthroscopy*, vol. 27, no. 8, pp. 1048–1054, 2011.

[14] T. R. Duquin, P. R. Chavan, and L. J. Bisson, "Innervation of the supinator muscle and its relationship to two-incision distal biceps tendon repair: an anatomic study," *Clinical Anatomy*, vol. 23, no. 4, pp. 413–419, 2010.

[15] J. N. Lawton, M. Cameron-Donaldson, P. E. Blazar, and J. R. Moore, "Anatomic considerations regarding the posterior interosseous nerve at the elbow," *Journal of Shoulder and Elbow Surgery*, vol. 16, no. 4, pp. 502–507, 2007.

[16] K. S. Matullo, N. L. Strasser, A. T. Bishop, A. Y. Shin, and B. T. Elhassan, "Delayed onset of posterior interosseous nerve palsy after a nonanatomic routing of a distal biceps repair: a case report," *Journal of Shoulder and Elbow Surgery*, vol. 19, no. 6, pp. e1–e5, 2010.

15

Gliosarcoma with Primary Skull Base Invasion

Quoc-Bao D. Nguyen,[1] Avital Perry,[2] Christopher S. Graffeo,[2] Cody L. Nesvick,[2] Aditya Raghunathan,[3] Mark E. Jentoft,[3] Brian P. O'Neill,[4] Padraig P. Morris,[5] Jonathan M. Morris,[5] and Jamie J. Van Gompel[2,6]

[1]*Texas A&M Health Science Center College of Medicine, Temple, TX, USA*
[2]*Department of Neurological Surgery, Mayo Clinic, Rochester, MN, USA*
[3]*Department of Laboratory Medicine and Pathology, Mayo Clinic, Rochester, MN, USA*
[4]*Department of Neurology, Mayo Clinic, Rochester, MN, USA*
[5]*Department of Radiology, Mayo Clinic, Rochester, MN, USA*
[6]*Department of Otolaryngology-Head and Neck Surgery, Mayo Clinic, Rochester, MN, USA*

Correspondence should be addressed to Jamie J. Van Gompel; vangompel.jamie@mayo.edu

Academic Editor: Fumiyuki Yamasaki

Gliosarcoma is an uncommon variant of glioblastoma, which commonly demonstrates dural attachment. However, skull base invasion is rarely seen with this entity. Herein, we report a 44-year-old female patient diagnosed with primary intracranial gliosarcoma extensively invading the skull base and muscles of mastication. She presented to our institution with a three-month history of difficult right jaw opening and retro-orbital pressure and one week of severe right-sided postauricular headache. Head CT demonstrated a 6 cm mass with marked bony erosion. Brain MRI at a one-week interval more clearly characterized tumor extension through the right orbit and muscles of mastication, with overall growth to 7 cm and worsening midline shift. The patient underwent a right frontotemporal craniotomy for gross total resection. Pathology confirmed the diagnosis of gliosarcoma, IDH-wildtype (WHO grade IV). Her postoperative course was uneventful and she was discharged at preoperative neurologic baseline. To our knowledge, this is the third reported case of a primary intracranial gliosarcoma with direct invasion of skull base, brain parenchyma, and extracranial compartment. However, this is the first report case of primary GS invading the surrounding musculature and orbit. This case report highlights the rapid aggressiveness of gliosarcomas and further a prior undescribed radiographic and anatomic finding of skull base invasion with this entity.

1. Introduction

Gliosarcoma (GS) is a rare variant of glioblastoma (GB), characterized by a biphasic tissue pattern, with alternating areas of glial and mesenchymal differentiation [1]. GS comprise 2–8% of all GB, are known to have a worse prognosis than GB, and have high prevalence in the 5th and 6th decades of life with a 2 : 1 male predilection—although isolated cases of congenital GS have been reported [1–5]. GS typically appear as rapidly growing, heterogeneously enhancing intra-axial masses comparable to GB with a temporal predominance [4, 6]. At resection, GS are observed as a firm, often times well-circumscribed, superficial lesion, with meningeal adhesions. GS invading the skull base with accompanying extracranial extension has not been previously documented in primary GS. We report the first case of primary intracranial GS with diffuse, multicompartment invasion of the surrounding skull base, brain parenchyma, orbit, and muscles of mastication, alongside a review of the relevant literature. This presentation would expand the radiographic differential in patients with lesions such as this.

2. Case Presentation

A 44-year-old woman presented with difficulty opening her right jaw, swelling in the right cheek and temple region, and

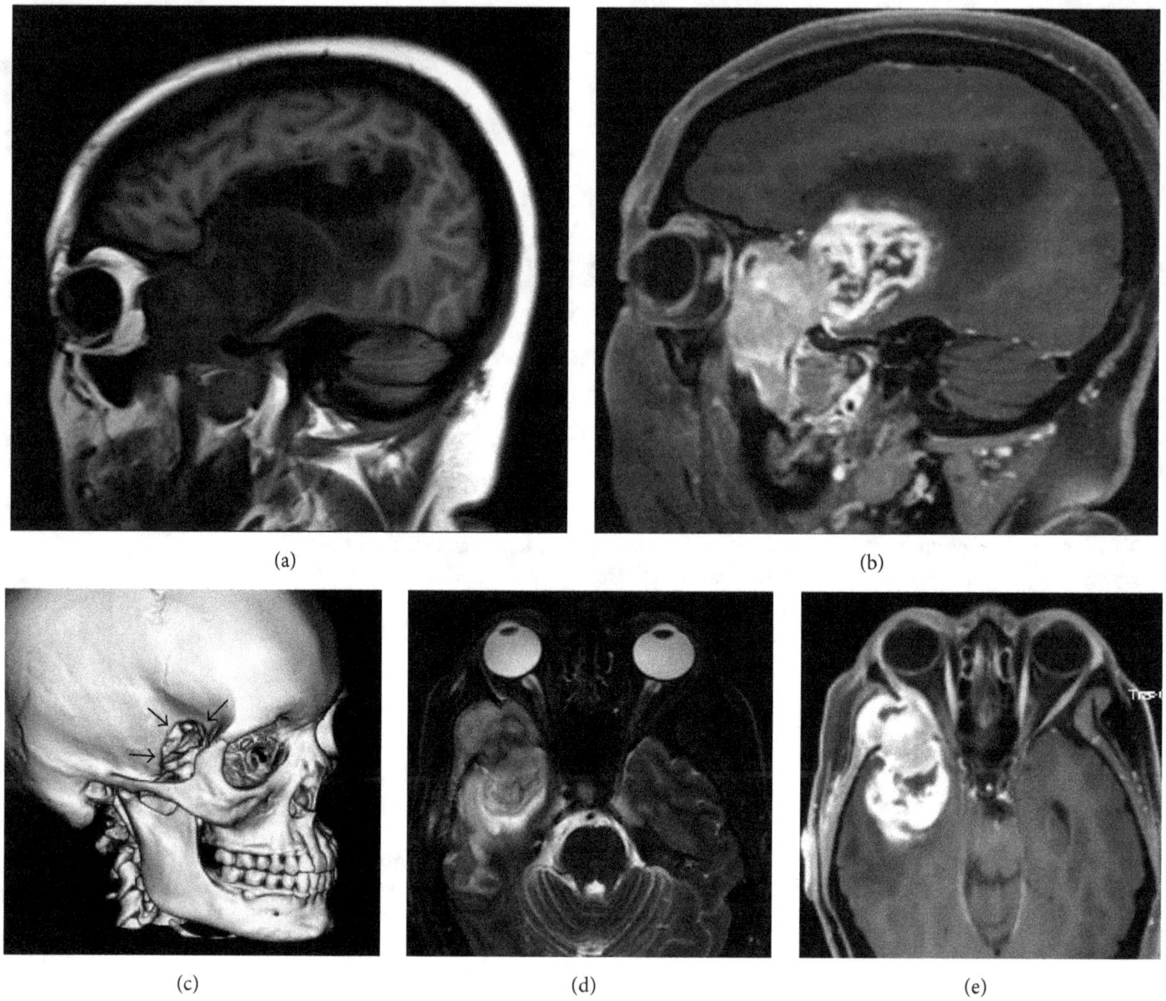

Figure 1: MRI and CT findings prior to surgery. (a) Sagittal T1-weighted imaging (T1WI) demonstrated a heterogeneous T1 hypointense mass involving a majority of the anterior temporal lobe with associated mass effect and surrounding vasogenic edema. Tumor extends through the greater wing of the sphenoid into the infratemporal fossa. (b) Sagittal postgadolinium T1WI demonstrates avid heterogeneous enhancement. The anterior portion in the soft tissues solidly enhances and intracranially has central necrosis. (c) 3D reconstruction from head CT demonstrates aggressive destruction of the greater wing of the sphenoid. (d) Axial FSE T2-weighted imaging demonstrates the mass to be heterogeneous iso/hypointense tumor with surrounding vasogenic edema suggesting increasing cellularity. (e) Axial postgadolinium T1WI demonstrates avid heterogeneous enhancement with central necrosis intracranially.

right retro-orbital pressure. She had no history of radiation therapy or tobacco use. Family history was significant for multiple malignancies, including second- and third-degree relations with leukemia, prostate cancer, breast cancer, and ovarian cancer. She denied any family history of neurologic disease—including central nervous system neoplasms.

A presumed diagnosis of sinusitis was made, and a short course of steroids and antibiotics was initiated. Three months later, the patient's symptoms had not improved but rather had expanded to include severe headache and retroauricular pain with cervical radiation, as well as V2 distribution paresthesia. She presented to an outside emergency department, where head CT identified a 6 cm right temporal lobe mass growing through and destroying the greater wing of the sphenoid bone and invading into the infratemporal fossa. She was subsequently referred to our institution for further work-up and treatment.

On examination, the patient was noted to have a firm right temporal mass, mild right proptosis, and right V2 paresthesias, but no other appreciable neurologic deficits. Brain MRI demonstrated marked growth, approximately 1 cm, over the one-week interval, with increased midline shift, mass effect, and vasogenic edema. The extracranial extension was better delineated with clear extension into the orbit, maxillary sinus, and invasion of the right pterygoid, masseter, and temporalis muscles (Figure 1). CT-guided biopsy of the temporal extracranial component was performed and histopathology revealed a tumor consistent with high-grade glioma versus GS, and an expedited operative resection was recommended.

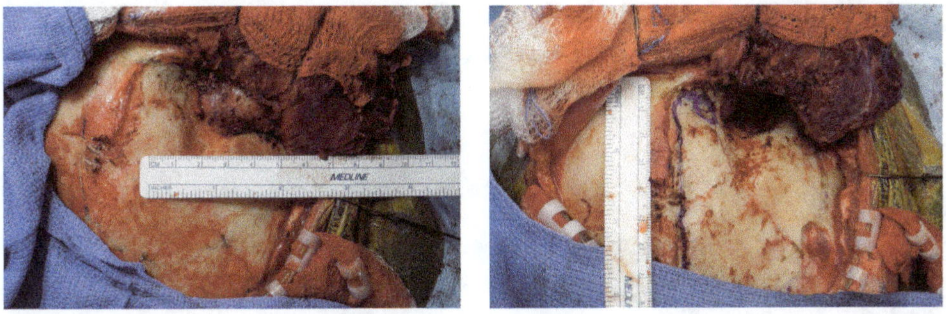

(a) (b)

FIGURE 2: Intraoperative photos of the firm, encapsulated tumor penetrating through the temporal bone and involving the temporalis muscle, (a) before and (b) after debulking the tumor extracranially.

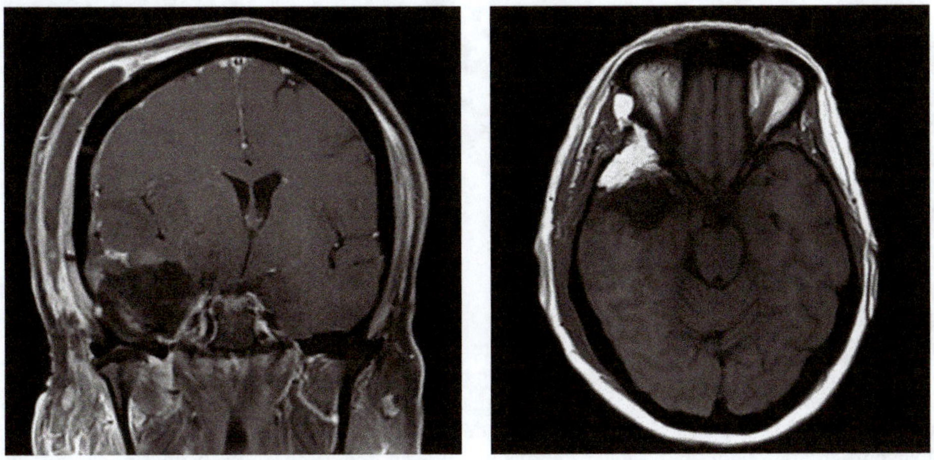

(a) (b)

FIGURE 3: Postoperative T1-weighted gadolinium-enhanced MRI of the brain. Both (a) coronal and (b) axial sequences confirm gross total resection of all enhancing tumor. New hyperintensity appreciated at the anterior right temporal pole identifies abdominal fat graft placed during reconstruction.

The patient was taken to the operating room for a right frontotemporal craniotomy, subtemporal exploration, tumor resection, and temporal lobectomy. During exposure, a firm and encapsulated tumor invasive through the temporal bone was encountered below the temporalis muscle (Figure 2(a)), which was debulked extracranially throughout infratemporal fossa and dissected off the periorbita, isolating the intracranial components (Figure 2(b)). After elevation of the frontotemporal bone flap and opening of the dura, the posterior tumor margin was identified and noted to be infiltrating adjacent cortex. An anterior temporal lobectomy with partial resection of the superior temporal gyrus and sparing of the mesial structures was completed to remove all intraparenchymal tumor and expose the portion invasive through the skull base at the inferomedial triangle between V1 and V2. The remaining bone was then drilled away and the lateral wall of the cavernous sinus was mobilized, exposing the lateral tumor margin and allowing for a gross total resection, including resection of all involved dura. The skull base was repaired in layers with pericranium, DuraGen, and abdominal fat graft.

The procedure was well tolerated and the patient recovered without complaints of jaw motion difficulties or new facial numbness. Routine MRI performed on postoperative day one revealed no evidence of residual enhancing tumor (Figure 3), and the patient was dismissed from the hospital on postoperative day three. Follow-up included close clinical and radiographic evaluations, as well as an adjuvant treatment plan of external beam radiation, 76 Gy in 30 fractions.

Pathology revealed a malignant neoplasm with variable morphology and extensive infiltration of adjacent fibroadipose and muscle tissue. Gliofibrillary cytoplasmic processes and cerebral parenchymal investment consistent with infiltrative glioma were widely observed, with foci of necrosis surrounded by vaguely pseudopalisading tumor cells (Figure 4(a)). The infiltrative glioma areas were also noted to alternate with mesenchymal-pattern areas of fibrotic stroma comprised of tumor cells with elongated, spindle-shaped nuclei (Figure 4(b)). Other characteristic GB features included positive immunohistochemical staining for glial fibrillary acid protein, which was notably absent from mesenchymal-predominant regions (GFAP, Figure 4(c)). In

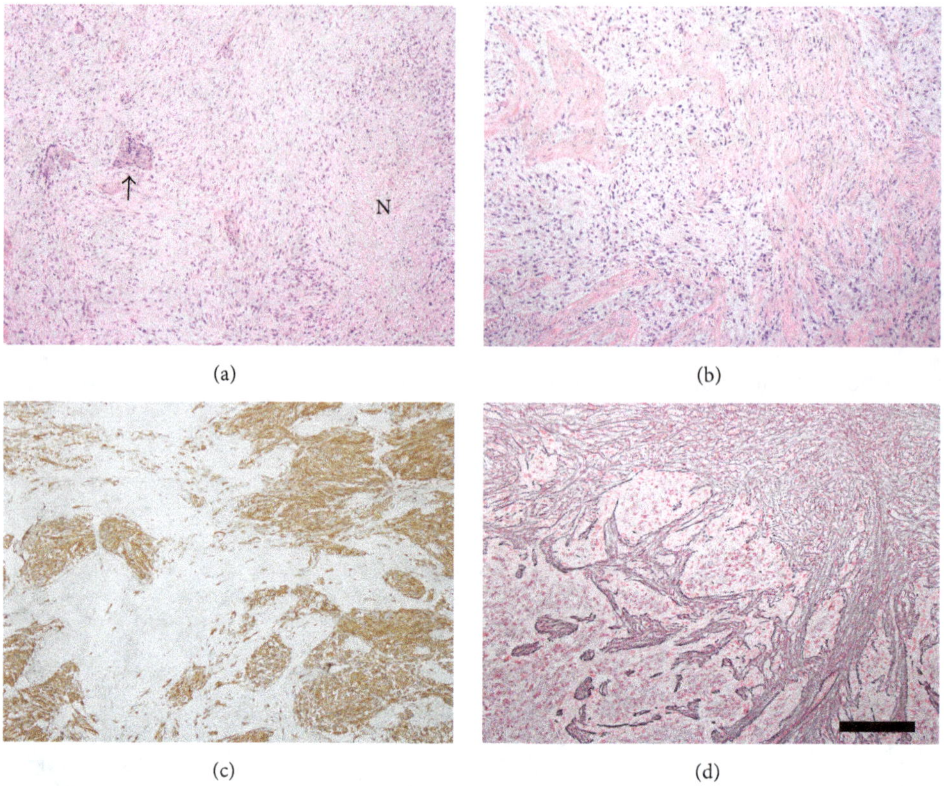

FIGURE 4: (a) The hematoxylin and eosin-stained histological sections showed an infiltrating glioma containing microvascular proliferation (arrow) and foci of necrosis surrounded by vaguely pseudopalisading tumor cells ("N"), diagnostic of glioblastoma. (b) Other areas showed a malignant mesenchymal component admixed with the glioblastoma. (c) The GFAP stain highlights the glial component and is negative in the mesenchymal component. (d) In contrast, the reticulin stain demonstrates extensive pericellular deposition of collagen fibers in the mesenchymal component only and is negative in the glial component. These findings support the diagnosis of gliosarcoma (all images at 100x magnification; scale bar = 300 μm).

parallel, reticulin staining showed a dense pericellular deposition pattern in mesenchymal regions and was negative in GFAP-positive areas (Figure 4(d)). Malignant cells were negative for mutant IDH1-R132H protein, with retained ATRX expression and no *IDH1* or *IDH2* mutation detectable by pyrosequencing. Methylguanine-DNA methyltransferase (*MGMT*) promoter methylation was not detected by a methylation-specific PCR-based assay.

3. Discussion

Primary GS is an uncommon tumor and in its prototypical form rarely extends beyond the dura in the absence of preceding radiation or craniotomy. Specific invasion of the skull base is exquisitely rare for primary GS, with three prior cases appearing in the literature [7–9], two of which involved both the skull base and either the surrounding parenchyma or extracranial soft tissue [8, 9]. We report the first case of primary intracranial GS with multicompartment invasion of the adjacent parenchyma, skull base, extracranial soft tissues, and orbit.

Literature review for case reports was completed by searching PubMed using keywords "gliosarcoma" together with "extracranial" or "skull base." Initial search, primary review, and secondary bibliographic review identified 29 publications from 1985 to 2013. Six of these were confirmed cases of GS with involvement of the skull base [7–12]. Four reported secondary invasive GS in the setting of previously resected and radiated primary GB (Schuss et al. 2011, Murphy et al. 1985, Maeda et al. 2010, and Oberndorfer et al. 2013); two cases of primary GS with involvement of multicompartment infiltration were identified (Borota et al. 2006 and Sade et al. 2006). Based on the six confirmed cases of GS involving the skull base and our case report, headache was the most common presenting symptoms ($n = 6$, 86%); proptosis was not previously observed, whereas cranial neuropathies, papilledema, and mass effect were inconsistently reported.

Although the number of studies available for comparison is small, MRI characteristics of GS invading skull base appear to be consistent. They typically demonstrate heterogeneous, peripheral enhancement attributable to frequent tumor hemorrhage and internal necrosis, with a corresponding predominance of peritumoral cytotoxic edema that may obscure clear radiographic differentiation at the tumor-parenchyma interface. Involvement of the infratemporal fossa or sphenoid sinus is common, with each occurring in roughly two-thirds of patients ($n = 5$, 71%). In the setting of primary GB, progression to GS after radiation occurred within 2–6 months. Mortality was high with only one patient surviving beyond 12 months; death is most frequently attributed to metastatic disease, including spread to the lungs and spine [9].

The mechanism of extradural and extracranial extension by GS remains unclear, although the most important barrier to tumor dissemination is thought to be the dura, which plays a role in the containment of glial and other related CNS malignancies [13]. Several candidate mechanisms for invasion of the skull and meninges by astrocytomas were proposed by Kawano et al. [14], who listed three key possibilities: via perivascular or dural slits, along the cranial or spinal nerves, or through direct destruction of the cranial architecture. Still other plausible mechanisms were advanced by Shenoy and Raja, who theorized dural necrosis resulting from a combination of disrupted blood supply and bone invasion [15].

Although GS treatment falls within the broader paradigm of GB management, several studies have reported that temozolomide does not significantly impact overall survival [16, 17]. One recent retrospective study of 75 patients with GS has reported that neither temozolomide-based chemoradiation nor adjuvant chemotherapy was superior to radiotherapy alone [18]. Correspondingly, they recommended surgery with adjuvant radiation at a minimum dose of 54 Gy as standard-of-care therapy for GS. In our presented case, 76 Gy of adjuvant radiation was administered.

Sequencing and comparative genomic hybridization studies have helped elucidate differences between GB and GS, although their results are limited by the lack of randomized studies or molecular data, both of which are attributable to the rarity of GS [4]. Notwithstanding, limited but stepwise discoveries are optimizing treatment protocols, as in the specific example of GS frequently lacking the overexpression of epidermal growth factor receptor (EGFR) seen in IDH-wildtype GB, which challenges the utility of anti-EGFR modalities in GS treatment [19]. Still other studies of the molecular alterations in GS have found a high incidence of TP53 mutations, as well as rare EGFR and IDH mutations [20, 21]. Further study of the molecular mechanisms underlying GS development and spread is required to better understand the natural history and optimal treatment of these lethal tumors.

4. Conclusion

To our knowledge, this is the first reported case of a primary intracranial GS with direct invasion of the skull base, brain parenchyma, extracranial compartment, and orbit. This case report illustrates how rapid and aggressive the natural history of GS can be. Further this case report adds to the radiographic differential of a mass involving the soft tissues, bone, and intra-axial compartments beyond aggressive meningioma, metastasis, primary bone neoplasm, or sarcoma. Although GS is rare and similar to GB, the higher mortality of GS and notable molecular differences between GS and GB urge the need for specialized treatment modalities beyond mild alterations of standard GB treatment.

Abbreviations

GB: Glioblastoma
GS: Gliosarcoma.

References

[1] D. N. Louis, A. Perry, G. Reifenberger et al., "The 2016 World Health Organization Classification of Tumors of the Central Nervous System: a summary," *Acta Neuropathologica*, vol. 131, no. 6, pp. 803–820, 2016.

[2] E. Galanis, J. C. Buckner, R. P. Dinapoli et al., "Clinical outcome of gliosarcoma compared with glioblastoma multiforme: North Central Cancer Treatment Group results," *Journal of Neurosurgery*, vol. 89, no. 3, pp. 425–430, 1998.

[3] O. R. I. Hocwald, D. McFadden, H. Osiovich, and C. Dunham, "Congenital gliosarcoma: detailed clinicopathologic documentation of a rare neoplasm," *Pediatric and Developmental Pathology*, vol. 12, no. 5, pp. 398–403, 2009.

[4] K. R. Kozak, A. Mahadevan, and J. S. Moody, "Adult gliosarcoma: epidemiology, natural history, and factors associated with outcome," *Neuro-Oncology*, vol. 11, no. 2, pp. 183–191, 2009.

[5] N. Ono, M. Nakamura, H. K. Inoue, M. Tamura, and M. Murata, "Congenital gliosarcoma; so-called sarcoglioma," *Child's Nervous System*, vol. 6, no. 7, pp. 416–420, 1990.

[6] A. E. Romero-Rojas, J. A. Diaz-Perez, L. M. Ariza-Serrano, D. Amaro, and A. Lozano-Castillo, "Primary gliosarcoma of the brain: radiologic and histopathologic features," *The Neuroradiology Journal*, vol. 26, no. 6, pp. 639–648, 2013.

[7] P. Schuss, C. T. Ulrich, P. N. Harter, D. S. Tews, V. Seifert, and K. Franz, "Gliosarcoma with bone infiltration and extracranial growth: case report and review of literature," *Journal of Neuro-Oncology*, vol. 103, no. 3, pp. 765–770, 2011.

[8] O. C. Borota, D. Scheie, B. Bjerkhagen, E. A. Jacobsen, and K. Skullerud, "Gliosarcoma with liposarcomatous component, bone infiltration and extracranial growth," *Clinical Neuropathology*, vol. 25, no. 4, pp. 200–203, 2006.

[9] B. Sade, R. A. Prayson, and J. H. Lee, "Gliosarcoma with infratemporal fossa extension. Case report," *Journal of Neurosurgery*, vol. 105, no. 6, pp. 904–907, 2006.

[10] D. Maeda, T. Miyazawa, T. Toyooka, and K. Shima, "Temporal gliosarcoma with extraneural metastasis: case report," *Neurologia Medico-Chirurgica*, vol. 50, no. 4, pp. 343–345, 2010.

[11] M. N. Murphy, J. A. Korkis, F. C. Robson, and A. A. Sima, "Gliosarcoma with cranial penetration and extension to the maxillary sinus," *Journal of Otolaryngology*, vol. 14, no. 5, pp. 313–316, 1985.

[12] S. Oberndorfer, A. Wöhrer, J. A. Hainfellner et al., "Secondary gliosarcoma with massive invasion of meninges, skull base, and soft tissue, and systemic metastasis," *Clinical Neuropathology*' vol. 32, no. 6, pp. 522–524, 2013.

[13] P.-H. Pedersen, G. J. Rucklidge, S. J. Mørk et al., "Leptomeningeal tissue: a barrier against brain tumor cell invasion," *Journal of the National Cancer Institute*, vol. 86, no. 21, pp. 1593–1599, 1994.

[14] N. Kawano, K. Yada, Y. Ogawa, and K. Sasaki, "Spontaneous transdural extension of malignant astrocytoma. Case report," *Journal of Neurosurgery*, vol. 47, no. 5, pp. 766–770, 1977.

[15] S. N. Shenoy and A. Raja, "Spontaneous transdural spread of glioblastoma with atypical presentation," *British Journal of Neurosurgery*, vol. 19, no. 1, pp. 61–65, 2005.

[16] O. Damodaran, J. Van Heerden, A. K. Nowak et al., "Clinical management and survival outcomes of gliosarcomas in the era of multimodality therapy," *Journal of Clinical Neuroscience*, vol. 21, no. 3, pp. 478–481, 2014.

[17] G. V. Walker, M. R. Gilbert, S. S. Prabhu, P. D. Brown, and M. F. McAleer, "Temozolomide use in adult patients with gliosarcoma: an evolving clinical practice," *Journal of Neuro-Oncology*, vol. 112, no. 1, pp. 83–89, 2013.

[18] J. Castelli, L. Feuvret, Q. C. Haoming et al., "Prognostic and therapeutic factors of gliosarcoma from a multi-institutional series," *Journal of Neuro-Oncology*, vol. 129, no. 1, pp. 85–92, 2016.

[19] R. M. Reis, D. Konu-Lebleblicioglu, J. M. Lopes, P. Kleihues, and H. Ohgaki, "Genetic profile of gliosarcomas," *The American Journal of Pathology*, vol. 156, no. 2, pp. 425–432, 2000.

[20] D. Cachia, C. Kamiya-Matsuoka, J. J. Mandel et al., "Primary and secondary gliosarcomas: clinical, molecular and survival characteristics," *Journal of Neuro-Oncology*, vol. 125, no. 2, pp. 401–410, 2015.

[21] J. E. Oh, T. Ohta, N. Nonoguchi et al., "Genetic alterations in gliosarcoma and giant cell glioblastoma," *Brain Pathology*, vol. 26, no. 4, pp. 517–522, 2016.

16

Cholangiocarcinoma Arising from a Type VI Biliary Cyst: A Case Report

İlkay Çamlıdağ,[1] Mehmet Selim Nural,[1] Murat Danacı,[1] İlhan Karabıçak,[2] and Kağan Karabulut[2]

[1]*Department of Radiology, Ondokuz Mayıs University, Kurupelit, 55139 Samsun, Turkey*
[2]*Department of General Surgery, Ondokuz Mayıs University, Kurupelit, 55139 Samsun, Turkey*

Correspondence should be addressed to İlkay Çamlıdağ; ilkayozaydin@hotmail.com

Academic Editor: Vincent Low

Cystic dilatations of the cystic duct which are suggested as type VI biliary cysts are very rare and many of them go unrecognized or are confused with other cysts until the operation although they are obvious on imaging studies. They can present with fusiform or saccular dilatations and can be accompanied by common bile duct dilatations. It is important to identify these cysts as they share the same characteristics as the other biliary cyst types and can be complicated with malignancy. We herein present a very unusual case of a cholangiocarcinoma arising from a type VI biliary cyst in a 58-year-old female patient and review the literature. The patient presented with jaundice, weight loss, and abdominal pain. On imaging, the cystic duct and common bile duct were fusiformly dilated and had a wide communication. There was a mass filling the distal parts of both ducts. The patient was urgently operated on after perforation following ERCP. Histopathology was compatible with a type VI biliary cyst and an associated cholangiocarcinoma.

1. Introduction

Choledochal cysts are congenital cystic dilatations of any portion of the bile ducts which are not associated with a tumor, stone, or inflammation as the cause of the dilatation [1]. Traditionally, biliary cysts have been classified into five main types by Todani et al. [2]. However, cystic dilatation of the cystic duct is not included in this classification. Congenital cystic duct cysts are extremely rare with a very limited number of cases in the literature. They are regarded as "type VI biliary cysts" and the term was first proposed by Serradel et al. [3]. It is well known that there is an association of bile duct adenocarcinoma and biliary cysts [4]. Adenocarcinoma arising from a type VI biliary cyst is extremely rare with only one reported case in the literature [5]. Herein, we aimed to present the imaging findings of an adenocarcinoma arising from a type VI biliary cyst which is the second case in the literature to our knowledge and review the literature.

2. Case Report

A 58-year-old female was referred to our hospital from a local hospital. She had complaints of abdominal pain, jaundice for the last two months, and weight loss. On clinical examination, she had slight icteric sclera and tenderness in the right upper quadrant on palpation. Laboratory studies showed markedly elevated hepatic enzymes. Aspartate transaminase, alanine transaminase, and gamma-glutamyl transferase levels were 259, 412, and 1289 IU/L, respectively. Bilirubin levels were slightly elevated with a direct bilirubin level of 1.2 mg/dL and total bilirubin level of 2.61 mg/dL. Other blood tests were unremarkable. On subsequent ultrasound examination, cystic and choledochal ducts were dilated. There was a polypoid mass at the junction of cystic and choledochal duct. The patient underwent magnetic resonance cholangiopancreatography (MRCP) for better delineation of the ultrasonography findings. On MRCP, cystic duct was fusiformly dilated having a wide opening to the common bile duct which was

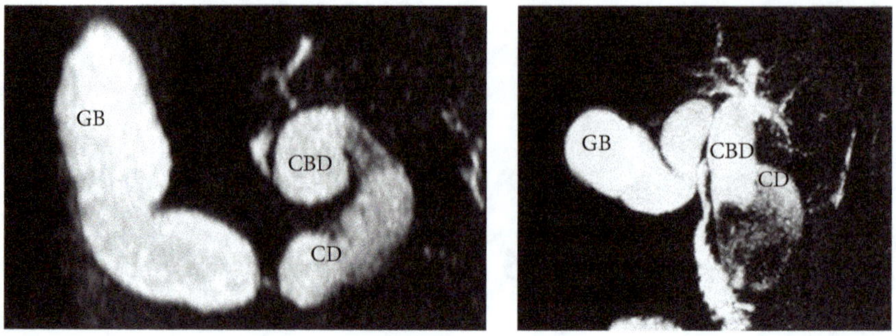

(a) (b)

Figure 1: A 58-year-old female with type VI biliary cyst and associated cholangiocarcinoma. (a, b) Axial and coronal MRCP images show fusiformly dilated cystic duct (CD) with a wide opening to the common bile duct (CBD) which is also fusiformly dilated. Intrahepatic bile ducts are slightly dilated in the centre. There is a hypointense, heterogeneous mass filling distal parts of both the cystic and choledochal ducts (GB: gallbladder).

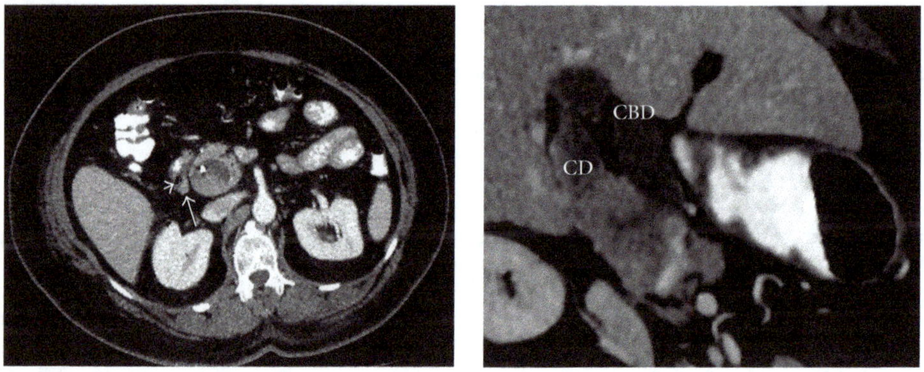

(a) (b)

Figure 2: CT examination performed with the suspicion of perforation following ERCP. (a) Axial contrast enhanced CT image shows intraperitoneal free air (short arrow) and periduodenal contrast extravasation (long arrow) suggesting perforation. (b) Multiplanar reconstructed CT image shows fusiform cystic dilatation of the cystic duct having a wide opening to the extrahepatic bile duct which is also fusiformly dilated and the enhancing mass.

also fusiformly dilated. There was a hypointense, heterogeneous mass filling the distal parts of both ducts. Intrahepatic bile ducts were minimally dilated in the central part but were in normal caliber in the remainder (Figure 1). An endoscopic retrograde cholangiopancreatography (ERCP) procedure was performed for mass sampling. ERCP confirmed the findings of MRCP. After the procedure, the patient complained of severe abdominal pain and underwent computed tomography (CT) which showed free intra-abdominal air and periduodenal contrast leakage (Figure 2(a)) consistent with perforation along with the other findings (Figure 2(b)). There was no sign of lymphadenopathy or distant metastasis on CT. The patient urgently underwent Whipple procedure. It was not until then that all the findings of fusiform dilatation of the cystic and choledochal ducts were interpreted as a cystic duct cyst which was proposed as a type VI biliary cyst. On histopathological examination, there was a polypoid mass which was characterized by atypical epithelial cells lining a fibrovascular core extending from the cyst wall that was lined by columnar epithelium (Figure 3). The histopathological diagnosis of the polypoid mass was consistent with cholangiocarcinoma. To our knowledge, this is the second case of cholangiocarcinoma arising from a type VI biliary cyst.

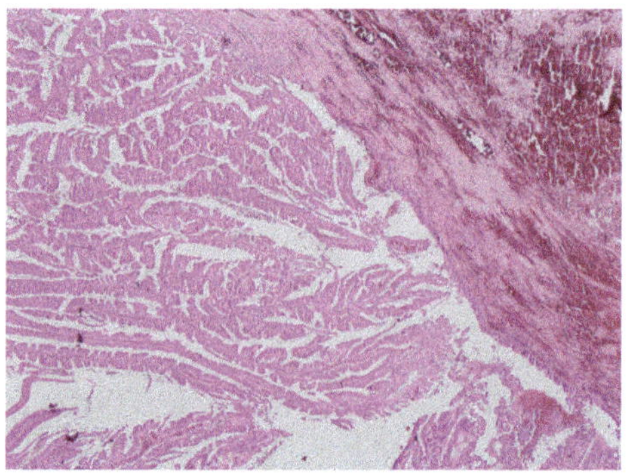

Figure 3: Atypical epithelial cells lining a fibrovascular core extending from the cyst wall that is lined by columnar epithelium are seen on the histopathological specimen.

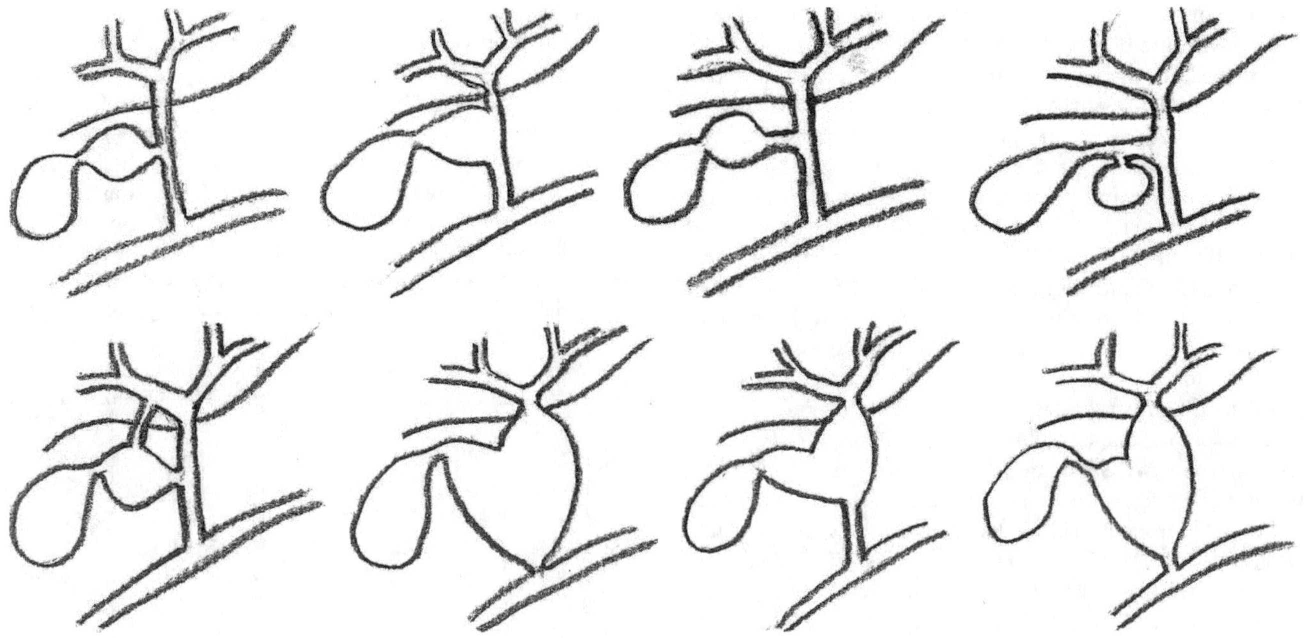

FIGURE 4: Schematic illustration of the type VI biliary cysts reported in the literature to date.

3. Discussion

Biliary cysts are cystic dilatations of the bile ducts and are rarely seen with an incidence of 1 : 100000 to 150000 in western countries and an increased incidence of 1 : 1000 in Asian population. It comprises 1% of all benign biliary diseases [4]. Traditionally, biliary cysts are classified into five categories as described by Todani et al. Type I is cyst of the CBD; type II is a cystic diverticulum of the extrahepatic bile duct; type III is a cyst in the intraduodenal portion of the common bile duct; type IV refers to multiple cysts in the intra- and extrahepatic biliary tract; and type V is single or multiple cysts in the intrahepatic ducts alone which is known as Caroli disease [2]. Although not included in this classification of biliary cysts, cystic dilatation of the cystic duct can also be encountered; however, it is extremely rare with very limited number of reports in the literature mainly consisting of single case reports and only one review to our knowledge [5]. Serradel et al. were the first to propose calling these cysts as type VI biliary cysts [3]. Due to very little acquaintance with the condition, diagnosis is challenging with most of the cases being undiagnosed as our case or misdiagnosed as other types [3, 6, 7]. The correct diagnosis was made intraoperatively in most of the cases in the literature [8].

Type VI biliary cyst can be encountered in different forms. The cystic dilatation can be limited to the cystic duct either fusiform or saccular without any associated findings in the other bile ducts [3, 5, 6, 9, 10] or can be accompanied by fusiform common bile duct dilatation with varying size of communication between the cyst and dilated CBD (see [5, 10, 11], Figure 4).

The most common theory for the development of biliary cysts is the anomalous pancreaticobiliary junction (APBJ). In the APBJ the biliary and pancreatic duct join proximal to the sphincter of Oddi forming a long common channel that causes the pancreatic enzymes to flow upstream into the bile duct resulting in the weakening of the CBD wall and leads to the formation of a cyst. However, not all biliary cysts are accompanied by APBJ and APBJ is also encountered in the absence of biliary cysts. So, more than one mechanism must be responsible for the occurrence of biliary cysts [1].

Presenting features and complications of cysts of the cystic duct are similar to other types of biliary cysts. They might be asymptomatic and incidentally detected or present with varying degrees of abdominal pain, jaundice, and complications such as cholangitis, calculus disease, and malignancy with the last one being the most serious and feared one [1, 4]. Most of the reported cases of biliary cyst associated cancers are cholangiocarcinomas arising from the cyst itself. However, they also can arise from the gallbladder or anywhere else in the biliary ducts especially in the presence of APBJ [1, 12, 13]. To our knowledge, there is only one reported case of cholangiocarcinoma in the literature arising from a type VI biliary cyst reported by Maheshwari et al. [5]. In their case, cholangiocarcinoma arose from a saccular type cystic duct cyst. The information of the presence of APBJ was not given. In our case, the mass originated from the fusiformly dilated cystic and common bile ducts and there was no evidence of APBJ. Two more cases of type VI biliary cyst related cholangiocarcinoma arising from the gallbladder without any APBJ [10] and left hepatic bile duct in the presence of APBJ have also been reported [12].

Radiological imaging is very useful in the diagnosis of biliary cysts. Ultrasonography (USG) is the modality of choice for initial evaluation and frequently provides enough information to make the diagnosis of a biliary cyst. In case of a dilated nonvascular cystic structure near the porta hepatis, attempt should be made to delineate its connection and relationship with the biliary tract and the gallbladder. However, USG may fail to depict these relationships as it is operator-dependent and sensitivity is decreased in the presence of overlying bowel gas and inflammatory conditions. ERCP is the gold standard in the diagnosis of biliary cysts but it is invasive, always requires sedation, and comes with inherent risks such as pancreatitis, perforation, hemorrhage, contrast allergy, cholangitis, and biliary sepsis. Given its relatively moderate risk profile and lower cost, MRCP should be the diagnostic test of choice when preoperatively evaluating biliary cysts and their associated anomalies. MRCP is equivalent to ERCP in determining biliary cyst type and is helpful in diagnosing related pancreaticobiliary anomalies, cholangiocarcinoma, and choledocholithiasis. ERCP should be used when MRCP inadequately visualizes the terminal common bile duct or the pancreaticobiliary junction or when a therapeutic procedure is needed. A multidetector computed tomography (MDCT) with reformatted imaging is another important technique which has the ability to demonstrate the anatomic details of the biliary tree and the ABPJ. It can show the presence of an associated cancer and is useful for staging. The disadvantages are high-dose radiation exposure and contrast agent administration especially in children [1, 4, 5, 9, 13].

Preferred treatment for type VI biliary cysts is the surgical excision as for the other types. Early and proper diagnosis is important to avoid complications and choose the appropriate surgical method. Cholecystectomy and transection of the cystic duct are sufficient in the presence of a narrow common duct junction. However, in the presence of a wide opening to the common bile duct, hepaticoduodenostomy or hepaticojejunostomy should be performed [7, 11].

In conclusion, we had a very typical but unrecognized case of type VI biliary cyst with obvious findings on all imaging modalities. Because of the unfamiliarity with the condition, the cysts were interpreted as dilatations secondary to mass obstruction. However, disproportionate and only mild dilatation of the central intrahepatic bile ducts should have warned us that it was not result of obstruction as they would be much more dilated given the degree of the extrahepatic bile duct dilatation. We think that increased familiarity with cystic duct cysts is crucial as early treatment can prevent complications like inflammation and more importantly malignancy. We think that cystic duct cysts should officially be included in the Todani et al. classification as type VI biliary cyst with all its subtypes because it has all the characteristics of the other biliary cysts in terms of clinical findings and complications.

References

[1] K. L. Hae, J. P. Seong, H. Y. Bum, A. L. Lee, H. M. Jong, and W. C. Yun, "Imaging features of adult choledochal cysts: a pictorial review," *Korean Journal of Radiology*, vol. 10, no. 1, pp. 71–80, 2009.

[2] T. Todani, Y. Watanabe, M. Narusue, K. Tabuchi, and K. Okajima, "Congenital bile duct cysts. Classification, operative procedures, and review of thirty-seven cases including cancer arising from choledochal cyst," *The American Journal of Surgery*, vol. 134, no. 2, pp. 263–269, 1977.

[3] A. F. S. Serradel, E. S. Linares, and R. H. Goepfert, "Cystic dilatation of the cystic duct: a new type of biliary cyst," *Surgery*, vol. 109, no. 3, pp. 320–322, 1991.

[4] B. Jabłońska, "Biliary cysts: etiology, diagnosis and management," *World Journal of Gastroenterology*, vol. 18, no. 35, pp. 4801–4810, 2012.

[5] P. Maheshwari, "Cystic malformation of cystic duct: 10 cases and review of literature," *World Journal of Radiology*, vol. 4, no. 9, pp. 413–417, 2012.

[6] W. E. Bode and J. B. Aust, "Isolated cystic dilatation of the cystic duct," *The American Journal of Surgery*, vol. 145, no. 6, pp. 828–829, 1983.

[7] E. S. Chan, E. D. Auyang, and E. S. Hungness, "Laparoscopic management of a cystic duct cyst," *Journal of the Society of Laparoendoscopic Surgeons*, vol. 13, no. 3, pp. 436–440, 2009.

[8] U. De, S. Das, and S. Sarkar, "Type VI choledochal cyst revisited," *Singapore Medical Journal*, vol. 52, no. 5, pp. e91–e93, 2011.

[9] C. Goya, M. S. Arslan, A. Yavuz et al., "A rare anomaly of biliary system: MRCP evidence of a cystic duct cyst," *Case Reports in Radiology*, vol. 2014, Article ID 291071, 4 pages, 2014.

[10] J.-H. Yoon, "Magnetic resonance cholangiopancreatography diagnosis of choledochal cyst involving the cystic duct: report of three cases," *British Journal of Radiology*, vol. 84, no. 997, pp. e18–e22, 2011.

[11] T. K. Loke, S. H. Lam, and C. S. Chan, "Choledochal cyst: an unusual type of cystic dilatation of the cystic duct," *American Journal of Roentgenology*, vol. 173, pp. 619–620, 1999.

[12] R. Noun, R. Sayegh, C. Tohme-Noun, K. Honein, T. Smayra, and N. Aoun, "Extracystic biliary carcinoma associated with anomalous pancreaticobiliary junction and cysts," *Journal of Hepato-Biliary-Pancreatic Surgery*, vol. 13, no. 6, pp. 577–579, 2006.

[13] R. Sugita, "Magnetic resonance evaluations of biliary malignancy and condition at high-risk for biliary malignancy: current status," *World Journal of Hepatology*, vol. 5, no. 12, pp. 654–665, 2013.

17

Recurrent Enlarging Mesenteric Desmoid Tumor following Remote Surgical Resection

Connie Hapgood[1] and Allison DeLong[2]

[1]*Department of Radiology, Memorial University, St. John's, NL, Canada*
[2]*Faculty of Medicine, Memorial University, St. John's, NL, Canada*

Correspondence should be addressed to Connie Hapgood; chapgood@hotmail.com

Academic Editor: Atsushi Komemushi

Intra-abdominal desmoid tumors are commonly associated with genetic syndromes such as familial polyposis coli. Radiological cross imaging studies such as CT and MRI are used in the preoperative work-up of such tumors. Postoperatively, CT and MRI are useful in the assessment of recurrent desmoid tumors. MRI is more accurate in tissue characterization. Where possible, surgical resection remains the standard first-line treatment. For patients where surgery is not possible, or the resection margins are not clear, other forms of treatment are possible. These include hormonal and nonhormonal options. We present a case of a recurrent sporadic intra-abdominal (mesenteric) desmoid tumor. Such an entity is rare with few cases reported in the literature. Treatment options regarding intra-abdominal desmoid tumors will be discussed.

1. Introduction

Desmoid tumors are deep-seated monoclonal myofibroblastic tumors that account for approximately 0.03% of all neoplasms [1–3]. Desmoid tumors are histologically benign and will not metastasize; however they can display an aggressive growth pattern. Desmoid tumors can be grouped as extra-abdominal, within the abdominal wall, or intra-abdominal, extra-abdominal being the most common [4]. Desmoid tumors can occur sporadically; however they are most commonly associated with familial adenomatous polyposis (FAP) syndrome [4]. Such predisposing factors as prior surgery or trauma and high estrogen states have also been associated with the development of desmoid tumors. Abdominal wall desmoids are often associated with scar tissue. Intra-abdominal desmoid tumors tend to be associated with a diagnosis of FAP. Sporadic desmoid tumors are rarely intra-abdominal, most commonly occurring in the extremities. Desmoid tumors tend to have a high rate of recurrence even with total local resection. Sporadic desmoid tumors tend to reoccur less frequently in comparison to desmoid tumors associated with FAP [5]. Clinical presentation varies depending on the size and location of the tumor. Most patients are asymptomatic. Intra-abdominal desmoid tumors can be associated with abdominal pain and bowel obstruction.

2. Case Report

47-year-old female presented to our Emergency department in 2012. She complained of progressive intermittent abdominal pain. Clinical exam revealed bilateral pitting edema and an elevated jugular venous pressure, with no history of familial polyposis or colorectal cancer. Laboratory work-up was noncontributory. CT revealed an ill-defined hypoattenuating solid mass in the small bowel mesentery (Figure 1), with slight displacement of adjacent small bowel loops and mild enhancement.

The mass was resected surgically along with a right hemicolectomy and pathology reported it as a desmoid tumor. Mass was noted to have clear margins on pathology. No additional treatment was given. The patients immediate postoperative course was uneventful.

Four years later, the patient returned to the Emergency department with a small bowel obstruction. There was no additional change in medical history. CT was repeated

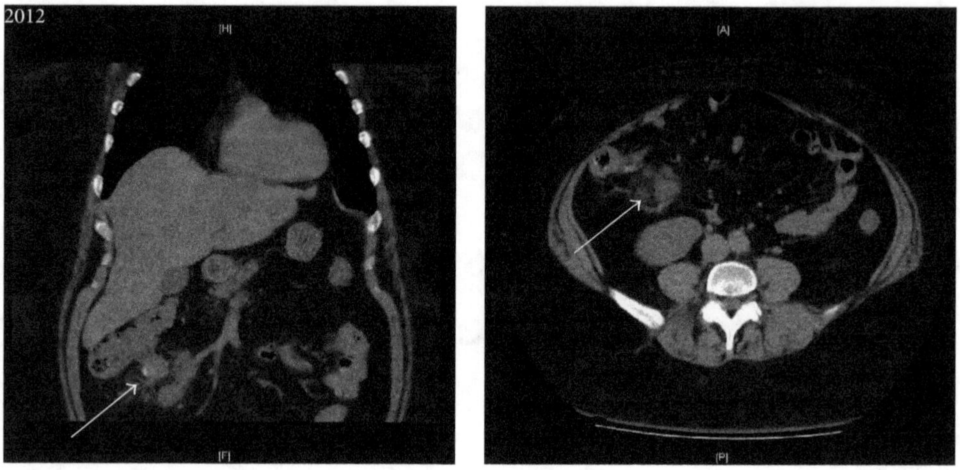

(a) (b)

FIGURE 1: 2012 Coronal enhanced (a) and axial enhanced (b) CT showing hypovascular solid mass (white arrow) in the mesentery of the right lower quadrant.

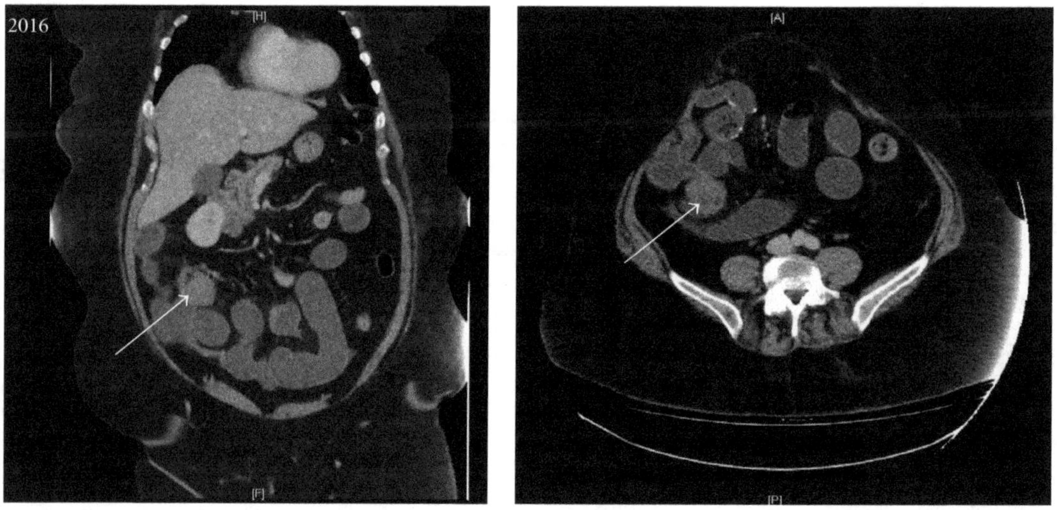

(a) (b)

FIGURE 2: Coronal enhanced (a) and axial enhanced (b) CT performed 4 years later, showing recurrent hypovascular solid mass (white arrow) in the mesentery of the right lower quadrant.

showing a recurrent irregular solid hypoattenuating mass in the mesentery of the right lower quadrant (Figure 2). The mass was located in close proximity to adjacent loops of ileum. The small bowel was distended with little gas in the colon consistent with a small bowel obstruction.

MRI advised for further characterization of the right lower mesenteric mass. MRI (Figure 3) shows the mesenteric mass to be of heterogenous signal intensity on T2 weighted imaging, low in signal of T1 before contrast and slight enhancement after contrast. The findings suggest desmoid recurrence in the right lower quadrant.

In the four-month interval between most recent scans the mass had grown significantly from 5 × 4 cm on CT to 8 × 7 cm on MR (Figures 2 and 3, resp.). The patient underwent another laparotomy for definitive diagnosis. On surgical resection, the margins of the mass were noted to push against the edge of the serosal peritoneum. The mass was adherent to small bowel and involved 25–30 cm of the small bowel mesentery but was mobile.

On gross pathology, the mass was noted to be adherent to small bowel and firm. The mass was circumscribed and measured 9.2 × 7.3 × 7.2 cm. Focal areas of hemorrhage were noted near the periphery. The tumor did not invade surrounding fat or bowel (Figure 4). Microscopically the lesion was composed of fibroblasts arranged in sweeping fascicles (Figure 5). No atypia or pleomorphism was identified. Beta-catenin was diffusely positive (Figure 6).

Following surgical resection, no adjuvant therapy was administered. Follow-up with radiological imaging was planned.

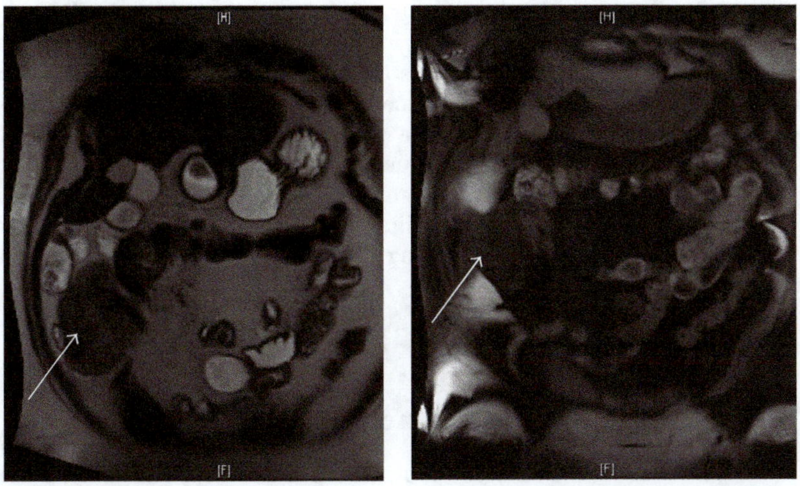

(a) T2 weighted (b) T1 weighted, fat sat before contrast (c) T1 weighted, fat sat after contrast

FIGURE 3: MRI T2 sequence (a), T1 unenhanced sequence (b), and T1 enhanced sequence (c), performed four months following most recent CT. This shows a solid mass (white arrow) of mixed signal intensity on T2, with mild enhancement, in the mesentery of the right lower quadrant that has increased in size from most recent CT.

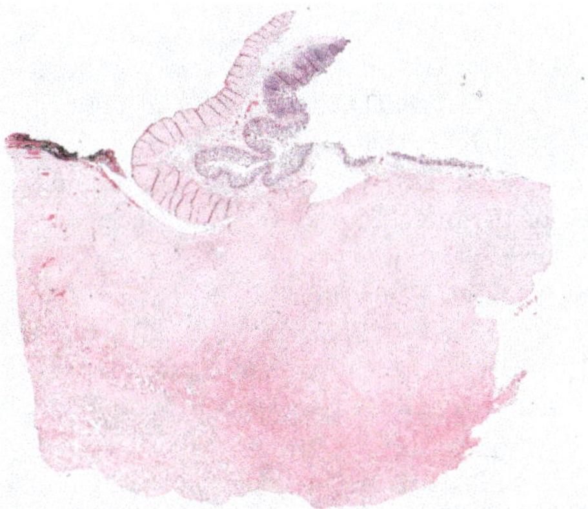

FIGURE 4: Low power view of the lesion in relation to the mucosa and muscular layer of the small bowel. The pink area at the bottom half of the image is all tumor.

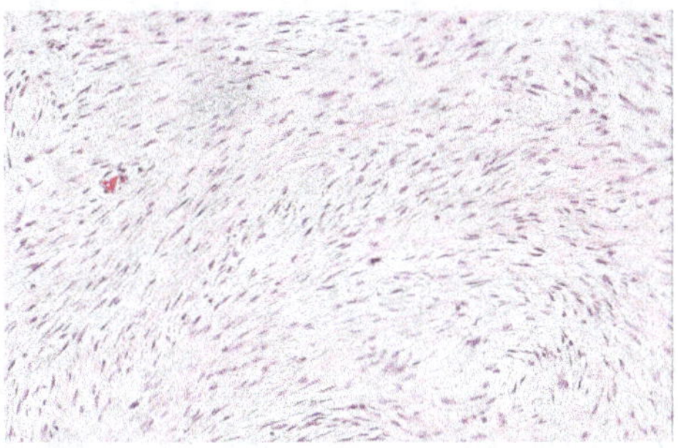

FIGURE 5: Medium power view (×20) is H&E stain of the tumor showing spindle cells (fibroblasts in sweeping fascicles).

3. Discussion

Desmoid tumors are exceedingly rare. Some identified risk factors include abdominal surgery/trauma, women of childbearing age (desmoid tumor growth is thought to be influenced by estrogen), and familial adenomatous polyposis/Gardner's Syndrome. Common presenting complaints are abdominal distention, pain, vomiting, and intestinal obstruction. However, most patients will present with a painless enlarging mass [3]. Intra-abdominal desmoid tumors are more commonly seen in patients with familial adenomatous polyposis. While sporadic desmoids more commonly present as an extra-abdominal mass [6, 7].

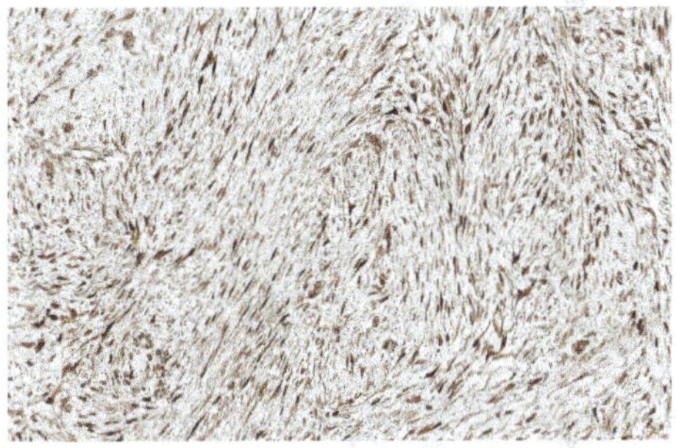

FIGURE 6: IHC stain for beta-catenin (×20) showing characteristic nuclear staining, confirming the diagnosis of fibromatosis.

On CT, desmoid tumors commonly appear as a well-circumscribed homogenous lesion isodense or hyperdense relative to muscle [8]. The CT characteristics are not pathognomonic of desmoid tumors. Other mesenteric masses such as gastrointestinal stromal tumors (GIST) can have a similar appearance. The differential for such a mesenteric mass on CT would also include carcinoid, leiomyoma, leiomyosarcoma, and lymphoma. CT is useful preoperatively to assess involvement of adjacent organs and vasculature. Desmoids on MRI are of low signal intensity of T1 images and will often demonstrate heterogeneity on T2 images [9]. MRI is a useful tool in tissue characterization, commonly used in the cases of desmoid tumor recurrence. Histologically the tissue obtained from a desmoid biopsy would appear as intertwining bundles of spindle cells within a collagen matrix [10]. Sporadic desmoid tumors are commonly associated with somatic mutations of the beta-catenin gene while desmoids associated with familial adenomatous polyposis coli often contain mutations in the APC gene [11].

The course of mesenteric fibroblastic tumors/desmoid tumors is often unpredictable. They can be indolent and spontaneously regress while others can be very aggressive with rapid growth and mass effect [12]. They do not metastasize but may recur. Some studies quote recurrence rates as high as 40% [2]. Close observation is an acceptable strategy for stable asymptomatic patients. Complete surgical resection with wide surgical margins (at least 1 cm) is often the first line therapy for resectable tumors [7]. However even with complete surgical resection margins, desmoid tumors may recur. Furthermore, surgery may be difficult depending on the patient's comorbidities or location. For instance, resection of mesenteric desmoid tumors is often associated with resection of bowel and mesenteric vasculature increasing the risk of postop comorbidities. Most patients require an individualized treatment approach. In our patient, no adjuvant therapy was offered following surgical resection. Margins were free of tumor. In patients where the desmoid tumor is infiltrative with vital structures involved, or margins are not free of tumor, additional therapy may be warranted. There are hormonal and nonhormonal options for medical management. Tamoxifen is often used in combination with NSAIDs (indomethacin or sulindac) [11, 12]. Tamoxifen is a selective ER modulator that acts by binding to ER receptors and inhibiting cell proliferation. Alternatively, the analog Raloxifene can be used with prior studies showing positive treatment results [13]. NSAIDS can have partial or complete response. Chemotherapy is reserved for people who have aggressive nonsurgical tumors or in patients who are highly symptomatic when other therapy regimes are not feasible or have failed. Chemotherapy is typically given in doses individualized to the patient based upon a team approach. Furthermore, in patients who are not a candidate for surgery, tyrosine kinase inhibitor may be an option for treatment. Radiation treatment is an option, reserved mainly for extra-abdominal tumors due to the risk of radiation induced injury to intra-abdominal structures, for example, radiation induced enteritis.

4. Conclusion

Sporadic intra-abdominal tumors occur much less frequently when compared to intra-abdominal desmoid tumors associated with familial polyposis coli. Most sporadic tumors are extra-abdominal in location. Management of intra-abdominal desmoid tumors involves a multidisciplinary team approach. Asymptomatic patients are commonly closely observed for disease progression. Resection remains the first line of treatment. Hormonal and nonhormonal treatments remain an option in patients where resection is not feasible or in those where disease free margins are not achieved. Disease free survival following resection depends on tumor size (>5 cm), extra-abdominal location, margin resection status, and history of recurrence [6]. The recommendation for surveillance is imaging every 3–6 months for the first 2-3 years, then annually [2]. Sporadic desmoid fibromatosis of the mesentery is a rare occurrence. In our case, the recurrent tumor size was 9 cm, the excision margins were clear, and an immunohistochemical analysis of beta-catenin was positive. No additional adjuvant treatment initiated at this time; the patient is on long term clinical and radiological imaging surveillance.

Acknowledgments

The authors Would like to thank Dr. Altaf Taher, Divisional Chief Department of Pathology at Eastern Health, St. John's, NL, for providing the pathology slides.

References

[1] B. N. Anandaravi, C. D. Jagadish Kumar, P. S. Sreejith, M. Mayur, and U. R. S. Roopa, "Giant aggressive mesenteric fibromatosis-A case report," *Journal of Clinical and Diagnostic Research*, vol. 9, no. 2, pp. PD07–PD08, 2015.

[2] C. Escobar, R. Munker, J. O. Thomas, B. D. Li, and G. V. Burton, "Update on desmoid tumors," *Annals of Oncology*, vol. 23, no. 3, pp. 562–569, 2012.

[3] L. Amaadour, Z. Benbrahim, K. Benhayoune, L. Chbani, S. Arifi, and N. Mellas, "Sporadic desmoid tumor of the small bowel mesentery in a male patient: a case report and literature review," *Journal of Cancer Therapy*, vol. 5, no. 11, pp. 1000–1004, 2014.

[4] P. Misiak, Ł. Piskorz, S. Wcisło, S. Jabłoński, and M. Brocki, "Giant mesentery fibromatosis presenting as acute abdomen - Case report," *Wspolczesna Onkologia*, vol. 17, no. 5, pp. 468-469, 2013.

[5] K. Kovacevic, D. Obad-Kovacevic, and J. Popic-Ramac, "Sporadic giant intra-abdominal desmoid tumor: a radiological case report. molecular and clinical oncology," *Molecular and Clinical Oncology*, vol. 6, pp. 896–898, 2017.

[6] G. A. Efthimiopoulos, D. Chatzifotiou, M. Drogouti, and G. Zafiriou, "Primary asymptomatic desmoid tumor of the mesentery," *American Journal of Case Reports*, vol. 16, pp. 160–163, 2015.

[7] M. H. Nieuwenhuis, M. Casparie, L. M. H. Mathus-Vliegen, O. M. Dekkers, P. C. W. Hogendoorn, and H. F. A. Vasen, "A nation-wide study comparing sporadic and familial adenomatous polyposis-related desmoid-type fibromatoses," *International Journal of Cancer*, vol. 129, no. 1, pp. 256–261, 2011.

[8] S. C. Faria, R. B. Iyer, A. Rashid, L. Ellis, and G. J. Whitman, "Desmoid tumor of the small bowel and the mesentery," *American Journal of Roentgenology*, vol. 183, no. 1, p. 118, 2004.

[9] J. Casillas, G. J. Sais, J. L. Greve, M. C. Iparraguirre, and G. Morillo, "Imaging of intra- and extraabdominal desmoid tumors," *Radiographics*, vol. 11, no. 6, pp. 959–968, 1991.

[10] R. Lopez, N. Kemalyan, H. S. Moseley, D. Dennis, and R. M. Vetto, "Problems in diagnosis and management of desmoid

tumors," *The American Journal of Surgery*, vol. 159, no. 5, pp. 450–453, 1990.

[11] J. H. Howard and R. E. Pollock, "Intra-abdominal and abdominal wall desmoid fibromatosis," *Oncology and Therapy*, vol. 4, no. 1, pp. 57–72, 2016.

[12] M. Santos, A. Rocha, V. Martins, and M. Santos, "Desmoid tumours in familial adenomatous polyposis: Review of 17 patients from a portuguese tertiary center," *Journal of Clinical and Diagnostic Research*, vol. 10, no. 10, pp. PC01–PC05, 2016.

[13] F. Tonelli, F. Ficari, R. Valanzano, and M. L. Brandi, "Treatment of desmoids and mesenteric fibromatosis in familial adenomatous polyposis with raloxifene," *Tumori Journal*, vol. 89, no. 4, pp. 391–396, 2003.

18

Malignant Tumours Mimicking Complicated Appendicitis and Discovered upon Follow-Up after Percutaneous Drainage: A Case of Two Patients

Sharandran Chandra Mohan, Krishna Mohan Gummalla, and Martin Weng Chin H'ng

Diagnostic Radiology Department, Tan Tock Seng Hospital, 11 Jalan Tan Tock Seng, Singapore 308433

Correspondence should be addressed to Sharandran Chandra Mohan; sharandran@gmail.com

A ademic Editor: Vincent Low

The conservative management of periappendiceal abscesses is gaining favour due to decreased morbidity and improved clinical outcomes for patients. Occasionally however an abscess can mask underlying sinister pathology. In this article, we highlight two cases of appendiceal adenocarcinoma that were initially diagnosed as periappendiceal abscesses and managed conservatively with percutaneous drainage. We also discuss clinical and imaging features that may assist with identifying a hidden malignancy when presented in these situations.

1. Introduction

Patients presenting with periappendiceal abscesses are generally treated conservatively [1]. A drain is inserted under radiological guidance until the abscess resolves. Periappendiceal abscesses are usually due to acute appendicitis. However, appendiceal malignancy may also present with periappendiceal abscesses and it becomes difficult to differentiate between these two. Periappendiceal abscess due to malignancy can be recurrent or persistent despite drain insertion. Follow-up is advised after drain insertion, as once the abscess resolves there may be unmasking of an underlying malignancy.

Approximately 20 patients underwent image guided drainage in our institution for periappendiceal collections between 2013 and 2015 (2 years). We present two cases where the initial diagnosis was periappendiceal abscess due to acute appendicitis and a drain was inserted. There was persistent abscess collection despite drainage in these cases and subsequent histology revealed an underlying malignancy.

2. Case Report

2.1. Case 1. A 76-year-old man presented with a one-week history of intermittent fever, nausea, and right iliac fossa (RIF) pain. Initial CT scan performed at an external centre showed a large irregular collection in the RIF, compatible with an abscess, likely from a perforated appendix. He was referred to our institution and underwent CT-guided drainage of the collection (Figure 1). The amount of drainage gradually resolved and the tube was removed after 18 days.

An outpatient CT scan performed one month after the drainage for recurrent symptoms revealed a persistent abscess in the retrocaecal region, now extending to involve the pelvic side wall and iliopsoas muscles (Figure 2). The patient was managed with a repeat drainage of the primary collection.

Another follow-up in the general surgery clinic showed persistent symptoms and continuous drain output, and he underwent an extended right hemicolectomy approximately 3 months from the date of initial presentation. Intraoperative findings revealed a large, polypoid caecal tumour with a 2 cm defect and contained abscess posteriorly extending into the lateral abdominal wall, close to the iliac crest. Histology confirmed this to be a mucinous adenocarcinoma.

2.2. Case 2. A 49-year-old lady presented to our emergency department with a one-week history of fever and localised RIF pain. CT scan performed on admission delineated a dilated and ill-defined appendix with focal perforation at

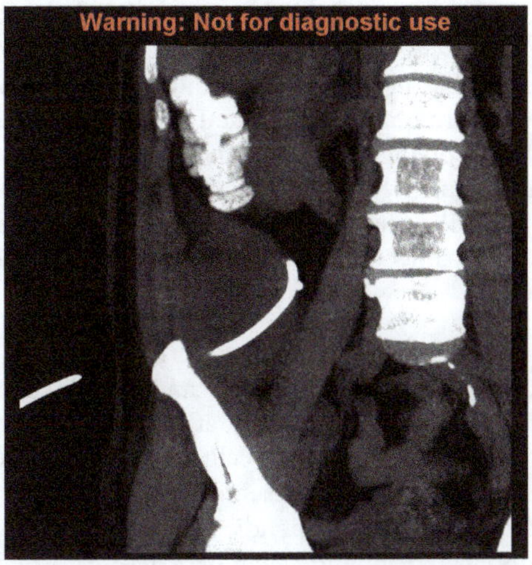

FIGURE 1: Coronal reconstruction demonstrating a drainage tube within the appendiceal collection.

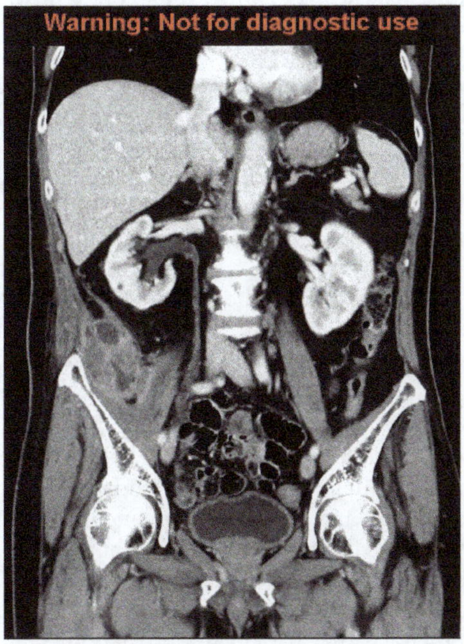

FIGURE 2: Coronal reconstruction demonstrating a persistent abscess in the retrocaecal region, with new extension to involve the pelvic side wall and iliopsoas muscles.

its tip (Figure 3). There was an adjacent abscess with surrounding fat-stranding as well as reactive thickening of the caecum and terminal ileum with prominent ileocolic lymph nodes. The patient was initially treated conservatively with intravenous antibiotics.

She represented approximately 2 weeks later due to worsening symptoms. Repeat CT scan (Figure 4) demonstrated a stable collection and CT-guided drainage was performed. As the drain output progressively decreased, this tube was removed after 7 days.

She returned another two and a half months later for nonresolving symptoms. The repeat CT scan (Figure 5) revealed

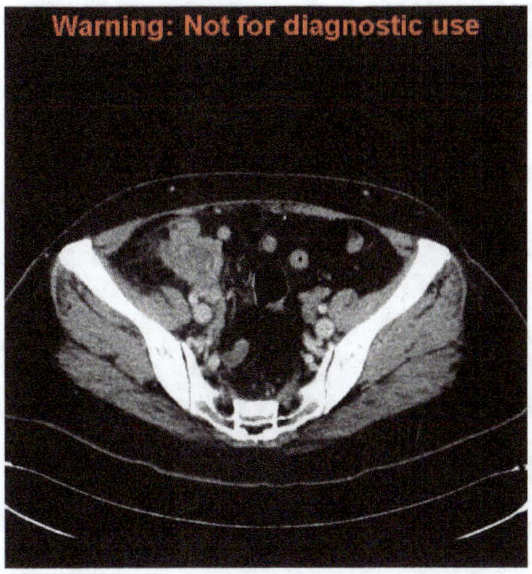

FIGURE 3: Thickened and inflamed appendix with a focal perforation of the tip with an adjacent abscess.

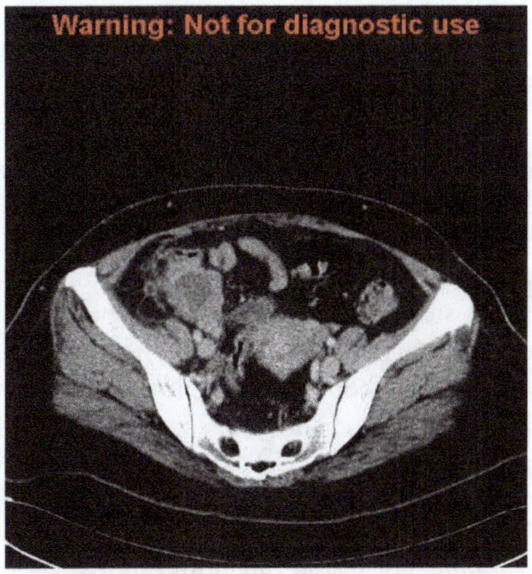

FIGURE 4: Repeat CT scan demonstrates a largely stable periappendiceal collection.

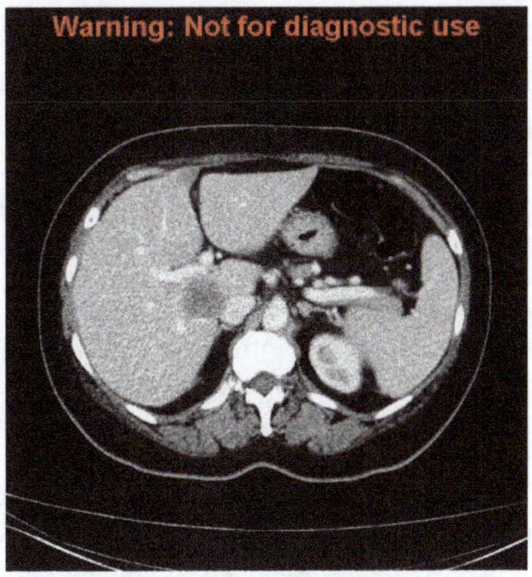

FIGURE 5: A new hypodense lesion in caudate lobe of the liver suspicious for metastasis.

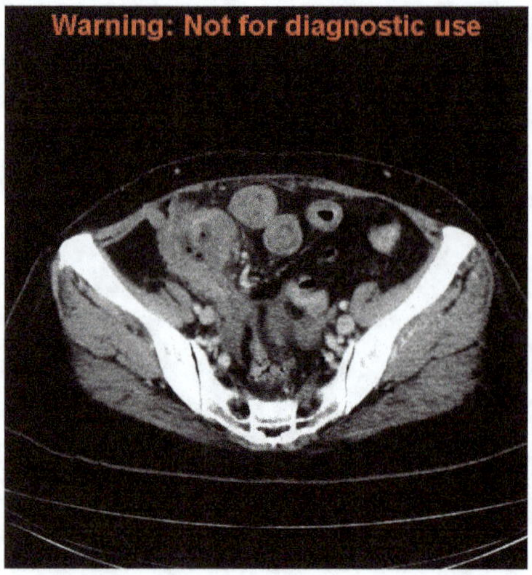

FIGURE 6: A persistent periappendiceal collection is again seen. New findings include small bowel obstruction as well as nodules adjacent to the collection and along the track of previous drain insertion.

an irregular lobulated mass with central necrosis at the ileocaecal junction associated with small bowel obstruction. New small soft-tissue nodules were observed adjacent to the mass and along the track of previous drain insertion. The adjacent mesenteric lymph nodes were enlarged and necrotic. A new hypodense lesion in the caudate lobe of the liver was also identified, suspicious for a metastasis (Figure 6).

The patient underwent an open right hemicolectomy with en bloc right salpingooophorectomy. Intraoperative findings revealed a mass involving and encasing the terminal ileum as well as involving the right fallopian tube, ovary, and ureter and extending into the pelvic side wall. A separate appendix was not identified within the mass. Multiple peritoneal nodules were evident in the omentum and as far up as the hepatic dome. The histology specimen was confirmed to be an adenocarcinoma.

3. Discussion

Acute appendicitis is the result of luminal obstruction. This is typically caused by faecolith or lymphoid hyperplasia and less frequently by foreign body impaction or parasites [2]. A small subset of acute appendicitis is caused by primary appendiceal malignancies such as carcinoid tumours, adenocarcinoma, Kaposi sarcoma, and lymphoma and less frequently due to metastases from breast or colonic tumours [2, 3]. Perforation with abscess formation is an infrequent but important complication of appendicitis as it leads to increased morbidity and mortality [4].

CT scans are routinely performed nowadays both to diagnose acute appendicitis and to identify mimics such as right ureteric calculus, epiploic appendagitis, torsion of a Meckel's diverticulum, mesenteric adenitis, inflammatory bowel disease, colitis, gynaecological disorders, and right-sided diverticulitis [4].

Current literature supports nonsurgical management of appendiceal abscesses [1, 4, 5]. This reduces morbidity and mortality. Antibiotic therapy is the mainstay of treatment and percutaneous drainage is performed in cases where there is a large or nonresolving collection. In cases of periappendiceal abscess due to underlying malignancy, there can be recurrent or persistent collections despite drainage [3]. A decrease in the size of the collection may unmask the underlying mass lesion.

A case report by Fusari et al. described findings of acute appendicitis on a preoperative CT scan with a loculated fluid collection and lymphadenopathy adjacent to the appendix that was found to be a signet cell carcinoma on histology [6]. Jongsma and Puylaert presented a case in which a lesion initially thought to be an appendiceal abscess was later found to be a complicated appendiceal mucocoele [7]. Another case report by Fiume et al. describes a caecal adenocarcinoma presenting as an appendiceal abscess [8]. Our cases similarly illustrate two examples of appendiceal malignancy presenting as appendiceal abscesses which were both proven to be adenocarcinomas on histology.

Multiple case studies are available describing imaging findings of pathology at or near the appendix such as mucocoeles, mucinous epithelial neoplasms, soft-tissue masses with nonmucinous or colonic-type epithelial neoplasms, carcinoid tumours, and lymphoma causing diffuse mural thickening and dilation of the appendiceal lumen [9, 10]. These conditions may also result in abscesses, which are difficult to distinguish from those caused by perforated acute appendicitis. In patients with Crohn's disease, transmural inflammation and penetration of the bowel may also lead to abscess formation in the region of the terminal ileum [11].

Imaging alone however is inadequate for the follow-up of complicated appendicitis. There is evidence to support an early colonoscopy and an interval appendectomy in appropriate patients. A study by Lai et al. [12] showed that patients who had colon cancer associated with appendicitis had a higher stage and a greater incidence of distant metastasis. He recommended that patients older than 40 years should undergo an early colonoscopy to exclude the possibility of a coexistent colorectal cancer. Wright et al. [13] showed that appendiceal neoplasms were more frequent in patients undergoing an interval appendectomy after initial nonoperative management. This was most prevalent is patients above the age of 40, in whom 16% were found to have an underlying malignancy. They recommended an interval appendectomy as part of routine care and this view has been supported by other authors who have shared data showing that an interval appendectomy is a safe procedure [14].

Ethical Approval

Approval from our institutional review board is not required for a retrospective case report.

References

[1] B. Quartey, "Interval appendectomy in adults: a necessary evil," *Journal of Emergencies, Trauma, and Shock*, vol. 5, no. 3, pp. 213–216, 2012.

[2] A. Petroianu, "Diagnosis of acute appendicitis," *International Journal of Surgery*, vol. 10, no. 3, pp. 115–119, 2012.

[3] J. Tannoury and B. Abboud, "Treatment options of inflammatory appendiceal masses in adults," *World Journal of Gastroenterology*, vol. 19, no. 25, pp. 3942–3950, 2013.

[4] R. E. Andersson and M. G. Petzold, "Nonsurgical treatment of appendiceal abscess or phlegmon: a systematic review and meta-analysis," *Annals of Surgery*, vol. 246, no. 5, pp. 741–748, 2007.

[5] F. T. Drake, M. G. Florence, M. G. Johnson et al., "Progress in the diagnosis of appendicitis: a report from washington state's surgical care and outcomes assessment program," *Annals of Surgery*, vol. 256, no. 4, pp. 586–594, 2012.

[6] M. Fusari, N. Sorrentino, E. C. Bottazzi et al., "Primary signet ring cell carcinoma of the appendix mimicking acute appendicitis," *Acta Radiologica Short Reports*, vol. 1, no. 9, pp. 1–3, 2012.

[7] T. E. F. Jongsma and J. B. C. M. Puylaert, "Infection of a malignant appendiceal mucocele masquerading as an appendiceal abscess: Role of preoperative sonography and CT," *Journal of Clinical Ultrasound*, vol. 37, no. 4, pp. 236–238, 2009.

[8] I. Fiume, V. Napolitano, G. Del Genio, A. Allaria, and A. Del Genio, "Cecum cancer underlying appendicular abscess. Case report and review of literature," *World Journal of Emergency Surgery*, vol. 1, no. 1, article no. 11, 2006.

[9] P. J. Pickhardt, A. D. Levy, C. A. Rohrmann Jr., and A. I. Kende, "Primary neoplasms of the appendix: radiologic spectrum of disease with pathologic correlation," *RadioGraphics*, vol. 23, no. 3, pp. 645–662, 2003.

[10] K. E. Karzazi, P. Sanchez, P. A. C. García et al., Primary malignant neoplasms of the cecal appendix: classification, forms of presentation and MDCT findings, ECR, Educational Exhibit C-1527, 2014.

[11] R. J. Richards, "Management of abdominal and pelvic abscess in Crohn's disease," *World Journal of Gastrointestinal Endoscopy*, vol. 3, no. 11, pp. 209–212, 2011.

[12] H.-W. Lai, C.-C. Loong, L.-C. Tai, C.-W. Wu, and W.-Y. Lui, "Incidence and odds ratio of appendicitis as first manifestation of colon cancer: a retrospective analysis of 1873 patients," *Journal of Gastroenterology and Hepatology*, vol. 21, no. 11, pp. 1693–1696, 2006.

[13] G. P. Wright, M. E. Mater, J. T. Carroll, J. S. Choy, and M. H. Chung, "Is there truly an oncologic indication for interval appendectomy?" *The American Journal of Surgery*, vol. 209, no. 3, pp. 442–446, 2015.

[14] A. J. González-Sánchez, J. M. Aranda-Narváez, A. Titos-García, C. Montiel-Casado, and J. Santoyo-Santoyo, "Appendiceal inflammatory mass. Letter to the editor," *Journal of Gastrointestinal Surgery*, vol. 19, no. 4, p. 797, 2015.

19

Pyogenic Odontoid Osteomyelitis with Sinus Thrombosis

Rohit Aiyer,[1] Janice Hwang,[2] and Edward H. Yu[3]

[1]*Department of Psychiatry, Hofstra Northwell Health, Staten Island University Hospital, Staten Island, NY, USA*
[2]*Department of Radiology, Hofstra Northwell Health, Staten Island University Hospital, Staten Island, NY, USA*
[3]*Department of Neurology, Hofstra Northwell Health, Staten Island University Hospital, Staten Island, NY, USA*

Correspondence should be addressed to Rohit Aiyer; rohitaiyer@gmail.com

Academic Editor: Amit Agrawal

71/F presented with left sided headaches and neck pain with nuchal rigidity progressively worsening over 3 weeks with no other neurologic symptoms. Odontoid osteomyelitis with epidural abscess was discovered on further workup with neuroimaging. Concurrent jugular vein and transverse sinus venous thrombosis was also found and suspected to be secondary to the pyogenic odontoid osteomyelitis. Patient was treated with intravenous antibiotics for the osteomyelitis as well as intravenous heparin for the venous thrombosis. To our knowledge, this is the first case reported in literature of transverse sinus venous thrombosis secondary to odontoid osteomyelitis.

1. Introduction

Cervical vertebral osteomyelitis readily responds to conservative treatments if detected early but can lead to significant morbidity if fulminant due to adjacent infectious and inflammatory changes. Osteomyelitis affecting the cranium can lead to thrombosis of the subjacent cerebral venous sinus, often seen in untreated mastoiditis resulting in lateral or transverse sinus thrombosis [1]. Extracranial thrombosis of the internal jugular vein can result from adjacent oropharyngeal abscesses resulting in Lemierre's syndrome. We describe a patient presenting with spontaneous cervical osteomyelitis affecting the odontoid process with thrombosis of the adjacent internal jugular vein extending intracranially into cerebral sinuses.

2. Case Report

We present a 71/F presenting with a left occipital headache and neck pain progressing over 3 weeks. Pain was persistent and radiated down the left side of her neck. Vital signs were normal and physical examination was significant for nuchal rigidity with reproducible pain on head movement and limited range of motion. Cervical paraspinal muscles were tender to palpation without Spurling sign. There were no other neurologic deficits noted. Serologic testing revealed lymphocyte predominant leukocytosis (total WBC 16,500/mm^3; lymphocyte 1,110/mm^3, monocyte 350/mm^3, granulocyte 14,570/mm^3, eosinophils 10/mm^3, and basophils 20 mm^3). Inflammatory markers were elevated with erythrocyte sedimentation rate 120 mm/hr and c-reactive protein of 13.95 mg/dl.

MRI of the cervical spine revealed bone marrow edema within the C2 odontoid process with surrounding prevertebral and ventral epidural inflammation with an area of liquefaction posterior to the dens (Figures 1–3) suggestive of an infectious process. Magnetic resonance imaging (MRI, General Electric 3 Tesla) of the brain with and without gadolinium (DTPA) contrast revealed a near occlusive filling defect of the left sigmoid sinus extending into the left jugular vein (Figures 4–6). Enhancement of the prevertebral and ventral epidural space was suspicious for an epidural abscess. Magnetic resonance venography (MRV) revealed soft tissue signal with decreased flow suggestive of a thrombosis within the left sigmoid sinus and internal jugular vein (Figure 7). Echocardiogram and serial blood cultures were negative.

The patient was anticoagulated with intravenous unfractionated heparin with eventual conversion to long term oral anticoagulation with warfarin. Broad spectrum antibiotics

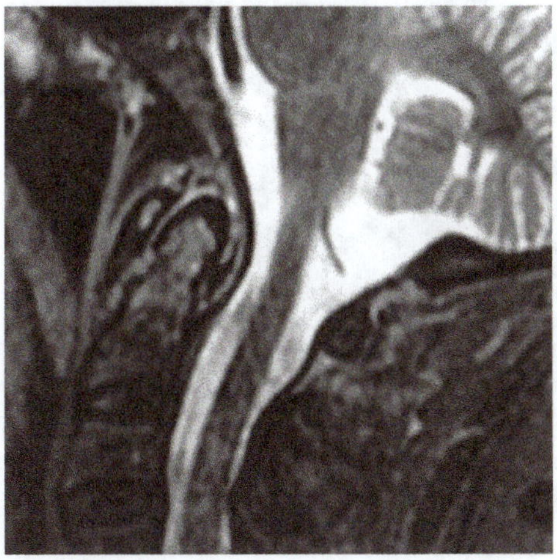

Figure 1: Sagittal STIR sequence demonstrating bone marrow edema within the C2 odontoid process. There are also high signal changes in the surrounding soft tissues reflecting related inflammation.

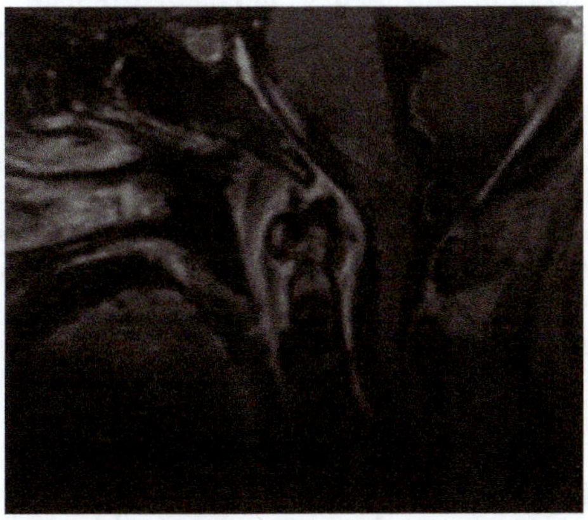

Figure 2: Sagittal postcontrast sequence demonstrating enhancement within the C2 odontoid process and surrounding prevertebral and epidural enhancing inflammatory soft tissue with liquefaction.

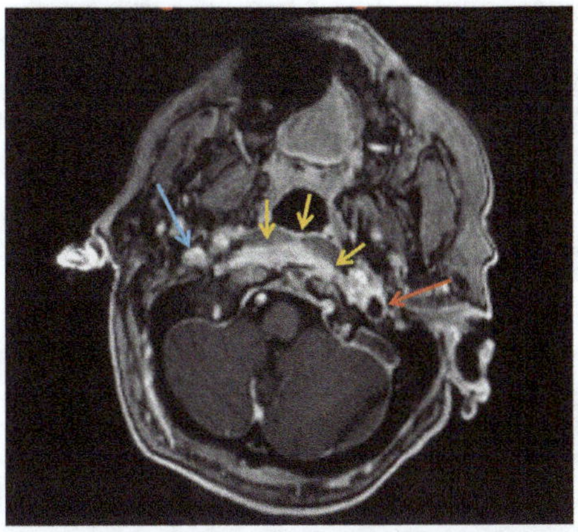

Figure 3: Postcontrast axial FSPGR sequence demonstrating filling defect within the left sigmoid sinus and proximal jugular vein (red arrows). Compare with the normal appearing right jugular vein (blue arrow). Also seen is inflammatory soft tissue in the prevertebral space (orange arrows) which extends into the epidural space behind the dens.

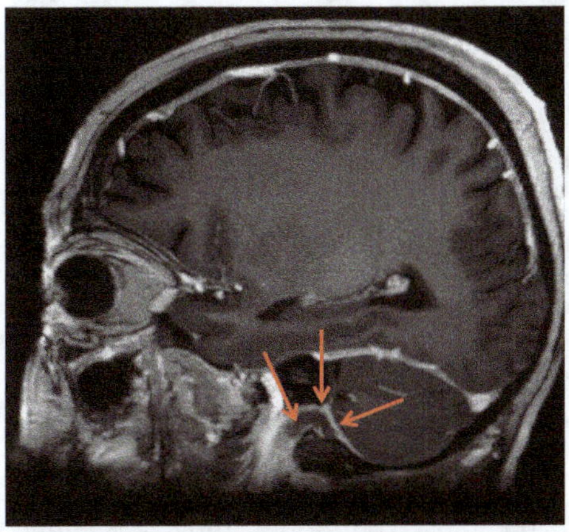

Figure 4: Sagittal reformatted postcontrast FSPGR images demonstrating filling defect within the left sigmoid sinus and proximal jugular vein. Arrow demonstrates thrombus within the distal sigmoid sinus and internal jugular vein.

were initiated and continued for 6 weeks. After 6 weeks of treatment, our patient had near complete resolution of cervical pain and headache with no significant neurologic deficits. Blood cultures remained negative throughout hospitalization.

3. Discussion

Vertebral osteomyelitis is less commonly associated with the cervical spine than with thoracic or lumbar segments accounting for only 12% of spinal osteomyelitis cases and is particularly rare affecting the odontoid process [2]. Cervical osteomyelitis occurs in 0.2–1.2 patients per 10,000 hospital admissions [3] with few cases involving the odontoid process specifically. Rheumatic destruction of the odontoid process is more common with the predominance of articular surfaces within the atlantoaxial articulation, which is distinct from other spinal cord segments [2]. While computed tomography (CT) is useful for locating areas of cortical bone destruction, prevertebral swelling, and delineation of abscesses [4], MRI remains the definitive study for early diagnosis of vertebral osteomyelitis with sensitivity of 95% and specificity of 90% [5]. T1 and T2 weighted sequences can also be used to differentiate complicated from uncomplicated osteomyelitis by examining involvement of the surrounding soft tissue.

Pathogenesis for vertebral osteomyelitis is usually due to local invasion of infectious organisms with progression to abscess formation through accumulation of pus in adjacent soft tissue spaces. Pyogenic osteomyelitis usually occurs by hematogenous spread in the absence of open trauma. Incidence of associated comorbid conditions includes diabetes mellitus in 24% of patients, followed by cancer (16%), intravenous drug users (10%), and corticosteroid treatment

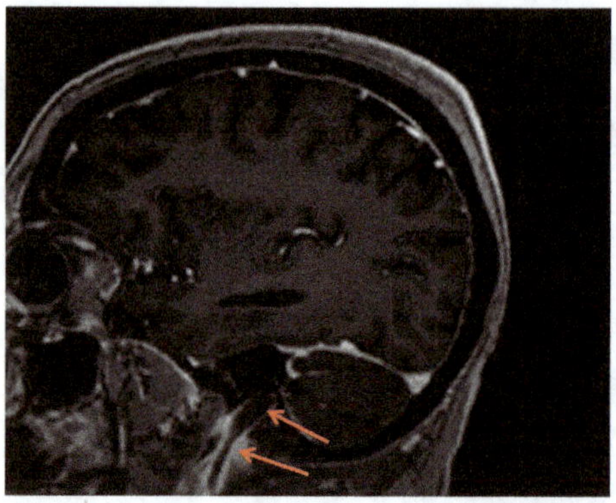

FIGURE 5: Sagittal reformatted postcontrast FSPGR images demonstrating filling defect within the left sigmoid sinus and a clearer view of the jugular vein. Arrow demonstrates thrombus within the distal sigmoid sinus and internal jugular vein.

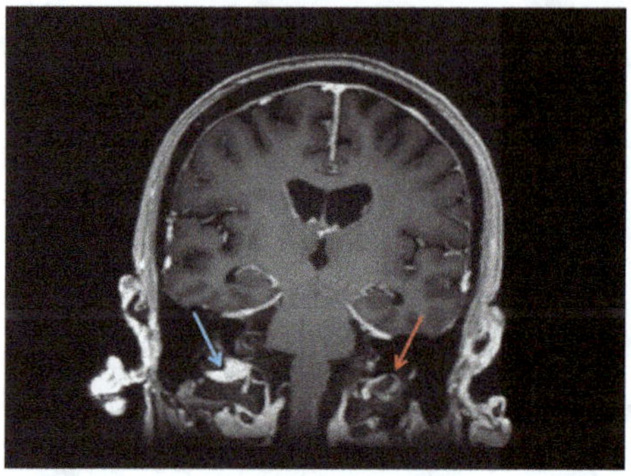

FIGURE 6: Coronal reformatted postcontrast FSPGR sequence demonstrating filling defect within the left sigmoid sinus. Blue arrow is demonstrating a normal right vein. Red arrow is demonstrating clot within the left vein.

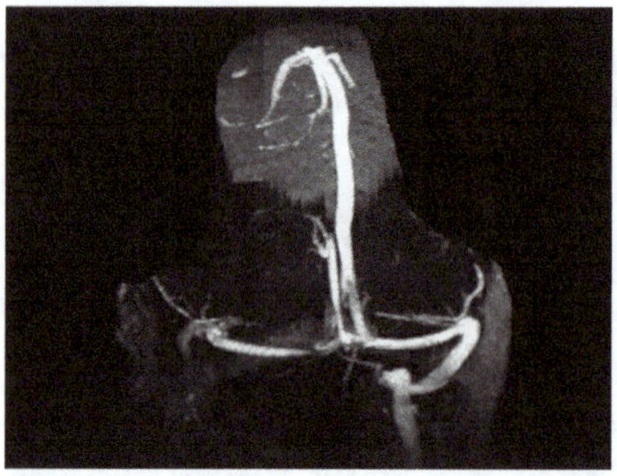

FIGURE 7: Time of flight MRV image demonstrating absence of signal within the left sigmoid sinus and proximal jugular vein.

(7%) [6]. The most common pathogen is *Staphylococcus aureus*, which accounts for 40–80% of all cases [7].

Cerebral venous thrombosis (CVT) has an annual incidence of 1 per 100,000 patients [8]. Risk factors for CVT include prothrombotic conditions, infections, and malignancy. More than one risk factor increases the risk of CVT with over half of all CVT patients having 2 or more risks factors and 13% with no risks [9]. Intracranial infections as a cause for CVT are relatively rare accounting for only 6–12% of all CVTs [9]. Sinus venous thrombosis associated with vertebral osteomyelitis is even more rare with scant literature showing correlation.

Vertebral osteomyelitis with CVT is uncommon likely due to anatomic factors since most infections are detected before extension into nonadjacent vertebral bodies or skull base. Neurologic complications from osteomyelitis often arise from epidural abscess formation and since the dura is tightly adherent to the foramen magnum separating intracranial dural space from the spinal thecal sac, epidural abscesses typically do not cross from thecal sac intracranially. Infection can spread through hematogenous means since both arterial and venous systems span both intracranial and spinal segments. Vertebral osteomyelitis in high cervical segments such as the odontoid process can spread to adjacent soft tissue resulting in adherence of fibrin, blood, and platelets producing thrombosis which can extend intracranially into the sigmoid and transverse sinus as in our patient.

Mortality and dependency rates of CVT remain high with an estimated 15% of cases resulting in death or significant disability [9]. Complications occur in the form of venous infarcts and early detection leads to more favorable outcomes with early initiation of anticoagulation to prevent progression of thrombosis with resultant venous infarcts. Treatment for osteomyelitis requires long term intravenous antibiotics and possible surgical excision of epidural abscesses or empyema if present. Osteomyelitis affecting the odontoid process is rare and special consideration should be made when treating these infections since it is well situated to cause cerebral venous thrombosis due to continuity between of the internal jugular vein with cerebral venous sinuses. Since these two entities require very different treatment approaches, CVT as a potential cause for neurologic complication should be assessed in any patient with high cervical infections.

References

[1] V. Biousse, A. Ameri, and M.-G. Bousser, "Isolated intracranial hypertension as the only sign of cerebral venous thrombosis," *Neurology*, vol. 53, no. 7, pp. 1537–1542, 1999.

[2] S. Noguchi, K. Yanaka, Y. Yamada, and T. Nose, "Diagnostic pitfalls in osteomyelitis of the odontoid process: Case report," *World Neurosurgery*, vol. 53, no. 6, pp. 573–579, 2000.

[3] M. Wiedau-Pazos, G. Curio, and C. Grüsser, "Epidural abscess of the cervical spine with osteomyelitis of the odontoid process," *The Spine Journal*, vol. 24, no. 2, pp. 133–136, 1999.

[4] T. J. Limbird, G. W. Brick, H. J. Boulas, and R. W. Bucholz, "Osteomyelitis of the odontoid process," *Journal of Spinal Disorders & Techniques*, vol. 1, no. 1, pp. 66–74, 1988.

[5] P. J. Reid and P. J. Holman, "Iatrogenic pyogenic osteomyelitis of C-1 and C-2 treated with transoral decompression and delayed posterior occipitocervical arthrodesis: Case report," *Journal of Neurosurgery: Spine*, vol. 7, no. 6, pp. 664–668, 2007.

[6] M. Doutchi, P. Seng, A. Menard et al., "Changing trends in the epidemiology of vertebral osteomyelitis in Marseille, France," *New Microbes and New Infections*, vol. 7, pp. 1–7, 2015.

20

Inferior Vena Cava Duplication: Incidental Case in a Young Woman

Danilo Coco,[1] Sara Cecchini,[2] Silvana Leanza,[3] Massimo Viola,[1] Stefano Ricci,[2] and Roberto Campagnacci[3]

[1]*Department of Surgery, Card. G. Panico Hospital of Tricase, 73039 Tricase, Italy*
[2]*Department of Radiology, INRCA Hospital of Ancona, 60125 Ancona, Italy*
[3]*Department of Surgery, C. Urbani Hospital of Jesi, 60035 Jesi, Italy*

Correspondence should be addressed to Danilo Coco; webcostruction@msn.com

Academic Editor: Salah D. Qanadli

A case of a double inferior vena cava (IVC) with retroaortic left renal vein, azygos continuation of the IVC, and presence of the hepatic portion of the IVC drained into the right renal vein is reported and the embryologic, clinical, and radiological significance is discussed. The diagnosis is suggested by multidetector computed tomography (MDCT), which reveals the aberrant vascular structures. Awareness of different congenital anomalies of IVC is necessary for radiologists to avoid diagnostic pitfalls and they should be remembered because they can influence several surgical interventions and endovascular procedures.

1. Introduction

The first case of inferior vena cava duplication (IVCD) was described in 1916 in a male subject dissected during an autopsy by Lucas in London [1]. As reported in the literature, the incidence of IVCD is 1.5% (range 0.2%–3%), with intraoperative findings between 0.2% and 0.6% [2–4]. Although congenital anomalies of the IVC cases are usually clinically silent and often detected incidentally by imaging, these venous anomalies may have important relevance during retroperitoneal surgery and venous interventional radiologic procedures [5]. We present one case of a double inferior vena cava (IVC) with retroaortic left renal vein, azygos continuation of the IVC, and presence of the hepatic portion of the IVC drained into the right renal vein, demonstrated by a multidetector computed tomography (MDCT).

2. Case Report

A 42-year-old woman with abdominal pain in right quadrant was referred to our radiology department for abdominal multidetector computed tomography (MDCT) examination. Abdominal MDCT (BrightSpeed Elite Select, GE Medical System) was performed before and after administration of intravenous contrast medium (150 mL of nonionic contrast material containing 320 mg of iopromide per milliliter) with 16 × 1.25 mm slice collimation, 1.25 mm slice thicknesses. 2D and 3D postprocessing images, such as multiplanar reformation (MPR) and volume rendering (VR) images, were obtained on the workstation for better visualization of vascular structures.

MDCT showed double IVC below the renal veins. Both IVC were formed from the respective common iliac veins and ran upwards bilaterally to the abdominal aorta as far as the renal veins. The left IVC terminated on the left renal vein. The left renal vein crossed posterior to the aorta to join the right IVC. The right IVC, once receiving the left and right renal veins, ran upwards as a single vein continuing superiorly as the azygos vein within the retrocrural space. The azygos vein drained into superior vena cava in the right paratracheal space. The hepatic veins drained into a stump of the hepatic segment of the IVC, which opened cranially into the right atrium and caudally drained into the right renal vein, at the confluence with right IVC (Figures 1(a)–1(g)).

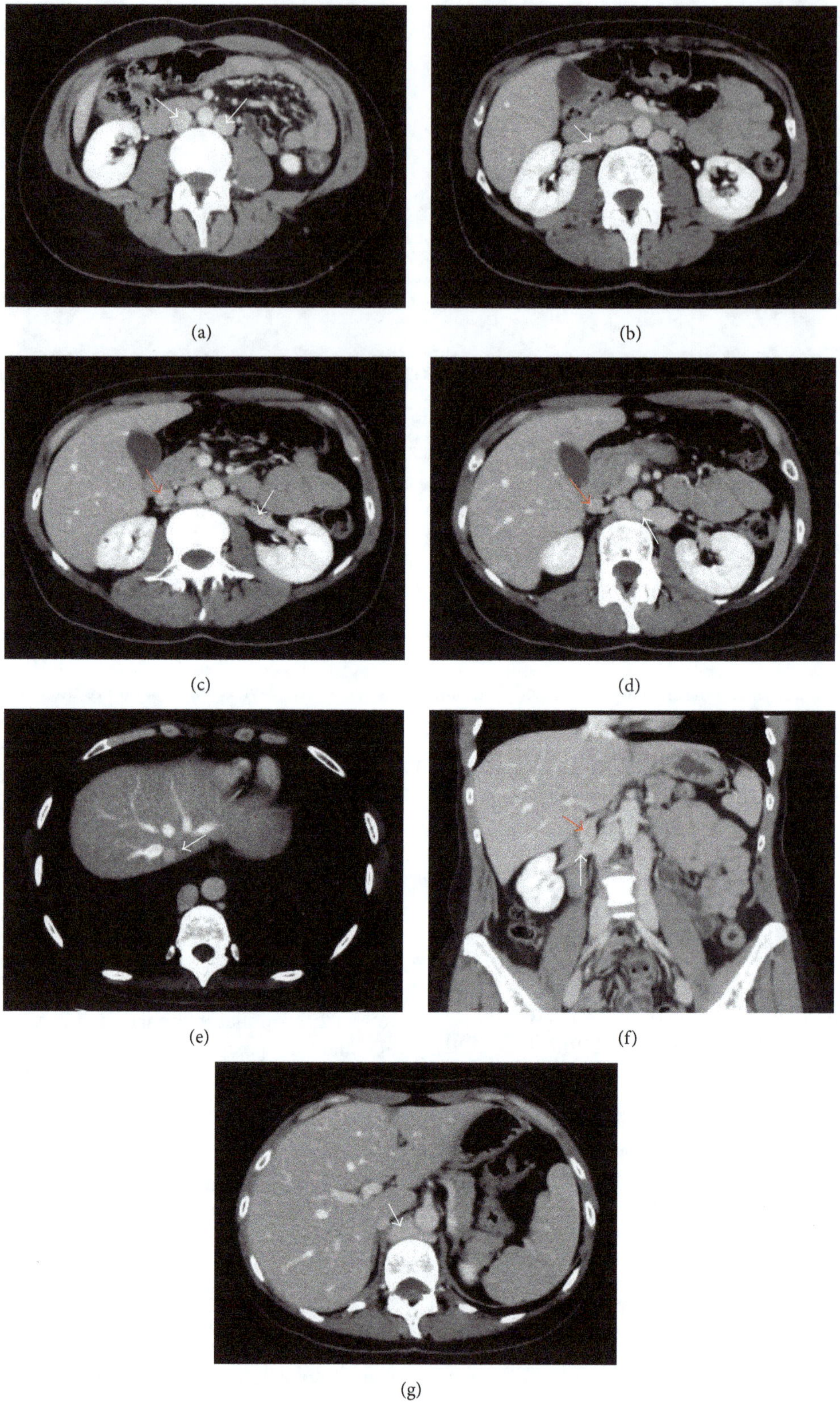

FIGURE 1: (a) CT axial images that presented from caudal to cranial sections show double IVC (arrows) below the renal veins. (b) The right IVC receives the right renal vein (arrow). (c) The left IVC receives the left renal vein (white arrow); presence of the hepatic portion (red arrow) of the IVC in the CT section before draining into the right renal vein. (d) The left renal vein (white arrow) crosses posterior to the aorta to join the right IVC; continuation of hepatic segment (red arrow). (e) The hepatic veins drain into a hypoplastic hepatic segment (arrow) of the IVC. (f) Coronal MPR image shows the hypoplastic hepatic segment (red arrow) draining into the right renal vein (white arrow), at the confluence with the right IVC. (g) The right IVC continues cephalad as the azygos vein (arrow) within the retrocrural space.

3. Discussion

The normal IVC is composed of four segments: hepatic, suprarenal, renal, and infrarenal. It derives from a complex embryogenic process beginning at the sixth week of gestation and involving three pairs of primitive veins (posterior cardinal, subcardinal, and supracardinal veins) that appear and regress anastomozing in the final IVC. In particular, the postcardinal veins appear and remain in the pelvis as the common iliac veins, the right supracardinal vein persists to form the infrarenal IVC, and the right subcardinal vein persists to develop into the suprarenal segment by formation of the subcardinal-hepatic anastomosis while the left subcardinal vein and the left supracardinal vein regress completely [2, 4, 6]. The renal segment develops from the anastomosis between the subcardinal and supracardinal veins while the hepatic segment derives from the right vitelline vein [6, 7].

An alteration of one step of this process determines at least 14 different anatomic anomalies of the IVC and many classification systems have been proposed to group these variants. As reported by Bass, major anomalies are double IVC (with a prevalence of 0.2–3%), left IVC (0.2–0.5%), retroaortic left renal vein (2.1%), circumaortic left renal vein (8.7%), and absence of the hepatic segment of the IVC with azygos continuation of the IVC (0.6% of cases).

The duplication of IVC results from persistence of the right and the left supracardinal veins [8, 9]. Recognition of IVCD is clinically relevant during retroperitoneal surgery or vascular interventional procedures in order to avoid recurrent pulmonary embolism following placement of an IVC filter [10].

The retroaortic left renal vein results from regression of the anterior intersubcardinal (sopra-subcardinal) anastomosis and persistence of the posterior intersupracardinal anastomosis so that a single renal vein passes posterior to the aorta. The clinical significance is in preoperative planning prior to nephrectomy. The presence of retroaortic left renal vein may also cause clinical symptoms such as abdominal pain and hematuria.

Azygos continuation of the IVC has also been named absence of the hepatic segment of the IVC with azygos continuation. The embryologic basis is the failure to form the right subcardinal, hepatic anastomosis.

It is important to be aware of anatomy of this variation in planning cardiopulmonary bypass, in catheterizing the heart, and in the differential diagnosis of right-sided paratracheal mass or retrocrural and paravertebral lymphadenopathy [11–15].

As described in the literature, in some case, more than one variation can coexist as double IVC with retroaortic right renal vein and hemiazygos continuation of the IVC, duplication of the inferior vena cava with azygos continuation, and retroaortic left renal vein and iliac vein variations. Particularly Bass et al. describe the possibility of double IVC with retroaortic left renal vein and azygos continuation of the IVC [6, 16].

The case we describe has a complex combination of these venous variations, which is extremely rare to find together in a patient.

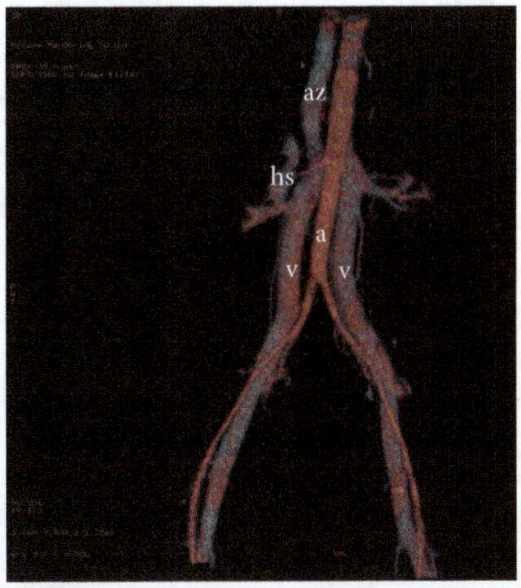

FIGURE 2: VR image coronal reconstruction shows double IVC (v), azygos continuation of the right IVC (az), and the hypoplastic hepatic segment (hs) of the IVC draining into the right IVC and the aorta (a).

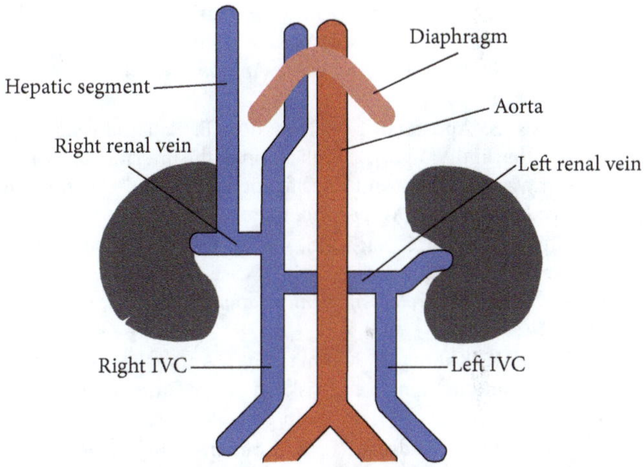

FIGURE 3: Schematic figure illustrating double IVC with a retroaortic left renal vein, azygos continuation, and the presence of a hypoplastic hepatic portion of the IVC, drained into the right renal vein.

In fact in the same patient double IVC with a retroaortic left renal vein, azygos continuation of the IVC, and the presence of a hypoplastic hepatic segment of the IVC coexist the last one is drained into the right renal vein, at the confluence with right IVC, probably due to an incomplete atrophy of the right subcardinal vein (Figures 2 and 3). Therefore, with the partial atrophy of the prerenal division of the IVC, the blood returning from the lower extremities is partially shunted from the supracardinal system through the suprasubcardinal anastomosis to the retrocrural azygos vein, which is derived from the thoracic segment of the right supracardinal vein and partially shunted to the hepatic segment of the IVC through the residual prerenal segment.

Although the presence of combination of these venous variations in a patient is extremely rare, it should be recognized in order to eliminate the risk for severe hemorrhage during abdominal and thoracic surgeries or the risk for recurrent embolism during the placement of an IVC filter in vascular interventional procedures. In addition, awareness of the different anomalies of the IVC is necessary for radiologists to prevent misinterpretation of aberrant vessels as paravertebral lymph node enlargement and mediastinal masses.

Multidetector CT technique is the preferred method for imaging the congenital vascular anomalies of IVC since it is less costly, less invasive than conventional angiography, fast, easily applicable, and reliable in terms of identification of thoracoabdominal vascular structures. In fact MDCT imaging enables the acquisition of high-spatial-resolution volumetric image data during a single breath hold with the possibility of two-dimensional (2D) and three-dimensional (3D) image after processing, which allows the visualization of complex vascular malformations in an understandable way.

References

[1] M. F. Lucas, "A case of double inferior vena cava," *Journal of Anatomy*, vol. 51, pp. 69–70, 1916.

[2] A. Banerjee, S. Maharana, I. A. Kumar, and P. Jhansi, "Duplication of the inferior vena cava-report of a rare congenital variation," *International Journal of Anatomical Variations*, vol. 5, pp. 141–143, 2012.

[3] K. Natsis, S. Apostolidis, G. Noussios, E. Papathanasiou, A. Kyriazidou, and V. Vyzas, "Duplication of the inferior vena cava: anatomy, embryology and classification proposal," *Anatomical Science International*, vol. 85, no. 1, pp. 56–60, 2010.

[4] H. Chen, S. Emura, S. Nagasaki, and K.-Y. Kubo, "Double inferior vena cava with interiliac vein: a case report and literature review," *Okajimas Folia Anatomica Japonica*, vol. 88, no. 4, pp. 147–151, 2012.

[5] S. Shindo, K. Kubota, A. Kojima et al., "Anomalies of inferior vena cava and left renal vein: risks in aortic surgery," *Annals of Vascular Surgery*, vol. 14, no. 4, pp. 393–396, 2000.

[6] J. E. Bass, M. D. Redwine, L. A. Kramer, P. T. Huynh, and J. H. Harris Jr., "Spectrum of congenital anomalies of the inferior vena cava: cross-sectional imaging findings," *Radiographics*, vol. 20, no. 3, pp. 639–652, 2000.

[7] D. Pineda, N. Moudgill, J. Eisenberg, P. DiMuzio, and A. Rao, "An interesting anatomic variant of inferior vena cava duplication: case report and review of the literature," *Vascular*, vol. 21, no. 3, pp. 163–167, 2013.

[8] R. J. Babaian and D. E. Johnson, "Major venous anomalies complicating retroperitoneal surgery," *Southern Medical Journal*, vol. 72, no. 10, pp. 1254–1258, 1979.

[9] R. Mathews, P. A. Smith, E. K. Fishman, and F. F. Marshall, "Anomalies of the inferior vena cava and renal veins: embryologic and surgical considerations," *Urology*, vol. 53, no. 5, pp. 873–880, 1999.

[10] B. Senecail, C. Lefevre, H. Person, and P. Meriot, "Radiologic anatomy of duplication of the inferior vena cava: a trap in abdominal imaging. A report of 8 cases," *Surgical and Radiologic Anatomy*, vol. 9, no. 2, pp. 151–157, 1987.

[11] Y. Tohno, S. Tohno, C. Azuma et al., "One case of the double inferior venae cavae found in a Japanese man," *Journal of Nara Medical Association*, vol. 57, no. 6, pp. 193–197, 2006.

[12] H.-G. Xue, C.-Y. Yang, M. Asakawa, K. Tanuma, and H. Ozawa, "Duplication of the inferior vena cava associated with other variations," *Anatomical Science International*, vol. 82, no. 2, pp. 121–125, 2007.

[13] H. S. Sürücü, K. M. Erbil, Ç. Tastan, and N. Yener, "Anomalous veins of the retroperitoneum: clinical considerations," *Surgical and Radiologic Anatomy*, vol. 23, no. 6, pp. 443–445, 2002.

[14] S. Morita, M. Higuchi, N. Saito, and N. Mitsuhashi, "Pelvic venous variations in patients with congenital inferior vena cava anomalies: classification with computed tomography," *Acta Radiologica*, vol. 48, no. 9, pp. 974–979, 2007.

[15] S. Ginaldi, V. P. Chuang, and S. Wallace, "Absence of hepatic segment of the inferior vena cava with azygous continuation," *Journal of Computer Assisted Tomography*, vol. 4, no. 1, pp. 112–114, 1980.

[16] A. Ahmetoglu and A. Cansu, "Duplication of the inferior vena cava with azygos continuation, retroaortic left renal vein and iliac vein variations," *Bratislavské Lekárske Listy*, vol. 113, no. 7, pp. 448–450, 2012.

21

MRI Findings of Syndrome of Acute Bilateral Symmetrical Basal Ganglia Lesions in Diabetic Uremia: A Case Report

Xin Cao,[1] Qiang Fang,[2] and Hao Shi[3]

[1]*Medical College, Shandong University, Jinan, Shandong 250012, China*
[2]*Medical College, Taishan Medical University, Tai'an, Shandong 271000, China*
[3]*Department of Medical Imaging, Qianfoshan Hospital Affiliated to Shandong University, Jinan, Shandong 250014, China*

Correspondence should be addressed to Hao Shi; hansenschie@163.com

Academic Editor: Samer Ezziddin

The syndrome of acute bilateral basal ganglia lesions is an uncommon clinical occurrence exhibiting acute onset of movement abnormalities, which can be seen almost exclusively among patients with chronic renal failure, especially in the setting of concurrent diabetes mellitus. Symmetrical lesions located in basal ganglia demonstrated in MRI are typical manifestation of this syndrome. Our study includes routine MRI examination, MRS, 3D-ASL, and SWI findings, which have been rarely reported and will contribute to diagnosing more cases about this syndrome.

1. Introduction

The syndrome of acute bilateral basal ganglia lesions is an illness which has been rarely reported so far. It is Wang and his colleagues who first found this syndrome in three patients back in 1998 [1]. Patients with this syndrome often present with several typical clinical symptoms including gait disturbance, dysarthria, and Parkinson-like tremor. Bilateral basal ganglia lesions were found in an Asian patient presented in this study suffering from end-stage diabetic nephropathy on dialysis and showing clinical signs of gait disturbance, dysarthria, and involuntary movements.

2. Case Report

A 49-year-old Chinese female was admitted to the hospital with gait disturbance, dysarthria, and involuntary movement of limbs for 10 days, with a history of edema in both lower extremities for 10 years, hypertension for almost 8 years, and diabetes mellitus for 2 years. Seven years ago when her serum creatinine level reached 2300 μmol/L, she began taking regular hemodialysis treatments twice a week and then three years later this increased to three times a week due to her restless legs syndrome (RLS) secondary to chronic renal failure. Besides, she had polycystic kidney disease and hyperparathyroidism. There was no previous history of movement disorders and family history of this kind. Clinical examination revealed her highest blood pressure to be 200/100 mmHg. Generalized chorea was noted mainly on the extremities. Laboratory results showed elevated concentrations of blood urea nitrogen (BUN) of 33.6 mg/dL and creatinine (Cr) of 5.4 mg/dL, serum potassium of 6.1 mmol/L, and parathyroid hormone of 1457 pg/mL. Axial brain MRI revealed symmetric edema in the bilateral basal ganglia, which exhibited hypointensity on T1-weighted images (Figure 1(a)) and hyperintensity on both T2-weighted images (Figure 1(b)) and fluid-attenuated inversion recovery (FLAIR) images (Figure 1(c)). Diffusion-weighted imaging (DWI) demonstrated slightly higher inhomogeneous signals in the involved regions (Figure 1(d)). Concurrently, increased apparent diffusion coefficient (ADC) values were demonstrated in the periphery compared with normal brain tissue (Figure 1(e)), indicating vasogenic edema rather than cytotoxic edema. Follow-up MRI of brain was performed 3

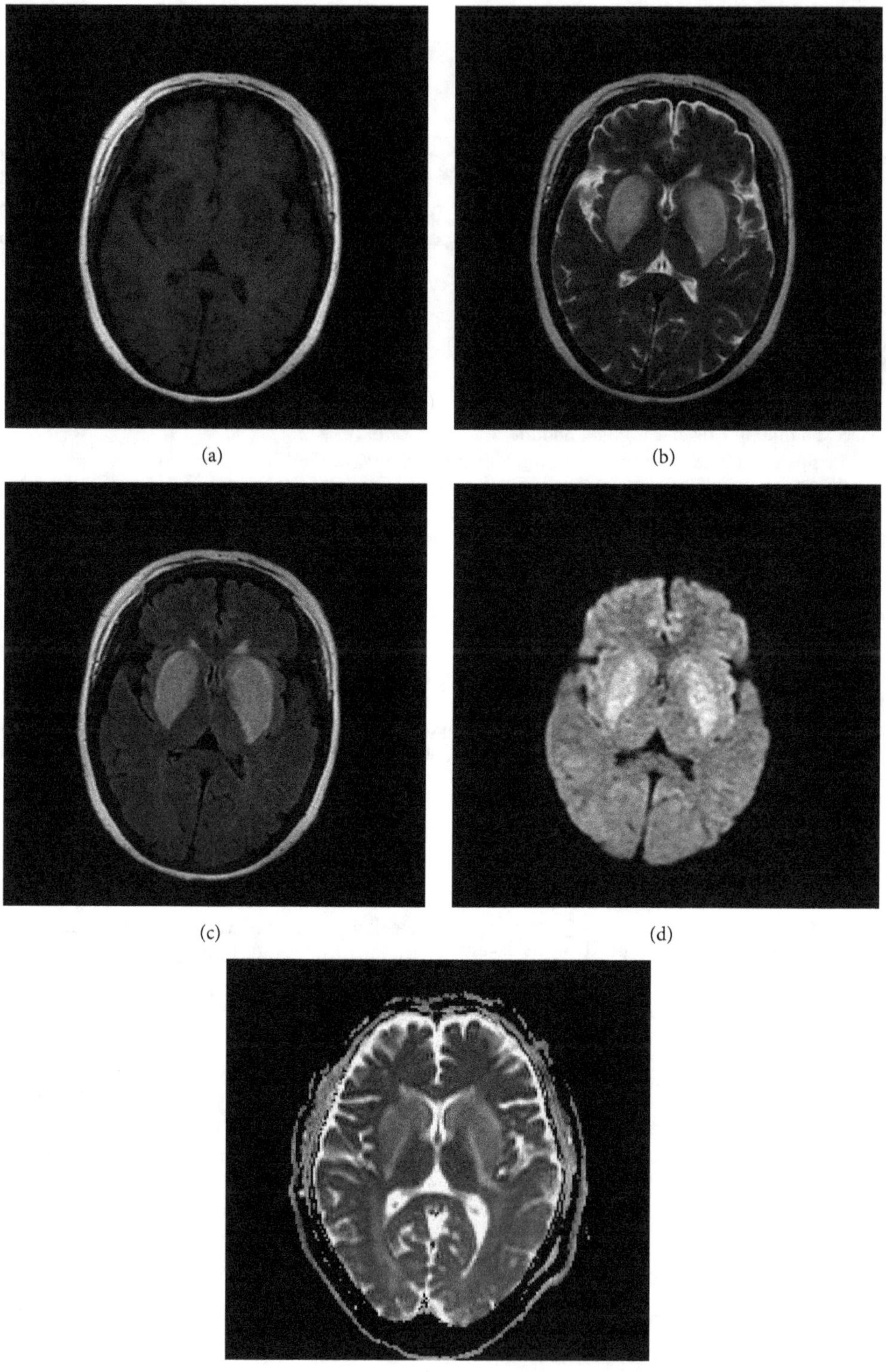

FIGURE 1: (a) Axial brain MRI showed symmetric hypointensity in the bilateral basal ganglia on T1-weighted images. (b, c) Axial brain MRI showed symmetric hyperintensity in the focal region on T2-weighted images and FLAIR images. (d) Diffusion-weighted imaging revealed slightly higher inhomogeneous signals in the involved regions. (e) ADC map revealed that the ADC value of the involved regions is not low.

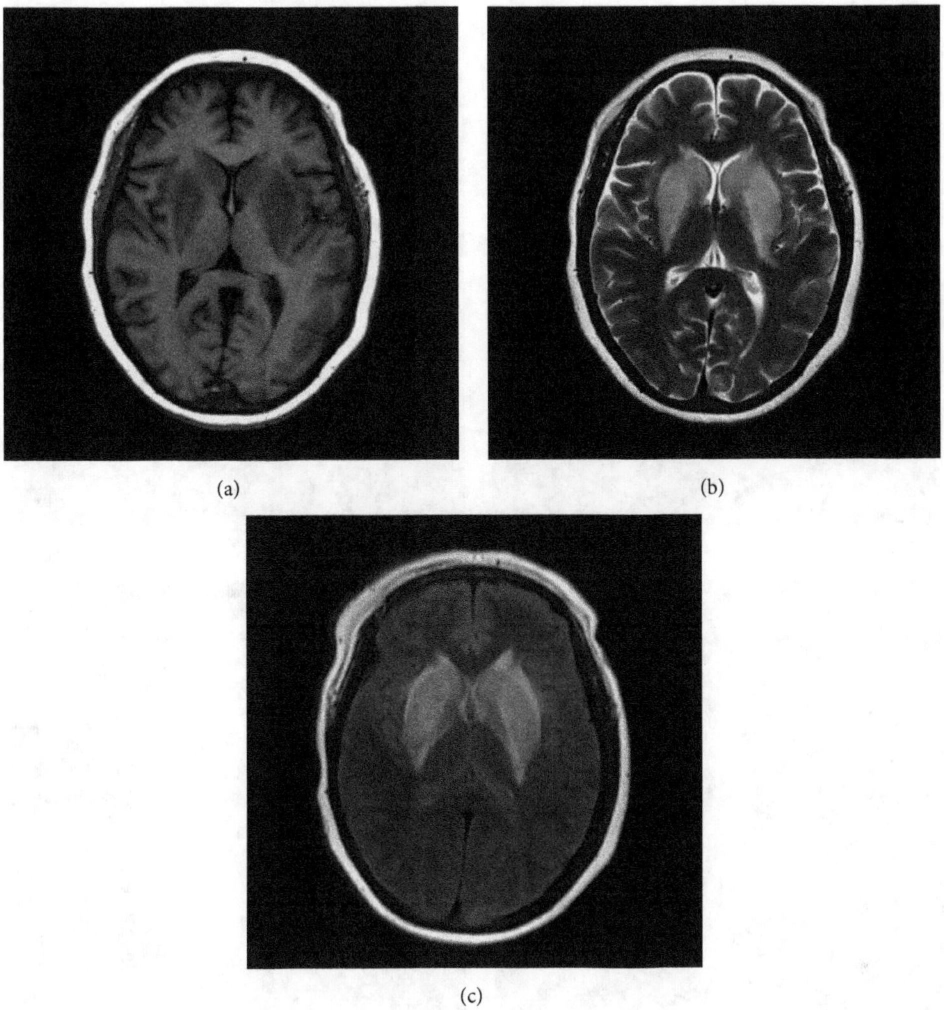

FIGURE 2: (a, b) The lesions extended in both T1WI and T2WI after 3 weeks. (c) FLAIR images showed demyelination around bilateral ventricles and lacunar infarctions.

weeks later, which showed lesions worsened and extended in both T1WI (Figure 2(a)) and T2WI (Figure 2(b)). Simultaneously, MR imaging revealed demyelination around bilateral ventricles and lacunar infarctions in FLAIR (Figure 2(c)). MR angiography showed atherosclerotic alterations of small brain vessels. Proton (1H) MR spectroscopy (MRS) (Figures 3(a) and 3(b)) with region of interest pinpointed on the left basal ganglia lesion displayed a decrease of N-acetylaspartate (NAA) peak and lactate (Lac) doublet. 3D-ASL results (Figure 3(c)) reflected the local perfusion condition, and the increased regional cerebral blood flow (rCBF) suggested hyperperfusion in the corresponding lesion area. Some dotted low signals were noted in the susceptibility weighted imaging (SWI) findings (Figure 3(e)). After two months, we were surprised to find that the abnormal signals of the lesions totally disappeared when we scanned her again, and this demonstrated that the acute bilateral basal ganglia lesions are reversible. The reports have been approved by the Institutional Review Board with patient informed consent.

3. Discussion

Acute movement disorders associated with isolated bilateral basal ganglia lesions have been recognized in patients with end-stage renal disease, particularly in the setting of diabetic nephropathy. Of the 24 cases reviewed by Li et al. [2], gait disturbance (76%), dysarthria (71%), and bradykinesia (47%) were the most common neurologic features. Tremor and rigidity, which are typical of parkinsonism, were noted in only 19% and 38% of all patients, respectively [2]. The neuroradiological abnormalities of patients with uremic encephalopathy are often seen in the cortical rather than bilateral basal ganglia regions [3]. Symmetric bilateral basal ganglia lesions on neuroimaging can be probably caused by carbon monoxide intoxication, hypoxia, toxins, metabolic disorders, small vessel vasculitis, or infection, but these lesions usually do not regress spontaneously [4]. Initial spontaneous improvement of the clinical symptoms and regression of the neuroimaging changes in this syndrome are common [5]. However, in this case, the condition of our patient worsened after three

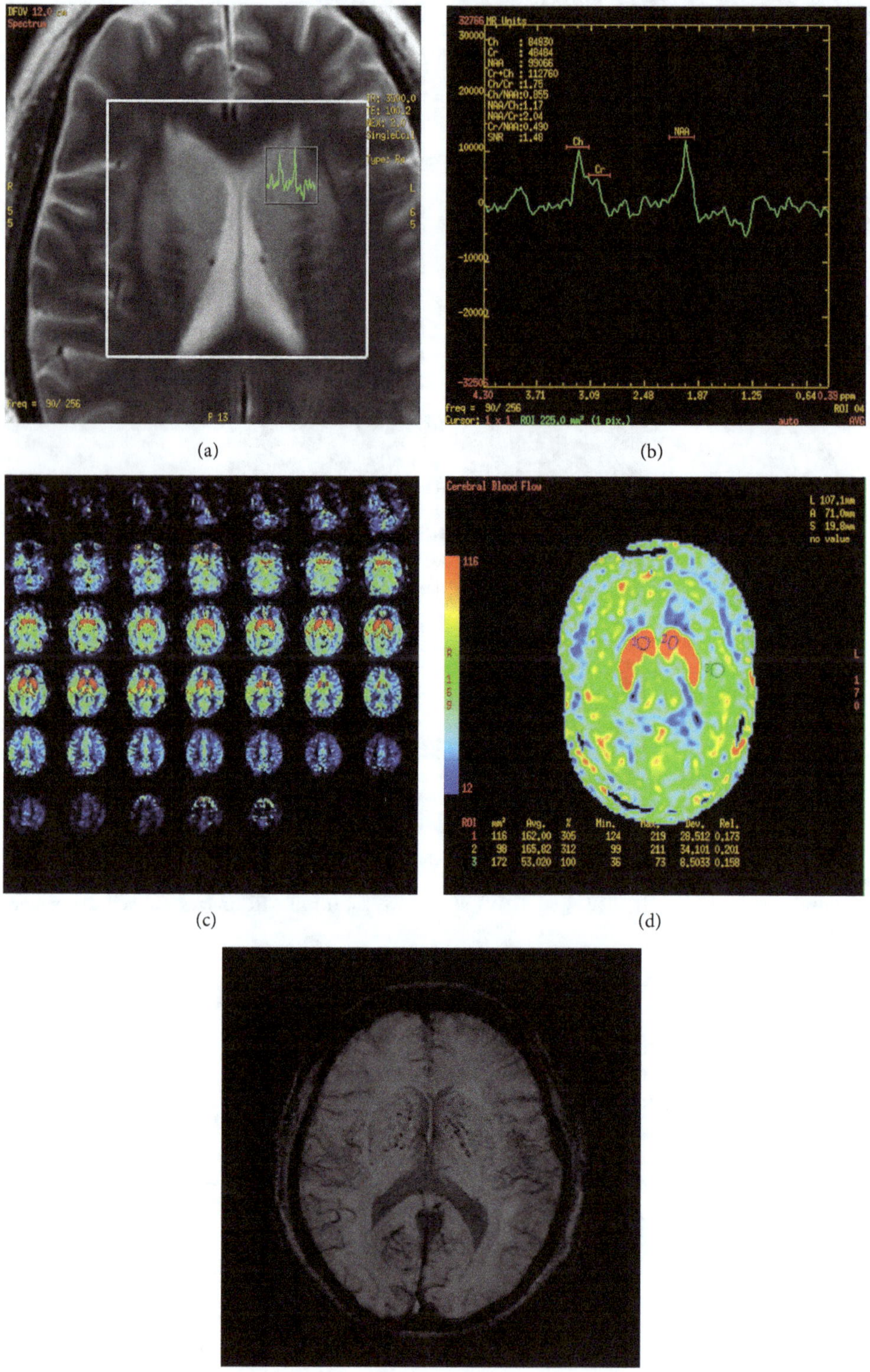

Figure 3: (a, b) MRS with region of interest pinpointed on the left basal ganglia lesion displayed a decrease of NAA/Cr value (2.04) and lactate doublet was detected. (c, d) 3D-ASL showed hyperperfusion in the lesion area and the rCBF was more than 160 mL/(100 g∗min). (e) SWI findings indicated old microbleeds and hemosiderin deposition.

weeks owing to her poor long-term prognosis. Therefore, we believe that the chances of recovery are closely related to the treatment of diabetic uremia.

DWI can be used to identify whether the bilateral ganglia lesions are caused by vasogenic edema or cytotoxic edema. In this case, the ADC maps revealed increased water mobility in the involved regions, which indicates that the edema in this syndrome is not cytotoxic in nature, but increased interstitial fluid from breakdown of autoregulation, and we held similar views to Lee et al. [6]. Nevertheless, some small regions of cytotoxic edema can also be detected in the central parts by DWI. These features, observed also by Kim and his colleagues, indicate that some regions in the basal ganglia lesions are undergoing irreversible cytotoxic damage [7]. The basal ganglia especially globus pallidus have sufficient mitochondrion and blood supply and are susceptible to a wide range of toxins and metabolic changes. The vasogenic edema caused by worsening renal condition and long-term diabetes led to the opening of endothelial tight junctions, autoregulatory dysfunction in small vessels, and disturbance of tissue homeostasis. Thus, being exposed to uremic toxins for a long time will be detrimental to the basal ganglia.

Proton (1H) MR spectroscopy showed a declining NAA peak and a rising lactate peak inside the lesions, which suggests decreased neuron and glucose utilization failure. Our findings coincided with the research of Dicuonzo et al. [8]. In addition, reduced uptake of glucose in the bilateral basal ganglia was demonstrated in two cases by Wang et al., on 18F-fluorodeoxyglucose positron emission tomography (FDG-PET) examination, and the energy use failure is considered to be either dysregulation of the cerebral circulation or lower brain cell activity [9].

3D-ASL findings in the syndrome of acute bilateral basal ganglia lesions have never been reported to date. We found that the rCBF was more than 160 mL/(100 g∗min) in bilateral basal ganglia lesions regions, while the rCBF was less than 60 mL/(100 g∗min) in normal cerebral tissue (Figure 3(d)). Our results were inconsistent with Lin [3] who deemed that the pathophysiological mechanism was acute cerebral hypoperfusion. Whether the perfusion condition remains unchanged or fluctuated since the acute phase is unknown. Patients with this syndrome may have microangiopathic changes and endothelium-dependent dysfunction, which will further induce focal destructive endothelial lesions and the breakdown of blood brain barrier [6]. Under these circumstances, the blood perfusion will likely increase and the rCBF will even be overestimated. Moreover, when the basal ganglia were further exposed to highly elevated uremic or metabolic toxins, the regional cellular metabolism may have been disturbed, or functional disturbance in smooth muscle cells of vessels of the basal ganglia may have been induced, which will ultimately lead to vasodilatation and focal hyperemia [6].

Susceptibility weighted imaging (SWI) is based on the blood oxygen level dependent effect, and it is exquisitely sensitive to paramagnetic substances, such as deoxygenated blood, blood products, iron, and calcium. Some dotted low signals were noted in the bilateral basal ganglia lesions regions, which indicated old microbleeds and hemosiderin deposition instead of calcifications. It may be related to endothelial cell injury and cerebral tiny vessel hemorrhage associated with diabetes mellitus. Focal hyperemia and vascular atherosclerosis may also increase permeability of blood brain barrier.

There are some other theories proposed by other researchers lacking solid evidence. For example, Sheu et al. assumed that changes in hemodynamics caused by hemodialysis are the primary reason for this injury [10]. Park et al. thought that thiamine deficiency can lead to cellular hypoxia and extrapyramidal motor dysfunction due to the blocking of the citric acid cycle [11]. Anyhow, the etiology of such lesions must be multifactorial.

In conclusion, we report the first patient with syndrome of acute bilateral basal ganglia lesions of SWI and 3D-ASL. Although the definitive treatment is uncertain, it is imperative to correct uremic toxins and metabolic derangement in time. The enhanced awareness on this field and the development of neuroimaging will gradually form a full picture of this syndrome.

References

[1] H.-C. Wang, P. Brown, and A. J. Lees, "Acute movement disorders with bilateral basal ganglia lesions in uremia," *Movement Disorders*, vol. 13, no. 6, pp. 952–957, 1998.

[2] J. Y. Z. Li, T. Y. Yong, R. Sebben, E. Khoo, and A. P. S. Disney, "Bilateral basal ganglia lesions in patients with end-stage diabetic nephropathy," *Nephrology*, vol. 13, no. 1, pp. 68–72, 2008.

[3] J.-J. Lin, "Generalized chorea in the syndrome of acute bilateral basal ganglia lesions in patients with diabetic uremia," *Journal of Clinical Neuroscience*, vol. 18, no. 9, pp. 1266–1268, 2011.

[4] J. C. Anderson, M. M. Costantino, and T. Stratford, "Basal ganglia: anatomy, pathology, and imaging characteristics," *Current Problems in Diagnostic Radiology*, vol. 33, no. 1, pp. 28–41, 2004.

[5] H.-C. Wang and S.-J. Cheng, "The syndrome of acute bilateral basal ganglia lesions in diabetic uremic patients," *Journal of Neurology*, vol. 250, no. 8, pp. 948–955, 2003.

[6] E. J. Lee, J.-H. Park, Y. K. Ihn, Y. J. Kim, S. K. Lee, and C. S. Park, "Acute bilateral basal ganglia lesions in diabetic uraemia: diffusion-weighted MRI," *Neuroradiology*, vol. 49, no. 12, pp. 1009–1013, 2007.

[7] T.-K. Kim, S. I. Seo, J. H. Kim, N. J. Lee, and H. Y. Seol, "Diffusion-weighted magnetic resonance imaging in the syndrome of acute bilateral basal ganglia lesions in diabetic uremia," *Movement Disorders*, vol. 21, no. 8, pp. 1267–1270, 2006.

[8] F. Dicuonzo, R. D. Fede, A. Salvati et al., "Acute extrapyramidal disorder with bilateral reversible basal ganglia lesions in a diabetic uremic patient: diffusion-weighted imaging and spectroscopy findings," *Journal of the Neurological Sciences*, vol. 293, no. 1-2, pp. 119–121, 2010.

[9] H.-C. Wang, J. L. Hsu, and Y.-Y. Shen, "Acute bilateral basal ganglia lesions in patients with diabetic uremia: an FDG-PET study," *Clinical Nuclear Medicine*, vol. 29, no. 8, pp. 475–478, 2004.

22

Perfusion Imaging in Autoimmune Encephalitis

Deepak Vallabhaneni,[1] Muhammad Atif Naveed,[2,3] Rajiv Mangla,[3] Awss Zidan,[4] and Rashi I. Mehta[3,5]

[1]*Department of Internal Medicine, SUNY Upstate Medical University, Syracuse, NY, USA*
[2]*Department of Radiology, Shaukat Khanum Memorial Cancer Hospital, Lahore, Pakistan*
[3]*Department of Radiology, SUNY Upstate Medical University, Syracuse, NY 13210, USA*
[4]*Department of Neurology, SUNY Upstate Medical University, Syracuse, NY, USA*
[5]*Department of Radiology, West Virginia University, Morgantown, WV, USA*

Correspondence should be addressed to Rajiv Mangla; manglarajiv@yahoo.com

Academic Editor: Paul Sijens

Encephalitis is characterized by inflammation of brain tissue and has various infectious and noninfectious causes. CSF analysis and MRI usually reveal inflammatory changes although sometimes brain imaging may be normal. Autoimmune encephalitis is caused by antibodies against neuronal synaptic receptors, surface proteins, or intracellular proteins. In this case report, we present a 65-year-old female who presented with a fall and altered mental status. Workup for infectious etiologies was negative and MRI of the brain displayed focal restricted diffusion with corresponding T2-FLAIR hyperintensity involving gray matter structures, making the diagnosis unclear. CT perfusion of the brain demonstrated increased cerebral blood volume and cerebral blood flow in the left parietooccipital gray matter, with corresponding normal mean transit time. Following treatment failure with acyclovir, antibiotics, and steroids, the patient was found to be positive for GAD65 antibodies and diagnosed with autoimmune encephalitis. Symptoms markedly improved with plasmapheresis. Autoimmune encephalitis rarely causes restricted diffusion and this is the first case report to describe corresponding hyperperfusion on CT perfusion study.

1. Introduction

Encephalitis is characterized by inflammation of brain tissue, causing symptoms such as headache, fever, altered mental status, seizures, and/or focal neurologic deficits. CSF analysis and MRI usually reveal the findings of inflammatory changes although normal findings are not uncommon. Etiologies of encephalitis are diverse, but autoimmunity has been increasingly identified. Autoimmune encephalitis is caused by antibodies against neuronal synaptic receptors and surface or intracellular proteins [1]. Despite the severity of symptoms that such antibodies can entail, immunotherapy has been shown to be highly effective [2]. Clinical signs specifically pointing to autoimmune encephalitis include subacute memory loss, psychiatric symptoms, and sleep disturbance [3]. Conversely, infectious features such as fever, vomiting, and MRI contrast enhancement are rarely seen in autoimmune encephalitis [4]. As a diagnosis of exclusion, it is important to rule out infectious etiology as well as malignant, metabolic, and toxic etiologies before arriving at the diagnosis of autoimmune encephalitis [3]. Subsequently, a search for autoreactive antibodies ensues in both serum and CSF [3]. EEG findings may include slow activity focally or as background, with or without epileptiform discharges. On imaging, MRI can range from normal to T2-FLAIR scattered hyperintensities [3].

2. Case Report

A 65-year-old female, with previous medical history of diabetes mellitus, stroke, hypertension, hypokalemia, and bipolar disorder, presented with gradually progressive subacute alteration of mental status manifesting as fluctuating awareness and impairment of cognitive functions including memory, language, and processing. Simultaneously, she

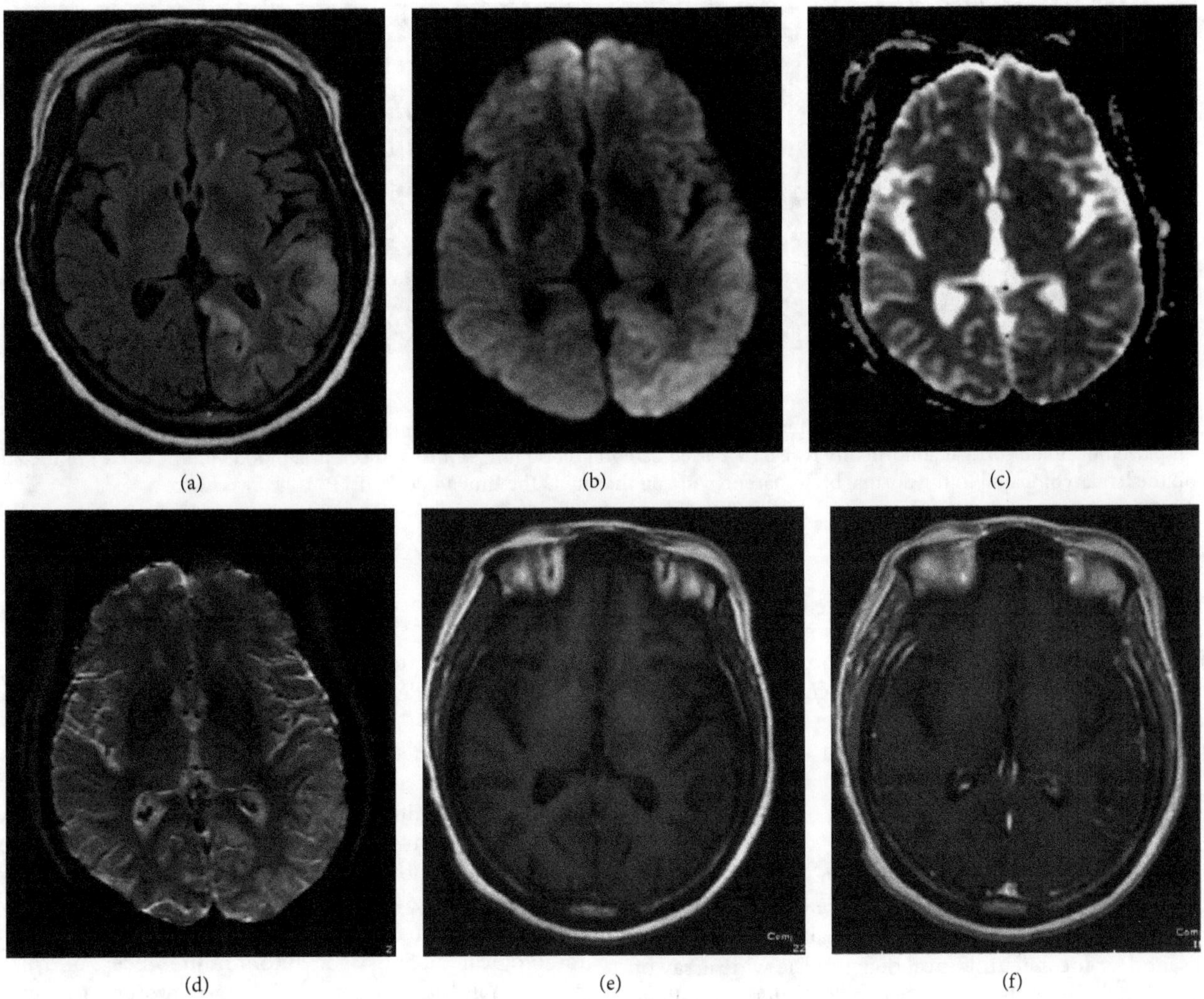

FIGURE 1: 64-year-old female with confusion, right lower extremity weakness, and questionable encephalitis. Axial FLAIR MR image (a) shows increased signal intensity and gyriform swelling in the cortex and subcortical white matter of the left parietooccipital lobe and a focus in the left thalamus. Diffusion weighed (b) and attenuation diffusion coefficient, ADC, MR images (c) reveal mild decreased diffusivity. No susceptibility artifact or contrast enhancement is observed on axial susceptibility weighted image, SWI (d), and axial T1 weighted (e) and axial T1 weighted postgadolinium images (f), respectively.

developed motor deficits leading to repetitive falls and right hemiparesis. Spasticity with involuntarily posturing later ensued. Initial CSF analysis revealed mild monocytic pleocytosis, with no identified bacterial, viral, or fungal pathogens. The patient was monitored closely for convulsive and/or nonconvulsive seizures during the time of her admission by three-day video EEG monitoring, and three spot EEGs, all within 10 days of the CT perfusion, and none of them demonstrated the transformation of the epileptogenic discharges into seizures. There was no change in mental status or neurological examination to suggest emergence of seizures on the day of CT perfusion. MRI of the brain showed left parietooccipital cortical swelling with decreased diffusivity and abnormal hyperintense signal on T2- FLAIR sequences, suggesting encephalitic etiology (Figure 1). CT perfusion of the brain showed increased cerebral blood volume (CBV) and cerebral blood flow (CBF) and corresponding decreased time to peak (TTP) in the left parietooccipital cortex as compared to the contralateral normal brain tissue (Figure 2). Empiric treatment with steroids did not lead to significant improvement. Serum, and then later CSF, paraneoplastic epilepsy panel was positive for GAD65 antibodies with high titers (serum 1068 nmol/L, normal <= 0.02). The lab evaluation was performed at Mayo Medical Laboratories which suggest a cutoff of 20 nmol/L for major neurologic disease.

All other antibodies were tested negative in serum and CSF in a full antibody workup (Mayo panel). The search for a causative tumor by full-body CT scans at the time of the presentation and then one year later was negative. A concomitant elevation of Thyroid Peroxidase antibodies occurred transiently and then resolved. Immunomodulating treatment with plasmapheresis resulted in definite, yet incomplete, improvement. Subsequent CSF analysis revealed increased GAD65 antibodies 1.83 nmol/l, normal <= 0.02. Due to incomplete clinical improvement, immunosuppression with Rituximab was initiated. Five months later, the

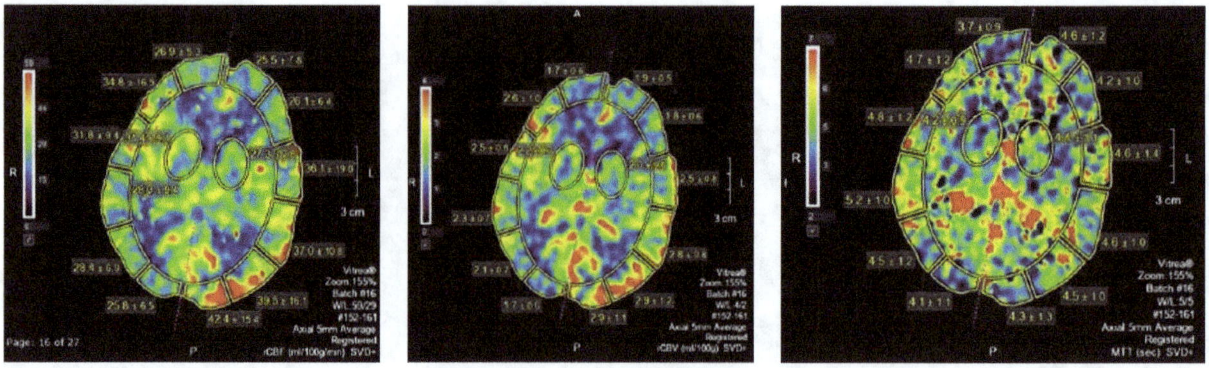

(a) (b) (c)

FIGURE 2: CT perfusion was performed 10 days after the initial MRI imaging. The postprocessed CT perfusion maps in axial plane at the level of the left parietooccipital cortical abnormality reveal increased cerebral blood flow (CBF) and cerebral blood volume (CBV) in the affected cortex on the left as compared to the normal brain parenchyma on the right. The time to peak (TTP) is decreased.

patient had recurrence of right-sided weakness and gait problems along with new right-sided sensory loss with MRI displaying worsening of the left parietooccipital lesion. At the time of this manuscript, the patient continues to show clinical improvement from her original presentation but with persistent significant disability.

3. Discussion

Autoimmune encephalitis can present in both adults and children [5]. The clinical manifestations are variable and may include prodromal symptoms, headache, altered mentation, seizures, and/or focal neurological deficits. The wide array of manifestations frequently leads to a diverse differential diagnosis with a myriad of investigative imaging studies. A variety of neuronal antibodies have been identified in autoimmune encephalitides. The vast majority of these encephalitides share some clinical and radiological features, although some uniqueness exists based on the location of the underlying immune response [6].

Glutamic acid decarboxylase (GAD) is an intracellular enzyme that is present at the terminal synaptic levels and catalyzes the synthesis of gamma-aminobutyric acid, the major inhibitory neurotransmitter in the CNS [7]. The anti-GAD antibodies typically cause a form of autoimmune encephalitis with classic temporal lobe lesions on MR imaging with the expected clinical findings of limbic encephalitis, and/or additional features of stiff person syndrome with early and prominent development of seizures [6].

This case demonstrates certain distinct clinical and radiological findings. First, this patient presented with extralimbic encephalitis based on the MRI findings, and the correlating EEG, which is atypical for GAD65 autoimmune encephalitis, which is frequently limbic in location [8]. Brain MRI showed cortical restricted diffusion which pathophysiologically signifies cytotoxic edema limiting water content in cells [9]. Second, the presence of hyperperfusion on CT perfusion exam of the brain with corresponding decreased diffusivity and T2-FLAIR hyperintensity in the cortex of the left parietooccipital lobe was observed. A very recent case report (in December 2017) has also found increased cerebral blood flow on arterial spin labelling in in anti-NMDA receptor encephalitis [10]. This case illustrates similar findings in anti-GAD encephalitis with CT perfusion. It has also been reported that perfusion imaging can demonstrate abnormality in autoimmune encephalitis even before the lesions are identifiable on conventional MRI sequences. The exact mechanism of focal increased perfusion in autoimmune encephalitis is not known but possibility of loss of cerebral vascular autoregulation has been suggested. In conclusion, this case demonstrates the utility of perfusion imaging in radiological diagnosis of autoimmune encephalitis, which may enable earlier diagnosis, more prompt therapy, and improved patient outcome.

References

[1] T. Armangue, M. Petit-Pedrol, and J. Dalmau, "Autoimmune encephalitis in children," *Journal of Child Neurology*, vol. 27, no. 11, pp. 1460–1469, 2012.

[2] E. Lancaster, E. Martinez-Hernandez, and J. Dalmau, "Encephalitis and antibodies to synaptic and neuronal cell surface proteins," *Neurology*, vol. 77, no. 2, pp. 179–189, 2011.

[3] B. Kalman, "Autoimmune encephalitides: A broadening field of treatable conditions," *The Neurologist*, vol. 22, no. 1, pp. 1–13, 2017.

[4] E. Lancaster, "The diagnosis and treatment of autoimmune encephalitis," *Journal of Clinical Neurology*, vol. 12, no. 1, pp. 1–13, 2016.

[5] J. Dalmau, E. Lancaster, E. Martinez-Hernandez, M. R. Rosenfeld, and R. Balice-Gordon, "Clinical experience and laboratory investigations in patients with anti-NMDAR encephalitis," *The Lancet Neurology*, vol. 10, no. 1, pp. 63–74, 2011.

[6] B. Kelley, S. Patel, H. Marin, J. Corrigan, P. Mitsias, and B. Griffith, "Autoimmune encephalitis: pathophysiology and imaging review of an overlooked diagnosis," *American Journal of Neuroradiology*, vol. 38, no. 6, pp. 1070–1078, 2017.

[7] C. S. Pinal and A. J. Tobin, "Uniqueness and redundancy in GABA production," *Perspectives on developmental neurobiology*, vol. 5, no. 2-3, pp. 109–118, 1998.

[8] M. P. Malter, C. Helmstaedter, H. Urbach, A. Vincent, and C. G. Bien, "Antibodies to glutamic acid decarboxylase define a form of limbic encephalitis," *Annals of Neurology*, vol. 67, no. 4, pp. 470–478, 2010.

[9] O. Ozbek, O. Koç, Y. Paksoy, K. Aydin, and A. Nayman, "Epstein-Barr virus encephalitis: Findings of MRI, MRS, diffusion and perfusion," *The Turkish Journal of Pediatrics*, vol. 53, no. 6, pp. 680–683, 2011.

[10] J. R. Sachs, M. E. Zapadka, G. S. Popli, and J. H. Burdette, "Arterial spin labeling perfusion imaging demonstrates cerebral hyperperfusion in anti-NMDAR encephalitis," *Radiology Case Reports*, vol. 12, no. 4, pp. 833–837, 2017.

23

Traumatic Haemorrhagic Cervical Lymphadenopathy with Underlying Infectious Mononucleosis

George Rahmani and Sarah Power

Department of Radiology, Beaumont Hospital, Dublin, Ireland

Correspondence should be addressed to George Rahmani; george.rahmani@gmail.com

Academic Editor: Lorenzo Monfardini

A 16-year-old male presented to the Emergency Department with a painful 3 × 3 cm left-sided neck swelling six hours following blunt trauma to the neck from a heavy swinging door. A CT angiogram was performed which revealed a large haemorrhagic lymph node as well as generalised cervical lymphadenopathy. The patient was eventually diagnosed with infectious mononucleosis. This case report describes a rare case of traumatic haemorrhagic cervical lymphadenopathy with an underlying diagnosis of infectious mononucleosis.

1. Introduction

Patients with infectious mononucleosis most commonly present with a triad of fever, lymphadenopathy, and pharyngitis [1]. Splenomegaly can also occur and these patients have an increased risk of traumatic splenic rupture [2]. Lymphadenopathy as a result of trauma is quite rare with only a handful of case reports in the literature [3, 4]. Haemorrhagic lymphadenopathy classically occurs in the core of necrotic lymph nodes that are affected by malignancy, either primary malignancy, as in lymphoma, or secondary metastasis [5]. Haemorrhagic lymphadenopathy has also been described in other conditions such as primary al amyloidosis [6]. We describe a case of haemorrhagic cervical lymphadenopathy following blunt force trauma to the neck in a patient with an underlying diagnosis of infectious mononucleosis.

2. Case

A 16-year-old male presented to the Emergency Department with a painful 3 × 3 cm left-sided neck swelling six hours following blunt trauma to the neck from a heavy swinging door. His vital signs were normal and he was alert and orientated in time, place, and person. His neurological examination was unremarkable. The swelling was nonpulsatile, but given the history of rapid growth, a computed tomography (CT) angiogram was performed. It did not demonstrate any vascular injury but revealed significant bilateral cervical lymphadenopathy, largest on the left side, level II measuring 4 × 3.4 × 2.5 cm, with mixed density suggestive of either a necrotic lymph node or, given the history of trauma and rapid swelling, haemorrhage into the lymph node (Figure 1). Of note, the lymphadenopathy showed signs of hypervascularity which was more in keeping with an infectious aetiology (Figures 2 and 3). The patient denied symptoms of weight loss or night sweats but complained of minor fatigue in recent weeks.

An ultrasound scan was performed to further characterise the lymphadenopathy, which demonstrated heterogeneous internal echoes with absent colour Doppler flow in the anterior aspect of the lesion (Figures 4 and 5). Ultrasonography also demonstrated generalised hypervascular cervical lymphadenopathy, again reflective of an infectious aetiology (Figure 6). A CT thorax did not demonstrate lymphadenopathy elsewhere.

A full blood count revealed a mild leucocytosis (12.8×10^9; normal range $4–11 \times 10^9$) with elevated monocytes (1.26×10^9; normal range $0.2–1.0 \times 10^9$). Of note, the lymphocyte count of 3.83×10^9 was within normal limits ($1.00–4.00 \times 10^9$) and

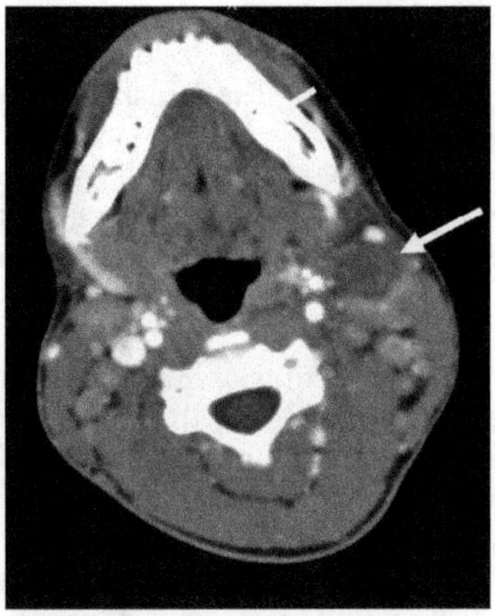

FIGURE 1: Axial CT angiogram showing bilateral cervical lymphadenopathy, the largest of which measures 4 × 3.4 × 2.5 cm (arrow). The posterior portion of the node demonstrates arterial phase enhancement while the anterior portion does not demonstrate it. This mixed density mass has the appearance of a necrotic or haemorrhagic lymph node.

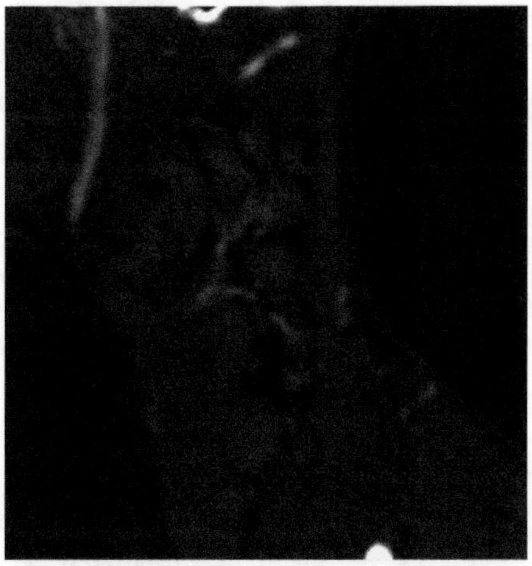

FIGURE 2: Sagittal CT angiogram demonstrating extensive hypervascularity of lymph nodes in the left neck.

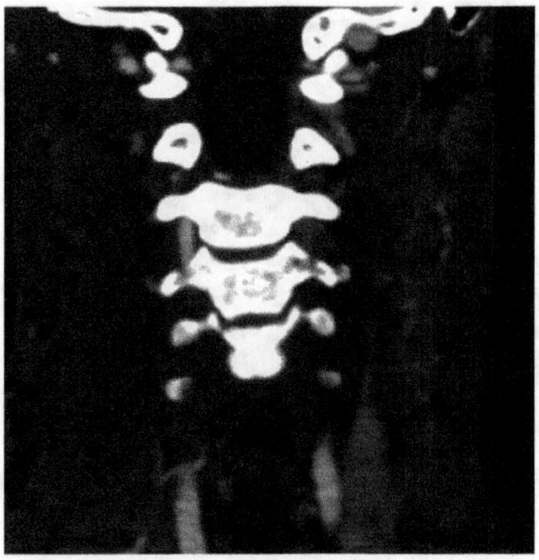

FIGURE 3: Coronal CT angiogram of the neck demonstrating extensive hypervascularity of cervical lymph nodes bilaterally which are more pronounced on the left side.

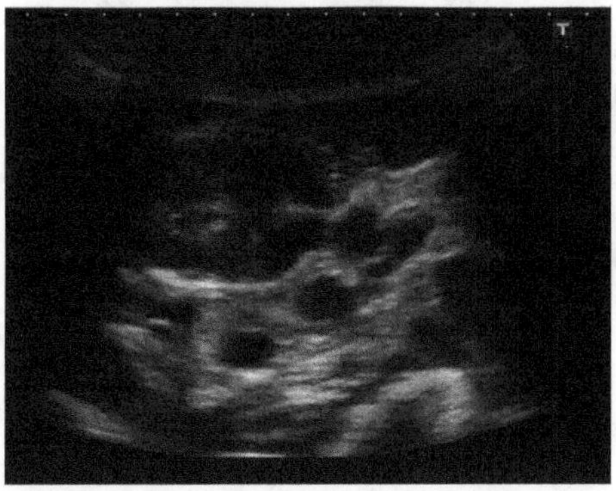

FIGURE 4: Ultrasound scan showing an enlarged left cervical lymph node with heterogeneous echogenicity.

additional microscopy did not demonstrate a disproportionate increase in atypical lymphocytes. The patient's coagulation profile was also normal.

A monospot test was positive for the presence of heterophile antibodies and further serological testing was carried out which detected the presence of IgM and IgG antibodies to the Epstein-Barr viral capsid antigen (VCA). Serological testing was negative for *Cytomegalovirus*, *Toxoplasma gondii*, *Treponema pallidum*, and hepatitis B and hepatitis C. Testing for IgG to Epstein-Barr nuclear antigen (EBNA) was also negative which helped to rule out a previous EBV infection.

In light of positive EBV serology and generalised hypervascular cervical lymphadenopathy, a diagnosis of infectious mononucleosis was made. Given the recent history of trauma, the left-sided neck swelling was determined to be a haemorrhagic lymph node. To the best of our knowledge, this is the first report of traumatic haemorrhagic cervical lymphadenopathy with an underlying diagnosis of infectious mononucleosis.

3. Discussion

Infectious mononucleosis, commonly referred to as "glandular fever," is one of the most common causes of prolonged illness in young adults. It is the manifestation of primary Epstein-Barr virus infection, which is latent in approximately 90% of the population [1]. The vast majority of people that have been exposed to EBV are asymptomatic. Approximately one-third of young adults will develop symptoms, of which the triad of fever, lymphadenopathy, and pharyngitis is found in 50% of cases [7, 8]. Other physical manifestations of infectious mononucleosis include splenomegaly, hepatomegaly, or palatal petechiae, which are each present in approximately 10% of cases [1]. The diagnosis is confirmed by serology; the presence of heterophile antibody is used as a rapid screening test with a sensitivity of 70–90% and specificity of 96–99% with rare false positives occurring in conditions such as viral hepatitis and *Cytomegalovirus* infection [9]. Testing for the

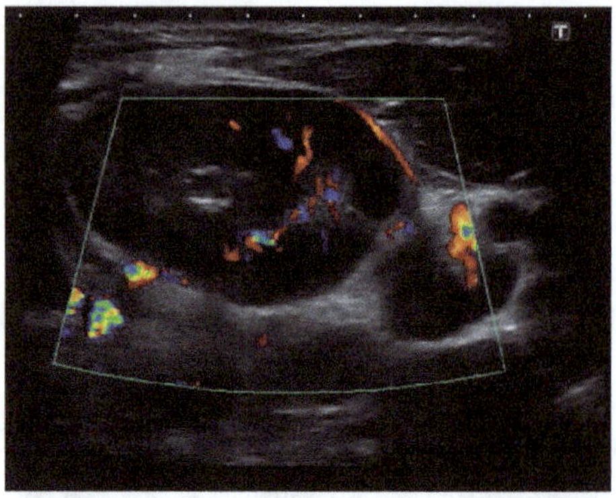

Figure 5: Ultrasound scan of the lesion in question showing colour Doppler flow in the posterior aspect of the lesion only.

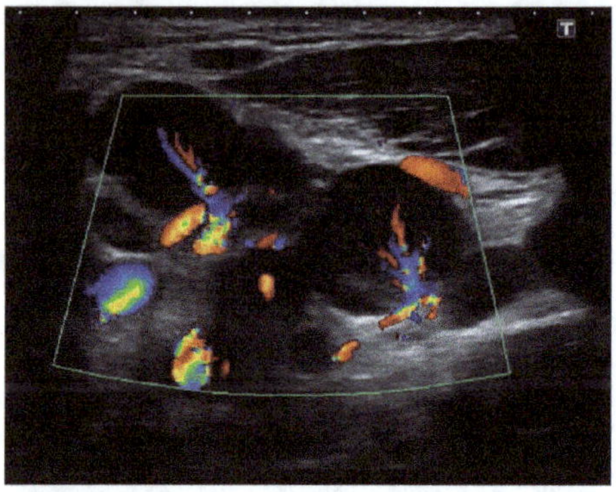

Figure 6: Ultrasound scan showing increased colour Doppler flow through enlarged left cervical lymph nodes.

presence of IgG and IgM antibodies to the Epstein-Barr VCA is more sensitive and specific for infectious mononucleosis and these antibodies are usually present by the time the disease has manifested clinically. Anti-VCA IgM remains in the circulation for approximately 1-2 months, while anti-VCA IgG will persist for life. The presence of IgG to EBNA suggests past EBV infection and in the context of positive serology is suggestive of reactivation of latent EBV.

Proliferation of mononuclear cells causes lymphadenopathy associated with infectious mononucleosis and can mimic other more serious underlying conditions, such as lymphoma. In some rare cases, these lymph nodes have been reported to contain geographic areas of necrosis and infarction [3, 10]. With regard to trauma, a case of lymph node infarction due to chronic trauma in the knee of a healthy patient has been previously described, mimicking synovial sarcoma on MRI [4]. In this case, the patient did not have underlying lymphadenopathy, and there was a history of chronic minor traumas, rather than an acute precipitory event.

The differential diagnosis for cervical lymphadenopathy would include other infectious aetiologies including viruses such as cytomegalovirus and herpes simplex virus, bacterial infections and mycobacterium infections like tuberculosis, and *Mycobacterium avium*-intracellulare complex infections. Malignancy is an important differential that must be ruled out including lymphoma and metastases from head and neck tumours. Other neoplastic lesions can cause cervical lymphadenopathy including Castleman disease and Kaposi sarcoma.

In our case, the appearance of the lymph node on CT and ultrasound was that of a heterogeneous soft tissue mass with absence of blood flow/contrast enhancement in the anterior portion. The differential diagnosis for the appearance of such a lesion was that of a necrotic or haemorrhagic lymph node. While cases of lymph node necrosis have been previously described in cases of infectious mononucleosis, given the acute history of trauma and the rapid appearance of the swelling, traumatic haemorrhage into the underlying abnormal lymph node is a more likely diagnosis. It may be that the mechanism of such an injury is likened to traumatic splenic rupture in the context of splenomegaly in response to EBV infection [2]. To the best of our knowledge, this is the first report of traumatic haemorrhagic cervical lymphadenopathy leading to an underlying diagnosis of infectious mononucleosis.

References

[1] J. I. Cohen, "Epstein-Barr virus infection," *The New England Journal of Medicine*, vol. 343, no. 7, pp. 481–492, 2000.

[2] I. M. Rutkow, "Rupture of the spleen in infectious mononucleosis: a critical review," *Archives of Surgery*, vol. 113, no. 6, pp. 718–720, 1978.

[3] M. Kojima, S. Nakamura, S. Sugihara, N. Sakata, and N. Masawa, "Lymph node infarction associated with infectious mononucleosis: Report of a case resembling lymph node infarction associated with malignant lymphoma," *International Journal of Surgical Pathology*, vol. 10, no. 3, pp. 223–226, 2002.

[4] R. Sinha, M. Sharma, and F. W. Smith, "Post-traumatic lymph node infarction in the knee mimicking synovial sarcoma," *Injury Extra*, vol. 37, no. 9, pp. 334–337, 2006.

[5] A. W. Bazemore and D. R. Smucker, "Lymphadenopathy and malignancy," *American Family Physician*, vol. 66, no. 11, pp. 2103–2110, 2002.

[6] J. P. Hanley, F. R. MacLean, J. L. Evans et al., "Hemorrhagic lymphadenopathy as a presenting feature of primary AL amyloidosis," *Pathology*, vol. 32, no. 1, pp. 21–23, 2000.

[7] K. F. Macsween and D. H. Crawford, "Epstein-Barr virus - Recent advances," *The Lancet Infectious Diseases*, vol. 3, no. 3, pp. 131–140, 2003.

[8] R. J. Hoagland, "The incubation period of infectious mononucleosis," *American Journal of Public Health and the Nation's Health*, vol. 54, pp. 1699–1705, 1964.

[9] F. Elgh and M. Linderholm, "Evaluation of six commercially available kits using purified heterophile antigen for the rapid diagnosis of infectious mononucleosis compared with Epstein-Barr virus-specific serology," *Clinical and Diagnostic Virology*, vol. 7, no. 1, pp. 17–21, 1996.

[10] M. Kojima, S. Nakamura, H. Itoh, Y. Yamane, S. Miyawaki, and N. Masawa, "Lymph node lesion in infectious mononucleosis showing geographic necrosis containing cytologically atypically B-cells. A case report," *Pathology - Research and Practice*, vol. 200, no. 1, pp. 53–57, 2004.

24

Sarcoid of the Upper Humerus Found Incidentally on MR Images Obtained for Work-Up of Rotator Cuff Tear Where Compromised Tissue Quality Was a Concern for Surgical Success

Tanner R. Henrie[1] and John G. Skedros[2,3,4]

[1] *Tulane University School of Medicine, New Orleans, LA, USA*
[2] *The University of Utah Department of Orthopaedic Surgery, Salt Lake City, UT, USA*
[3] *Utah Orthopaedic Specialists, Salt Lake City, UT, USA*
[4] *Intermountain Medical Center, Salt Lake City, UT, USA*

Correspondence should be addressed to John G. Skedros; jskedrosmd@uosmd.com

Academic Editor: Isao Ito

Sarcoidosis is an idiopathic systemic inflammatory disorder characterized histologically by noncaseating granulomas. The pathogenesis likely includes genetic, immunologic, and environmental factors. The lungs, skin, and eyes are most commonly affected. Although bone involvement is possible, sarcoidosis of the humerus is rare, with few cases reported. Furthermore, we are unaware of any reports of sarcoidosis of the upper humerus with a coexisting rotator cuff tear. We report the case of a 50-year-old female with sarcoidosis of the humerus and a coexisting tear of the supraspinatus tendon. Her medical history includes type 2 diabetes, depression, and fatigue. She had chronic shoulder pain that worsened after her dog jerked on the leash. Radiographs were grossly normal. Subsequent magnetic resonance imaging (MRI) demonstrated a possible small full-thickness rotator cuff tear. Multiple rounded lesions were also noted within the proximal humerus. A biopsy demonstrated noncaseating granulomas, confirming the diagnosis of sarcoidosis. There was concern that her sarcoid lesions would compromise bone quality, limiting options for surgical repair of her rotator cuff tear. However, it was determined that her lesion did not involve cortical bone, and surgery was performed. During surgery, the supraspinatus tendon was found to be partially torn and was treated with arthroscopic debridement and acromioplasty. An excellent result was ultimately achieved after her rheumatologist started adalimumab injections. This case demonstrates that there can be a rare incidental finding of osseous sarcoid lesions in the upper humerus where the bone might be compromised in the location of a planned rotator cuff repair.

1. Introduction

Grunewald et al. [1] described sarcoidosis as a systemic inflammatory disorder characterized by tissue infiltration by mononuclear phagocytes and lymphocytes with associated noncaseating granuloma formation. The proposed pathogenesis includes a combination of genetic, immunologic, and environmental factors [2]. Although the etiology of sarcoidosis remains uncertain, there is a growing body of evidence suggesting a relationship between sarcoidosis and an infectious process [2, 3].

Lung involvement is the most common manifestation of sarcoidosis, being present in over 90% of patients [4]. The skin and eyes are also commonly affected [5, 6]. Bone involvement in sarcoidosis is uncommon, affecting roughly 1–13% of patients [5, 6]. However, bone involvement may be underestimated, as approximately 38% of patients with sarcoidosis demonstrate radionuclide bone scan abnormalities [7]. Bone lesions may cause pain, but are typically asymptomatic [8]. The more commonly affected bones are small tubular bones of the appendicular skeleton, while axial bones are typically spared [6]. Osseous sarcoid may affect

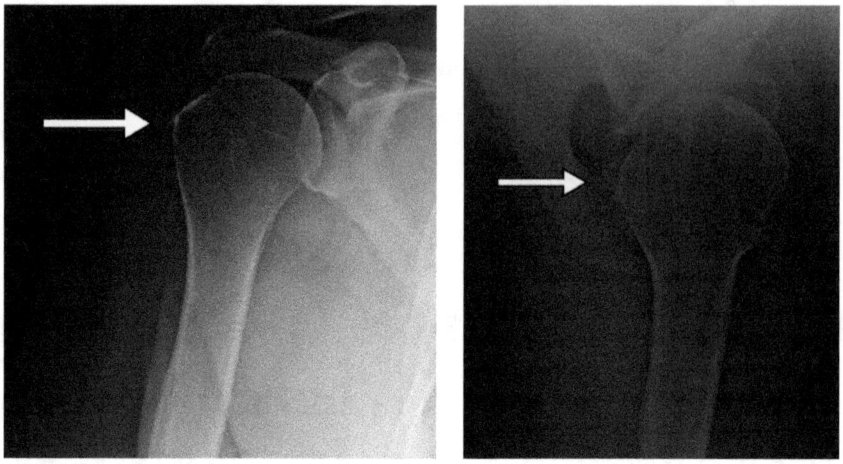

(a) (b)

FIGURE 1: Radiographs with no distinct bone lesions noted. However, subtle decrease in trabecular bone density adjacent to the greater tuberosity is noted in (a) near the arrow tip. The arrows also indicate mild calcific tendinitis.

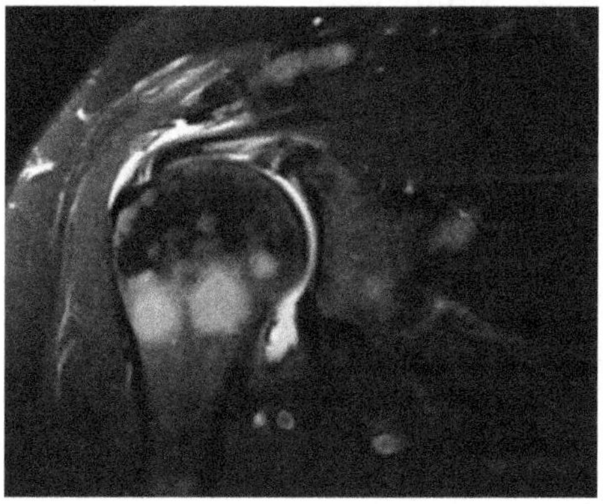

FIGURE 2: MRI demonstrating sarcoid lesions of the humerus.

the hands, feet, tibia, skull, and vertebrae, among other bones. It typically causes nonspecific osteolytic lesions that can mimic neoplasms (e.g., osteoblastoma, metastases, or multiple myeloma), osteomyelitis, or bone cysts [5, 8–12].

Sarcoidosis of the humerus is rare and only a few cases have been reported [7–9, 11, 13–15]. We report a rare case where sarcoidosis of the upper humerus was found incidentally with an MRI scan that was obtained for work-up of a rotator cuff tear.

2. Case Presentation

A 50-year-old female (BMI = 35) presented to our clinic in Salt Lake City, Utah, USA, with a chief complaint of right shoulder pain. She has a history of non-insulin-dependent diabetes, hypertension, anxiety, depression, and fatigue. Her medications included hydroxyzine for anxiety, ibuprofen for joint pains, lisinopril for hypertension, and pioglitazone tablets and liraglutide (Victoza®; Novo Nordisk A/S, Bagsvaerd, Denmark) subcutaneous injections for diabetes. She had a several-year history of intermittent low-grade right shoulder pain that was attributed to subacromial bursitis. This had been treated with subacromial corticosteroid injections and physical therapy, which only gave moderate pain relief.

Her right shoulder pain worsened acutely in April 2016 after her dog jerked on the leash, almost causing her to fall. Radiographs obtained one month later demonstrated a hooked acromion and subtle decrease in trabecular bone density adjacent to the greater tuberosity, but no distinct bone lesions were noted (Figure 1). The subtle decrease in trabecular bone was considered to possibly reflect disuse osteopenia associated with a long-standing rotator cuff tear [16–18]. Subsequent MRI with intra-articular contrast was obtained which demonstrated what was interpreted as a small full-thickness tear of the supraspinatus tendon. The MR images also revealed multiple quasi-circular lesions within the proximal humerus that were suggestive of metastases or multiple myeloma (Figure 2). Bone lesions were also in close proximity to the insertion of the supraspinatus tendon.

Ten days prior to the radiographs, she had an unrelated skin biopsy of a facial lesion that was diagnosed as sarcoidosis. A biopsy of the humeral lesions seen on MRI revealed noncaseating granulomatous inflammation, confirming osseous sarcoid of the humerus (Figure 3). Additionally, mediastinal

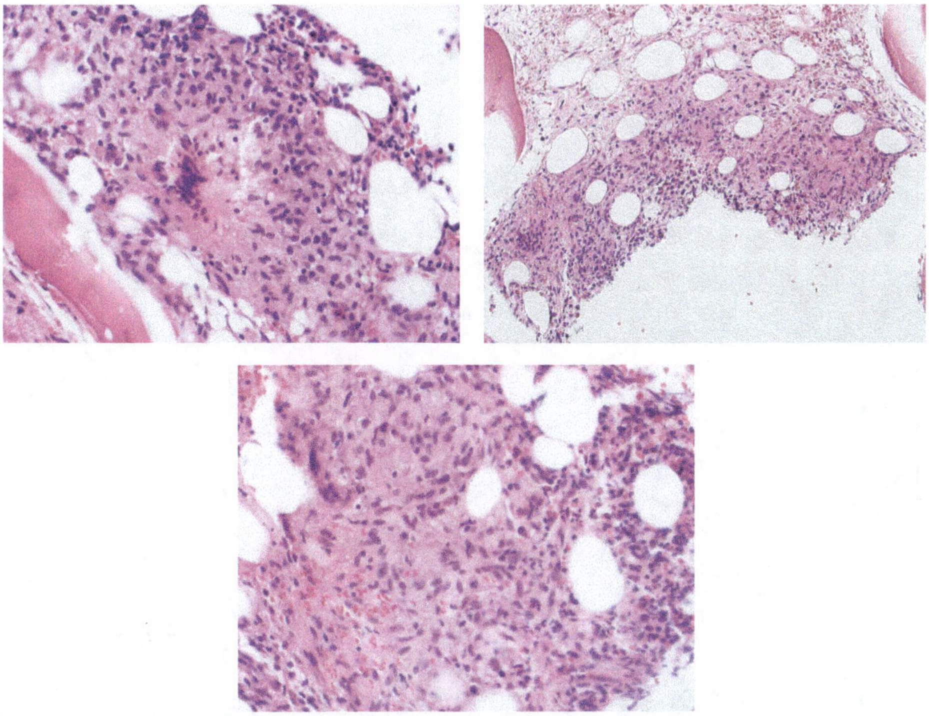

Figure 3: Biopsy of humeral lesions demonstrating noncaseating granulomas.

and hilar adenopathy seen on a subsequent chest computed tomography (CT) were consistent with the diagnosis of sarcoidosis.

With osseous sarcoid lesions, there is concern that pathologic disturbances in bone architecture could make surgical repair involving cortical bone difficult [19]. For example, Ungprasert et al. [20] reported an increased incidence of fragility fracture in the proximal humerus in patients with sarcoidosis of the humerus. However, given that our patient's humeral lesions involved cancellous bone, while cortical bone was spared, we concluded that the lesions were not a contraindication to a standard surgical repair of the rotator cuff tear. This is because only a small amount of cortical bone needs to be removed during the repair of a small rotator cuff tear [18, 21]. However, larger tears and/or cases with more invasive sarcoid lesions might require advanced repair techniques [22, 23]. This was not a concern in our patient's case because during surgery only a low-grade partial tear was found. Surgical treatment was done by JGS and included arthroscopic debridement, bursectomy, and acromioplasty [24, 25]. The shavings from the surgical procedure were not obtained for histological analysis. However, the tissues did not appear to be grossly abnormal.

Despite being enrolled in a physical therapy program at two weeks after surgery, she had an unusually prolonged recovery because of flares of pain in addition to shoulder stiffness. Treatment for this included a one-time seven-day course of an oral corticosteroid on a tapered dose schedule (methylprednisolone tablets; Medrol® dose pack; Pfizer Inc., New York, USA). Because the improvement with this was less than satisfactory, two sets of subacromial and glenohumeral corticosteroid injections (Depo-Medrol injectable suspension; Pfizer Inc., New York, USA) were administered two months apart [26]. Supervised physical therapy was also continued.

Because of continuing shoulder and generalized pain flares coupled with a great sense of fatigue, the patient consulted with a rheumatologist who prescribed adalimumab (Humira®, AbbVie Inc., North Chicago, Illinois, USA) subcutaneous injections once every other week. Adalimumab is a tumor necrosis factor-alpha (TNF-α) inhibitor that was selected over other first-line therapies for sarcoidosis because of its greater effect on sarcoidosis-associated fatigue [27]. Our patient reported that the adalimumab injections greatly improved her fatigue and thereby enhanced her ability to participate in physical therapy. At final postoperative follow-up at 48 months after her shoulder surgery the patient reported that she had an excellent result that included complete pain relief and restoration of full range of motion and strength.

3. Discussion

Sarcoidosis of the humerus is exceptionally rare, and few cases have ever been reported. To our knowledge, sarcoidosis of the humerus with a coexisting rotator cuff tear has not been reported. Importantly for this case, osseous sarcoidosis can compromise normal bone architecture and lead to pathologic fractures, thus potentially complicating surgical procedures [19]. However, our patient had a successful surgical debridement of her rotator cuff tear despite bony involvement of her sarcoidosis.

One of the challenges in diagnosing osseous sarcoidosis is that while bony lesions may cause pain, most patients are asymptomatic [8, 19]. Whether or not our patient's shoulder

Table 1: Radiological findings of sarcoid of the humerus.

Authors	Patient demographics	Presentation	Past medical history	Radiological findings	Diagnosis	Management
Mehrotra et al. 2011	59-year-old woman	Left facial palsy after coryzal illness, otherwise asymptomatic	Facial nerve palsy	Radiographs: lytic lesions in the humerus CT thorax/abdomen: low attenuation liver lesions and widespread vertebral, rib, pelvic lytic lesions	Biopsy	Did not receive steroids, has been stable for one year. Still has facial palsy.
Chaudhry and Richardson 2006	50-year-old man	Two-month history of right shoulder pain and mildly decreased mobility	Pulmonary sarcoidosis for eight years	Radiograph: faint sclerotic lesion in the inferomedial humeral head MRI: abnormal marrow signal intensity in the medial humeral head. Low signal intensity on both T1- and T2-weighted images. STIR image demonstrated a hyperintense signal focus within the marrow without cortical involvement CT: focal area of mild sclerosis in the inferomedial humeral head 99mTc radionuclide scan: mild uptake in the humeral head	Biopsy	Did not receive steroids (history of psychiatric side effects) and was treated with radiotherapy. His symptoms later improved.
Yachoui et al. 2015	58-year-old Caucasian woman	Six months of intermittent shoulder pain that eventually became constant	Hypertension, tonsillectomy	Radiograph: normal MRI: high signal intensity on T2 fat suppressed sequence, intermediate intensity on T1-weighted imaging with postcontrast enhancement in humeral metaphysis CT: hilar and mediastinal adenopathy PET: numerous areas of increased activity	Biopsy	Their patient improved after a course of prednisone and hydroxychloroquine.
Henrie and Skedros 2018	50-year-old woman	Several-year history of intermittent low-grade right shoulder pain, which worsened acutely after her dog jerked on the leash	Diabetes, hypertension, anxiety, depression, and fatigue	Radiograph: normal MRI: multiple lytic bone lesions of humerus	Biopsy	Did not receive steroids (contraindicated given history of diabetes). Received prolonged physical therapy and adalimumab injections.

pain was in fact due mostly to subacromial bursitis or underlying sarcoidosis, or a combination of the two, is uncertain. Another challenge in the diagnosis of osseous sarcoidosis is that these lesions might not appear on radiographs, and more sensitive imaging modalities like MRI are needed to make the diagnosis. MRI of sarcoidosis in long bones typically demonstrates abnormal foci of low signal intensity on T1-weighted images and high signal intensity on T2-weighted images [7]. Involvement of cortical bone is less likely in these long bone lesions [7, 14, 19]. Lack of cortical involvement may explain why many sarcoid lesions remain undiagnosed with radiographs in most cases. Mehrotra et al. [13] reported the case of a 59-year-old woman with sarcoidosis of the humerus that appeared as lytic lesions on radiographs. However, detection on radiographs is the exception, and MRI appears to be the most sensitive modality for detecting bone involvement [9].

Chaudhry and Richardson [7] described a case of a 50-year-old male with a history of pulmonary sarcoidosis who had increased uptake in his upper right humerus on a 99mTc radionuclide scan. An initial radiograph of the shoulder was read as normal. MRI showed an abnormal lesion in the proximal medial humeral head. A biopsy revealed non-caseating granulomas, confirming osseous sarcoidosis. This patient had previously developed psychotic side effects from corticosteroid therapy (route of administration not stated) and was therefore treated with radiotherapy. His symptoms later improved. He did not have a rotator cuff tear or other shoulder pathology, and he did not have shoulder surgery (other than the biopsy).

Yachoui et al. [15] reported the case of a 58-year-old Caucasian woman who initially presented with intermittent shoulder pain that eventually became constant. A plain radiograph of the shoulder was normal. However, MRI demonstrated irregular signal in the upper humeral metaphysis. A subsequent CT scan demonstrated hilar and mediastinal adenopathy. Positron emission tomography (PET) with 18F-fluorodeoxyglucose (18F-FDG) showed numerous areas of increased activity, which was suspicious for metastatic cancer. Histological examination of one of the lesions revealed small granulomas with epithelioid cells, consistent with osseous sarcoidosis. Their patient improved after a course of prednisone and hydroxychloroquine.

Similar to these cases, our patient's radiograph was unremarkable, and follow-up MRI showed multiple lytic bone lesions of the humerus that were concerning for metastases or multiple myeloma, as sarcoidosis can mimic these conditions [5, 8–12]. Additionally, biopsy in each case revealed histological findings consistent with sarcoidosis. These, as well as additional cases, are compared in Table 1.

4. Conclusion

In summary, we report a rare case of sarcoidosis of the upper humerus. The novel aspect of our case was that sarcoid lesions were found incidentally with MR images obtained to evaluate the patient's shoulder for a rotator cuff tendon tear. Notably, the integrity of the bone was not compromised to the point that surgery could not be performed, and our patient had arthroscopic debridement of a concurrent partial rotator cuff tear. The presence and locations of the sarcoid lesions did not influence the surgical procedure because they did not involve the cortical bone and tendon repair was not needed because the tear was partial. The excellent outcome that was ultimately achieved was facilitated by prolonged physical therapy and adalimumab injections. Follow-up at 48 months demonstrated full recovery from her rotator cuff tear and no residual symptoms in her shoulder.

Acknowledgments

The authors thank Vickie Martin for assistance with patient care.

References

[1] J. Grunewald, P. Spagnolo, J. Wahlström, and A. Eklund, "Immunogenetics of disease-causing inflammation in sarcoidosis," *Clinical Reviews in Allergy & Immunology*, vol. 49, no. 1, pp. 19–35, 2015.

[2] E. S. Chen and D. R. Moller, "Etiologies of sarcoidosis," *Clinical Reviews in Allergy & Immunology*, vol. 49, no. 1, pp. 6–18, 2015.

[3] C. Fang, H. Huang, and Z. Xu, "Immunological evidence for the role of mycobacteria in sarcoidosis: A meta-analysis," *PLoS ONE*, vol. 11, no. 8, Article ID e0154716, 2016.

[4] R. P. Baughman and E. E. Lower, "A clinical approach to the use of methotrexate for sarcoidosis," *Thorax*, vol. 54, no. 8, pp. 742–746, 1999.

[5] J. P. Buteau, E. D. Asuaje, É. Rousseau et al., "The great mimicker: an extensive bone sarcoidosis," *European Journal of Nuclear Medicine and Molecular Imaging*, vol. 42, no. 2, pp. 364-365, 2015.

[6] D. Talmi, S. Smith, and M. E. Mulligan, "Central skeletal sarcoidosis mimicking metastatic disease," *Skeletal Radiology*, vol. 37, no. 8, pp. 757–761, 2008.

[7] S. Chaudhry and M. L. Richardson, "Imaging findings in sarcoid of the humerus," *Radiology Case Reports*, vol. 1, no. 4, Article ID 30253, pp. 154–158, 2006.

[8] M. C. Iannuzi, B. A. Rybicki, and A. S. Tierstein, "Sarcoidosis," *The New England Journal of Medicine*, vol. 357, pp. 2153–2165, 2007.

[9] H. Kuzyshyn, D. Feinstein, S. L. Kolasinski, and H. Eid, "Osseous sarcoidosis: a case series," *Rheumatology International*, vol. 35, no. 5, pp. 925–933, 2015.

[10] A. M. Brandy-García, I. Cabezas-Rodriguez, L. Caminal-Montero, C. Suarez-Cuervo, and P. Redondo-Buil, "Sarcoidosis mimicking lytic osseous metastases," *Cleveland Clinic Journal of Medicine*, vol. 84, no. 10, pp. 753-754, 2017.

[11] E. Bargagli, C. Olivieri, F. Penza et al., "Rare localizations of bone sarcoidosis: Two case reports and review of the literature," *Rheumatology International*, vol. 31, no. 11, pp. 1503–1506, 2011.

[12] S. S. Nijjar and W. D. Leslie, "A case of skeletal sarcoidosis imitating skeletal metastases on bone scintigraphy," *Canadian Medical Association Journal*, vol. 178, no. 2, pp. 153-154, 2008.

[13] P. Mehrotra, M. Muller, B. Higgins, and I. Zammit-Maempel, "An unusual cause of widespread lytic bone lesions caused by sarcoidosis," *Journal of Radiology Case Reports*, vol. 5, no. 9, pp. 1–7, 2011.

[14] S. L. Moore, A. Teirstein, and C. Golimbu, "MRI of sarcoidosis patients with musculoskeletal symptoms," *American Journal of Roentgenology*, vol. 185, no. 1, pp. 154–159, 2005.

[15] R. Yachoui, B. J. Parker, and T. T. Nguyen, "Bone and bone marrow involvement in sarcoidosis," *Rheumatology International*, vol. 35, no. 11, pp. 1917–1924, 2015.

[16] E. R. Cadet, J. W. Hsu, W. N. Levine, L. U. Bigliani, and C. S. Ahmad, "The relationship between greater tuberosity osteopenia and the chronicity of rotator cuff tears," *Journal of Shoulder and Elbow Surgery*, vol. 17, no. 1, pp. 73–77, 2008.

[17] Y. Jiang, J. Zhao, M. T. van Holsbeeck, M. J. Flynn, X. Ouyang, and H. K. Genant, "Trabecular microstructure and surface changes in the greater tuberosity in rotator cuff tears," *Skeletal Radiology*, vol. 31, no. 9, pp. 522–528, 2002.

[18] D. C. Meyer, S. F. Fucentese, B. Koller, and C. Gerber, "Association of osteopenia of the humeral head with full-thickness rotator cuff tears," *Journal of Shoulder and Elbow Surgery*, vol. 13, no. 3, pp. 333–337, 2004.

[19] B. Crawford, F. Badlissi, and S. A. Lozano Calderón, "Orthopaedic considerations in the management of skeletal sarcoidosis," *Journal of the American Academy of OrthopaedicSurgeons*, vol. 26, no. 6, pp. 197–203, 2018.

[20] P. Ungprasert, C. S. Crowson, and E. L. Matteson, "Risk of fragility fracture among patients with sarcoidosis: a population-based study 1976–2013," *Osteoporosis International*, vol. 28, no. 6, pp. 1875–1879, 2017.

[21] P. St. Pierre, E. J. Olsons, J. J. Elliott, K. C. O'Hair, L. A. McKinney, and J. Ryan, "Tendon-healing to cortical bone compared with healing to a cancellous trough: A biomechanical and histological evaluation in goats," *The Journal of Bone & Joint Surgery*, vol. 77, no. 12, pp. 1858–1866, 1995.

[22] L. K. Postl, V. Braunstein, R. Von Eisenhart-Rothe, and C. Kirchhoff, "Footprint reconstruction in a rotator cuff tear associated cyst of the greater tuberosity: Augmented anchorage," *Archives of Orthopaedic and Trauma Surgery*, vol. 133, no. 1, pp. 81–85, 2013.

[23] W. Z. Burkhead Jr., J. G. Skedros, P. J. O'Rourke, W. A. Pierce, and T. C. Pitts, "A novel double-row rotator cuff repair exceeds strengths of conventional repairs," *Clinical Orthopaedics and Related Research*, no. 461, pp. 106–113, 2007.

[24] H. Ellman, "Diagnosis and treatment of incomplete rotator cuff tears," *Clinical Orthopaedics and Related Research*, no. 254, pp. 64–74, 1990.

[25] N. K. Donohue, A. R. Prisco, and S. I. Grindel, "Pre-operative corticosteroid injections improve functional outcomes in patients undergoing arthroscopic repair of high-grade partial-thickness rotator cuff tears," *Muscle, Ligaments and Tendons Journal*, vol. 7, no. 1, pp. 34–39, 2017.

[26] J. G. Skedros, M. G. Adondakis, A. N. Knight, and M. B. Pilkington, "Frequency of shoulder corticosteroid injections for pain and stiffness after shoulder surgery and their potential to enhance outcomes with physiotherapy: a retrospective study," *Pain and Therapy*, vol. 6, no. 1, pp. 45–60, 2017.

[27] C. Atkins and A. M. Wilson, "Managing fatigue in sarcoidosis - A systematic review of the evidence," *Chronic Respiratory Disease*, vol. 14, no. 2, pp. 161–173, 2017.

25

A Rare Finding of Falciform Ligament Thrombosis as a Sequel of Acute Pancreatitis

H. Q. C. Lim, X. W. J. Lee, and N. Mathias

Hairmyres Hospital, Glasgow G75 8RG, UK

Correspondence should be addressed to H. Q. C. Lim; cryslim@doctors.org.uk

Academic Editor: Vincent Low

Falciform ligament (remnant of umbilical vein) is an anatomical structure that connects the liver to the anterior abdominal wall. This case reports a rare clinical presentation of falciform ligament thrombosis as a consequence of acute gallstone pancreatitis, in a patient with noncirrhotic liver. A 55-year-old female with a history of cholelithiasis was admitted with abdominal pain. Biochemistry profile showed hyperamylasemia and deranged liver function tests. Computerized Tomography (CT) revealed a 3 cm attenuated structure that can be traced up to the left portal vein, which represents an acute thrombosis of the falciform ligament. The patient was treated with Tinzaparin and subsequently anticoagulated. She subsequently had a laparoscopic cholecystectomy and made an uneventful recovery. We suspect that pancreatitis caused thrombophlebitis subsequently leading to recanalization and thrombosis of the umbilical vein. Falciform ligament thrombosis is a rare and poorly described complication following pancreatitis which clinicians and radiologists should be aware of.

1. Introduction

The falciform ligament of the liver is a fibrous remnant of the obliterated umbilical vein [1, 2]. The umbilical vein and artery play a vital role during fetal growth. These structures allow the exchange of materials between fetal and maternal circulation. The umbilical vein divides into two structures at the liver (ductus venosus and a branch that communicates with the hepatic portal vein). During fetal development, the majority of oxygenated blood travels via the umbilical vein into the ductus venosus that subsequently drains into the inferior vena cava [2]. When renal, pulmonary, and digestive functions begin to function at birth, the umbilical vein collapses and remains as the falciform ligament.

Pancreatitis can potentially cause both systemic and local complications. Diseases involving the falciform ligament are extremely rare and recanalization of the umbilical vein has only been described in patients with portal hypertension [3]. We describe an unusual case report of isolated falciform ligament thrombosis as a sequel of acute pancreatitis.

2. Case Presentation

A 55-year-old female presented with a one-day history of colicky pain in the epigastric and right upper quadrant area with associated vomiting. The pain did not resolve with regular cocodamol 8/500 mg (2 tablets). She has a background of cholelithiasis and her symptoms were described as similar. She has no history of pancreatitis. She is a nonsmoker and consumes nine units of alcohol per week. There is no family history of bleeding or clotting disorders. Her only regular medication is hormone replacement therapy *(estradiol, norethisterone)*.

On admission, her basic observations were normal: temperature (36.8°C), blood pressure (117/79 mmHg), heart rate (73 beats per minute), and alert and oriented. Abdominal examination revealed point tenderness in the right upper quadrant, no organomegaly, or peritonism.

Admission laboratory investigations revealed deranged liver function tests: alanine aminotransferase (ALT) (275 U/L), bilirubin (54 umol/L), hyperamylasemia (1900 U/L), normal alkaline phosphatase (80 U/L), normal C-reactive protein (<6 mg/L), and raised white cell count (18×10^9/L). Abdominal ultrasound revealed cholelithiasis with no evidence of common bile duct obstruction. The patient was subsequently treated for gallstone pancreatitis with intravenous fluid therapy and analgesia.

Three days after admission, she had episodes of pyrexia (temperature 38.2°C) with elevated inflammatory markers

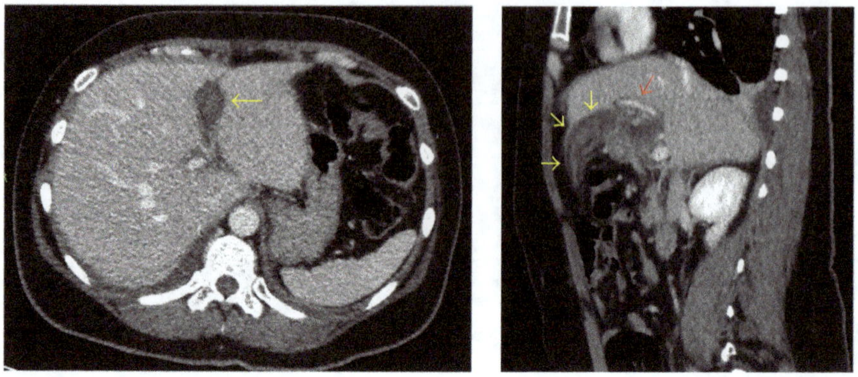

(a) (b)

Figure 1: Abdominal axial (a) and sagittal (b) CT scan showing thrombosed falciform ligament (yellow arrows) with patent left portal vein (red arrow).

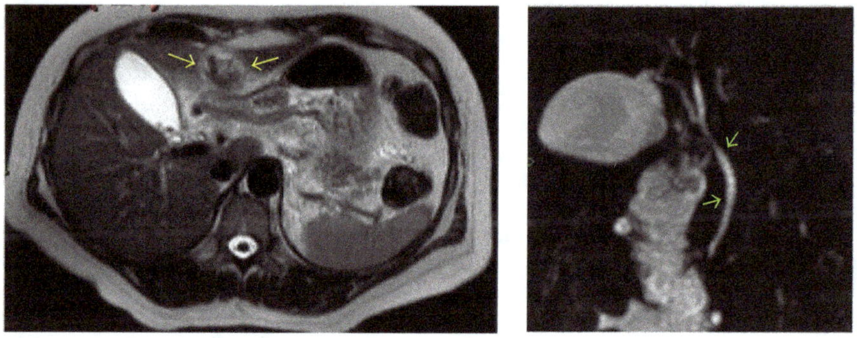

(a) (b)

Figure 2: MRCP (magnetic resonance cholangiopancreatography). Axial view (a) showing thrombosed falciform ligament (yellow arrows). Projective coronal view (b) showing patent bile duct with no stones (green arrows).

(C-reactive protein 255 mg/L and white cell count 19 × 10^9/L). She was started on intravenous antibiotics empirically (Amoxicillin 1 g three times a times a day, Metronidazole 500 mg three times a day, and Gentamicin as per weight and renal function) to treat possible biliary sepsis and/or necrotizing pancreatitis. Liver function tests had improved with bilirubin 20 umol/L, ALT 81 U/L, and amylase of 143 U/L. Computerized Tomography (CT) scan of her abdomen and pelvis with contrast (Figure 1) was performed to confirm our diagnosis but instead it revealed a thin-walled gall bladder, stranding adjacent to the pancreatic tail and a 3 cm reduced attenuation structure, which was thought to represent an acute thrombosis of the umbilical vein. There was no evidence of collection. Magnetic resonance cholangiopancreatography (MRCP) (Figure 2) was subsequently performed which confirmed the above findings and no biliary duct stones were identified. Intravenous antibiotics were immediately discontinued as per protocol as no source of sepsis was found from imaging.

Patient coagulation parameters (prothrombin time, partial thrombin time, International Normalized Ratio, platelets, and fibrinogen) were normal since admission. A thrombophilia screen was subsequently carried out and was normal. She was treated with Tinzaparin 12000 units (treatment dose) and was discharged home after a week with warfarin (target INR of 2.0–3.0) for a target period of 6 months and hormone replacement therapy discontinued.

Four months after her hospital admission, she had a second episode of pancreatitis (hyperamylasemia of 1819 U/L). CT scan of the abdomen and pelvis with contrast (Figure 3) demonstrated ongoing cholecystitis with a resolving falciform ligament thrombosis. Laparoscopic cholecystectomy was carried out uneventfully and operative cholangiogram revealed no stones in the common bile duct (CBD). Histology of the gall bladder revealed features of chronic cholecystitis with multiple yellow mulberry stones ranging from 3 to 8 mm in diameter. A MRCP scan (Figure 4) was carried out 8 weeks after procedure and revealed no biliary duct stones or strictures and a complete resolution of falciform ligament thrombosis.

3. Discussion

Isolated umbilical vein thrombosis in the adult population is a rare occurrence. To the best of our knowledge, there have been no reported cases in the literature. Incidental isolated umbilical vein thrombosis in neonates has occurred as a consequence following umbilical vein catheterisation [4, 5].

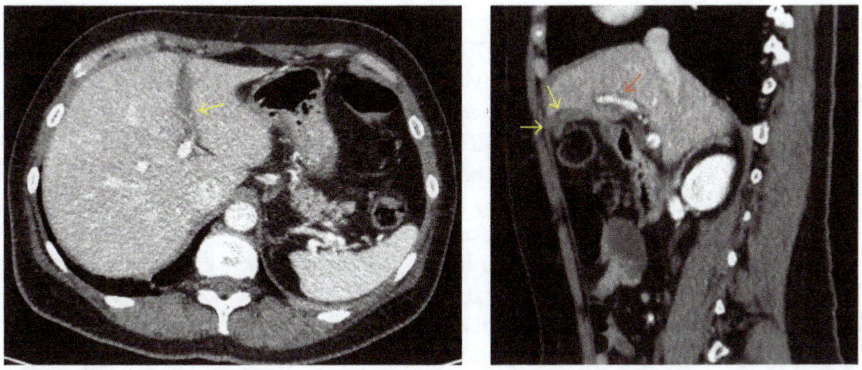

(a) (b)

FIGURE 3: Abdominal axial (a) and sagittal (b) CT scan showing resolution of falciform ligament thrombosis (yellow arrows) with patent left portal vein (red arrow).

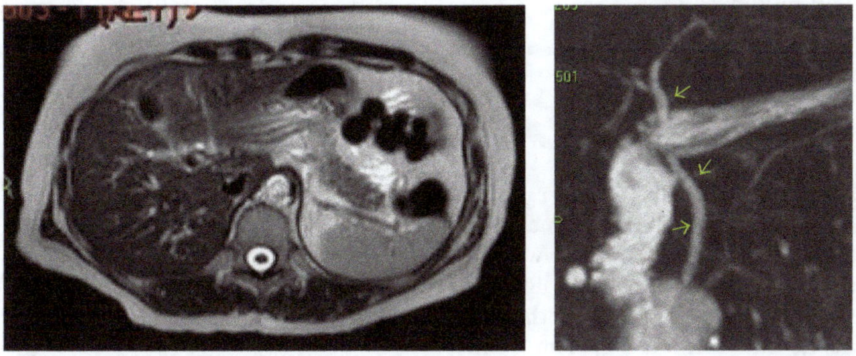

(a) (b)

FIGURE 4: MRCP axial view (a) showing postcholecystectomy and resolved falciform ligament thrombosis. Projective coronal view (b) showing patent bile duct (green arrows).

Pancreatitis is an inflammatory process and is well documented to potentially cause venous and arterial vascular complications. These complications are also noted to be more common in alcohol induced, necrotizing, and chronic pancreatitis [6]. Studies have stated that venous thrombosis following pancreatitis is frequent and typically manifests as splanchnic vein thrombosis (SVT), predominantly involving splenic vein (SpIV) [7]. This thrombosis frequently resolves spontaneously after the resolution of inflammatory disease. Clinically, SVT in pancreatitis is becoming more common with advancement of imaging technology. One recent meta-analysis demonstrated that 13.6% of pancreatitis had SVT, 6.2% had portal vein thrombosis (PVT), 11.2% had SplV thrombosis (SplVT), and 2.7% had mesenteric vein thrombosis (MVT). It also identified that the prevalence of SVT in pancreatitis in Europe reached 16.9%, which is the highest among the three continents compared (Europe, America, and Asia) [8].

The causes of PVT can be primarily classified into either local causes or systemic prothrombotic states. Various reports [9–11] described PVT following pancreatitis; however acute recanalization of the paraumbilical vein is rare. The umbilical vein however has been speculated to spontaneously recanalize during portal hypertension to serve as a hepatofugal, decompressing collateral [12]. The peculiarity of this case presentation is based on the fact there has been acute thrombosis of the falciform ligament in a noncirrhotic liver with a patent portal venous system.

We suspect that this patient may have thrombophlebitis secondary to pancreatitis rather than an infective source. This has been supported by radiological and biochemical findings (CT describing no evidence of cholecystitis and improving liver function tests). The paraumbilical vein originates from the umbilical portion of the left portal vein in the falciform ligament and proceeds to the umbilicus and periumbilical veins [13]. We hypothesise that the effects of pancreatitis in this patient was thrombophlebitis which may have spread via the portal venous system into the falciform ligament subsequently leading to spontaneous recanalization and acute thrombosis.

At present, review of the previous studies and case reports outlined that both CT and MRI can be used for diagnosis. However, its appearance on both imaging modalities varies with the thrombus age. Acute clot appears hypodense or isodense to adjacent liver structures on CT while showing as high intensity signals on both T1 and T2 weighted MRI sequences. MRI has been noted to be the most sensitive imaging modality for the detection of PVT but its appearance is once again dependant on thrombus age and specific MRI sequence. As time progresses, there is a loss of T2 weighted signal on MRI [9, 14].

We extrapolated treatment recommendations from cases [15–18] of PVT following pancreatitis and treated her with early anticoagulation therapy. There has been no evidence to suggest that initial thrombolysis should be given in preference to anticoagulation for patient with PVT and anticoagulation did not increase the risk of bleeding. However, there have been reported cases where thrombolysis has been shown to be effective only when initial anticoagulation therapy has failed [10]. We agree with other studies [10, 11] and recommend that anticoagulant therapy should be given for only six months and continued only if an underlying thrombophilia has been identified in umbilical vein thrombosis.

4. Conclusion

In conclusion, falciform ligament thrombosis is a rare and poorly differentiated complication following pancreatitis which both clinicians and radiologists should be aware of. In this setting, it is important to exclude falciform ligament thrombosis as a differential diagnosis in a patient with ongoing abdominal pain despite adequate management of the pancreatitis. The acute diagnosis can be well demonstrated on both contrast CT and MRI, and we recommend early anticoagulation to allow recanalization.

References

[1] K. L. Moore, A. F. Dalley, and A. M. R. Agur, *Clinically Oriented Anatomy*, Wolters Kluwer/Lippincott Williams & Wilkins, Philadelphia, Pa, USA, 6th edition, 2010.

[2] G. J. Tortora and B. Derrickson, "Principles of Anatomy & Physiology," in *International Student*, pp. 862–865, Wiley, Hoboken, NJ, USA, 13th edition.

[3] Z. T. Ozkececı, M. Ozsoy, B. Celep, A. Bal, and C. Polat, "A rare cause of acute abdomen: an isolated falciform ligament necrosis," *Case Reports in Emergency Medicine*, vol. 2014, Article ID 570751, 3 pages, 2014.

[4] J. M. Scott, "Iatrogenic lesions in babies following umbilical vein catheterization," *Archives of Disease in Childhood*, vol. 40, no. 212, pp. 426–429, 1965.

[5] P. Rubabaza and R. J. Persadie, "Two Cases of Umbilical Vein Thrombosis, One With Associated Portal Vein Thrombosis," *Journal of Obstetrics and Gynaecology Canada*, vol. 30, no. 4, pp. 338–343, 2008.

[6] W.-S. Park, H.-I. Kim, B.-J. Jeon, S.-H. Kim, and S.-O. Lee, "Should anticoagulants be administered for portal vein thrombosis associated with acute pancreatitis?" *World Journal of Gastroenterology*, vol. 18, no. 42, pp. 6168–6171, 2012.

[7] N. A. Nadkarni, S. Khanna, and S. S. Vege, "Splanchnic venous thrombosis and pancreatitis," *Pancreas*, vol. 42, no. 6, pp. 924–931, 2013.

[8] W. Xu, X. Qi, J. Chen, C. Su, and X. Guo, "Prevalence of splanchnic vein thrombosis in pancreatitis: a systematic review and meta-analysis of observational studies," *Gastroenterology Research and Practice*, vol. 2015, Article ID 245460, 23 pages, 2015.

[9] R. J. Foster and G. W. Cowell, "Acute paraumbilical vein recanalization: an unusual complication of acute pancreatitis," *BJR—case reports*, vol. 1, no. 1, p. 20150021, 2015.

[10] G. J. M. Webster, A. K. Burroughs, and S. M. Riordan, "Portal vein thrombosis—new insights into aetiology and management," *Alimentary Pharmacology & Therapeutics*, vol. 21, no. 1, pp. 1–9, 2005.

[11] D.-C. Valla and B. Condat, "Portal vein thrombosis in adults: pathophysiology, pathogenesis and management," *Journal of Hepatology*, vol. 32, no. 5, pp. 865–871, 2000.

[12] J. Aagaard, L. I. Jensen, T. I. Sørensen, U. Christensen, and F. Burcharth, "Recanalized umbilical vein in portal hypertension," *American Journal of Roentgenology*, vol. 139, no. 6, pp. 1107–1110, 1982.

[13] H. R. Parvey, B. Raval, and C. M. Sandler, "Portal vein thrombosis: imaging findings," *American Journal of Roentgenology*, vol. 162, no. 1, pp. 77–81, 1994.

[14] L. R. Warren, M. D. Chandrasegaram, D. J. Madigan, P. M. Dolan, E. L. Neo, and C. S. Worthley, "Falciform ligament abscess from left sided portal pyaemia following malignant obstructive cholangitis," *World Journal of Surgical Oncology*, vol. 10, article no. 278, 2012.

[15] B. Condat, F. Pessione, M. Helene Denninger, S. Hillaire, and D. Valla, "Recent portal or mesenteric venous thrombosis: increased recognition and frequent recanalization on anticoagulant therapy," *Hepatology*, vol. 32, no. 3, pp. 466–470, 2000.

[16] B. Condat, F. Pessione, S. Hillaire et al., "Current outcome of portal vein thrombosis in adults: risk and benefit of anticoagulant therapy," *Gastroenterology*, vol. 120, no. 2, pp. 490–497, 2001.

[17] Y. Chawla, A. Duseja, and R. K. Dhiman, "Review article: the modern management of portal vein thrombosis," *Alimentary Pharmacology & Therapeutics*, vol. 30, no. 9, pp. 881–894, 2009.

[18] X. Qi, V. de Stefano, H. Li, J. Dai, X. Guo, and D. Fan, "Anticoagulation for the treatment of portal vein thrombosis in liver cirrhosis: a systematic review and meta-analysis of observational studies," *European Journal of Internal Medicine*, vol. 26, no. 1, pp. 23–29, 2015.

26

Mediastinal Hibernoma: A Rare Case with Radiologic-Pathologic Correlation

Maxine Darke, Anil Dasyam, Matthew Then, Kavita Varma, Amir A. Borhani, and Rakesh Varma

University of Pittsburgh Medical Center, 200 Lothrop Street, Pittsburgh, PA 15213, USA

Correspondence should be addressed to Rakesh Varma; varmark@upmc.edu

Academic Editor: Atsushi Komemushi

Hibernomas, especially located in the mediastinum, are extremely rare benign tumors, which are important to consider in the differential diagnosis of a heterogeneously enhancing mass with areas of fat attenuation on imaging of an often incidentally discovered mass. Other common possibilities in the differential include malignant tumors, such as liposarcoma, hence histopathology is usually required to confirm the diagnosis. Hibernomas often follow the distribution of sites of persistence of brown fat in adults, and intrathoracic locations are unusual. We present a very rare case of a mediastinal hibernoma in a 53-year-old woman. She presented to the emergency department with severe, progressive right neck and shoulder pain with radiation down her arm and was found to have a right apical posterior mediastinal mass on imaging. Initial radiographs of the shoulder showed a soft tissue mass within the apical right hemithorax. Further imaging with CT revealed a well circumscribed, heterogeneously enhancing mass with areas of fat attenuation. Pathology confirmed the diagnosis of mediastinal hibernoma, and the mass was completely excised. Fourteen months after surgery, the patient had a normal chest radiograph, and thirty-two months after surgery, she remains asymptomatic.

1. Introduction

Hibernomas are rare, benign tumors composed of brown fat. Hibernomas can occur in multiple sites, including the head, neck, trunk, and extremities. Only a few mediastinal hibernomas have previously been documented in literature. These tumors enhance heterogeneously and often contain macroscopic fat, which can result in misdiagnosis as liposarcoma. While imaging can provide useful clues, the diagnosis needs histopathologic confirmation. We present a very rare case of a mediastinal hibernoma with excellent radiology-pathology correlation.

2. Case Presentation

A 53-year-old woman with no significant past medical history presented to the emergency department with a ten-day history of progressive, severe right neck and shoulder/scapular pain that was worse with movement and radiated down her right arm to her fingers. NSAIDs, range of motion exercises, and trigger point injections had provided only minimal relief. She denied recent trauma, had no infectious symptoms, and reported no smoking history.

Right shoulder radiographs revealed a right superior mediastinal mass (Figure 1). Further imaging with contrast enhanced CT showed a 7.2 cm well demarcated, heterogeneously enhancing mass with areas of fat attenuation and some prominent internal vessels within the right superior, posterior mediastinum (Figure 2). The mass anteriorly abutted the brachiocephalic artery and trachea but did not invade adjacent structures. A cervical spine MRI obtained for cervical radiculopathy symptoms partially included the mass, which was heterogeneous, hyperintense to muscle on both T1 and T2 weighted sequences with a few internal flow voids, and showed moderate loss of signal with fat saturation (Figure 3).

Mesenchymal neoplasms, lymphoma, and teratoma were considered in the differential diagnosis based on imaging. Microscopically, the CT-guided biopsy showed multivacuolated and granular eosinophilic cells with small centrally located nuclei consistent with hibernoma. No lipoblasts or

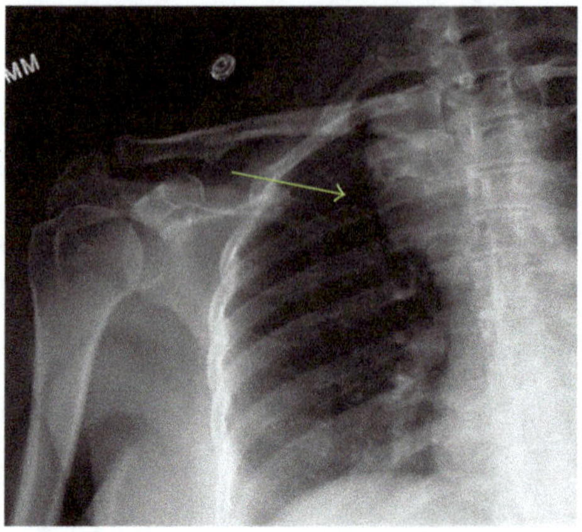

FIGURE 1: Frontal radiograph of the right shoulder shows a superior mediastinal mass (green arrow) within the right hemithorax.

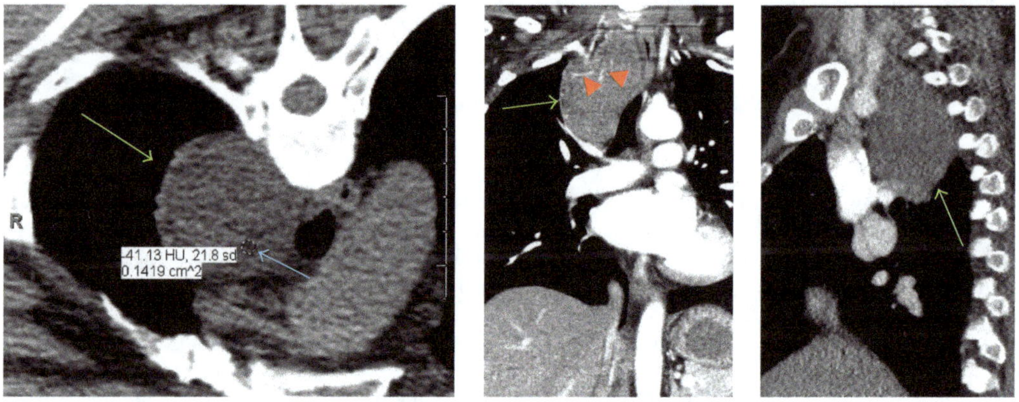

(a) (b) (c)

FIGURE 2: Contrast enhanced axial CT (a) with coronal (b) and sagittal (c) CT reconstructions of the chest demonstrating a well circumscribed, heterogeneously enhancing mass (green arrows) with areas of fat attenuation (blue arrow pointing to ROI in (a)) and a few mildly prominent internal vessels (red arrow heads in (b)) within the superior, posterior right mediastinum.

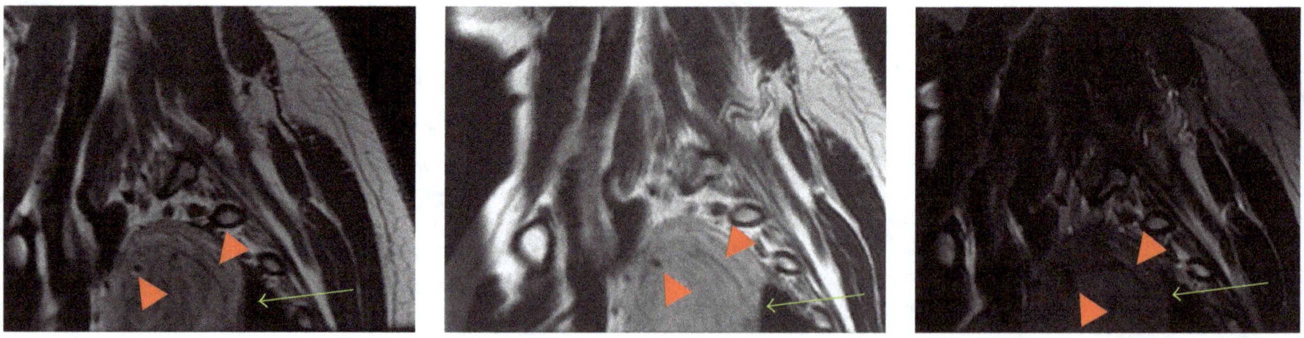

(a) (b) (c)

FIGURE 3: Sagittal T1 (a), T2 (b), and fat saturation T2 (c) weighted images from the cervical spine MRI show a heterogeneous, T1, and T2 hyperintense mass (green arrows in (a) and (b)) with a few internal flow voids (red arrow heads in (a), (b), and (c)) and moderate loss of signal with fat saturation (green arrow in (c)).

cytologic atypia was seen to suggest liposarcoma. Due to the unusual location, large size, and possible mass effect on adjacent structures, total excision was performed by a right video-assisted thoracoscopy. The surgeon described a dense, fatty, lobulated mass located in the posterior mediastinum with extension into the lower neck and without direct invasion of surrounding structures. The resection specimen measured 8 × 5 × 3 cm. Grossly, it was described as a circumscribed, yellow to tan, lobulated mass (Figure 4). Histologic sections demonstrated cytologically bland brown

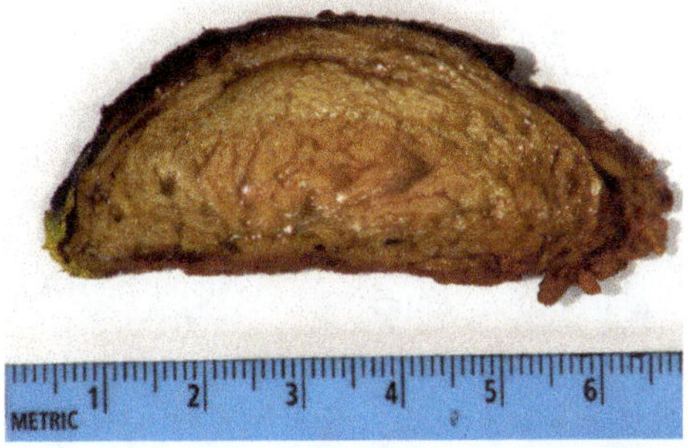

FIGURE 4: The cut surface of the gross specimen shows a circumscribed, yellow to tan, lobulated mass.

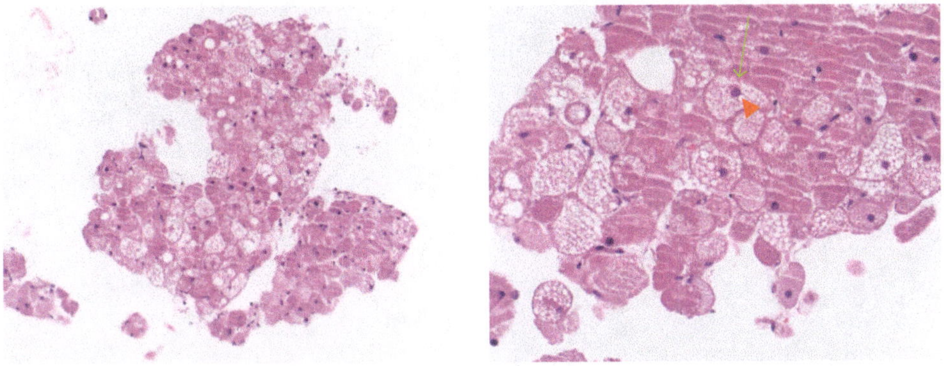

(a) (b)

FIGURE 5: H&E, 40x (a) and 200x (b), respectively, demonstrating sheets of cells resembling brown fat. The higher power examination revealing well demarcated granular, multivacuolated eosinophilic cells (green arrow in (b)) with small centrally placed nuclei (red arrow head in (b)).

fat cells with abundant granular cytoplasm identical to the preoperative biopsy (Figure 5). Due to their classic histomorphologic features, most hibernomas can readily be diagnosed without the use of ancillary studies. Cytogenetic studies have demonstrated rearrangements of 11q13; however, amplification of MDM2 should prompt consideration of an atypical lipomatous tumor/well differentiated liposarcoma. The patient was discharged on the second postoperative day.

On follow-up, the patient had transient right vocal cord paralysis, likely due to the close proximity of the resected mass to the recurrent laryngeal nerve, with return of full vocal cord mobility about one month after surgery. No CT evidence of recurrence was seen on a chest CT four months after surgery, and a chest radiograph fourteen months after surgery was normal. Thirty-two months after surgery, the patient remains asymptomatic.

3. Discussion

Tumors composed of brown fat are called hibernomas, a term that originated due to the similarity to brown fat in hibernating animals [1]. Hibernomas are rare, benign, and slow growing and are often asymptomatic incidental findings on imaging or physical exam [2, 3].

Since these tumors are hypothesized to arise from tiny remnants of fetal brown fat, it is logical that common sites for hibernomas are areas known to contain brown fat in adults [1, 3]. In the largest review of 170 hibernomas, the most common locations were the thigh and the shoulder. Intrathoracic hibernomas, including the mediastinum and pleura, only accounted for 0.065% (11/170) of those cases [4]. In 2004, only the fourth mediastinal hibernoma was reported in the world literature [3]. Therefore, our case of a hibernoma in the posterior mediastinum is extremely rare and demonstrates excellent radiologic-pathologic correlation.

It is important to recognize hibernomas from imaging and pathology as benign tumors, not to be confused with malignant tumors like liposarcomas. On CT, hibernomas are well circumscribed, heterogenous lesions with mixed low attenuation fatty components and enhancing soft tissue components. It is essential to note that hibernomas are hypervascular, a key imaging differentiation from liposarcomas [2, 5]. On MRI, hibernomas are often hyperintense on T1 and T2 weighted images with loss of some signal on fat suppression images; striking contrast enhancement and flow voids on T2 weighted images are other MR features that can be identified [1, 5]. Despite the tumor's hypervascularity, Papathanassiou et al. reported no complications from core needle biopsy in their series [6].

Gross pathology is typically described as a tan colored, well-defined, soft, lobulated mass that can be encapsulated [2]. Histology commonly reveals multivacuolated fat cells that contain small centrally located nuclei; atypia should not be present [4]. The tan color of the mass is due to the combination of hypervascularity and high mitochondria content. The four histologic variants include typical, which is most common, myxoid, lipoma-like, and spindle cell [2]. Positive staining for S-100 is a typical, but nonspecific, feature with 85% (17/20) of cases in one study reported as positive [4]. Pathologic features that are worrisome for liposarcoma include lack of vascularity, cellular atypia, and irregular septa [1].

Although the masses are most commonly asymptomatic, they can grow to large sizes and become symptomatic. Therefore, treatment with complete surgical resection is common. Incomplete excision can lead to local recurrence of the tumor [6]. Overall, prognosis is excellent. There are no known cases of hibernoma metastases or malignant transformation [2, 5].

Ethical Approval

IRB approval for case reports is not required at our institution.

References

[1] A. C. da Motta, D. E. Tunkel, W. H. Westra, and D. M. Yousem, "Imaging findings of a hibernoma of the neck," *American Journal of Neuroradiology*, vol. 27, no. 8, pp. 1658–1659, 2006.

[2] M. D. Murphey, J. F. Carroll, D. J. Flemming, T. L. Pope, F. H. Gannon, and M. J. Kransdorf, "Benign musculoskeletal lipomatous lesions," *Radiographics*, vol. 24, no. 5, pp. 1433–1466, 2004.

[3] A. Baldi, M. Santini, P. Mellone et al., "Mediastinal hibernoma: a case report," *Journal of Clinical Pathology*, vol. 57, no. 9, pp. 993–994, 2004.

[4] M. A. Furlong, J. C. Fanburg-Smith, and M. Miettinen, "The morphologic spectrum of hibernoma: a clinicopathologic study of 170 cases," *The American Journal of Surgical Pathology*, vol. 25, no. 6, pp. 809–814, 2001.

[5] B. P. Little, F. J. Fintelmann, M. Mino-Kenudson, M. Lanuti, J.-A. O. Shepard, and S. R. Digumarthy, "Intrathoracic hibernoma: a case with multimodality imaging correlation," *Journal of Thoracic Imaging*, vol. 26, no. 1, pp. W20–W22, 2011.

[6] Z. G. Papathanassiou, M. Alberghini, S. Taieb, C. Errani, P. Picci, and D. Vanel, "Imaging of hibernomas: a retrospective study on twelve cases," *Clinical Sarcoma Research*, vol. 1, no. 1, article 3, 2011.

27

Pulmonary Embolism Originating from a Hepatic Hydatid Cyst Ruptured into the Inferior Vena Cava: CT and MRI Findings

Necdet Poyraz,[1] Soner Demirbaş,[2] Celalettin Korkmaz,[2] and Kürşat Uzun[2]

[1]*Department of Radiology, Meram Faculty of Medicine, Necmettin Erbakan University, Konya 42080, Turkey*
[2]*Department of Pulmonary Disease, Meram Faculty of Medicine, Necmettin Erbakan University, Konya 42080, Turkey*

Correspondence should be addressed to Necdet Poyraz; necdetpoyraz@gmail.com

Academic Editor: Salah D. Qanadli

Pulmonary embolism due to hydatid cysts is a very rare clinical entity. Hydatid pulmonary embolism can be distinguished from other causes of pulmonary embolism with contrast-enhanced computed tomography (CECT) and magnetic resonance imaging (MRI). MRI especially displays the cystic nature of lesions better than CECT. Here we report a 45-year-old male patient with the pulmonary embolism due to ruptured hydatid liver cyst into the inferior vena cava.

1. Introduction

Cystic echinococcosis (CE), or cystic hydatidosis, is a complex, chronic parasitic disease with a cosmopolitan distribution. Human CE remains highly endemic in pastoral communities,particularly in regions of South America, the Mediterranean littoral, Eastern Europe, the Near and Middle East, East Africa, Central Asia, China, and Russia [1–3]. Cystic echinococcosis is caused by the larval stage (metacestode) of *Echinococcus granulosus* in sheep raising areas with close contact to dogs. Organisms that reach the gastrointestinal system go to the liver via the portal vein and then to the right heart and to the lung via the pulmonary artery and may reach the spleen, muscles, central nervous system, or eye via systemic circulation [1, 2, 4]. In humans, 75% of HCs are seen in the liver, 15% in the lungs, and 10% in other anatomical locations. The cardiovascular system may also be involved in less than 2% of the cases [4].

We report a case of a 45-year-old man with hydatid cyst embolization to the pulmonary arteries mimicking the clinical presentation of acute pulmonary embolism.

2. Case Presentation

A 45-year-old male patient was referred to our clinic with symptoms of chest pain and dyspnea at rest. There was no history of cardiovascular diseases. Physical examination was unremarkable. Electrocardiogram traces demonstrated a sinus tachycardia. The D-dimer test was normal. From past medical history, he had cystic echinococcosis in the liver two years ago, but the patient refused surgical intervention and for this reason he was given medical treatment with albendazole alone. Since then he did not have check-up. A pulmonary embolism was clinically suspected. Chest radiography showed several nodules in the lower lung zones. The CECT revealed a typical HC with the size 63 × 53 mm, containing peripherally aligned small cysts, adjacent to the inferior vena cava in the liver as CE 3a cyst following the WHO classification (Figure 1). In the lower lobe segmental branches of the pulmonary arteries bilaterally, multiple cystic nodules that caused luminal widening consistent with emboli were observed (Figure 2). A cyst that caused a filling defect was noted in the lumen of the inferior vena cava (Figure 3). Pleural effusion was present in the right hemithorax. The patient did not have any predisposing factors of thromboembolic diseases or any findings of deep vein thrombosis in the lower extremities. The thoracic MRI performed to confirm the findings revealed septation in the liver and HC containing multiple daughter vesicles aligned peripherally, and the cystic structure of the emboli inside the inferior vena cava and pulmonary arteries was shown on MR images (Figure 4).

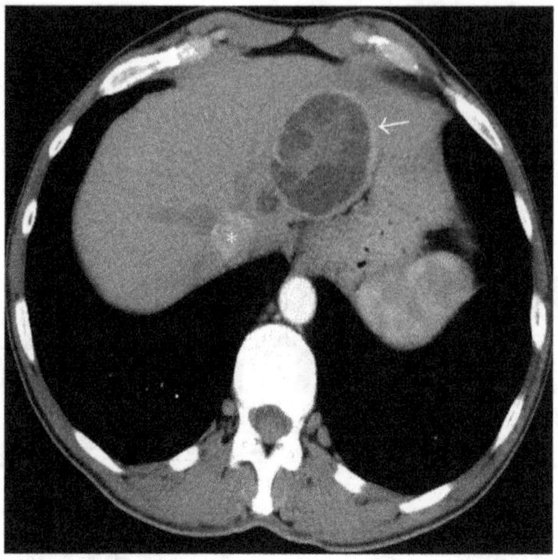

FIGURE 1: Contrast-enhanced CT scan reveals typically hydatid liver cyst as CE 3a cyst following the WHO classification (arrow) adjacent to the IVC (asterisk).

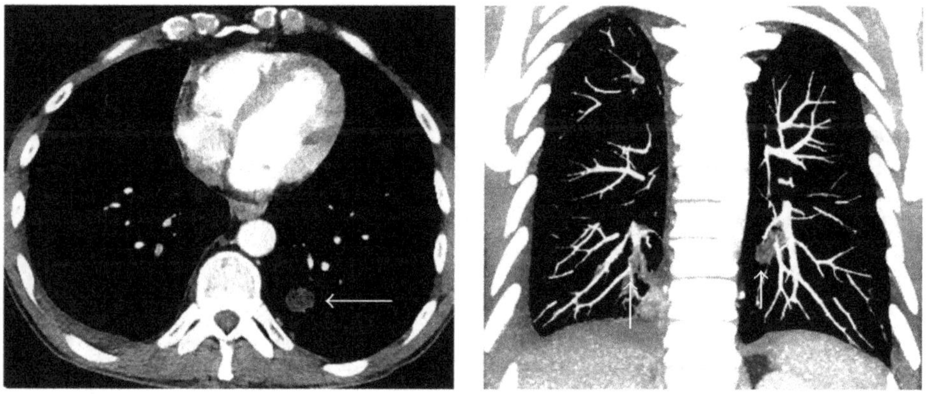

(a) (b)

FIGURE 2: Axial contrast-enhanced CT scan (a) and coronal MIP image (b) show multiple cystic nodules in the inferior pulmonary arteries (arrows).

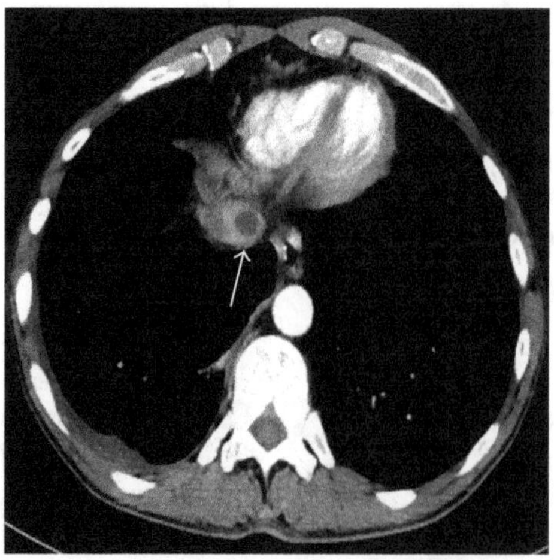

FIGURE 3: Contrast-enhanced CT scan shows a fluid attenuation round lesion, daughter cyst, within the IVC (arrow).

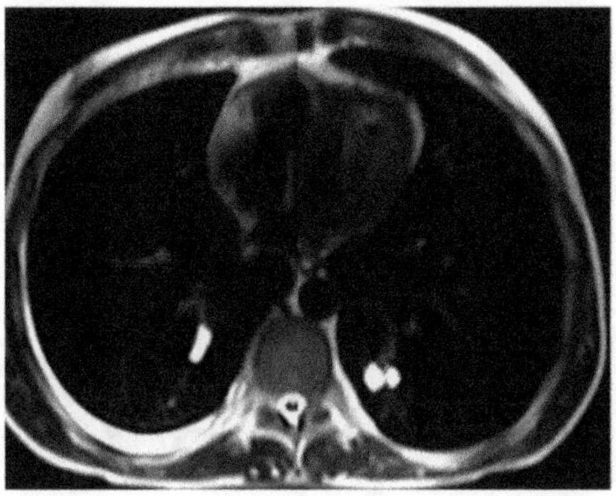

(a)

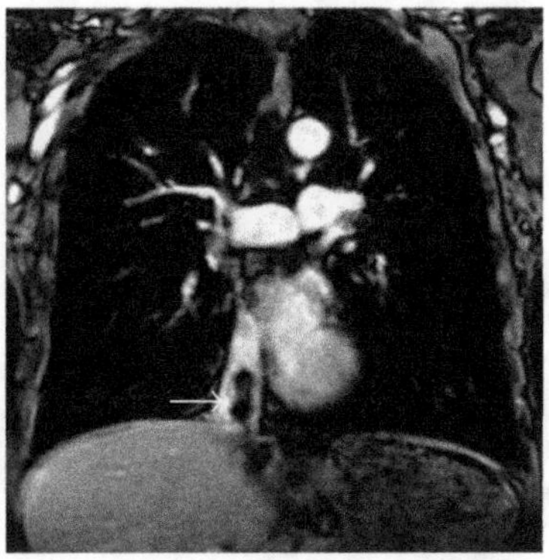

(b)

FIGURE 4: Axial T2-weighted MRI shows hyperintense cystic nodules in the lower lobe segmental pulmonary arteries bilaterally (a). Contrast-enhanced T1-weighted Vibe sequence coronal MRI shows contrast filling defect within the IVC due to ruptured liver hydatid cyst (b) (arrow).

3. Discussion

Pulmonary or systemic embolisms caused by HCs are rare complications. Hepatic echinococci may open to the inferior vena cava, and daughter vesicles may cause embolisms in the pulmonary arteries. Sometimes cardiac HC can rupture directly into the pulmonary arteries [4, 5]. In these cases, a clinical presentation similar to acute pulmonary thromboembolism with coughing, hemoptysis, and chest pain develops [5]. These cysts might mechanically block blood flow. When supportive blood nutrition is provided by bronchial arteries, the pulmonary artery obstruction caused by slow-growing cysts may remain asymptomatic. Finally, the progression of the disease may cause symptoms like dyspnea, hemoptysis, and chest pain, and anaphylactic shock may develop due to leakage of the hydatid cyst fluid. Early diagnosis with imaging studies and treatment are the main aspects of preventing complications [6–8].

The diagnosis of HC pulmonary embolism can be made with clinical and radiological findings. On CECT, cysts causing focal widening of the lumen of arteries and not enhancing with contrast appear homogenous and hypodense at fluid density. MRI displays the cystic nature of lesions better than CECT [9]. The presence of HC inside the heart or liver (as in our case) makes the diagnosis easier. In our case, CECT and MRI successfully revealed the lower lobe pulmonary artery segmental branches bilaterally and the daughter vesicles of the cystic embolisms inside the inferior vena cava [6, 10].

Other reasons of intraluminal filling defects such as pulmonary thromboembolism and primary arterial tumors should also be considered in the differential diagnosis. Primary arterial tumors are more aggressive and enhance with contrast [7, 8].

In limited cases of pulmonary embolism caused by HCs surgery is recommended [6]. Our patient refused surgery; therefore, he was discharged on oral albendazole therapy and is still being followed up.

In conclusion, incorrect and unnecessary treatments can be avoided by distinguishing pulmonary emboli secondary to HCs from pulmonary thromboembolisms.

References

[1] R. Morar and C. Feldman, "Pulmonary echinococcosis," *European Respiratory Journal*, vol. 21, no. 6, pp. 1069–1077, 2003.

[2] I. Beggs, "The radiology of hydatid disease," *American Journal of Roentgenology*, vol. 145, no. 3, pp. 639–648, 1985.

[3] E. Brunetti, P. Kern, and D. A. Vuitton, "Expert consensus for the diagnosis and treatment of cystic and alveolar echinococcosis in humans," *Acta Tropica*, vol. 114, no. 1, pp. 1–16, 2010.

[4] I. Pedrosa, A. Saíz, J. Arrazola, J. Ferreirós, and C. S. Pedrosa, "Hydatid disease: radiologic and pathologic features and complications," *Radiographics*, vol. 20, no. 3, pp. 795–817, 2000.

[5] S. Bayraktaroglu, N. Ceylan, R. Savaş, S. Nalbantgil, and H. Alper, "Hydatid disease of right ventricle and pulmonary arteries: a rare cause of pulmonary embolism—computed tomography and magnetic resonance imaging findings," *European Radiology*, vol. 19, no. 8, pp. 2083–2086, 2009.

[6] Y. Namn and P. D. Maldjian, "Hydatid cyst embolization to the pulmonary artery: CT and MR features," *Emergency Radiology*, vol. 20, no. 6, pp. 565–568, 2013.

[7] V. Akgun, B. Battal, B. Karaman, F. Ors, O. Deniz, and A. Daku, "Pulmonary artery embolism due to a ruptured hepatic hydatid cyst: clinical and radiologic imaging findings," *Emergency Radiology*, vol. 18, no. 5, pp. 437–439, 2011.

[8] M. F. Damiani, P. Carratù, I. Tatò, H. Vizzino, C. Florio, and O. Resta, "Recurrent pulmonary embolism due to echinococcosis secondary to hepatic surgery for hydatid cysts," *Journal of Computer Assisted Tomography*, vol. 36, no. 5, pp. 534–535, 2012.

[9] M. Stojkovic, K. Rosenberger, H.-U. Kauczor, T. Junghanss, and W. Hosch, "Diagnosing and staging of cystic echinococcosis: how do CT and MRI perform in comparison to ultrasound?" *PLoS Neglected Tropical Diseases*, vol. 6, no. 10, Article ID e1880, 2012.

[10] D. Herek and N. Karabulut, "CT demonstration of pulmonary embolism due to the rupture of a giant hepatic hydatid disease," *Clinical Imaging*, vol. 36, no. 5, pp. 612–614, 2012.

28

Rosai-Dorfman Disease: Rare Pulmonary Involvement Mimicking Pulmonary Langerhans Cell Histiocytosis and Review of the Literature

Rashid AL Umairi[1], **Danielle Blunt,**[2] **Wedad Hana,**[3]
Matthew Cheung,[2] **and Anastasia Oikonomou**[1]

[1]*Department of Medical Imaging, Sunnybrook Health Sciences Centre, University of Toronto, Toronto, ON, Canada*
[2]*Department of Medicine, Sunnybrook Health Sciences Centre, University of Toronto, Toronto, ON, Canada*
[3]*Department of Anatomic Pathology, Sunnybrook Health Sciences Centre, University of Toronto, ON, Canada*

Correspondence should be addressed to Rashid AL Umairi; alumairi1@yahoo.com

Academic Editor: Atsushi Komemushi

Rosai-Dorfman disease (RDD), also known as sinus histiocytosis with massive lymphadenopathy, is a rare nonmalignant lymphohistiocytic proliferative disorder. We report a patient with RDD who presented with multiple skin lesions, pulmonary involvement, and CT manifestations mimicking Langerhans cell histiocytosis, which improved after initiation of corticosteroid treatment.

1. Introduction

Rosai-Dorfman disease (RDD), also known as sinus histiocytosis with massive lymphadenopathy, is a rare nonmalignant lymphohistiocytic proliferative disorder, described for the first time by Rosai and Dorfman in 1969 [1]. The disease typically manifests as painless, massive lymphadenopathy that frequently affects cervical lymph nodes and is accompanied by fever, leukocytosis, increased erythrocyte sedimentation rate, and hypergammaglobulinemia [2]. Although the disease commonly affects lymph nodes, extranodal involvement, either isolated or associated with lymph node involvement, has been reported in up to 43% of cases including skin, soft tissue, nasal cavity, bone, orbit, intrathoracic structures, central nervous system, breast, urogenital tract, and gastrointestinal tract [3–13]. We report a case of RDD with multiple skin lesions and pulmonary CT manifestations mimicking Langerhans cell histiocytosis, which improved after initiation of corticosteroid treatment.

2. Case Report

A 65-year-old male, smoker with a history of type 2 diabetes mellitus, hypertension, and hyperlipidemia, started to notice slowly growing lesions in his left cheek, posterior left shoulder, and left upper arm. The lesions were not tender or itchy. There was no history of shortness of breath. On physical examination, an indurated 10 × 10 cm lesion arising on the left cheek was identified (Figure 1). Similar lesions were also identified in the right upper arm measuring 2 × 3 cm and posterior left shoulder measuring 5 × 5 cm. No palpable lymphadenopathy or organomegaly was noted. Subsequent biopsy and microscopic examination of the left cheek skin lesion revealed an infiltrate formed by sheets of foamy macrophages surrounded by a dense plasma cell infiltrate and lymphocytes with scattered neutrophils. There was focal granuloma formation. Special stains for organism were negative. Immunohistochemical studies showed diffuse staining of the histiocytes for S100 protein and CD68. They were negative of CD1a, ruling out histiocytosis X. The lymphocytes were a mixture of T and B cells. The plasma cell infiltrate was polyclonal and was confirmed by in situ hybridization for kappa and lambda. The combination of findings was consistent with cutaneous Rosai-Dorfman disease. CT scan of the chest was performed, which showed bilateral thin and mildly thick-walled pulmonary cysts. Some of them were rounded and some demonstrated bizarre shapes

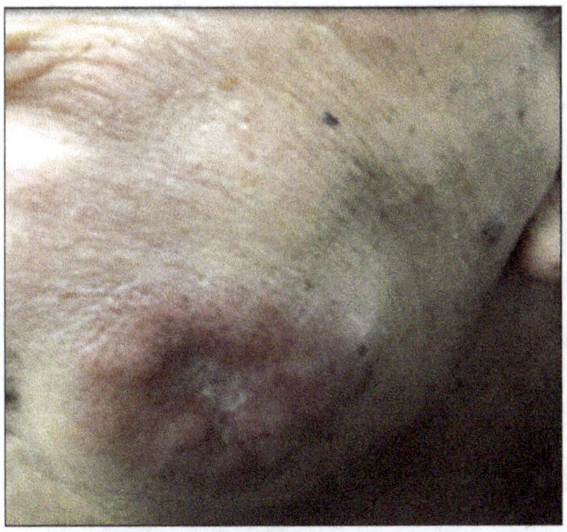

FIGURE 1: Heterogeneous pink plaque localized to the left cheek.

with multiloculation and internal septations. There were also numerous ground-glass nodules ranging from 1-2 mm up to a few centimeters. The findings had a characteristic upper lung zone predominance sparing the lung bases and the anteromedial parts of the middle lobe and lingula (Figure 2). There was no intrathoracic lymphadenopathy and no pleural effusion. Initially, the skin lesion at the cheek was treated with radiotherapy (1500 cGy in 5 fractions); however, there was only minimal response. The patient was started on 50 mg oral prednisone daily, which resulted in improvement of the skin lesions. However, treatment with prednisone was complicated by worsening of diabetes and peripheral edema and hence was stopped. A follow-up chest CT five months later showed complete resolution of the ground-glass nodules and persistence of the lung cysts (Figure 3).

3. Discussion

Rosai-Dorfman disease (RDD) is a rare nonmalignant histiocytic/phagocytic cell proliferative disorder, which typically presents in childhood and early adulthood with male predominance and a higher incidence in African-Americans [2, 6]. The histiocytic disorders are classified based on the cell origin. For instance, RDD and Langerhans cell histiocytosis (LCH) are both abnormal proliferation of histiocytic/phagocytic cells; however, they are different entities. RDD is monocytic/macrophage proliferative disorder, whereas LCH is dendritic cell proliferation disorder [14, 15].

The etiology of Rosai-Dorfman disease remains unknown and different etiologies have been proposed including viral infection and immune dysfunction. A proposed mechanism is cytokine activation following HHV6 or EBV infection leading to activation and accumulation of histiocytes, which is supported by the expression of HHV-6 antigens in abnormal histiocytes from RDD patients [2, 6, 8, 16].

Patients with Rosai-Dorfman disease typically present with fever and massive painless cervical lymphadenopathy. Extranodal involvement, either isolated or associated with lymph node involvement, has been reported in up to 43% of cases [2, 17]. Our patient had no abnormally enlarged intrathoracic or intra-abdominal lymphadenopathy. Approximately 10% of the patients have skin lesions, with 3% having disease only detectable in the skin. Skin lesions usually are xanthoma-like, yellowish, or reddish-brown plaques or nodules that can ulcerate. Our patient presented with slowly growing skin lesions on his left cheek, posterior left upper shoulder, and left upper arm (Figure 1). Intrathoracic lymphadenopathy is the most common intrathoracic manifestation in RDD, reported in 66% of patients in one case series (21). In that study, mediastinal adenopathy was the most common location of intrathoracic lymphadenopathy seen in 5 out of 21 patients. Less common findings included pleural effusion and interstitial infiltration with peripheral and basal predominance, while honeycombing and cystic changes were minimal or absent [18]. Intrathoracic manifestations of Rosai-Dorfman disease have rarely been reported in the literature, in less than 3% of cases, characterized by pulmonary nodules, pleural effusion, cystic changes, and interstitial lung disease. However, no details are available about the interstitial findings [19–21]. Ji et al. reported a case with Rosai-Dorfman disease presenting with left lower lobe mass [22]. Park et al. reported a case of Rosai-Dorfman disease with mediastinal and hilar lymph nodes and bilateral irregular nodular and patchy ground-glass opacities [23]. CT chest of our patient showed bilateral pulmonary cysts and numerous ground glass nodules of variable size ranging from a few millimeters to a few centimeters with characteristic upper lobe predominance and sparing of the lung bases and anteromedial parts of the middle lobe and lingula. There was no intrathoracic lymphadenopathy or pleural effusion. The chest CT findings were identical to the expected radiological features for pulmonary Langerhans cell histiocytosis [20]. However, the biopsy of the concomitant skin lesion confirmed the histological diagnosis of RDD. There was no histologic biopsy of the pulmonary lesions; however it would be less likely, although not excluded, that the pulmonary lesions would be histologically consistent with Langerhans cell histiocytosis when the skin lesion showed Rosai-Dorfman disease.

The diagnosis of RDD is based on a combination of clinical findings and characteristic histological features. The two classical histological features include scattered histiocytes with emperipolesis, which represent histiocytic phagocytosis of intact plasma cells, lymphocytes, and cellular debris as well as expression of S100 protein, CD14, CD68, and CD1c and absence of staining for CD1a and MHC-2 (which are both positive for Langerhans-type dendritic cells). The differential diagnosis includes Langerhans cell histiocytosis, lymphoma, immunoglobulin G4-related interstitial lung disease, and Erdheim-Chester disease. Our patient had a biopsy of his skin lesion, which showed focal granulomas formation with histiocytes positive for S100 protein and CD68 and negative for CD1a, confirming RDD and excluding pulmonary Langerhans cell histiocytosis. Cartin-Ceba and his group reported two patients with lung parenchymal findings and lung biopsy-proven Rosai-Dorfman disease. The first patient had bilateral intestinal infiltrates and the second patient had bilateral subpleural reticulation with scattered areas of ground glass opacities and tiny cysts. Histopathologic findings revealed interstitial thickening due to abnormal

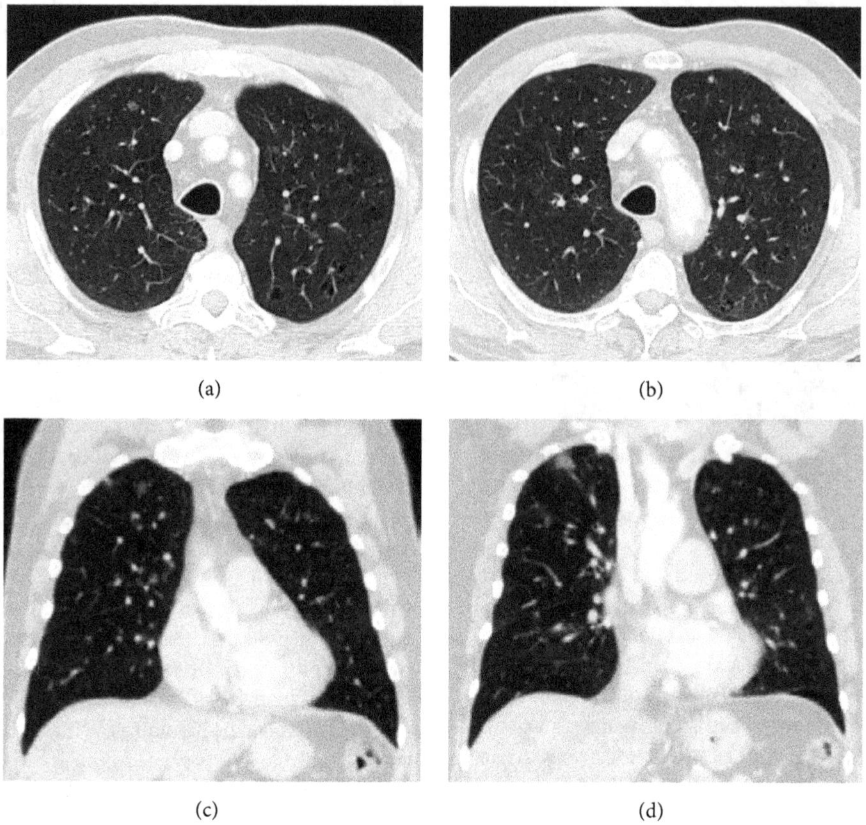

FIGURE 2: Selected axial and coronal HRCT images on lung windows show bilateral pulmonary cysts. Some of them are rounded and some demonstrate bizarre shapes with multiloculation and internal septations. There are also bilateral ground-glass nodules ranging from 1-2 mm up to a few centimeters. The findings are upper lobe predominant and spare the lung bases.

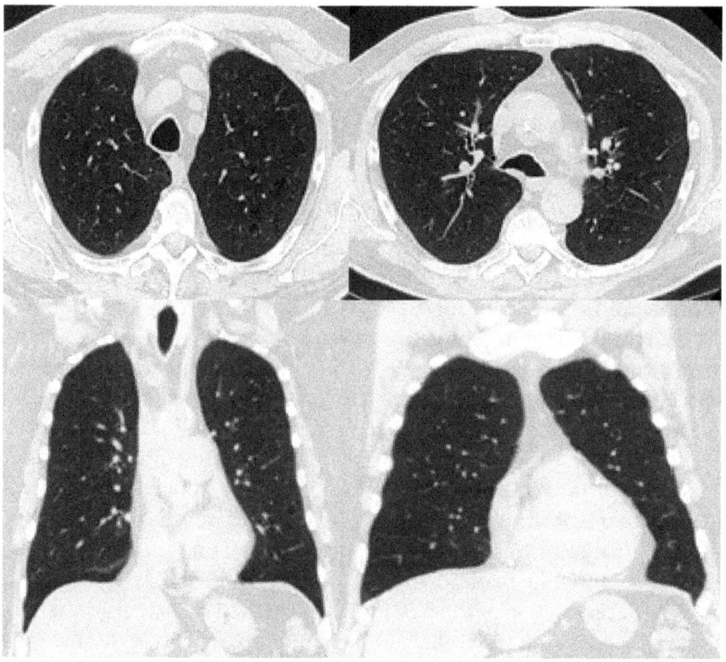

FIGURE 3: Follow-up HRCT images at the same level and planes as Figure 2 show resolution of the ground-glass nodules with persistent lung cysts.

histiocytic collections and associated mixed inflammatory infiltrates [18].

RDD is a self-limiting disease; however, fatality has been rarely reported due to massive adenopathy, involvement of different organs, anemia, and immunological abnormalities [24]. Approximately 50% of the patients require no treatment and spontaneous remission has been reported in approximately 20% of the cases [14, 25, 26]. Treatment is preserved for symptomatic patients or patients with vital organ or system involvement. If patients require treatment, surgery is an appropriate option for localized disease with complete remission reported in RDD cases involving the CNS treated with surgery only [27, 28]. Steroids, chemotherapy, and radiation therapy have been used for systemic disease or in cases of extensive organ involvement with varying degree of success [2, 27, 28]. Our patient had local radiotherapy to the skin lesion with no significant response. Subsequent oral prednisone was associated with improvement of the skin lesion and resolution of the ground-glass nodules.

4. Conclusion

We present a case with a skin lesion histologically confirmed as Rosai-Dorfman disease (RDD) and pulmonary CT pattern identical to pulmonary Langerhanss cell histiocytosis. Familiarity with this rare pulmonary CT manifestation of RDD along with the appropriate clinical findings may raise suspicion and accurate diagnosis of this rare type of histiocytosis.

Disclosure

The authors declare that there has been no significant financial support for this work that could have influenced its outcome. They confirm that the manuscript has been read and approved by all named authors and that there are no other persons who satisfied the criteria for authorship but are not listed. They further confirm that the order of authors listed in the manuscript has been approved by all of them. They also confirm that they have given due consideration to the protection of intellectual property associated with this work and that there are no impediments to publication, including the timing of publication, with respect to intellectual property. In so doing, they confirm that they have followed the regulations of their institutions concerning intellectual property.

References

[1] J. Rosai and R. F. Dorfman, "Sinus histiocytosis with massive lymphadenopathy. A newly recognized benign clinicopathological entity," *Archives of Pathology & Laboratory Medicine*, vol. 87, no. 1, pp. 63–70, 1969.

[2] S. Dalia, E. Sagatys, L. Sokol, and T. Kubal, "Rosai-Dorfman disease: tumor biology, clinical features, pathology, and treatment," *Cancer Control*, vol. 21, no. 4, pp. 322–327, 2014.

[3] A. Ali and D. Mackay, "Rosai-Dorfman disease of the lung," *Thorax*, vol. 64, no. 10, pp. 908-909, 2009.

[4] R. A. Anders, J. N. Keith, and J. Hart, "Rosai-Dorfman disease presenting in the gastrointestinal tract," *Archives of Pathology & Laboratory Medicine*, vol. 127, no. 2, pp. E74–E75, 2003.

[5] A. I. Hida, S.-I. Yagi, Y. Obase et al., "Rosai-Dorfman disease presenting as a solitary mediastinal mass," *Pathology International*, vol. 59, no. 4, pp. 265–268, 2009.

[6] K. Hur, C. Liu, and J. A. Koempel, "Paranasal rosai-dorfman disease with osseous destruction," *Case Reports in Otolaryngology*, vol. 2017, Article ID 1453097, 4 pages, 2017.

[7] D. V. La Barge III, K. L. Salzman, H. R. Harnsberger et al., "Sinus histiocytosis with massive lymphadenopathy (Rosai-Dorfman disease): imaging manifestations in the head and neck," *American Journal of Roentgenology*, vol. 191, no. 6, pp. W299–W306, 2008.

[8] I. W. Lao, Y. Dong, and J. Wang, "Rosai-Dorfman disease of the pericardium: a case report and review of literature," *International Journal of Clinical and Experimental Pathology*, vol. 7, no. 6, pp. 3408–3412, 2014.

[9] H. Ma, Y. Zheng, G. Zhu, J. Wu, C. Lu, and W. Lai, "Rosai-Dorfman disease with massive cutaneous nodule on the shoulder and back," *Annals of Dermatology*, vol. 27, no. 1, pp. 71–75, 2015.

[10] K. O'Gallagher, L. Dancy, A. Sinha, and D. Sado, "Rosai-Dorfman disease and the heart," *Intractable & Rare Diseases Research*, vol. 5, no. 1, pp. 1–5, 2016.

[11] N. N. Paryani, L. C. Daugherty, M. I. O'Connor, and L. Jiang, "Extranodal Rosai-Dorfman disease of the bone treated with surgery and radiotherapy," *Rare Tumors*, vol. 6, no. 4, article 5531, pp. 132–134, 2014.

[12] C. B. Pham, L. V. Abruzzo, E. Cook, G. J. Whitman, and T. W. Stephens, "Rosai-Dorfman disease of the breast," *American Journal of Roentgenology*, vol. 185, no. 4, pp. 971-972, 2005.

[13] D. M. Walters, G. H. Dunnington, S. M. Dustin et al., "Rosai-Dorfman disease presenting as a pulmonary artery mass," *The Annals of Thoracic Surgery*, vol. 89, no. 1, pp. 300–302, 2010.

[14] J. Goupil de Bouille, A. de Muret, E. Diot et al., "Pulmonary manifestations revealing Rosai-Dorfman disease," *Sarcoidosis Vasculitis and Diffuse Lung Disease*, vol. 32, no. 3, pp. 275–277, 2015.

[15] B. E. Favara, A. C. Feller, M. Pauli et al., "The who committee on histiocytic/reticulum cell proliferations. Reclassification working group of the histiocyte society," *Medical and Pediatric Oncology*, vol. 29, no. 3, pp. 157–166, 1997.

[16] M. Luppi, P. Barozzi, R. Garber et al., "Expression of human herpesvirus-6 antigens in benign and malignant lymphoproliferative diseases," *The American Journal of Pathology*, vol. 153, no. 3, pp. 815–823, 1998.

[17] J. Rosai and R. F. Dorfman, "Sinus histiocytosis with massive lymphadenopathy: a pseudolymphomatous benign disorder. Analysis of 34 cases," *Cancer*, vol. 30, no. 5, pp. 1174–1188, 1972.

[18] R. Cartin-Ceba, J. M. Golbin, E. S. Yi, U. B. S. Prakash, and R. Vassallo, "Intrathoracic manifestations of Rosai-Dorfman disease," *Respiratory Medicine*, vol. 104, no. 9, pp. 1344–1349, 2010.

[19] E. Foucar, J. Rosai, and R. Dorfman, "Sinus histiocytosis with massive lymphadenopathy (Rosai-Dorfman disease): review of the entity," *Seminars in Diagnostic Pathology*, vol. 7, no. 1, pp. 19–73, 1990.

[20] J. Ahuja, J. P. Kanne, C. A. Meyer et al., "Histiocytic disorders of the chest: Imaging findings," *RadioGraphics*, vol. 35, no. 2, pp. 357–370, 2015.

[21] R. N. Rao, C. A. Moran, and S. Suster, "Histiocytic disorders of the lung," *Advances in Anatomic Pathology*, vol. 17, no. 1, pp. 12–22, 2010.

[22] H. Ji, B. Zhang, D. Tian, S. Wu, X. Wang, and Y. Zhu, "Rosai-Dorfman disease of the lung," *Respiratory Care*, vol. 57, no. 10, pp. 1679–1681, 2012.

[23] B.-H. Park, D. H. Son, M.-H. Kim, T. S. Shim, H. J. Lee, and J. Huh, "Rosai-dorfman disease: report of a case associated with igG4-related: Sclerotic lesions," *The Korean Journal of Pathology*, vol. 46, no. 6, pp. 583–586, 2012.

[24] J. Chen, H. Tang, B. Li, and Q. Xiu, "Rosai-Dorfman disease of multiple organs, including the epicardium: an unusual case with poor prognosis," *Heart & Lung*, vol. 40, no. 2, pp. 168–171, 2011.

[25] A. Pulsoni, G. Anghel, P. Falcucci et al., "Treatment of sinus histiocytosis with massive lymphadenopathy (rosai-dorfman disease): report of a case and literature review," *American Journal of Hematology*, vol. 69, no. 1, pp. 67–71, 2002.

[26] F. B. Lima, P. S. V. Barcelos, A. P. N. Constâncio, C. D. Nogueira, and A. A. Melo-Filho, "Rosai-Dorfman disease with spontaneous resolution: case report of a child," *Revista Brasileira de Hematologia e Hemoterapia*, vol. 33, no. 4, pp. 312–314, 2011.

[27] F. Forest, A. T. N'Guyen, J. Fesselet et al., "Meningeal Rosai-Dorfman disease mimicking meningioma," *Annals of Hematology*, vol. 93, no. 6, pp. 937–940, 2014.

[28] B. Y. Huang, H. Zhang, W. J. Zong, and Y. H. Sun, "Rosai-dorfman disease of rare isolated spinal involvement: report of 4 cases and literature review," *World Neurosurgery*, vol. 85, pp. 367.e11–367.e16, 2016.

29

CT and MRI Features of Pediatric-Aged Colloid Cysts: Report of Two Cases

Hidayatullah Hamidi, Fazel Rahman Faizi, Najibullah Rasouly, and Mer Mahmood Shah Hoshang

French Medical Institute for Children (FMIC), Kabul, Afghanistan

Correspondence should be addressed to Hidayatullah Hamidi; hedayatullah.hamidi@gmail.com

Academic Editor: Alberto Spalice

A 10-year-old boy with the history of headache, anorexia, and vomiting was referred to our department to undergo a brain CT scan. CT images demonstrated a well-defined, rounded, hyperdense lesion at the level of the foramen of Monro causing moderate dilatation of the lateral ventricles. An 11-year-old girl with a long history of a headache was also referred to undergoing a brain MRI. MR images demonstrated a well-defined round abnormal signal intensity lesion at the level of the foramen of Monro causing moderate dilatation of lateral ventricles. The findings from imaging perspective were consistent with the colloid cyst of the third ventricle. Therefore, the diagnosis of the colloid cyst was made.

1. Introduction

Colloid cysts are benign intracranial neoplasms constituting 1% of CNS tumors. They may be totally asymptomatic or may manifest with symptoms of raised intracranial pressure. The symptoms may be intermittent, self-limiting, and non-specifically apparent when the foramen of Monro is blocked temporarily by pendulous movement of the cyst or may be acute and severe presenting with acute hydrocephalus, brain herniation, and sudden death. They usually appear as hyperdense lesions on CT; however, they can manifest as isodense or hypodense lesions as well. The appearance of the lesion on MRI is variable on different sequences and is dependent on cholesterol and protein contents of the cyst.

2. Case Presentation

2.1. Case 1. A 10-year-old boy with the history of headache, anorexia, and vomiting was referred to Radiology Department of French Medical Institute for Children to undergo a brain CT scan. The CT scan was performed with 128 slices' Siemens scanner. Precontrast images demonstrated a well-defined, rounded, hyperdense lesion at the level of the foramen of Monro causing moderate dilatation of the lateral ventricles. No specks of calcification were appreciated in the cyst. No significant enhancement appeared after intravenous contrast injection (Figures 1(a) and 1(b)).

2.2. Case 2. Interestingly, an 11-year-old girl with a long history of headache was referred to undergoing a brain MRI. The MRI was performed with 1.5 Tesla Siemens machine.

A well-defined rounded abnormal signal intensity lesion was visualized at the foramen of Monro resulting in moderate acute hydrocephalus. The lesion was isointense to gray matter on T2WI and hyperintense on T1WI and FLAIR images. No drop of the signal was visualized in $T2^*$ GRE sequence to suggest intralesional hemorrhage. No diffusion restriction was noted. Subtle enhancement of the lesion was seen on postcontrast images (Figures 2 and 3).

The first case did not receive any surgical treatment and, after ten months of follow-up, he claimed that the symptoms have diminished. The second case was lost of follow-up.

3. Discussion

Colloid cysts are benign congenital tumors of the brain located in the anterosuperior part of the third ventricle comprising 1% of CNS tumors and occur in three individuals

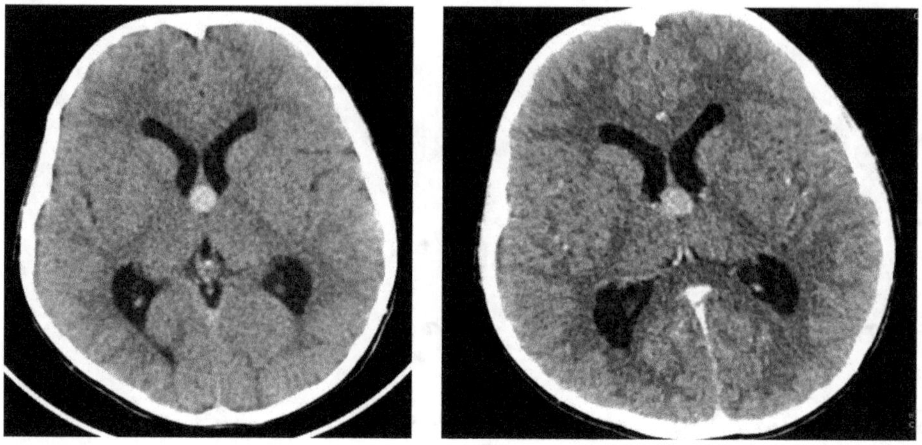

(a) (b)

Figure 1: (a) Nonenhanced axial section at the level of the foramen of Monro: a well-defined, round, hyperdense lesion causing mild prominence of bilateral lateral ventricles. (b) Contrast enhanced image shows no significant enhancement in the lesion.

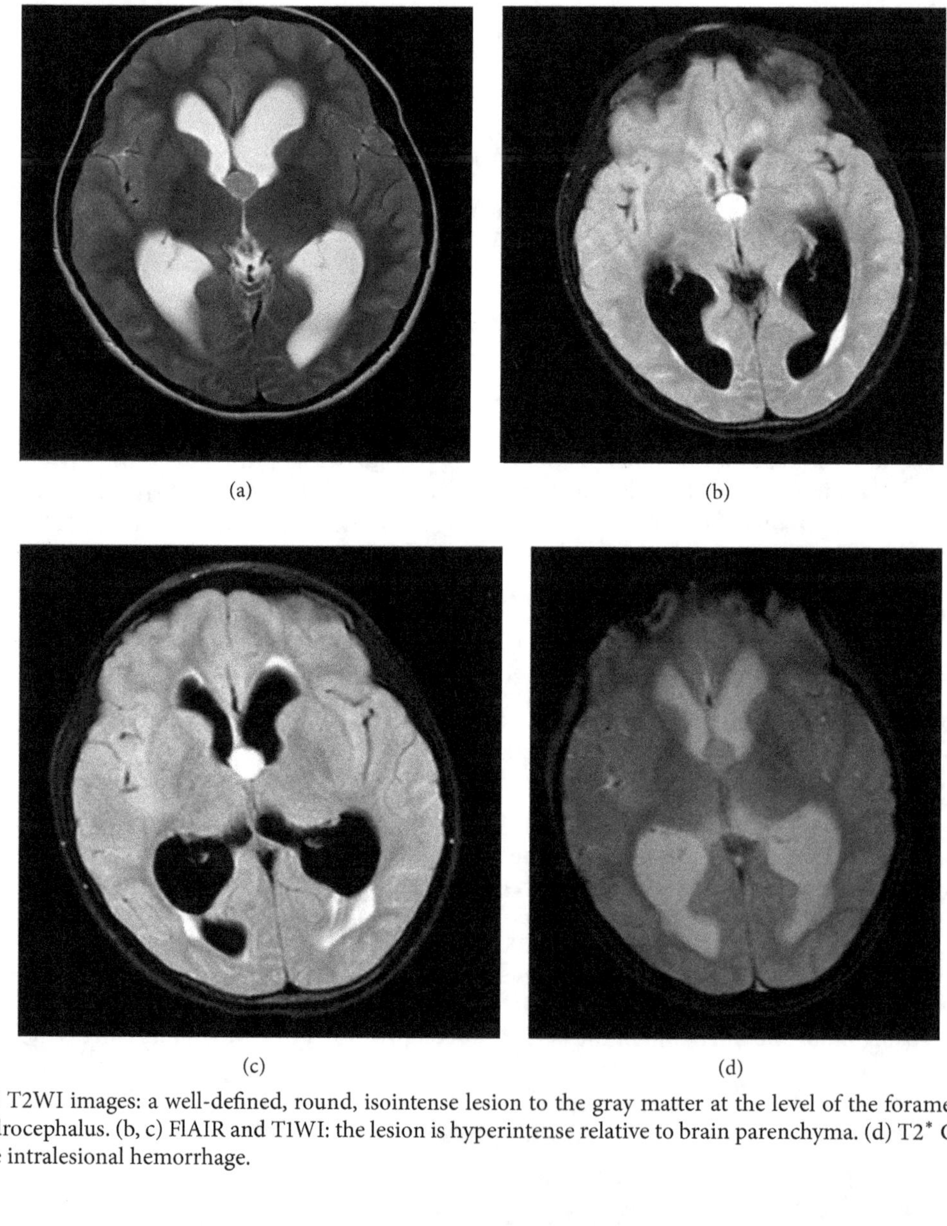

(a) (b)

(c) (d)

Figure 2: (a) Axial T2WI images: a well-defined, round, isointense lesion to the gray matter at the level of the foramen of Monro causing moderate acute hydrocephalus. (b, c) FlAIR and T1WI: the lesion is hyperintense relative to brain parenchyma. (d) T2* GRE images: no drop of signal to indicate intralesional hemorrhage.

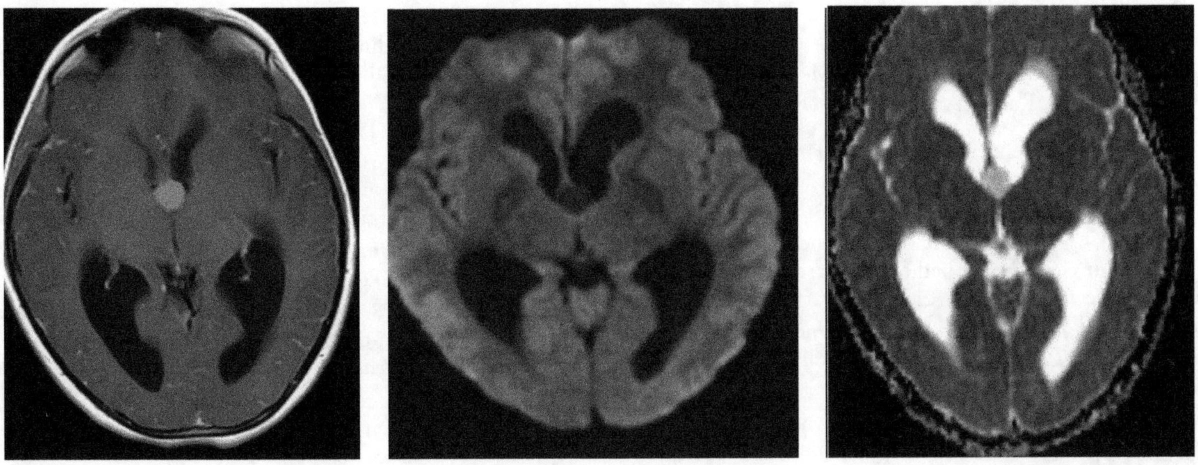

(a) (b) (c)

FIGURE 3: (a) TIWI + C: subtle enhancement after intravenous gadolinium injection. (b & c) No elevated diffusion pattern.

per million per year [1–4]. The age of onset is between 10 and 68 years of life with 68% occurring in third and fourth decades of life [5]. In our case, both patients were too young, in their early second decade of life.

In 1965, Shuangshoti et al. suggested that these cysts originate from neuroepithelium, like ependyma and choroid plexus, hence the term neuroepithelial cyst [6]; however, in 1992, Tsuchida et al. offered a nonneuroepithelial origin of colloid cyst, indicating its similarity to respiratory mucosa of the trachea and sphenoid sinus by using immunohistochemical techniques [7]. It has been postulated that colloid cysts and Rathke cleft cysts may present the same lesion in different locations [1, 8].

Colloid cysts are histologically benign and may be entirely asymptomatic, with no clinical symptom, and may be discovered incidentally. However, they may obstruct the foramen of Monro, raise intracranial pressure, and cause acute hydrocephalus [1, 2, 9].

3.1. Clinical Perspective. In symptomatic patients, headache is the presenting sign occurring in 68–100% of cases. It lasts seconds to minutes and initiates, is exacerbated, or terminates by a change in position [1, 3, 10]. Gait disturbances (47%) and short-term memory disturbances (37%) are the two other common symptoms; meanwhile, papilledema (47%) and ataxia (32%) are the most common signs [3]. The symptoms may be intermittent presenting when the foramen of Monro is obstructed by episodic pendulous movement of the cyst, though some may present with acute hydrocephalus, brain herniation, and sudden death [1, 3]. Acute hemorrhage within the cyst is a rare life-threatening condition due to the rapid development of obstructive hydrocephalus or exacerbating preexisting hydrocephalus which requires immediate diagnosis and surgical intervention [11, 12].

3.2. Imaging Workup. CT and MRI are both useful for diagnosis of the colloid cysts. On CT, they appear as round or oval shaped hyperdense lesions in the rostral aspect of the third ventricle; they may appear as isodense and hypodense lesions as well [1, 3]. On MRI, about 50% of colloid cysts are hyperintense on T1-weighted images and the rest are either isointense or hypointense with respect to the brain; on T2-weighted images, most colloid cysts are hypointense [1]. Isointense lesions may be difficult to identify on MRI; therefore, CT images are more useful [1, 3].

In a study performed by Sener NR, he claimed that colloid cyst had hypointense signal on DWI (on the b = 1000 sec/mm) which were apparently higher than cerebral parenchyma and lower than CSF. The diffusion MR imaging features of the colloid cyst are consistent with an elevated diffusion pattern [13].

Preoperative detection of the rare entity of hemorrhage within the cyst remains a challenge since these cysts usually appear hyperdense on CT images and hyperintense on T1W images. However, in isodense cysts, hyperdense areas may be visible inside the lesion representing acute hemorrhage on CT images [11, 12].

3.3. Treatment and Prognosis. Definitive treatment of colloid cyst is surgical excision, through an open craniotomy, endoscopy, or stereotactic aspiration of the cyst contents. However, treatment of asymptomatic patients is dependent upon a number of factors like the lesion size, the presence of hydrocephalus, the age of the patient, and medical conditions [3].

Surgical excision of colloid cyst is challenging due to its deep midline anatomical position [5].

4. Conclusion

Colloid cysts of the third ventricle are rare intracranial neoplasm and can affect young individuals. As surgical treatment of colloid cyst is challenging due to its deep midline anatomical position, it is better to treat young patients conservatively. One of our cases revealed diminishing symptoms after ten months of follow-up.

Additional Points

Place. The work is carried out in French Medical University for Children (FMIC), Kabul, Afghanistan.

References

[1] D. Armao, M. Castillo, H. Chen, and L. Kwock, "Colloid cyst of the third ventricle: imaging-pathologic correlation," *American Journal of Neuroradiology*, vol. 21, no. 8, pp. 1470–1477, 2000.

[2] A. Hassan, "Colloid cyst of brain," *Journal of the Liaquat University of Medical and Health Sciences*, vol. 5, no. 1, pp. 40–41, 2006.

[3] S. M. Joshi, K. K. Gnanalingham, P. Mohaghegh, A. Wilson, and A. Elsmore, "A case of familial third ventricular colloid cyst," *Emergency Medicine Journal*, vol. 22, no. 12, pp. 909–910, 2005.

[4] K. Opeskin, R. M. Anderson, and K. A. Lee, "Colloid cyst of the 3rd ventricle as a cause of acute neurological deterioration and sudden death," *Journal of Paediatrics and Child Health*, vol. 29, no. 6, pp. 476–477, 1993.

[5] K. I. Desai, T. D. Nadkarni, D. P. Muzumdar, and A. H. Goel, "Surgical management of colloid cyst of the third ventricle—a study of 105 cases," *Surgical Neurology*, vol. 57, no. 5, pp. 295–302, 2002.

[6] S. Shuangshoti, M. P. Roberts, and M. G. Netsky, "Neuroepithelial (colloid) cysts: pathogenesis and relation to choroid plexus and ependyma," *Archives of pathology*, vol. 80, pp. 214–224, 1965.

[7] T. Tsuchida, R. H. Hruban, B. S. Carson, and P. C. Phillips, "Colloid cysts of the third ventricle: immunohistochemical evidence for nonneuroepithelial differentiation," *Human Pathology*, vol. 23, no. 7, pp. 811–816, 1992.

[8] N. Graziani, H. Dufour, D. Figarella-Branger, A. Donnet, P. Bouillot, and F. Grisoli, "Do the suprasellar neurenteric cyst, the Rathke cleft cyst and the colloid cyst constitute a same entity?" *Acta Neurochirurgica*, vol. 133, no. 3-4, pp. 174–180, 1995.

[9] G. Wilms, "MR imaging of colloid cysts of the third ventricle," *American Journal of Neuroradiology*, vol. 22, no. 8, 2001.

[10] W. B. Young and S. D. Silberstein, "Paroxysmal headache caused by colloid cyst of the third ventricle: case report and review of the literature," *Headache*, vol. 37, no. 1, pp. 15–20, 1997.

[11] T. Beems, T. Menovsky, and M. Lammens, "Hemorrhagic colloid cyst: case report and review of the literature," *Surgical Neurology*, vol. 65, no. 1, pp. 84–86, 2006.

[12] R. Carrasco, J. M. Pascual, D. Medina-López, and A. Burdaspal-Moratilla, "Acute hemorrhage in a colloid cyst of the third ventricle: a rare cause of sudden deterioration," *Surgical Neurology International*, vol. 3, no. 1, article no. 24, 2012.

[13] R. N. Sener, "Colloid cyst: diffusion MR imaging findings," *Journal of Neuroimaging*, vol. 17, no. 2, pp. 181–183, 2007.

Diagnosis and Management of Spontaneous Lumbar Venous Retroperitoneal Hematoma in Setting of Deep Venous Thrombosis: A Case Report and Algorithm

Joseph Tseng,[1] Michael Leshen,[2] Todd Chapman,[3] Ryan Scott,[3] and Olga Kalinkin[3]

[1]*Department of Medicine, University of California Irvine School of Medicine, 333 City Boulevard West, Suite 400, Orange, CA 92868, USA*
[2]*Creighton University School of Medicine, Phoenix Regional Campus, 350 W Thomas Road, Phoenix, AZ 85013, USA*
[3]*Department of Radiology, St. Joseph's Hospital, 350 W Thomas Road, Phoenix, AZ 85013, USA*

Correspondence should be addressed to Michael Leshen; mal40015@creighton.edu

Academic Editor: Atsushi Komemushi

Retroperitoneal hematoma is rare and benefits from a systematic approach to prevent morbidity and mortality. Management of such bleeds is based upon patient stability, the cause (spontaneous or posttraumatic), and source (arterial or venous). Herein, the authors describe a diagnostic and management algorithm for retroperitoneal hemorrhage with an example of a rare lumbar venous bleed under the complicated clinical setting of deep venous thrombosis.

1. Introduction

Retroperitoneal hematoma is a well-known, but rare, clinical condition that can be potentially lethal. They are most frequently seen as a complication of interventions such as femoral artery catheterizations or abdominal trauma [1]. Retroperitoneal hemorrhage has a variety of etiologies that should be suspected in patients with significant groin, flank, abdominal, back pain, or hemodynamic instability following an interventional procedure. When this occurs in patients without any obvious precipitating factors, it is termed spontaneous retroperitoneal hemorrhage. Most often, these patients are anticoagulated or on hemodialysis. There is an incidence of 0.1% to 0.6% in patients receiving oral anticoagulants [2]. Despite having well-recognized clinical signs such as the Grey-Turner and Cullen signs, diagnosis of retroperitoneal hemorrhage is often delayed due to the manifestation of these signs late in the clinical course. Due to the ability of hemorrhage to rapidly exsanguinate and cause shock, the survival of the patient is dependent on rapid and accurate diagnosis.

Lumbar vein hemorrhage is rare. There have been reports of lumbar vein rupture as a complication of acute pancreatitis and a patient taking fondaparinux [3, 4]. However there has never been a report of this occurring in otherwise asymptomatic patients. In this case, bleeding was identified with CT and managed with the utilization of transcatheter venous embolization as a method of bleeding control. Here, we present a rare case of retroperitoneal hematoma formation secondary to a lumbar vein bleed in the setting of deep venous thrombosis and provide a diagnostic and management algorithm.

2. Case Report

A 58-year-old homeless male with a history of hypertension and prior venous thromboembolism presented to the emergency department (ED) for 1 week of weakness and fatigue. He denied any hemoptysis, dyspnea, chest pain, headache, nausea, and vomiting. Besides a heart rate of 113 bpm his physical exam was normal. His past medical history included type II diabetes. His past surgical history was significant for an infrarenal IVC filter placement 15 years ago that was still in place. He was unsure as to why it was initially placed. He had no known allergies and took atenolol,

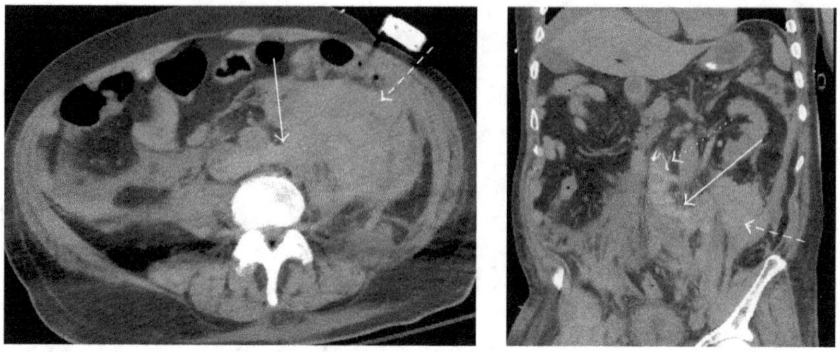

(a) (b)

Figure 1: (a) Initial noncontrast CT axial image demonstrated a large high density left retroperitoneal hematoma (dashed arrow) contiguous with left site of aorta and IVC (arrow). (b) Initial noncontrast CT coronal reformatted images demonstrated a large high density left retroperitoneal hematoma (dashed arrow) contiguous with high-attenuated tubular structure arising from the left side of IVC (arrow), likely a lumbar vein. There is an expansile appearance of infrarenal IVC. IVC filter above the left inferior renal vein is also appreciated (dotted arrow).

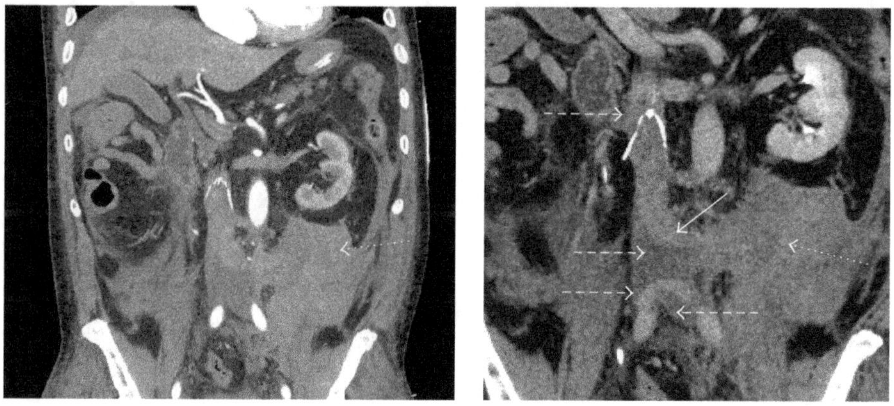

(a) (b)

Figure 2: (a) Subsequent contrast CT coronal reformatted image during arterial phase demonstrated no active aortic or arterial contrast extravasation associated with a high density large retroperitoneal hematoma (dotted arrow). (b) Contrast CT coronal reformatted image during delayed (120 sec) venous phase demonstrated hyperattenuated contrast material below the IVC filter contiguous with dilated left lumbar vein (arrow) extending to left retroperitoneal hematoma (dotted arrow). Nonocclusive hypoattenuated clots (dashed arrows) are present below the IVC filter along with an irregular contour of the distal left IVC. Small nonocclusive thrombi above the IVC filter tip and in the iliac veins are also appreciated (dashed arrows).

lisinopril, and metformin at home. He was not taking any oral anticoagulants. He had no family history of malignancies and bleeding disorders.

While in the ED the patient became unresponsive and ACLS was initiated and lasted for 11 minutes. The patient was intubated, resuscitated, and transferred to the intensive care unit. While in the ICU it was noted that the patient's hemoglobin dropped from 12.3 gm/dL to 6.8 gm/dL.

3. Differential Diagnosis

The differential diagnosis for acute anemia primarily includes blood loss and a wide variety of hemolytic processes such as microangiopathic hemolytic anemia, disseminated intravascular coagulation, sickle cell disease, and paroxysmal nocturnal hemoglobinuria just to name a few. Based on the patient's history and current clinical condition our initial concern was acute anemia secondary to blood loss and a noncontrast CT scan of the chest, abdomen, and pelvis was ordered.

4. Imaging Findings

The CT scan demonstrated a large, left-sided retroperitoneal hematoma contiguous with left site of aorta and IVC, mass effect on the bladder, and expansile appearance of IVC below the IVC filter (Figures 1(a) and 1(b)). Follow-up abdominal CT angiogram with arterial and venous phases excluded arterial etiology of retroperitoneal bleed and reveled nonocclusive IVC and bilateral common iliac vein thrombi slightly extended above the IVC filter. High attenuation left retroperitoneal hematoma was contiguous with left wall of infrarenal IVC and tubular left retroperitoneal structure of likely dilated left lumbar vein (Figures 2(a) and 2(b)). A follow-up CT angiogram of the chest was obtained due to the

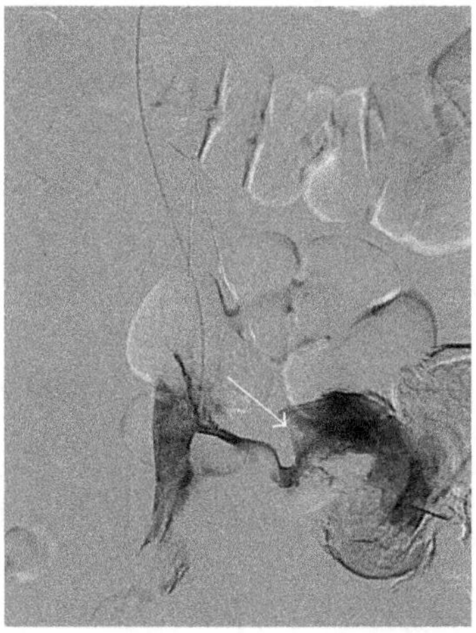

FIGURE 3: Selective catheter venogram reveals brisk active extravasation from a left lumbar vein into the left retroperitoneal hematoma (arrow).

presence of the thrombus proximal to the patient's IVC filter and revealed multiple subsegmental pulmonary emboli in the right lower lobe of the lung.

5. Treatment

The patient was referred to Interventional Radiology and an inferior venacavogram was performed. The right internal jugular vein was chosen as an access point due to operator preference and to avoid the large clot burden in the iliac veins and IVC. It was accessed with a micropuncture system, via ultrasound guidance. The micropuncture sheath was exchanged for a 5-French vascular sheath. An Omni Flush catheter was then advanced to the infrarenal IVC, distal to the patient's old IVC filter. Injection of contrast revealed brisk active extravasation from a left lumbar venous branch (Figure 3). This branch was then selectively embolized with Gelfoam slurry and multiple 0.035 embolic coils (Figures 4(a) and 4(b)). No residual extravasation was identified on postembolization venography.

The IVC above the filter was then selected and an inferior venacavogram was again performed, this time showing multiple filling defects compatible with venous thrombus, including thrombus at the superior aspect of the IVC filter, outside of the filter cone. Given the acute subsegmental pulmonary emboli noted on the previous CTA chest, as well as the contraindication to oral anticoagulation, the decision was made to deploy a suprarenal IVC filter (Figure 5). The patient tolerated the procedure well with no complications and his hemoglobin stabilized to 9.3 gm/dL.

Over the next two days the patient developed persistent scrotal pain, leg swelling, and pain. This was attributed to the patients extensive clot burden. Thrombectomy and infrarenal IVC filter retrieval were then performed in an attempt to alleviate the patients swelling. Due to the large size of the clots an AngioVac cannula and circuit were used. During the procedure a large portion of clot was removed from the patient's left superficial femoral vein through the IVC. However, the infrarenal IVC was unable to be retrieved. While recovering from the procedure the patient became tachycardic, hypoxic, and hypotensive and was readmitted to the ICU. The patient's instability was most likely due to a postprocedure pulmonary embolism secondary to thrombus disruption. However, no imaging was performed to confirm this suspicion. He was then stabilized and was placed on lovenox and with the intention to bridge to warfarin for outpatient management. His hemoglobin remained stable throughout the remainder of his hospitalization and he was discharged shortly thereafter. Unfortunately the patient was then lost to follow-up and the status of either IVC filter is unknown.

6. Discussion

This patient presented with a complicated clinical scenario; as he had a history of thromboembolic events, yet he was actively hemorrhaging into the retroperitoneum. Furthermore, the patient had a previous infrarenal IVC filter that was involved in an occlusive clot formation. IVC filter thrombosis has been reported in 3 to 30 percent of patients following filter placement [5]. While obstruction can be asymptomatic, it can often lead to lower extremity edema, increase the risk of other sequelae of venous insufficiency, and result in the development of collateral vessels that may serve as a route for recurrent embolization [1].

6.1. Spontaneous Retroperitoneal Hematoma from Lumbar Vein. Retroperitoneal hematoma is a rare clinical condition, with an incidence of 0.1%, and as high as 0.6% in patients receiving oral anticoagulation therapy. It is most frequently seen as a complication of interventions such as femoral artery catheterizations and pelvic or lumbar trauma. Retroperitoneal hemorrhage has a variety of etiologies that should be suspected in patients with significant groin, flank, abdominal, back pain, or hemodynamic instability following an interventional procedure. When bleeding happens without any obvious precipitating factors, it is termed spontaneous hemorrhage. Spontaneous hemorrhage occurs most frequently in patients who are anticoagulated or on hemodialysis [6].

The pathogenesis and pathophysiology of spontaneous retroperitoneal bleeding remain unclear, but it has been hypothesized that heparin or anticoagulation-induced immune microangiopathy may play a role. In this model, unrecognized minor trauma in the microcirculation in the presence of coagulation may lead to hemorrhage. This unrecognized trauma can be due to a variety of factors, such as vomiting, coughing, or even trauma secondary to participating in sports [6].

Lumbar vein hemorrhage is rare, and lumbar vein hemorrhage leading to a retroperitoneal hematoma has previously been unreported. Lumbar veins drain blood from the abdominal wall and vertebral venous plexus into the inferior vena cava, ascending lumbar veins, renal veins, or lumbar azygous vein. While there has been a reported case of lumbar vein rupture as a complication of acute pancreatitis, there has been no report of this occurring in otherwise asymptomatic patients [3].

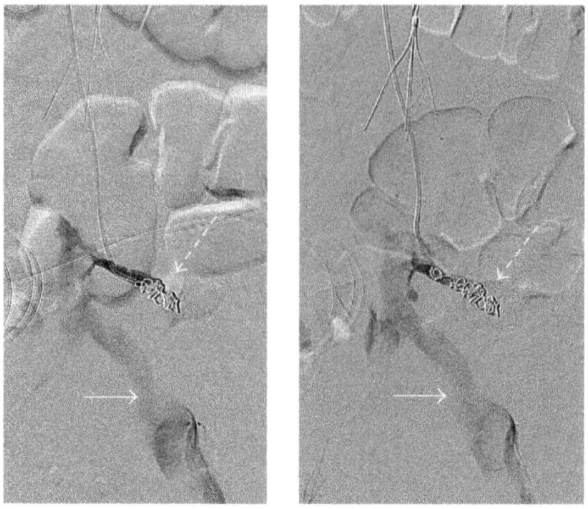

(a) (b)

FIGURE 4: Postembolization venography after Gelfoam and coil embolization (dashed arrow) showed no residual active extravasation from this branch. A nonocclusive thrombus in the common iliac vein is noted (arrow).

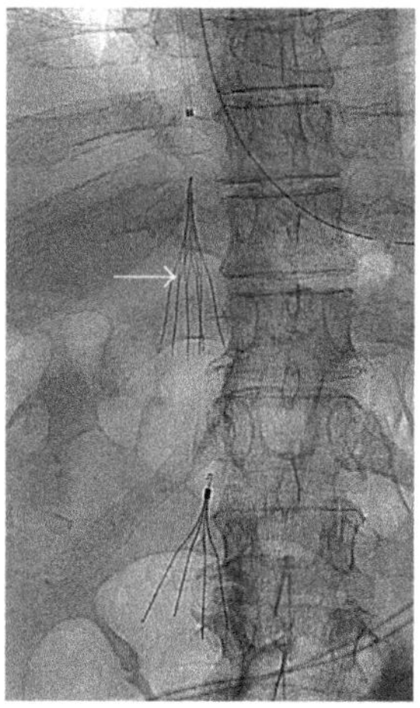

FIGURE 5: A final fluoroscopic spot view confirmed appropriate positioning of suprarenal IVC filter placement (arrow).

In our unique case we cannot completely rule out iatrogenic trauma secondary to CPR. It is possible that the chest compressions forced blood retrograde, below the filter. The thrombosed infrarenal IVC filter may have acted as a valve, slowing anterograde flow, increasing pressure in the lumbar vein, and causing it to rupture. However retroperitoneal bleeds due to CPR are extremely rare, with an incidence of 0.1% [7]. In addition to the low incidence of iatrogenic retroperitoneal hematomas secondary to CPR, the site of the lumbar vein hematoma in this patient was not near the area of chest compressions and thus makes it less likely to be the cause of the bleed.

6.2. Radiological Evaluation of Retroperitoneal Hematoma. The initial assessment of a patient with a suspected retroperitoneal hematoma requires evaluation for shock. Patients should forgo CT/CTA and go directly to angiography if there is high suspicion of a retroperitoneal hematoma and the patient has abnormal vital signs such as hypotension, tachycardia, decreased urine output, or altered mental status. If a patient is stable, then a more methodical radiological approach may be utilized (Figure 6). In our case, after noting a severe drop in the patient's hemoglobin a CT abdomen was ordered. Noncontrast CT revealed left retroperitoneal hematoma contiguous with the aorta, IVC, and retroaortic sentinel clot.

Identification of the etiology of bleeding is the next critical step for selection of intervention, whether it may be surgical, interventional radiological, or medical. Firstly, it must be determined whether the bleed is of arterial or venous origin. If the bleed is of arterial origin, the next step is to determine whether it is from the aorta or aortic branch. If the bleed is of venous origin, the next step is to determine whether it is from the inferior vena cava or other small veins.

A subsequent CT angiogram was performed, which excluded an aortic or arterial origin of bleeding. The large left retroperitoneal hematoma was contiguous with the IVC/lumbar vein and was highlighted by the sentinel clot. IVC thrombi below and above the IVC filter as well as the segmental pulmonary emboli in spite of the presence of the IVC filter were identified.

Arterial vascular bleeding requires immediate vascular intervention with coil embolization. A venous bleed with a large hematoma and slow contrast extravasation requires intervention. On the other hand, slow venous bleeding from small vessels can be managed with observation. The decision was then made to proceed with a catheter venous angiogram to identify the site of the venous bleed and to provide further management with insertion of an IVC filter. In the case of our patient the IVC filter was placed above the renal veins. It was previously thought that suprarenal IVC filters would increase the risk of renal vein thrombosis due to thrombus accumulation. However, several studies have shown there no increased risk associated with suprarenal IVC

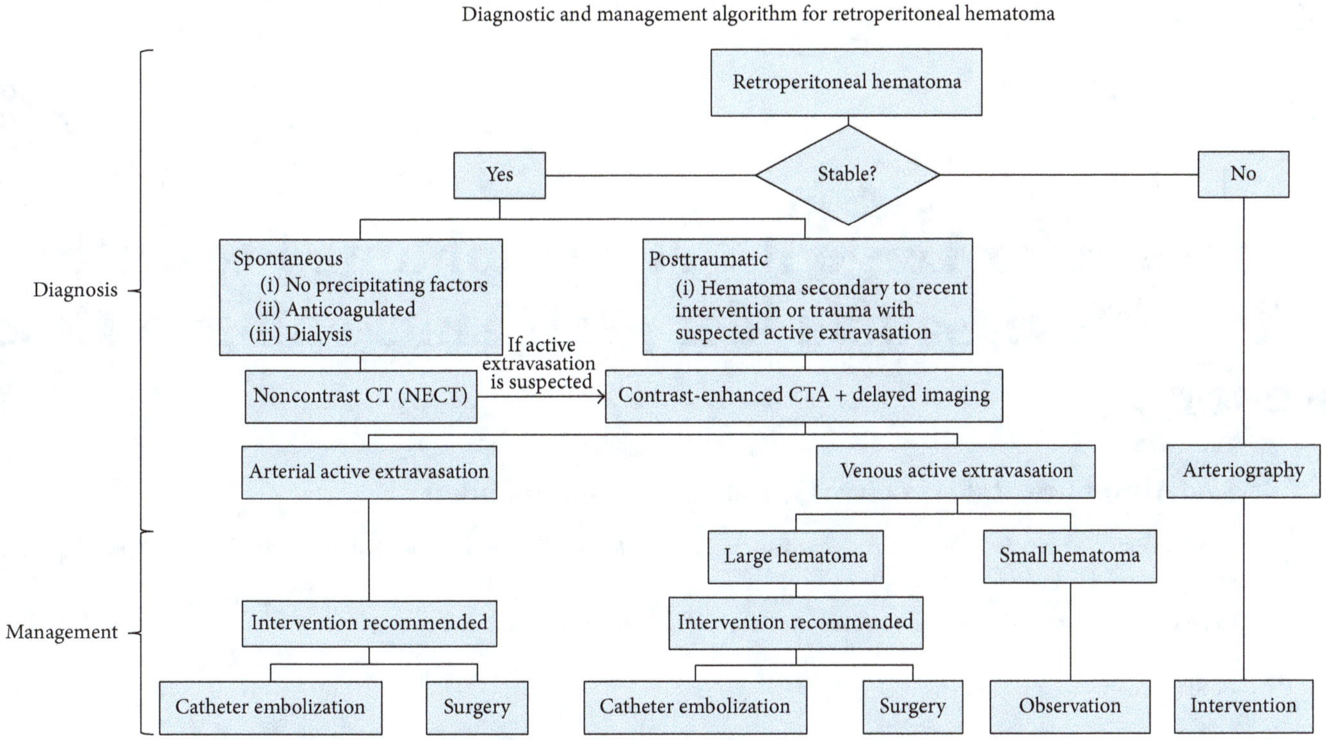

FIGURE 6: Diagnostic algorithm for evaluation of a retroperitoneal hematoma.

filters versus infrarenal IVC filters [8, 9]. The most common complication of suprarenal IVC filters is filter migration due to its variability of blood volume and venous return [10].

Additional Points

Learning Points. (1) Spontaneous retroperitoneal hematomas are a rare event that typically occurs in patients that are receiving anticoagulation or hemodialysis. (2) Retroperitoneal hematomas may benefit from an algorithm-based approach to management. (3) Management of pulmonary embolism or DVT can be complicated by active bleeding.

References

[1] P. F. Fedullo, L. J. Rubin, K. M. Kerr, W. R. Auger, and R. N. Channick, "The natural history of acute and chronic thromboembolic disease: the search for the missing link," *European Respiratory Journal*, vol. 15, no. 3, pp. 435–437, 2000.

[2] X. Estivill Pallejà, P. Domingo, J. Fontcuberta, and J. Félez, "Spontaneous retroperitoneal hemorrhage during oral anticoagulant therapy," *Archives of Internal Medicine*, vol. 145, no. 8, pp. 1531-1534, 1985.

[3] A. De Rosa, K. Oyewole, M. R. Hanief, and R. Vashisht, "A complication of acute pancreatitis: lumbar vessel rupture," *Internet Journal of Surgery*, vol. 22, no. 2, pp. 1–4, 2009.

[4] M. Fortina, S. Carta, E. O. Del Vecchio, E. Crainz, S. Urgelli, and P. Ferrata, "Retroperitoneal hematoma due to spontaneous lumbar artery rupture during fondaparinux treatment. Case report and review of the literature," *Acta Biomedica de l'Ateneo Parmense*, vol. 78, no. 1, pp. 46–81, 2007.

[5] D. M. Becker, J. T. Philbrick, and J. B. Selby, "Inferior vena cava filters. Indications, safety, effectiveness," *Archives of Internal Medicine*, vol. 152, no. 10, pp. 1985–1994, 1992.

[6] Y. C. Chan, J. P. Morales, J. F. Reidy, and P. R. Taylor, "Management of spontaneous and iatrogenic retroperitoneal haemorrhage: conservative management, endovascular intervention or open surgery?" *International Journal of Clinical Practice*, vol. 62, no. 10, pp. 1604–1613, 2008.

[7] J. P. Krischer, E. G. Fine, J. H. Davis, and E. L. Nagel, "Complications of cardiac resuscitation," *Chest*, vol. 92, no. 2, pp. 287–291, 1987.

[8] S. P. Kalva, C. Chlapoutaki, S. Wicky, A. J. Greenfield, A. C. Waltman, and C. A. Athanasoulis, "Suprarenal inferior vena cava filters: a 20-year single-center experience," *Journal of Vascular and Interventional Radiology*, vol. 19, no. 7, pp. 1041–1047, 2008.

[9] W. J. Matchett, M. P. Jones, D. R. McFarland, and E. J. Ferris, "Suprarenal vena caval filter placement: follow-up of four filter types in 22 patients," *Journal of Vascular and Interventional Radiology*, vol. 9, no. 4, pp. 588–593, 1998.

[10] H. Ni and L. L. Win, "Retrievable inferior vena cava filters for venous thromboembolism," *ISRN Radiology*, vol. 2013, Article ID 959452, 8 pages, 2013.

Intravascular Large B-Cell Lymphoma Presenting with Diffuse Gallbladder Wall Thickening: A Case Report

Sayf Al-Katib, Robert Colvin, and Farnoosh Sokhandon

Department of Diagnostic Radiology and Molecular Imaging, Oakland University William Beaumont School of Medicine, Beaumont Health, Royal Oak, MI, USA

Correspondence should be addressed to Sayf Al-Katib; sayf.al-katib@beaumont.org

Academic Editor: Soon Thye Lim

Intravascular large B-cell lymphoma is a rare subtype of extranodal diffuse B-cell lymphoma characterized by proliferation of neoplastic cells within the lumen of small and medium sized vessels. Clinical and imaging findings are nebulous as the intravascular subtype of lymphoma can involve a multitude of organs. Involvement of the gallbladder is extremely uncommon, and imaging findings can be easily confused for more prevalent pathologies. We report a case of intravascular large B-cell lymphoma in an 83-year-old male and review clinical presentation and imaging findings on CT, ultrasound, hepatobiliary iminodiacetic acid (HIDA) scan, and MRI. It is important for the radiologist to know about this disease as the imaging findings are atypical of other types of lymphoma, and this may lead to a delay in diagnosis and treatment.

1. Introduction

Intravascular large B-cell lymphoma is a rare subtype of extranodal diffuse B-cell lymphoma characterized by proliferation of neoplastic cells within the lumen of small and medium sized vessels. Clinical and imaging findings are nebulous as the intravascular subtype of lymphoma can involve a multitude of organs. Involvement of the gallbladder is extremely uncommon, and imaging findings can be easily confused for more prevalent pathologies. This case is a reminder of a rare but important diagnostic consideration in the setting of a diffusely thickened gallbladder wall.

2. Case Presentation

An 83-year-old Caucasian male with past medical history of hypertension, diabetes, and coronary artery disease presented to the emergency department with extreme fatigue, weakness, and disorientation. He reported a history of 10–15-pound weight loss over the previous month. Physical exam did not yield any focal signs. Laboratory evaluation revealed pancytopenia (Hgb 9.6 g/dL, WBC 3.0 bil/L, and platelets 169 bil/L) and increased liver function enzymes (AST 311 U/L, ALT 62 U/L, and ALP 237 U/L). The patient was admitted for generalized weakness and fatigue.

An unenhanced CT scan of the abdomen and pelvis obtained in the emergency department showed a nondistended gallbladder with diffuse wall thickening (Figure 1). A small calcified gallstone was identified in the neck of the gallbladder. Neither a soft tissue mass nor lymphadenopathy was present. Although acute cholecystitis was not a leading differential diagnosis based on the clinical presentation, HIDA scan was recommended based on the unexpected CT findings.

The patient developed worsening alteration of mental status, metabolic acidosis, further increase in liver function tests, and pancytopenia. D-dimer was elevated (1830 ng/mL). There was initially clinical concern for pulmonary embolism versus disseminated intravascular coagulation. Nuclear medicine testing with ventilation-perfusion (VQ) scan was performed and low probability for pulmonary embolism was found. Coagulation testing remained stable.

The HIDA scan revealed cystic duct patency (Figure 2). Subsequently, a targeted sonographic examination of the

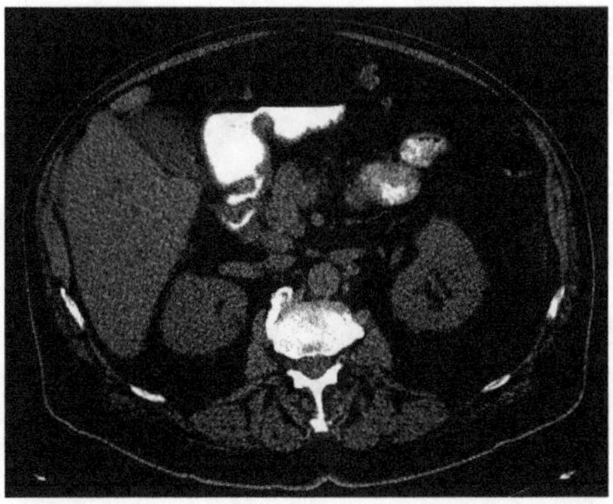

FIGURE 1: Axial unenhanced CT of the abdomen obtained at presentation shows a diffusely thickened and low attenuation gallbladder wall.

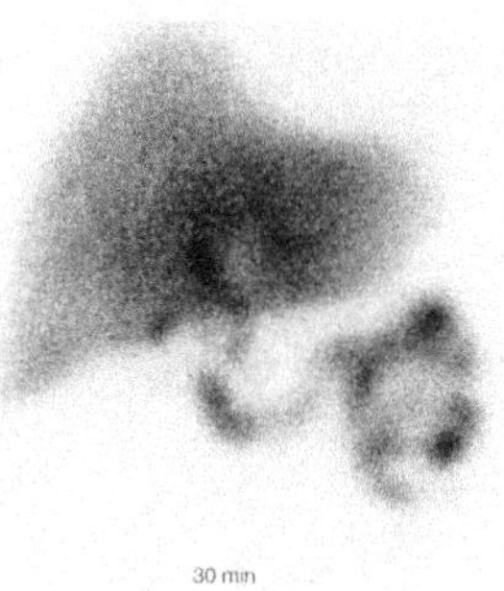

FIGURE 2: Image obtained during HIDA scan shows early filling of the gallbladder by 30 minutes which was confirmed on delayed 40- and 60-minute images.

right upper quadrant was performed to further characterize the nonspecific findings on the CT scan. This revealed diffuse gallbladder wall thickening measuring up to 8 mm. The gallbladder wall had a striated appearance with a central hypoechoic stripe surrounded by an echogenic band on either side (Figure 3). The sonographic Murphy's sign was negative. The gallbladder was decompressed and contained a few small stones. An MRI of the abdomen with contrast showed diffusely thickened gallbladder wall measuring up to 12 mm with intramural increased signal intensity on T2 weighted images. Contrast enhanced T1 weighted sequences showed no abnormal enhancement or nodularity of the gallbladder wall. The gallbladder did contain a few small stones, but there was no luminal distention, pericholecystic fluid, or lymphadenopathy (Figure 4). Clinical concern further developed for septicemia with the gallbladder as the primary site of origin given the imaging findings. The patient underwent laparoscopic cholecystectomy.

Pathologic evaluation of the surgical specimen revealed findings of intravascular large B-cell lymphoma (IVLBCL), a rare variant of extranodal diffuse large B-cell lymphoma. Histologic evaluation with hematoxylin and eosin stain demonstrated diffuse gallbladder wall thickening with lymphatic ectasia (Figure 5). Several blood vessels in the subserosal fat showed infiltration with large, atypical lymphomatous cells.

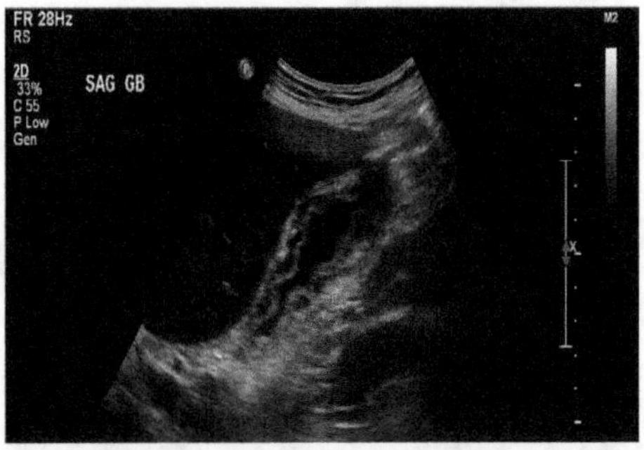

FIGURE 3: Grayscale longitudinal sonographic image of the right upper quadrant shows a decompressed gallbladder wall with diffuse wall thickening. The gallbladder wall has a striated appearance without increased vascularity.

The mucosa was uninvolved. These features explained all the imaging findings well in this particular case.

Flow cytometry of the peripheral blood revealed a small population of aberrant B-cells which correlate to the pathologic gallbladder wall findings. Subsequent bone marrow core biopsy and aspiration were performed. Pathologic evaluation demonstrated slight hypercellularity of the marrow and 10–15% involvement by diffuse large B-cell lymphoma. Immunohistochemical stain of bone marrow core biopsy sample was positive for CD79a, confirming B-cell origin.

Postoperatively, the patient's condition continued to deteriorate requiring respiratory support in the intensive care unit. He developed severe metabolic acidosis and hemodynamic instability. Given the patient's poor functional status and concomitant diagnosis of IVLBCL, the decision to withdraw supportive care was made by his family. The patient expired 7 days after initial presentation.

3. Discussion

Intravascular B-cell lymphoma is a highly aggressive form of extranodal B-cell lymphoma characterized by neoplastic cell growth within the lumen of small sized vessels [1]. It presents as a disseminated aggressive disease without focal mass or lymphadenopathy [2]. Neoplastic vascular involvement can affect all types of organs, such as bone marrow, CNS, skin, lung, adrenal gland, liver, kidney, spleen, thyroid, pituitary gland, and gastrointestinal tract [3]. In our patient, no additional lesions were identified in the base of the lungs, abdomen, or pelvis. No cross-sectional imaging was performed on the chest or brain during this hospitalization, so involvement of the lungs or brain cannot be excluded. Overall, findings in this case are consistent with secondary IVLBCL of the gallbladder wall. IVLBCL presenting with gallbladder symptoms is very rare with only a handful of cases described in the literature [4]. Common clinical presentation includes nonspecific systemic symptoms, such as fever of unknown origin, fatigue, deterioration of performance status, and neurological alteration.

This case highlights the diagnostic conundrum of IVLBCL. In our case, the patient experienced nonspecific intermittent altered mental status and fatigue without focal

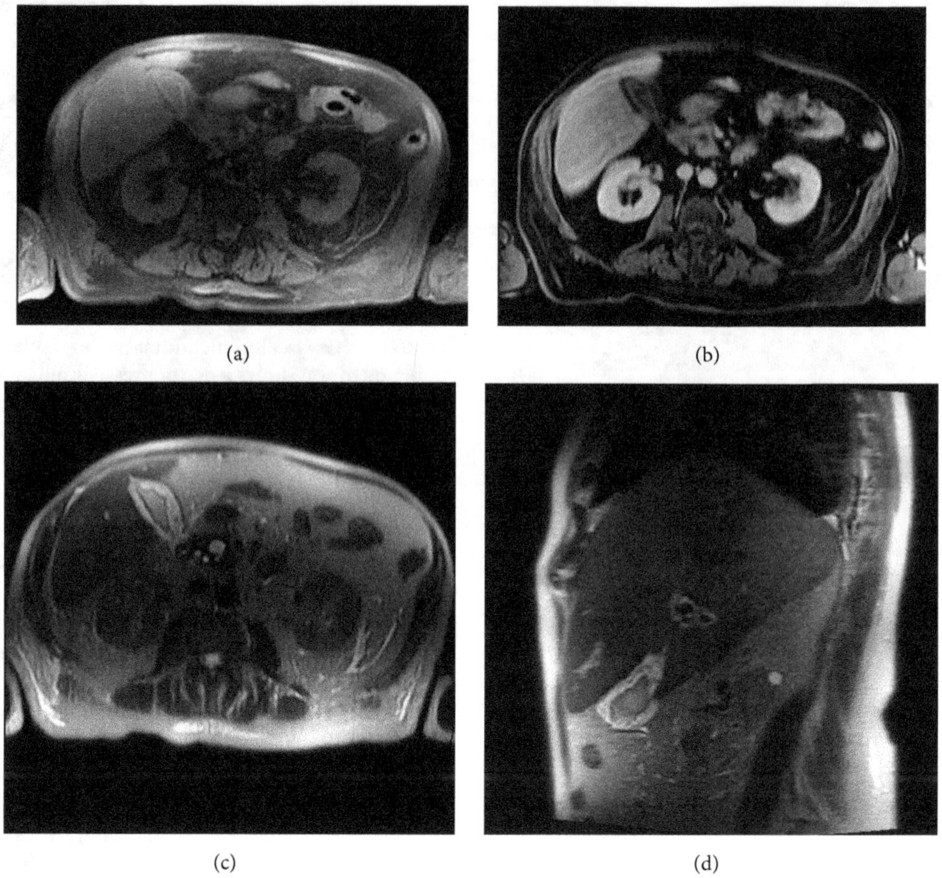

FIGURE 4: (a) Axial T1W-VIBE precontrast, (b) axial T1W-VIBE postcontrast, (c) axial T2W-fat suppressed, and (d) coronal T2W-fat suppressed sequences. MR images show diffuse gallbladder wall thickening with increased signal intensity on T2 weighted fat suppressed images. Postcontrast fat suppressed images demonstrate homogeneous mucosal enhancement with no transmural wall enhancement.

abdominal pain. Furthermore, imaging evaluation revealed only nonspecific findings of striated gallbladder wall thickening. The lack of lymphadenopathy in patients with IVLBCL also makes timely diagnosis challenging. Additionally, staging of this disease is difficult secondary to the lack of discrete mass.

To our knowledge, the multimodal imaging characteristics of IVLBCL affecting the gallbladder have not been described in the literature. Diffuse gallbladder wall thickening is nonspecific. It can be secondary to primary gallbladder pathology such as acute and chronic cholecystitis, adenomyomatosis, or gallbladder carcinoma [5]. It may also be a manifestation of a host of conditions extrinsic to the gallbladder such as hypoalbuminemia, congestive heart failure, hepatitis, renal failure, and physiologic contraction after a recent meal. A thickened gallbladder wall with a striated sonographic appearance (thick echogenic wall with a homogenous sonolucent central band) is more characteristic of benign noninflammatory conditions [6].

MRI evaluation is helpful in characterizing gallbladder wall thickening as those cases which show early and prolonged enhancement tend to be malignant whereas benign etiologies generally have less rapid and prolonged enhancement [7]. However, our case did not follow this concept. With vessel occlusion by intravascular neoplastic cells, one would expect to find decreased postcontrast enhancement as seen in our case. The lack of a focal mass, lymphadenopathy, and postcontrast enhancement make for an unusual imaging constellation for lymphoma [8]. While findings of neurologic alteration, pancytopenia, and elevated liver function studies have been described in cases of IVLBCL, they are not specific [3]. Additional potentially useful imaging, not obtained in this case, includes diffusion weighted imaging and positron emission tomography (PET). Diffusion weight imaging (DWI) would likely show abnormally restricted diffusion due to the presence of high grade malignant cells. PET would likely show increased FDG activity as with large B-cell lymphoma elsewhere. Unfortunately, these findings overlap with acute cholecystitis and would not help in distinguishing lymphoma from acute inflammation.

IVLBCL is a highly aggressive neoplastic proliferation of B-cells within medium and small sized vessels. The clinical and laboratory findings are not specific, and the diagnosis is often delayed. Furthermore, the imaging findings

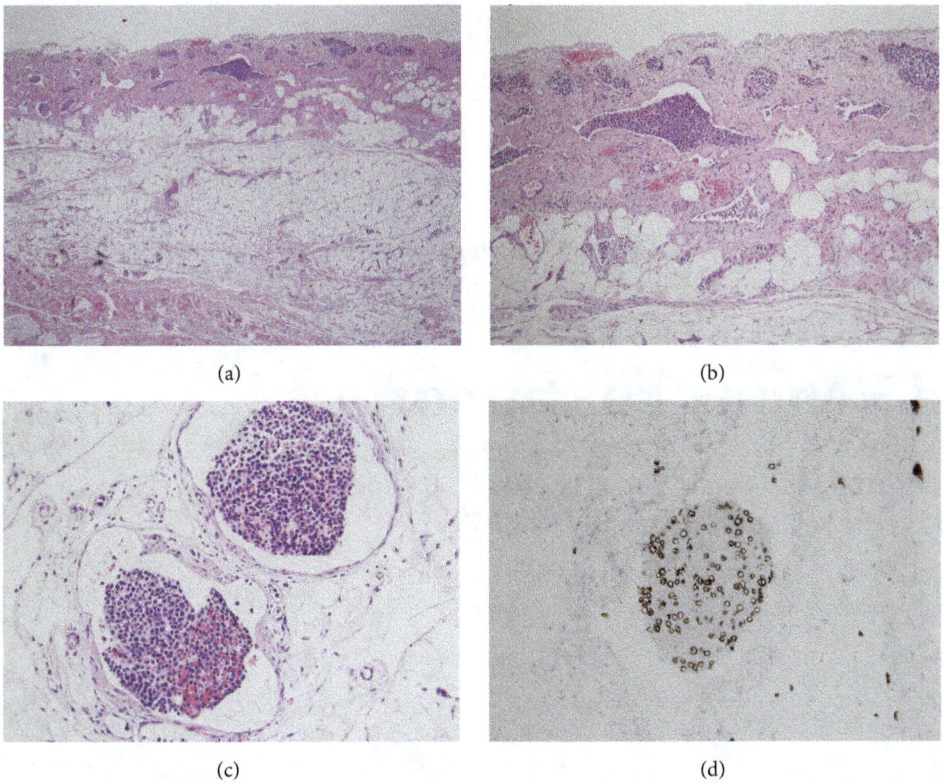

FIGURE 5: Microscopic images show gallbladder wall thickening and lymphatic ectasia. Several blood vessels in the subserosal fat are infiltrated with large, atypical lymphomatous cells. The mucosa is uninvolved. Immunohistochemical stain with CD79a confirms B-cell origin.

in our case highlight the diagnostic challenge of IVLBCL. The lack of a focal mass, lymphadenopathy, and abnormal contrast enhancement misleadingly point to a nonneoplastic process. Furthermore, diffuse gallbladder wall thickening with a trilaminar appearance is most characteristic of benign noninflammatory conditions, which would not prompt tissue diagnosis. A benign condition such as diffuse adenomyomatosis with numerous Rokitansky-Aschoff sinuses could be considered, but this case had no cystic changes and the trilaminar appearance of the gallbladder would be an unusual imaging finding. Although no diagnostic imaging features of IVLBCL exist, with increased awareness, the antemortem identification of this elusive diagnosis may be suggested.

Authors' Contributions

Sayf Al-Katib is the primary author of this manuscript. Robert Colvin was a contributing author and assisted in write-up and editing. Farnoosh Sokhandon is a contributing author and provided guidance in the write-up.

References

[1] K. Shimada, T. Kinoshita, T. Naoe, and S. Nakamura, "Presentation and management of intravascular large B-cell lymphoma," *The Lancet Oncology*, vol. 10, no. 9, pp. 895–902, 2009.

[2] Q. Shen, X. Duan, W. Feng et al., "Intravascular large B-cell lymphoma: report of three cases and analysis of the mTOR pathway," *International Journal of Clinical and Experimental Pathology*, vol. 4, no. 8, pp. 782–790, 2011.

[3] T. Murase, M. Yamaguchi, R. Suzuki et al., "Intravascular large B-cell lymphoma (IVLBCL): a clinicopathologic study of 96 cases with special reference to the immunophenotypic heterogeneity of CD5," *Blood*, vol. 109, no. 2, pp. 478–485, 2007.

[4] X. Duan, A. Lapus, R. E. Brown, and L. Chen, "Intravascular large B-cell lymphoma presenting as cholecystitis and pancytopenia: case report with literature review," *Annals of Clinical and Laboratory Science*, vol. 41, no. 3, pp. 262–266, 2011.

[5] A. C. Van Breda Vriesman, M. R. Engelbrecht, R. H. M. Smithuis, and J. B. C. M. Puylaert, "Diffuse gallbladder wall thickening: Differential diagnosis," *American Journal of Roentgenology*, vol. 188, no. 2, pp. 495–501, 2007.

[6] R. H. Cohan, B. S. Mahony, J. D. Bowie, C. Cooper, M. E. Baker, and F. F. Illescas, "Striated intramural gallbladder lucencies on US studies: Predictors of acute cholecystitis," *Radiology*, vol. 164, no. 1, pp. 31–35, 1987.

[7] K. Yoshimitsu, H. Honda, K. Kaneko et al., "Dynamic MRI of the gallbladder lesions: Differentiation of benign from malignant," *Journal of Magnetic Resonance Imaging*, vol. 7, no. 4, pp. 696–701, 1997.

[8] T. Yamamoto, M. Kawanishi, H. Yoshiba, E. Kanehira, and H. Itoh, "Primary non-Hodgkin's lymphoma of the gallbladder," *American Journal of Roentgenology*, vol. 184, no. 3 Suppl, Article ID 15728033, pp. S86–S87, 2005.

32

Unilateral Thalamic Venous Infarction in an Infant: A Rare Presentation of Bilateral Deep Cerebral Venous Thrombosis

Katherine Chung,[1] **Umar Tariq**,[2] **Rabia M. Khan**,[2] **Thomas P. Nickles**,[2] **and Joseph H. Lock Jr.**[2]

[1]*Geisinger Commonwealth School of Medicine, Scranton PA 18510, USA*
[2]*Department of Radiology, Geisinger Medical Center, Danville PA 17821, USA*

Correspondence should be addressed to Katherine Chung; kchung@som.geisinger.edu

Academic Editor: Daniel P. Link

Cerebral venous thrombosis (CVT) may manifest as superficial cerebral venous thrombosis (SCVT) or deep cerebral venous thrombosis (DCVT). Of the two patterns, DCVT is less commonly observed, although it often results in greater morbidity and mortality due to involvement of the deep gray nuclei. It can present at any age and typically results in edema of the bilateral thalami, with occasional extension into the basal ganglia. Unilateral thalamic infarct is rare and results in an ambiguous imaging pattern. We present the clinical and neuroimaging profile of an acute unilateral thalamic venous infarct in an infant secondary to bilateral DCVT. Early recognition of this atypical pattern will facilitate accurate diagnosis and treatment, and obviate the need for unnecessary interventions.

1. Introduction

Cerebral venous thrombosis (CVT) may be subdivided into superficial cerebral venous thrombosis (SCVT) or deep cerebral venous thrombosis (DCVT). Thrombosis of the deep system occurs in only 10% of CVT [1]. The deep venous system includes the basal and internal cerebral veins, great cerebral vein (of Galen) and straight sinus, which drain the deep gray nuclei. Because of this anatomy, DVCT typically results in bilateral thalamic infarction, with occasional extension into the basal ganglia. DCVT has a greater morbidity and mortality compared to SCVT due to involvement of the deep gray nuclei. We present a unique case of acute unilateral thalamic infarct secondary to bilateral DCVT in a pediatric patient with imaging and clinical correlation.

2. Case Presentation

A 15-month-old male presented to the Emergency Department (ED) with sudden onset of right arm and leg weakness beginning 3 hours prior to admission. His clinical history included a viral illness 5 days prior to admission, with malaise, fever, vomiting, and diarrhea. Early in the course of that illness he was seen by a pediatrician who noted mild dehydration, and suggested oral rehydration and antipyretics. He was otherwise healthy, with up-to-date immunizations.

On arrival to the ED physical exam revealed flaccidity in right upper and lower extremities. X-rays of right upper extremity obtained to rule out trauma were negative. Lab results showed microcytic anemia with hemoglobin of 6 g/dL, and thrombocytosis, with a platelet count of 512,000. The remaining labs were normal. Computed tomography (CT) of the head without contrast showed hypodensity of the left thalamus (Figure 1). In addition, high attenuation was noted throughout the bilateral deep venous system, compatible with acute DCVT (Figure 1).

Anticoagulation therapy and IV hydration were initiated immediately after radiologic findings were discussed with the ED physician. The patient was transferred to the Intensive Care Unit of our tertiary pediatric hospital. Magnetic resonance imaging (MRI) of the brain demonstrated restricted diffusion in the central aspect of the thalamus, surrounded by vasogenic edema, compatible with acute venous infarction (Figure 2). No other parenchymal lesion was detected. Signal

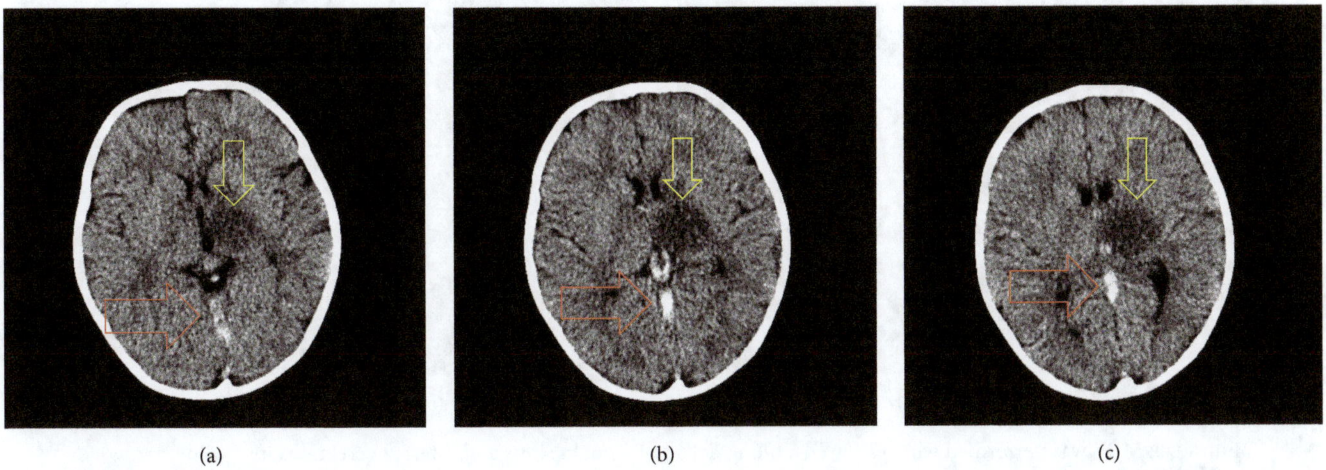

FIGURE 1: Axial noncontrast CT at the level of basal ganglia. These scans demonstrate dense clot sign which show a dark area (yellow arrows) where the infarct of the left thalamus is located due to thrombosis of internal cerebral veins and straight sinus (red arrows).

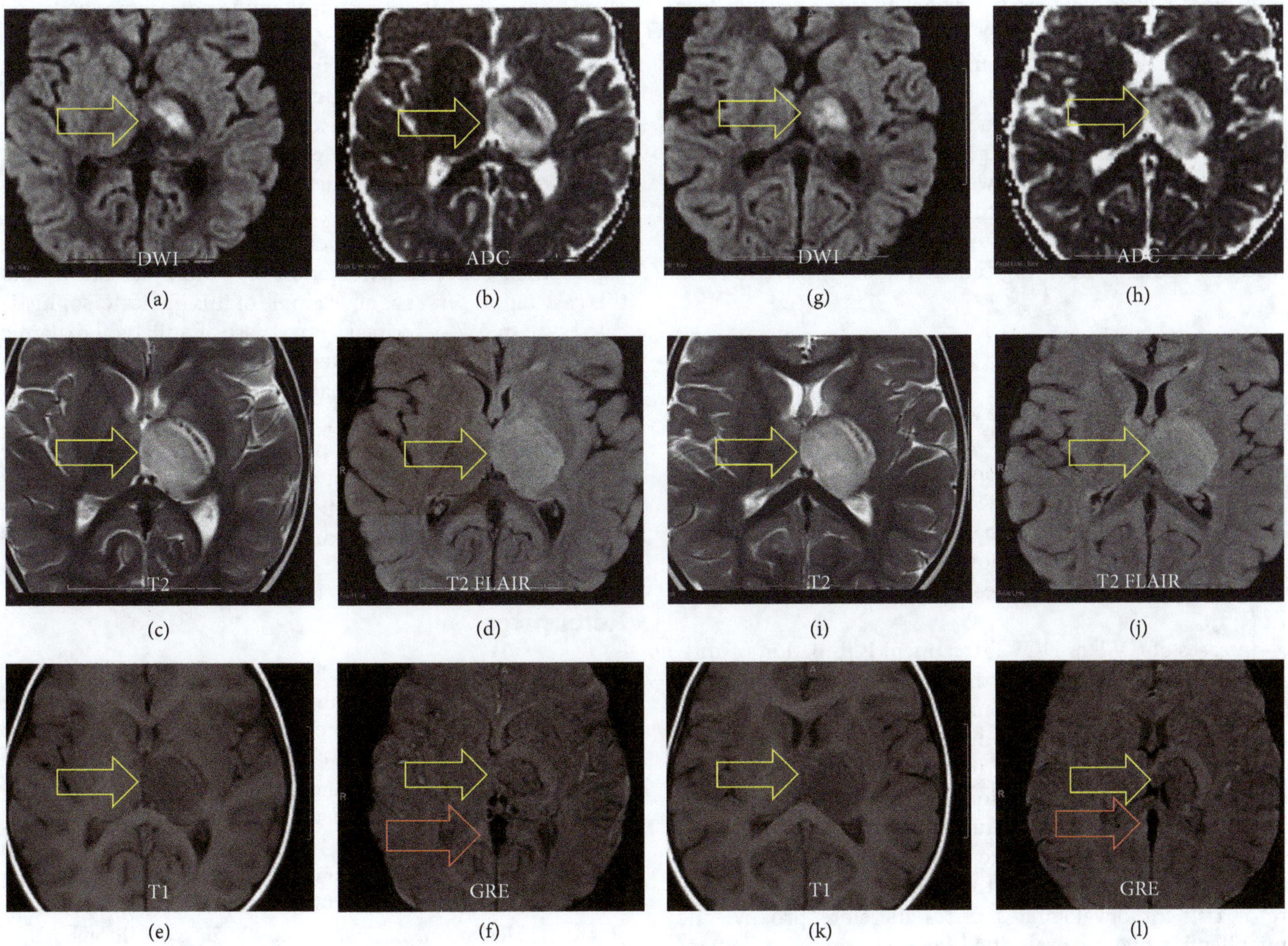

FIGURE 2: MRI obtained to confirm deep cerebral venous thrombosis and left thalamic infarction. DWI and ADC imaging ((a), (b), (g), and (h)) shows restricted diffusion in the anteromedial left thalamus without distinct territorial boundaries in relation to venous ischemia. T2 FLAIR hyperintensity ((c), (d), (i), and (j)) shows surrounding edema related to the infarction. GRE image (f) shows dark signal loss suggestive of petechial hemorrhage around the area of ischemia. GRE image (l) shows linear signal drop in the posteromedial surface of the left thalamus, highly suggestive of thrombus within a venous structure, likely part of the left internal cerebral vein.

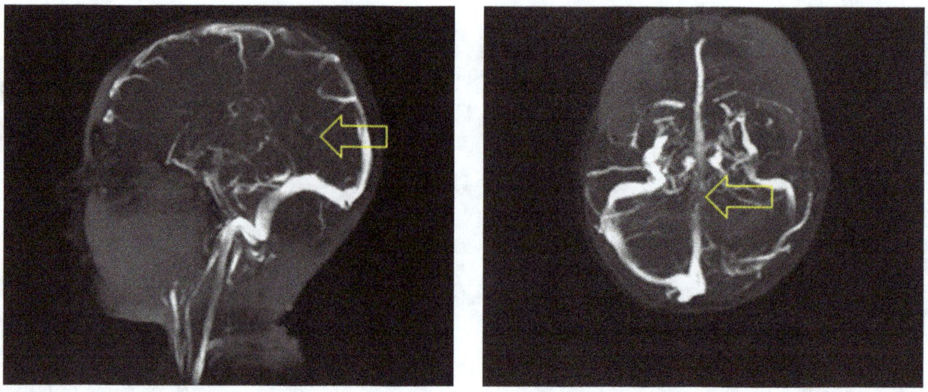

(a) (b)

Figure 3: MRV was performed which showed a filling defect of straight sinus and internal cerebral veins (yellow arrow).

changes within the deep venous system were compatible with acute intraluminal thrombus (Figure 2). MR venography confirmed lack of flow-related signal throughout the deep venous system (Figure 3).

The patient had a follow-up MR venography done two days later before discharge but was found to have no significant interval change with relatively stable venous infarct in the left thalamus and posterior limb of the internal capsule. No other follow-up imaging was done since. His symptoms resolved completely after six months of physical and speech therapy without residual symptoms. He is now being followed closely by pediatric neurology and hematology physicians.

3. Discussion

DCVT is a rare cause of stroke which may affect the pediatric or adult population. Multiple risk factors have been associated with CVT. Dehydration, infection, thrombocytosis, and trauma have been described in the pediatric population. Genetic predisposition, malignancy, inflammatory bowel disease, pregnancy, and medications are additional factors seen in adults [2]. Anemia is a recently validated risk factor for CVT [3].

In cases of CVT or DCVT, treatment is initiation of anticoagulant after imaging confirmation of intraluminal venous thrombosis. The figures demonstrate edema and ischemia in relation to acute venous thrombosis. In contrast to arterial ischemic lesions, those tend to regress, with good recoveries if successful recanalization is promptly obtained. Our patient received IV heparin infusion and later transitioned to enoxaparin (Lovenox). He also received 15 mL/kg of packed RBCs and ferrous sulfate due to anemia. Children with CVT are at risk for developing seizures therefore prophylactic antiepileptics may be prescribed for up to one year. Patient remained on lovenox for 6 months.

Multiple labs, including a hypercoagulability panel, and clinical testing were done to establish the etiology of the patient's infarction. However, all were unremarkable except for a low ferritin (2.4 ng/nl) and a hemoglobin of 6 g/dL; anemia was suggested as a possible cause for thrombosis. Our patient also had a preceding viral URI complicated by dehydration. These factors were described as the inciting events for CVT in the consultation note from pediatric neurology.

Unilateral thalamic infarction is rare, but has been reported in the setting of unilateral internal cerebral vein thrombosis [4]. Four such cases have been reported, with left sided thromboses more frequent than right [4, 5]. To the best of our knowledge, our case is the first report of a unilateral thalamic infarct in the setting of bilateral DCVT.

The cerebrovascular system is complex because of vast variation in collateral circulation and brain structures and this case report serves as an example of this intricate, sophisticated system. We described a novel case of unilateral thalamic infarction secondary to bilateral DCVT. Interestingly, of the few case reports, unilateral thalamic infarct has been reported more frequently on the left side, although an underlying anatomic basis has not been proposed. We believe that there could be a possible collateral venous circulation to the right thalamus that causes the left thalamic infarction the more common presentation in setting of DCVT.

References

[1] J. Linn, T. Pfefferkorn, K. Ivanicova et al., "Noncontrast CT in deep cerebral venous thrombosis and sinus thrombosis: Comparison of its diagnostic value for both entities," *American Journal of Neuroradiology*, vol. 30, no. 4, pp. 728–735, 2009.

[2] J. Stam, "Cerebral venous and sinus thrombosis: incidence and causes," *Advances in Neurology*, vol. 92, pp. 225–232, 2003.

[3] J. Coutinho, S. Zuurbier, A. Gaartman et al., "Association between anemia and cerebral venous thrombosis," *Stroke*, vol. 46, no. 10, pp. 2735–2740, 2015.

[4] K. A. Herrmann, B. Sporer, and T. Yousry, "Thrombosis of the internal cerebral vein associated with transient unilateral thalamic edema: a case report and review of the literature," *American Journal of Neuroradiology*, vol. 25, pp. 1351–1355, 2004.

[5] M. Rousseaux, M. Cabaret, T. Bernati, J. P. Pruvo, and M. Steinling, "Residual deficit of verbal recall in a left internal cerebral vein infarct," *Revue Neurologique*, vol. 154, no. 5, pp. 401–407, 1998.

33

Septic Embolic Stroke Followed by Hemorrhage and Brain Abscess in a Patient with Systemic Infections: A Case Report

Jama A. Mohamud,[1] Jingtao Wu,[2] Ye Jing ,[2] and Yu Wang[3]

[1]*Department of Medical Imaging, Subei People's Hospital of Jiangsu Province, Medical College of Yangzhou University, Yangzhou, China*
[2]*Department of Medical Imaging, Subei People's Hospital of Jiangsu Province, Yangzhou University, Yangzhou, China*
[3]*Department of Neurology, Subei People's Hospital of Jiangsu Province, Dalian Medical University, Dalian, Liaoning Province, China*

Correspondence should be addressed to Ye Jing; yzhyejing@163.com

Academic Editor: Amit Agrawal

We report a case of 50-year-old man with a severe acute ischemic stroke followed by intracerebral hemorrhage and brain abscess due to systemic infection. His initial intracranial radiographic findings were normal but three days later MRI scan of the brain revealed well-defined rounded cystic lesion on the T2-weighted and T1-weighted images in the right basal ganglia; the lesion presented an area of diffusion restriction on DWI; lately the lesion was confirmed to be an early stage of cerebral abscess. A week later the patient was noted to have worsening neurological status and left extremity weakness, and emergency brain CT scan revealed massive intracerebral hemorrhage in the right occipital lobe; he underwent intracranial hematoma evacuation surgery. The hematoma was removed successfully, and the systemic infections were treated with antibiotics.

1. Introduction

Ischemic stroke is life-threatening and severe medical condition requiring urgent and comprehensive evaluation. Systemic infections can increase the risk of ischemic stroke and may worsen ischemic stroke (IS) prognosis. Acute infections of different types constitute a risk factor for IS, particularly within one week of the event [1, 2]. We report here computed tomography (CT) and the magnetic resonance imaging (MRI) findings and serial image changes in a case of an acute ischemic stroke followed by intracerebral hemorrhage and brain abscess caused by systemic infection; to the best of our knowledge, this has not been reported in the literature before.

2. Case Report

A 50-year-old man with a past history of hypertension and diabetes was referred to our hospital after the onset of left-sided numbness and weakness for 5 hours. The patient had not any other past medical history other than hypertension and diabetes, and there was no family history of similar diseases. A preoperative computed tomography (CT) of the head and CT angiogram of the brain (CTA) scan on admission showed no abnormalities and vascular malformations (Figures 1(a) and 1(b)). He was transferred to the intensive care unit (ICU) for further investigations and treatment. He was given an intensive care such as oxygen therapy and lipid-lowering.

Initial examination at the time of admission showed a temperature of 39°C, blood pressure of 140/92 mmHg, and a regular heart rate of 78/minute. His Glasgow coma scale (GCS) score was 7, pupils were equal and reacting, and there was grade 3 power in the left limb and grade 5 in the right limb. Further laboratory examination showed a leukocyte count of 16.5 × 109/L, a hemoglobin level of 129 g/L, neutrophil count of 83.4%, blood gas of pH 7.463, PO2 88.4, PCO2 26.8, and glucose in urine 4+; his

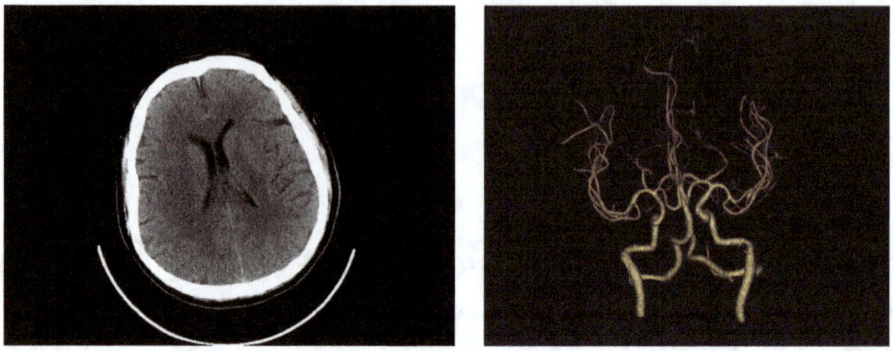

(a) (b)

FIGURE 1: Initially, (a) a noncontrast computed tomography (CT) and (b) a computed tomography angiography (CTA) of the head performed on at the time of the admission showed no abnormalities and vascular malformations.

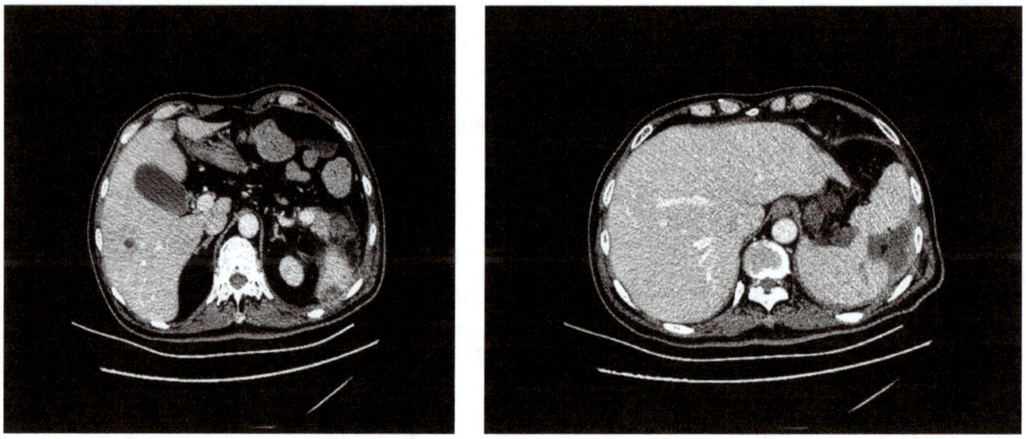

(a) (b)

FIGURE 2: A contrast-enhanced CT scan of abdomen showed (a) rounded hypodense lesion with central low attenuation in the right lobe of the liver (suggestive of liver abscess) and (b) hypodense splenic air-filled lesion with an irregular wall (suggestive of perisplenic infection).

hypersensitive c-reactive protein was 497.4 mg/L (normal < 3 mg/L). Echocardiography was performed showing a reduced compliance of left ventricle; the E-F slope of anterior mitral valve leaflet was decreased; otherwise, the size, structure, and movement of the heart were normal.

The patient was diagnosed with liver abscess, perisplenic and intracranial infection, and septicemia; a contrast-enhanced CT scan of the abdomen showed rounded hypodense lesion with central low attenuation in the right lobe of the liver and a hypodense splenic air-filled lesion with an irregular wall (Figure 2). Ultrasonically guided percutaneous drainage of the splenic cyst fluid was performed; approximately 65 ml of light yellow, murky fluid was removed. The blood cultures and splenic cyst drainage were positive with Klebsiella pneumoniae which were the primary source of septicemia.

On the third day in the hospital, magnetic resonance imaging (MRI) of the head showed high signal intensity on DW image and well-defined rounded cystic lesion on the T2-weighted and T1-weighted images involving in the right corona radiata and basal ganglia (Figure 3), although the lesion looks like that of an acute stroke but lately was confirmed to be early stage of cerebral abscess. On the seventh day, the patient was noted to have worsening neurological status and left extremity weakness and a repeat computed tomography (CT) scan revealed a right occipital lobe hematoma with blood loss of 40 ml (Figure 4). He was immediately admitted to the surgical ward to undergo an urgent intracranial hematoma evacuation surgery. During the first three postoperative days the patient was delirious; further MRI of the brain three days after operation showed multiple hemorrhagic lesions involving both cerebral hemispheres and cerebellum and a cystic lesion in the basal ganglia region (Figure 5).

On hospital day 34, the patient developed high-grade fevers accompanied by worsening neurological status. Contrast-enhanced CT of the head showed a well-defined lesion, with thin, ring-like enhancement pattern in the right basal ganglia with perilesional edema, which compressed right lateral ventricle with midline shift towards left and was given the possibility of brain abscess (Figure 6). The patient was treated conservatively with supportive care; he was given

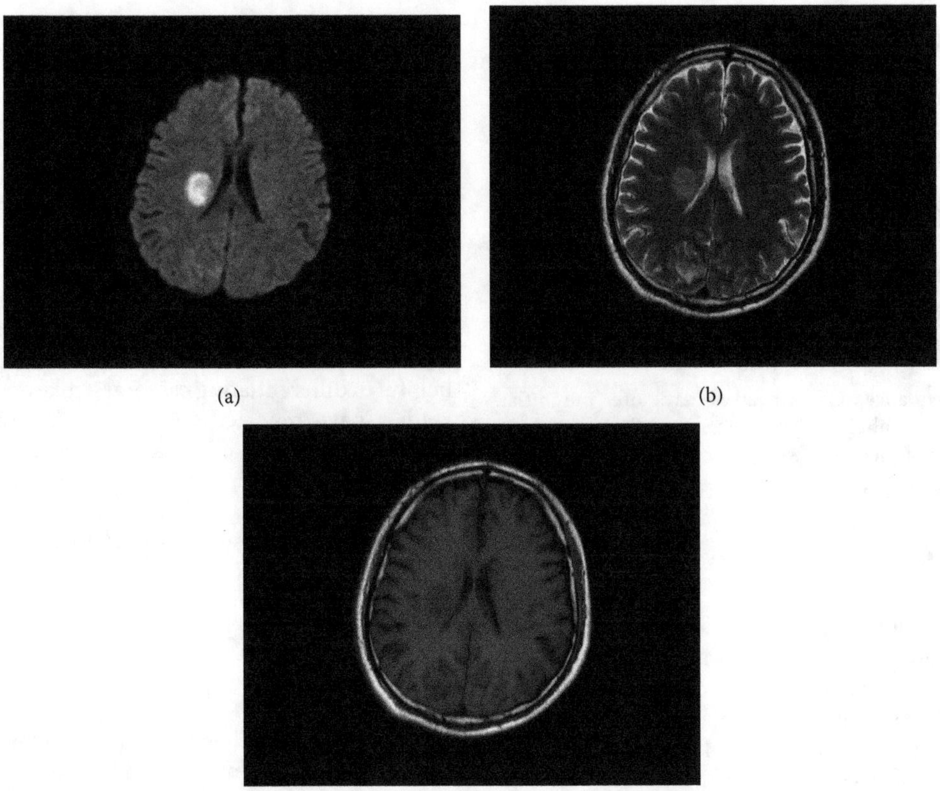

(a) (b) (c)

FIGURE 3: Brain MRI performed on the third day revealed (a) high signal intensity on DW image and (b, c) well-defined rounded cystic lesion on the T2-weighted and T1-weighted images involving in the right corona radiata and basal ganglia, compressing the right lateral ventricle with midline shift to left, suggestive of an early stage of brain abscess.

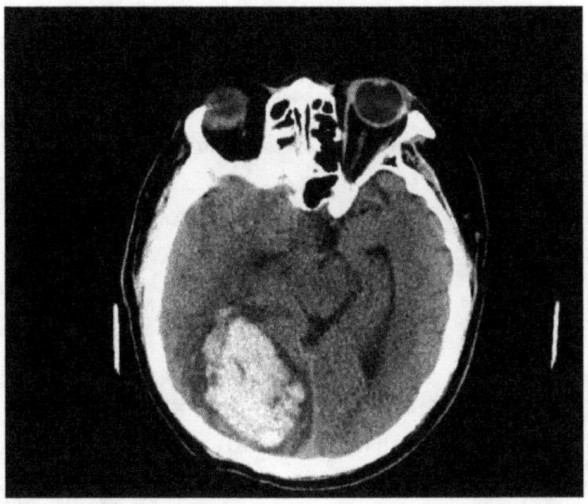

FIGURE 4: Noncontrast head CT performed on the 7th day demonstrates an acute hemorrhage in the right occipital lobe, with surrounding oedema and compressing the right lateral ventricle with midline shift to left.

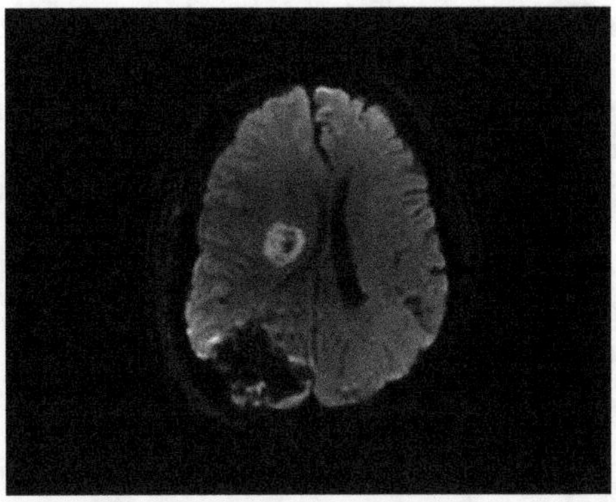

FIGURE 5: A contrast-enhanced MR imaging of brain performed three days after operation showed irregular mixed signal intensity on DWI with enhancement of its wall in the right occipital lobe and hyperintense lesion with small hypointense areas within in the basal ganglia region.

an antiplatelet and anti-infective therapy; the antibiotic drugs that he was given were included imipenem, linezolid, and vancomycin. He was discharged to home after two months in stable condition and slow improvement in his mental status but he still had some weakness on the left side of his body.

3. Discussion

Stroke has been defined as one of the most complicated pathologies; patients with stroke are at risk of developing a wide range of complications to their stroke, in particularly, stroke-associated infections increase the mortality and

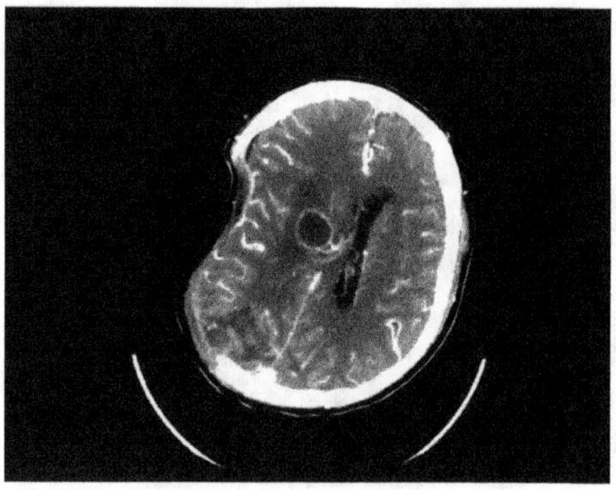

FIGURE 6: Contrast-enhanced CT of head 30 days after the initial ischemia showed a ring-enhancing cystic lesion in the right basal ganglia with perilesional oedema, which compressed right lateral ventricle with midline shift towards left suggestive of abscess.

morbidity rates [1]. Acute ischemic and hemorrhagic stroke followed by brain abscess during the same hospitalization period is a rare entity and association of these three life-threatening conditions may cause catastrophic result; it appears possible that acute infections of bacterial etiology, usually hepatic and of bacterial origin particularly in one week, may increase the risk factor for cerebral infarction in all age groups.

Septic embolic stroke usually results from vascular occlusion and corresponding degrees of ischemia and infarction, depending on vessel size, location, and collateral blood flow [3]. Cerebral arterial occlusion resulting in either infarction or transient ischemic attack accounts for 40–50% of central nervous system (CNS) complications of infective endocarditis [4]. The septic emboli are challenging because they involve three important cerebrovascular conditions: (a) cerebrovascular occlusions, (b) intracerebral abscess, and (c) arterial mycotic aneurysms. The main risk of neurologic complications is the absence of appropriate antibiotic therapy. It is important to note that most neurologic complications are already evident at the time of hospitalization or develop within a few days [5, 6].

The clinical course in the present case revealed unusual features and complex clinical manifestation. On his initial examinations, he was diagnosed with septicemia, liver abscesses, and perisplenic and intracranial infection indicating the presence of systemic infection and bacterial seeding in the body. *Klebsiella pneumoniae* was isolated from both the blood culture and splenic cyst drainage. Hence we hypothesize that hematogenous spread from the *K. pneumoniae* led to bacterial seeding of the ICH and the formation of the brain abscess, in the setting of impaired host defense mechanisms. The *k. pneumonia* bacteria entered the bloodstream and spread to the brain and thereby led to arterial thrombosis and the destruction of the vascular wall that resulted in right cerebral ischemia and the ICH; during the operation, we had seen multiple ruptured arterioles under the hematoma wall which was responsible for the bleeding vessels in the brain. This event illustrates that septic embolism can be considered as a cause of ischemic stroke and brain abscess in patients with a hepatic abscess.

Our patient was diabetic and hypertensive and did not have any other risk factors. Initial head CT scans done on admission time were normal. Three days later he developed acute ischemic stroke and brain abscess at different locations after an infectious complication. Cerebral abscesses are difficult to diagnose and they often mimic cerebral infarcts. In the earliest stages of cerebral abscess, a CT scan of the brain may be negative or it may show subtle nonspecific findings. However, MRI findings with a diffusion protocol are more helpful in differentiating cerebral stroke and abscess. Previous studies have reported that the formation of the cerebral abscess after a stroke is a rare event and serious condition that requires immediate recognition and treatment. However the need for having a high index of suspicion for septic stroke and cerebral abscess formation is necessary for early management, diagnosis, initiation of effective treatment, and prevention of significant morbidity and death [7, 8].

4. Conclusion

Intracranial hemorrhage after ischemic infarct due to septic emboli is a rare mechanism. *K. pneumoniae* is able to progress into severe bacterial infections leading to bloodstream infections and may lead to subsequent spread to brain parenchyma even in the absence of cyanotic heart disease. However, the recognition of infectious diseases and their risk factors for septic embolic stroke could be important for stroke prevention and may help to understand epidemiologic features of septic stroke.

References

[1] H. Emmez, A. Ö. Börcek, F. Doğulu, and N. Çeviker, "Ischemic stroke complicated by a brain abscess: A case report and review and review of the literature," *Turkish Neurosurgery*, vol. 17, no. 1, pp. 48–54, 2007.

[2] I. Y. Bova, N. M. Bornstein, and A. D. Korczyn, "Acute infection as a risk factor for ischemic stroke," *Stroke*, vol. 27, no. 12, pp. 2204–2206, 1996.

[3] S. P. Stawicki, M. S. Firstenberg, M. R. Lyaker et al., "Septic embolism in the intensive care unit," *International Journal of Critical Illness & Injury Science*, vol. 3, no. 1, pp. 58–63, 2013.

[4] C. Özbek, U. Yetkin, M. Bademci, N. Karahan, and A. Gürbüz, "Ring annuloplasty and successful mitral valve repair in a staphylococcal endocarditis case with bilobular saccular mycotic aneurysm at cerebral artery and frontal region infarction. Secondary to septic emboli," *Archives of Medical Science*, vol. 4, no. 1, pp. 94–99, 2008.

[5] Magnetic Resonance Imaging of the Brain and Spine (2 Volume Set) Fourth Edition.

[6] R. Sonneville, B. Mourvillier, L. Bouadma, and M. Wolff, "Management of neurological complications of infective endocarditis in ICU patients," *Annals of Intensive Care*, vol. 1, article 10, 2011.

34

Congenital Vitelline Band Causing Intestinal Obstruction in an Adult with a Double Inferior Vena Cava

Mihiri Wettasinghe,[1] Kumari Pussepitiya,[1] Bandula Samarasinghe,[2] and Nuwan Wickramasinghe[3]

[1]*Department of Radiology, Teaching Hospital, Peradeniya, Sri Lanka*
[2]*Department of Surgery, Faculty of Medicine, University of Peradeniya, Peradeniya, Sri Lanka*
[3]*Department of Community Medicine, Faculty of Medicine and Allied Sciences, Rajarata University of Sri Lanka, Saliyapura, Sri Lanka*

Correspondence should be addressed to Mihiri Wettasinghe; chamimw003@yahoo.com

Academic Editor: Vincent Low

Introduction. Vitelline artery remnants are rare causes of intra-abdominal bands leading to bowel obstruction. These bands may be associated with Meckel's diverticulum. Double inferior vena cava (IVC) is a rare presentation and is usually identified incidentally. *Case Presentation.* A sixty-year-old male presented with progressive vomiting for five days and he was clinically diagnosed with intestinal obstruction. Plain X-ray abdomen showed evidence of small bowel obstruction. CT scan of the abdomen revealed dilated small bowel loops with a small outpouching in the distal ileum with a band like structure attached to it. In the CT, left sided patent IVC draining into the left renal vein was identified. Left external iliac vein was in continuity with the left IVC. Left internal iliac vein was draining into the right IVC. Exploratory laparotomy revealed a Meckel's diverticulum with a band identified as the vitelline remnant attached to its apex and inserting at the anterior abdominal wall near the umbilicus. *Discussion.* Meckel's diverticulum with vitelline bands, although rare, should be borne in mind in adult patients with intestinal obstruction. Identification of this anomaly can be difficult in imaging studies. Presence of double IVC should be mentioned in the imaging findings to prevent possible catastrophic complications during surgery.

1. Introduction

Meckel's diverticulum is the commonest congenital anomaly in the gastrointestinal system, though being most often detected as an incidental finding. Incomplete obliteration of the omphalomesenteric duct is considered as the cause for this anomaly. However, apart from Meckel's diverticulum, there is a spectrum of anomalies that arise as a result of complete or incomplete obliteration of the omphalomesenteric duct. These include umbilicoileal fistula, omphalomesenteric duct sinus, omphalomesenteric duct cyst, and fibrous connection of the ileum to the umbilicus [1]. As the vitellointestinal duct connects the developing midgut to the yolk sac in the embryo, incomplete resorption of the obliterated vitelline duct results in fibrous band connecting the distal ileum to the umbilicus. Although, in the majority, Meckel's diverticulum does not lead to any complications, approximately 4% of the affected individuals develop complications related to Meckel's diverticulum including haemorrhage, perforation, diverticulitis, and obstruction [2]. Double IVC is also a rare presentation and is usually identified incidentally. The present case illustrates an old male presenting with intestinal obstruction due to vitelline band with a Meckel's diverticulum and incidental finding old double IVC in the same patient.

2. Case Presentation

A 69-year-old previously healthy male patient presented with a history of vomiting for five days' duration. The vomitus contained clear fluid initially, which later became brownish in colour. He had developed absolute constipation for three days. He had noticed gradual abdominal distension during

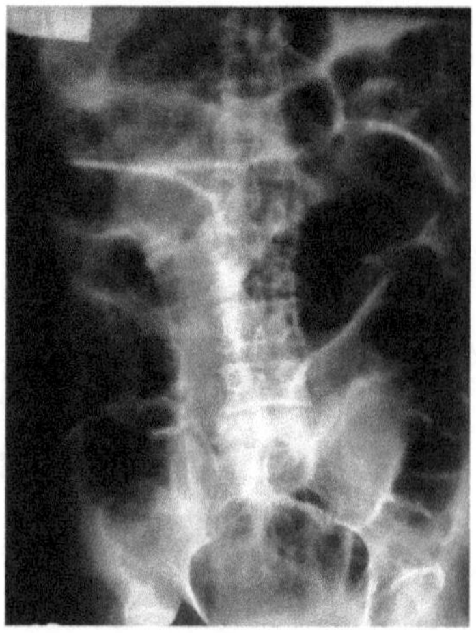

FIGURE 1: Supine X-ray abdomen showing dilated small bowel loops.

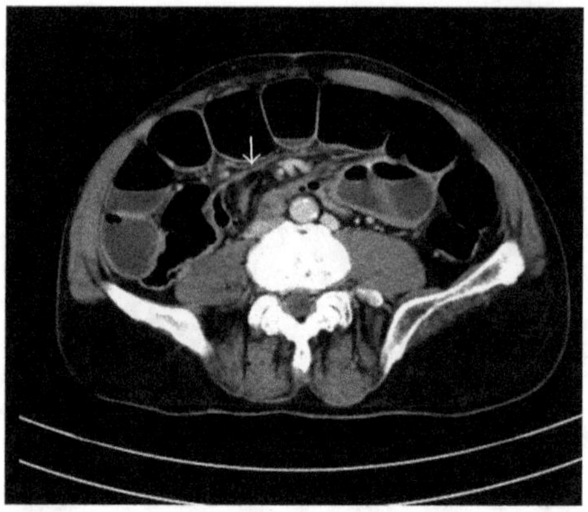

FIGURE 2: CT abdomen axial view showing band like structure extending from the distal ileum (white arrow).

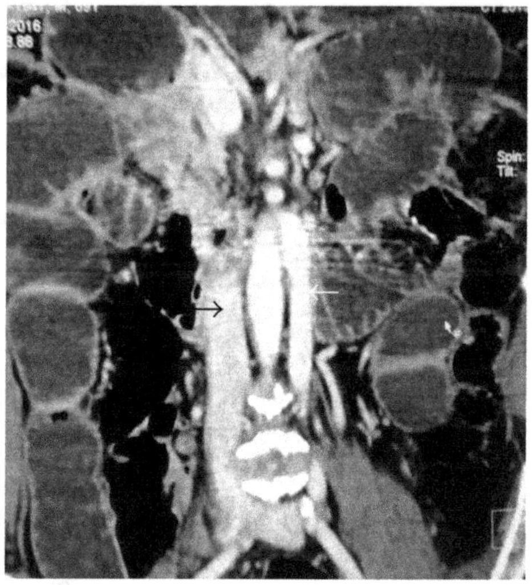

FIGURE 3: Coronal CT image showing double IVC with small left IVC (white arrow) and large caliber right IVC (black arrow).

this period. He had not undergone any abdominal surgeries in the past.

On examination, his abdomen was distended and there was mild tenderness in the lower abdomen. The examination of the respiratory system did not reveal any abnormalities. Biochemical investigations were unremarkable. With the clinical diagnosis of intestinal obstruction, he was referred for imaging studies.

2.1. X-Ray Abdomen. Plain X-ray abdomen was performed in the supine position and it revealed grossly distended small bowel loops with absent rectal gas (Figure 1). There was no pneumoperitoneum.

2.2. USS Abdomen. Ultrasound scan of the abdomen revealed fluid filled aperistaltic bowel loops. Central abdomen was distended and presence of bowel gas hindered evaluating the deeper structures. Pancreas appeared normal. There was no free fluid in the abdomen. Liver, spleen, and both kidneys were normal on ultrasound. The superior mesenteric artery appeared normal at the origin and showed normal colour and spectral flow pattern. The portal vein was normal.

2.3. CT Abdomen. CT abdomen showed grossly dilated jejunal and ileal loops. The appendix was identified separately. There were no fat strandings or fluid collections around the appendix. Distal ileal loops appeared collapsed. There was a soft tissue density band like structure extending from the collapsed ileal loops anteriorly (Figure 2).

However, its insertion site was not identified. There was no CT evidence of appendicitis. The cause for the small bowel obstruction was not identified on CT. However, as the patient had no previous surgeries, the possibility of a congenital band was highly suspected. The presence of a soft tissue density linear band led to the preoperative suspicion of a congenital band. Furthermore, Meckel's diverticulum was not considered on CT images.

There was a tubular retroperitoneal structure in the left side of the aorta which was extending up to the left renal vein. It was in continuity with the left external iliac vein and was identified as the left IVC. Right IVC was also noted. Left IVC was smaller in caliber than the right IVC (Figure 3).

Left internal iliac vein was seen crossing the midline to drain into the right common iliac vein (Figure 4).

3. Surgical Findings

Patient underwent exploratory laparotomy. There was a Meckel's diverticulum with fibrous band extending to the anterior abdominal wall (Figure 5). The size of the diverticulum was approximately 3 cm. The band was identified as the obliterated vitelline duct. The diverticulum was seen about 20 cm proximal to the ileocecal valve, arising from the antimesenteric border of the distal ileum. The small bowel loops were twisting around the band forming a volvulus, causing the small bowel obstruction. The band was resected and the obstruction was relieved.

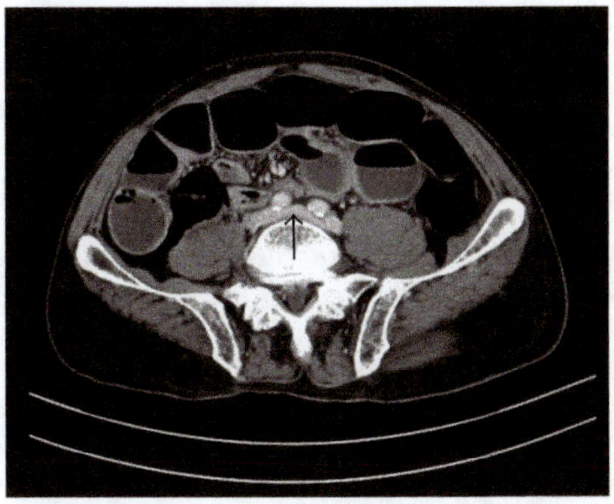

FIGURE 4: Left internal iliac vein draining to right common iliac vein (black arrow).

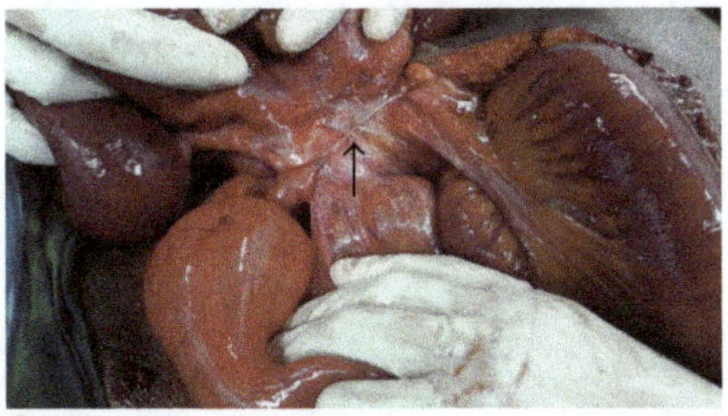

FIGURE 5: Fibrous band extending from Meckel's diverticulum to anterior abdominal wall (black arrow).

4. Discussion

Meckel's diverticulum is the result of incomplete obliteration of the vitelline or omphalomesenteric duct and is the commonest congenital anomaly of the gastrointestinal system [3]. It is located in the antimesenteric border of the distal ileum and is considered to be a true diverticulum [4]. As stated in the literature, intestinal obstruction secondary to Meckel's diverticulum is difficult to identify preoperatively [1] and this was seen in our patient as well.

Most of the instances, this anomaly is asymptomatic and the lifetime risk of developing complications is between 4% and 6% [5]. Furthermore, the presence of complications in elderly patients is even rare. Thus, developing small bowel obstruction from Meckel's diverticulum in an elderly person, as seen in our patient, is relatively rare. Haemorrhage, obstruction, and inflammation are considered to be the most frequent complications of Meckel's diverticulum and obstruction can be due to trapping of a bowel loop by a mesodiverticular band, a volvulus of the diverticulum around a mesodiverticular band, and intussusception [3, 4]. In our patient, the cause of obstruction was the vitelline band. Although a soft tissue density linear band was seen extending from the distal ileum, its insertion at the anterior abdominal wall was not identified. This could have been the reason for not diagnosing the vitelline band in the CT images.

Small intestine obstruction due to persistent vitelline-intestinal duct is extremely rare, especially in adult patients, and very few cases were reported in the literature [6]. Thus, age of the patient precluded preoperative diagnosis of Meckel's diverticulum and vitelline band. As these were not evident on CT images, definitive diagnosis for the cause of the obstruction was determined during the surgery. Although the cause for the obstruction is not clearly depicted in the CT images, early surgical intervention is vital in the management of these patients, as the cause for the obstruction is mechanical and delay in surgery would result in bowel ischaemia and gangrene.

Anatomical variation of the inferior vena cava occurs in 0.4–4% of the population [7]. Formation of IVC is a complex event that occurs in early embryonic life and adult form of IVC is the result of formation of series of anastomoses and regression of venous structures. Persistence of left supracardinal vein along with the right one leads to double IVC anomaly [7, 8]. Left IVC drains into left renal vein, which in turn drains into right IVC, forming a single suprarenal IVC. The left IVC may drain both the internal and external iliac veins in the left side. Sometimes, only the external iliac vein drains into left IVC and the internal iliac vein crosses the midline to drain into the right common iliac vein [9]. This variant was seen in our patient.

The importance of identifying the left IVC is that it can be mistaken for lymph node mass. It is also important to inform the referring surgeon regarding this anomaly to avoid catastrophic complications during surgery [10]. Although double IVC is known to be associated with a range of genitourinary abnormalities including horseshoe kidney, crossed fused ectopia, cloacal exstrophy, and retroaortic renal vein, none of these anomalies were seen in our patient [11]. There are reports on association between double IVC and congenital heart disease [12].

Reports on association of double IVC and congenital gastrointestinal anomalies are scarce. One case report was found in the literature stating duplication of inferior vena cava and malrotation of gut in the same patient [13]. However, meticulous literature search did not reveal any evidence on association between double IVC and congenital vitelline band.

5. Conclusion

In conclusion, although not common, Meckel's diverticulum should be borne in mind when elderly patients present with intestinal obstruction. Identification of this anomaly can be difficult in imaging studies. Presence of double IVC should be mentioned in the imaging findings as this will prevent catastrophic complications during surgery. It is important to communicate the presence of a double IVC to the operating surgeon, in order to avoid forceful interference during the surgical procedure.

Authors' Contributions

Mihiri Wettasinghe was involved in developing the concept, data collection, performing radiological investigations and interpretation which contributed to the diagnosis and patient management, and drafting the manuscript. Kumari

Pussepitiya was involved in data collection, performing radiological investigations and interpretation which contributed to the diagnosis and patient management. Bandula Samarasinghe was involved in patient management and drafting the manuscript. Nuwan Wickramasinghe was involved in developing the concept and drafting the manuscript. All the authors have read and approved the final manuscript.

Acknowledgments

Authors wish to acknowledge Dr. R. G. K. Nawarathna at Teaching Hospital, Peradeniya.

References

[1] A. D. Levy and C. M. Hobbs, "From the archives of the AFIP. Meckel diverticulum: radiologic features with pathologic correlation," *Radiographics*, vol. 24, no. 2, pp. 565–587, 2004.

[2] O. Tutar, M. Velidedeoglu, I. Yanik et al., "Computed tomography features of small bowel obstruction due to mesodiverticular band," *JBR-BTR*, vol. 97, no. 1, pp. 25–27, 2014.

[3] A. Sumer, O. Kemik, A. Olmez et al., "Small bowel obstruction due to mesodiverticular band of Meckel's diverticulum: a case report," *Case Reports in Medicine*, vol. 2010, Article ID 901456, 3 pages, 2010.

[4] J. Dumper, S. Mackenzie, P. Mitchell, F. Sutherland, M. L. Quan, and D. Mew, "Complications of Meckel's diverticula in adults," *Canadian Journal of Surgery*, vol. 49, no. 5, pp. 353–357, 2006.

[5] S. Sameer Mohiuddin, A. Gonzalez, and C. Corpron, "Meckel's diverticulum with small bowel obstruction presenting as appendicitis in a pediatric patient," *Journal of the Society of Laparoendoscopic Surgeons*, vol. 15, no. 4, pp. 558–561, 2011.

[6] N. K. Mahato, "Obliterated, fibrous omphalo-mesenteric duct in an adult without Meckel's diverticulum or vitelline cyst," *Romanian Journal of Morphology and Embryology*, vol. 51, no. 1, pp. 195–197, 2010.

[7] K. R. Saad, P. F. Saad, C. A. Amorim et al., "Duplication of the inferior vena cava: case report and a literature review of anatomical variation," *Journal of Morphological Sciences*, vol. 29, no. 1, pp. 60–64, 2012.

[8] B. Petik, "Inferior vena cava anomalies and variations: imaging and rare clinical findings," *Insights into Imaging*, vol. 6, no. 6, pp. 631–639, 2015.

[9] M. S. Shaaban, "Congenital anomalies of the inferior vena cava and iliac veins: a cross-sectional study by multi-detector computed tomography," *The Egyptian Journal of Radiology and Nuclear Medicine*, vol. 47, no. 3, pp. 883–890, 2016.

[10] A. Eldefrawy, M. Arianayagam, P. Kanagarajah, K. Acosta, and M. Manoharan, "Anomalies of the inferior vena cava and renal veins and implications for renal surgery," *Central European Journal of Urology*, vol. 64, no. 1, pp. 4–8, 2011.

[11] N. B. S. Mani, N. K. Venkataramu, P. Singh, and S. Suri, "Case report: duplication of IVC and associated renal anomalies," *Indian Journal of Radiology and Imaging*, vol. 10, no. 3, pp. 157–158, 2000.

[12] İ. Ertuğrul, V. Doğan, U. A. Örün, and S. Karademir, "A rare association: inferior vena cava anomalies and congenital heart diseases," *Turk Kardiyoloji Dernegi arsivi: Turk Kardiyoloji Derneginin Yayin Organidir*, vol. 43, no. 8, pp. 717–719, 2015.

[13] P. Shaha, A. Garg, K. Sahoo, N. Kothari, and P. Garg, "Duplication of inferior vena cava with associated anomalies: a rare case report," *Journal of Clinical and Diagnostic Research*, vol. 10, no. 3, pp. TD01–TD04, 2016.

Metastatic Renal Cell Carcinoma Presenting as Prolonged Pyrexia and Stauffer's Syndrome: Can a Routine Ultrasound Scan Fail to Detect a Renal Cell Carcinoma?

C. L. Fonseka,[1,2] A. G. T. A. Kariyawasam,[2] S. A. G. L. Singhapura,[2] C. M. de Silva,[2] T. E. Kanakkahewa,[2] I. G. T. M. Senarathna,[2] and C. K. Bodinayake[1,2]

[1]University Medical Unit, Teaching Hospital Karapitiya, Galle, Sri Lanka
[2]Department of Internal Medicine, Faculty of Medicine, University of Ruhuna, Sri Lanka

Correspondence should be addressed to C. L. Fonseka; lakmalfonseka@med.ruh.ac.lk

Academic Editor: Atsushi Komemushi

Background. Prolonged pyrexia and weight loss are recognised paraneoplastic manifestations of renal cell carcinoma (RCC). Stauffer's syndrome is a rarely described paraneoplastic manifestation, which is described early in the course of RCC. We report a patient who presented with unresolving fever with multiple pulmonary opacities with biochemical evidence of hepatic choleastasis and was later diagnosed to have metastatic RCC with Stauffer's syndrome. *Case Presentation.* We report a 54-year-old female who was investigated for a poorly resolving fever and recent weight loss for two months. During her course of illness, she developed bilateral multiple opacifications in the chest radiograph with negative pyogenic, mycobacterial microbiological studies. Despite intravenous antibiotics, her fever continued. She was found to have elevated alkaline phosphatase and gamma-glutamyl transferase and she underwent imaging with ultrasound scan of abdomen twice, which did not reveal demonstrable abnormalities. Later, contrast CT of abdomen and chest was performed and detected a renal cell carcinoma of the right upper pole of the kidney with multiple lung metastases, which was concluded as a metastatic RCC with paraneoplastic Stauffer's syndrome. *Conclusion.* Prolonged pyrexia with loss of weight and Stauffer's syndrome could be features to suggest renal cell carcinoma in the absence of positive microbiological studies. Isoechoic RCC could be missed in routine ultrasonography. When a RCC is suspected in the setting of a pyrexia of unknown origin, ultrasound with doppler or a contrast CT should be requested to aid diagnosis.

1. Background

Renal cell carcinoma (RCC) accounts for 2% of cancers worldwide. The incidence of RCC has risen over the past several decades largely due to incidental detection by imaging modalities such as CT scan, ultrasound, and MRI [1], in which the accuracy of diagnosis with CT scan amounts to greater than 95% [2]. The most common clinical presentations of RCC are hematuria (50-60%), abdominal pain (40%), and a palpable abdominal mass (30%); this classic triad of symptoms is present in less than 10% of cases [3]. Paraneoplastic manifestations of RCC, including hypercalcemia, polycythemia, hepatic dysfunction, amyloidosis, fever, and weight loss, are present in up to 20% of patients [4].

A paraneoplastic syndrome may be the initial clinical presentation of RCC in a significant number of patients, and recognition of these syndromes may facilitate early diagnosis. Most paraneoplastic syndromes associated with RCC remit after resection of the primary RCC or treatment of metastatic sites [4]. Hepatic panel abnormalities in the absence of hepatic metastasis, a condition known as Stauffer's syndrome, have been described as a paraneoplastic phenomenon classically in early-stage renal cell carcinoma (RCC) [5]. But Stauffer's syndrome has been anecdotally described with other cancers such as prostate cancer [6], bladder cancer [7], and pancreatic cancer [8] as well as bronchial malignancy [9].

Typical Stauffer's syndrome presents elevations in the enzymes aspartate transaminase (AST) and alanine transaminase (ALT) and alkaline phosphatase (ALP) without jaundice. However, atypical presentations with a jaundice component have also been described [10, 11]. The pathogenesis of Stauffer's syndrome is still incompletely elucidated. Blay et al.

found that interleukin-6 (IL-6) levels are elevated in patients with RCC as well as elevated alkaline-phosphatase, bilirubin, and gamma-glutamyl transferase (GGT), suggesting a probable IL-6 mediated process [12]. Biopsy from the liver in this syndrome typically shows cholestasis, sometimes with a mild inflammatory infiltrate. Surgical removal of the otherwise local cancer via nephrectomy leads to resolution of the hepatic abnormalities. In cases where there was a recurrence of cancer, this was heralded by the resurgence of the liver enzymes [13].

We report a patient with RCC who presented with prolonged pyrexia and multiple pulmonary opacities with hepatic cholestasis. RCC was missed in routine ultrasound scan but was later diagnosed by a contrast CT scan.

2. Case

A 54-year-old previously healthy female presented to the hospital with intermittent low-grade fever for two months with a mild dry cough. There was no associated pleuritic chest pain, shortness of breath, or hemoptysis. Accompanying anorexia and weight loss were pronounced. She gave a recent history of being investigated for right side loin pain, where she was managed as right renal calculus, which was evident with the ultrasound scan. But she did not have urinary symptoms or hematuria. Examination revealed a female who looked ill. She was averagely built but claimed that she has been overweight previously. She was afebrile and had mild pallor. There were no enlarged lymph glands. Respiratory system was clinically normal without pleural effusions or added sounds. She had regular pulse rate of 72 bpm and blood pressure of 120/80 mmHg. She had no hepatosplenomegaly or ballotable loin masses. She gave a history of being treated by several doctors with antibiotics for a possible infection.

Her complete blood count revealed normal white cell and platelet count. Her hemoglobin was $9.4 \times 103/\mu L$ with a normochromic normocytic anemia. Her inflammatory markers were significantly elevated with an ESR of 130 in the first hour and CRP of 124 u/l. Blood, urine, and sputum for pyogenic, mycobacterial, and fungal cultures were negative repeatedly, while the chest radiograph showed multiple bilateral opacities with small nodular lesions over all three zones of both lungs (Figure 1). Mantoux test revealed a wheal of 12 mm and the serology and cultures for melioidosis were negative. She had normal renal function tests with normal urine analysis. The liver functions revealed mildly elevated SGOT and SGPT (80/68 u/l) with markedly elevated ALP (417 U/L) and GGT (592 U/L). The total bilirubin was normal. Ultrasound scan of the abdomen was done twice and did not reveal a significant abnormality.

We empirically treated her for possible chest infection with intravenous antibiotics (ceftazidime) for two weeks. But neither the fever nor the inflammatory markers showed any response and the lung opacities were persistent. Next, we performed a contrast-enhanced computed tomography (CECT) of chest and abdomen. The CECT revealed a renal cell carcinoma of the right kidney (Figure 2) with multiple pulmonary metastasis (Figure 3).

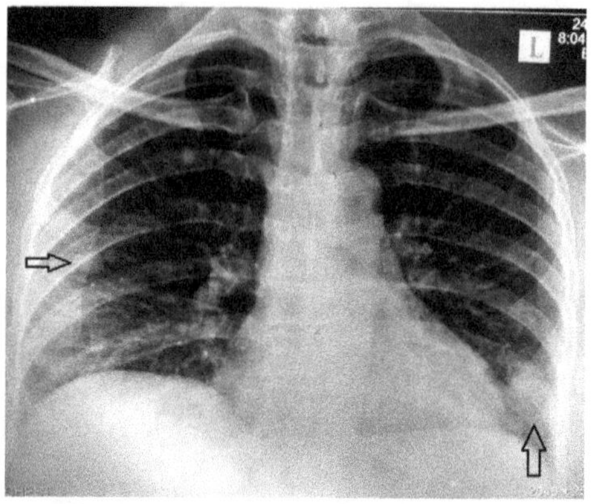

FIGURE 1: Bilateral multiple opacifications in chest radiograph.

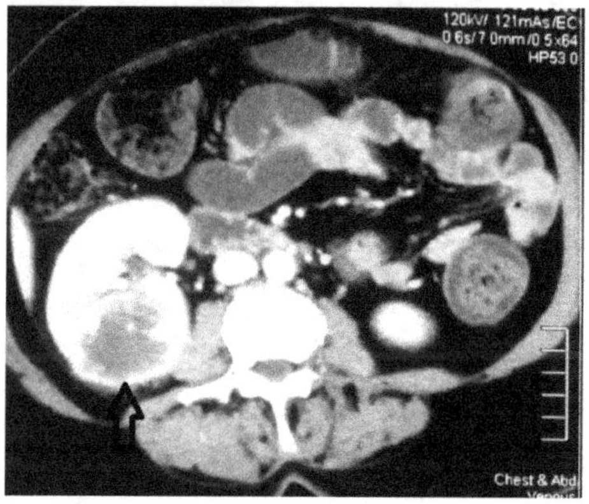

FIGURE 2: Renal cell carcinoma of the right kidney.

She was transferred for oncology care and was treated with oral Sunitinib, a multitargeted receptor tyrosine kinase inhibitor, in the hope of subsequent nephrectomy. With treatment, the hepatic abnormalities resolved.

3. Discussion

Pyrexia and Stauffer's syndrome are paraneoplastic features that usually occur early in patients with RCC and are reported in several case reports [13, 14]. There is a report where Stauffer's syndrome has presented with metastatic renal cell carcinoma [14]. Our patient had persistent fever with multiple bilateral opacifications, which directed us to exclude subacute bacterial endocarditis, pulmonary tuberculosis, and pulmonary melioidosis. But the patient showed a poor response to intravenous ceftazidime and also had negative mycobacterial studies. Possibility of cholestatic hepatitis was excluded by doing hepatitis serology and she did not have any hepatic metastasis or bile duct dilatation in imaging. After detection of multiple opacities with a repeated negative ultrasound imaging, these directed us to perform a CECT of chest and abdomen in view of looking for lymphoreticular malignancy. This revealed a renal cell carcinoma in the right kidney with multiple pulmonary metastases.

Our patient had a RCC that was missed in routine US leading to a delay in diagnosis. Ultrasonography (US) in

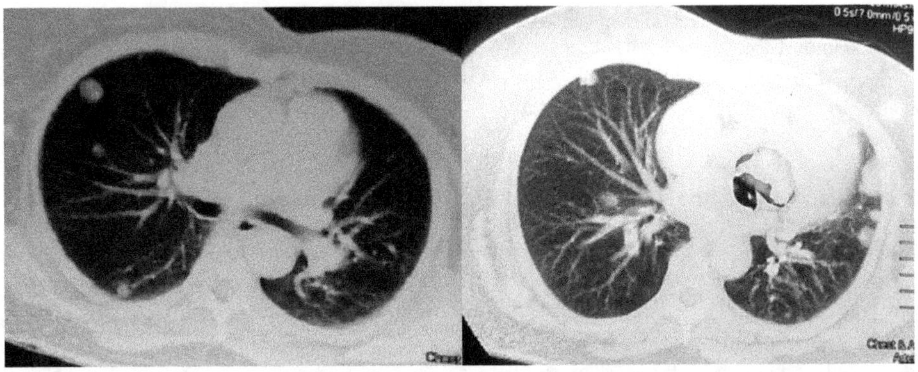

FIGURE 3: Bilateral pulmonary metastasis in middle and lower zones in CT of chest.

kidneys is usually useful in detecting solid from cystic masses with recent advanced US techniques. However, its use is still limited in detecting small lesion less than 10 mm and masses with similar echogenicity to the surrounding renal parenchyma. RCCs can have variable echogenic patterns that could be more echogenic, less echogenic, or isoechogenic. Isoechoic RCC may be difficult to detect with US, especially if it is small or displaces collecting system or gives rise to contour abnormalities. Also, isoechoic RCC can mimic normal anatomic structures or variants such as hypertrophy of ducts of Bertin [15]. Also, the tumour pseudocapsule can sometimes be visualised with ultrasound as a hypoechoic halo. Although this is a relatively specific sign, it is not particularly sensitive. Use of harmonic scanning has been reported to increase sensitivity to up to 85% [16]. Contrast-enhanced ultrasound may typically show heterogeneously hypervascular lesions in the arterial phase with early washout in the delayed phase [17]. Therefore, it should be emphasized that when there are isoechoic renal signals, US Doppler or other techniques in US could be used to detect increased and aberrant vascularity, which suggests the presence of a RCC. Also, calcifications in RCC could be mistaken for renal stones as in our case of an isoechoic RCC.

CT is optimal modality to detect RCC, and sometimes corticomedullary phases and nephrogenic phases are used to characterize the enhancement pattern of renal masses [15]. RCC can have variable densities in CT depending on areas of necrosis, hemorrhage, or calcifications. Rather than solid RCCs, cystic RCCs may show confusing radiographic patterns of malignancy and may be less specific than solid RCCs [18].

Therefore, radiographic imaging in RCC has certain pitfalls. The knowledge about these pitfalls is important to rectify these errors to arrive at an early diagnosis. Our patient had markedly elevated alkaline phosphatase and γ-glutamyl transferase with mild transaminitis. This case illustrates the importance of being familiar with Stauffer's syndrome in the background of prolonged fever, with a view to investigation for RCC.

4. Conclusion

Renal cell carcinoma can present as prolonged fever and Stauffer's syndrome even in an advanced stage of RCC with pulmonary metastasis. Ultrasonography can have certain pitfalls in detecting renal cell carcinoma. Isoechoic RCC could be missed in routine abdominal ultrasonography delaying diagnosis. CT scan would be a preferable choice in cases where obvious cause is unidentified in a setting of poorly resolving fever.

Authors' Contributions

C. L. Fonseka, A. G. T. A. Kariyawasam, S. A. G. L. Singhapura, I. G. T. M. Senarathna, and C. K. Bodinayake investigated the case. C. M. de Silva, T. E. Kanakkahewa, and C. K. Bodinayake planned radiological investigation and prepared the manuscript. All authors were involved in editing the content and approved the final version for publication.

References

[1] J. K. McLaughlin, L. Lipworth, and R. E. Tarone, "Epidemiologic Aspects of Renal Cell Carcinoma," *Seminars in Oncology*, vol. 33, no. 5, pp. 527–533, 2006.

[2] R. J. Zagoria, N. T. Wolfman, N. Karstaedt, G. C. Hinn, R. B. Dyer, and Y. M. Chen, "Radiology in the diagnosis and staging of renal cell carcinoma," *Crit Rev Diagn Imaging*, vol. 31, no. 1, pp. 81–115, 1990.

[3] R. J. Motzer, N. H. Bander, and D. M. Nanus, "Renal-Cell Carcinoma," *The New England Journal of Medicine*, vol. 335, no. 12, pp. 865–875, 1996.

[4] P. Gold, A. Fefer, and J. Thompson, "Paraneoplastic manifestations of renal cell carcinoma," *Semin Urol Oncol*, vol. 14, no. 4, pp. 216–222, 1996.

[5] M. Girotra, R. R. Abraham, M. Pahwa, and M. Arora, "Is Stauffer's syndrome an early indicator of RCC recurrence?" *ANZ Journal of Surgery*, vol. 80, no. 12, pp. 949-950, 2010.

[6] A. Karakolios, C. Kasapis, T. Kallinikidis, P. Kalpidis, and N. Grigoriadis, "Cholestatic Jaundice as a Paraneoplastic Manifestation of Prostate Adenocarcinoma," *Clinical Gastroenterology and Hepatology*, vol. 1, no. 6, pp. 480–483, 2003.

[7] J. Moreno-Palacios, H. Wingartz-Plata, P. Pardo-Belasteguigoitia, and J. Moreno-Aranda, "Stauffer syndrome in transitional cell carcinoma of the bladder," *Archivos Españoles de Urología*, vol. 64, no. 9, pp. 911–913, 2011.

[8] D. Harris and M. W. Saif, "Stauffer's syndrome in pancreatic cancer: first case report," *Cureus*, vol. 9, no. 5, 2017.

[9] P. Saintigny, J.-P. Spano, F. Tcherakian, M.-C. Pailler, and J.-L. Breau, "Non-metastatic intrahepatic cholestasis associated with bronchial adenocarcinoma," *Annales de Médecine Interne*, vol. 154, no. 3, pp. 171–175, 2003.

[10] M. Puga, E. Gonzalez-Ballina, and L. Rivas-Moral, "Stauffer's Syndrome Variant as an Unusual Case of Painless Jaundice," *Clinical Gastroenterology and Hepatology*, vol. 13, no. 9, pp. A25–A26, 2015.

[11] S. P. Dourakis, C. Sinani, M. Deutsch, E. Dimitriaclou, and S. J. Hadziyannis, "Cholestatic jaundice as a paraneoplastic manifestation of renal cell carcinoma," *European Journal of Gastroenterology & Hepatology*, vol. 9, no. 3, pp. 311–314, 1997.

[12] J.-Y. Blay, J.-F. Rossi, J. Wijdenes et al., "Role of interleukin-6 in the paraneoplastic inflammatory syndrome associated with renal-cell carcinoma," *International Journal of Cancer*, vol. 72, no. 3, pp. 424–430, 1997.

[13] G. P. Kranidiotis, P. T. Voidonikola, M. K. Dimopoulos, and M. I. Anastasiou-Nana, "Stauffer's syndrome as a prominent manifestation of renal cancer: A case report," *Cases Journal*, vol. 2, no. 1, 2009.

[14] A. Tomadoni, C. Garcia, M. Marquez, J. C. Ayala, and F. Prado, "Stauffer's syndrome with jaundice, a paraneoplastic manifestation of renal cell carcinoma: A case report," *Archivos Españoles de Urología*, vol. 63, no. 2, pp. 154–156, 2010.

[15] J. Kim, "Imaging findings of renal cell carcinoma," *Expert Review of Anticancer Therapy*, vol. 6, no. 6, pp. 895–904, 2006.

[16] G. Ascenti, M. Gaeta, C. Magno et al., "Contrast-enhanced second-harmonic sonography in the detection of pseudocapsule in renal cell carcinoma," *American Journal of Roentgenology*, vol. 182, no. 6, pp. 1525–1530, 2004.

[17] V. Duddalwar, "Contrast-Enhanced Ultrasound of the Liver and Kidney," *Update in Ultrasound, An Issue of Radiologic Clinics of North America, E-Book*, vol. 52, no. 6, p. 1177, 2015.

[18] P. Levy, O. Helenon, S. Merran et al., "Cystic tumors of the kidney in adults: radio-histopathologic correlations," *Journal de Radiologie*, vol. 80, no. 2, pp. 121–133, 1999.

36

Sacral Myeloid Sarcoma Manifesting as Radiculopathy in a Pediatric Patient: An Unusual Form of Myeloid Leukemia Relapse

Joana Ruivo Rodrigues,[1] **Manuel João Brito**,[2] **Rui Pedro Faria Pais**,[3] **and Sílvia Carvalho**[3]

[1]*Radiology Unit, Medical Imaging Department, Centro Hospitalar e Universitário de Coimbra, Coimbra, Portugal*
[2]*Pediatric Oncology Department, Hospital Pediátrico, Centro Hospitalar e Universitário de Coimbra, Coimbra, Portugal*
[3]*Neuroradiology Unit, Medical Imaging Department, Centro Hospitalar e Universitário de Coimbra, Coimbra, Portugal*

Correspondence should be addressed to Joana Ruivo Rodrigues; joana.ruivo130@gmail.com

Academic Editor: Amit Agrawal

Myeloid sarcoma (MS), granulocytic sarcoma or chloroma, is defined as a localized extramedullary mass of blasts of granulocytic lineage with or without maturation, occurring outside the bone marrow. MS can be diagnosed concurrently with acute myeloid leukemia (AML) or myelodysplastic syndrome (MDS). The authors report a case of sacral MS occurring as a relapse of myeloid leukemia in a 5-year-old girl who was taken to the emergency department with radiculopathy symptoms.

1. Introduction

In 1811, MS was described for the first time by Burns. Afterwards, in 1853, King called the disease chloroma due to its greenish appearance [1]. MS is frequently diagnosed in patients with recurrent AML. Immature myeloid cells or extramedullary proliferation of myeloblasts are present in MS [2]. The incidence of chloroma in AML is approximately 3–9.1% [3].

MS is an uncommon neoplastic condition [4, 5] and any organ system can be affected [1]. The soft tissue of the head, neck, skin, bone, and lymph nodes is usually affected [1]. Spinal MS of the sacrum is infrequent. Compressed spinal cord symptoms caused by an MS mass are unusual [1, 4]. Early diagnosis of MS is possible using enhanced Magnetic Resonance Imaging (MRI). This imaging technique can show the precise location and size of the lesion. Biopsy of the mass is required for a definitive MS diagnosis [4]. MS is a significant cause of morbidity among patients with leukemia.

In this paper, the authors describe the MRI findings and clinical manifestations of an uncommon case of spinal MS at the sacral level in a 5-year-old girl who presented with radiculopathy symptoms and had a previous history of AML.

2. Case Presentation

A 5-year-old girl with acute myeloid leukemia (AML) with t(8;21) underwent relatively standard AML chemotherapy, which consisted of 2 cycles of induction chemotherapy with daunorubicin, cytarabine, and etoposide, followed by 2 cycles of consolidation chemotherapy with high-dose cytarabine 3 gr/m^2 per dose ×6, in each cycle. Intrathecal therapy was also carried out. The patient was in remission by morphology and flow cytometry assessment after the first cycle and in molecular remission after the second cycle by flow cytometry assessment. Four months after the end of therapy, she presented progressive radicular pain of the lower right extremity and gait claudication. Neurological assessment revealed symmetrical depressed reflexes of the lower limbs and reduction of right knee extension. The posterolateral regions of the right buttock and thigh were painful to the touch. Laboratory evaluation showed normal blood counts. The imaging study evaluation with an MRI of the spine revealed a soft tissue intracanalar epidural mass located from L5 to S4, which extended through multiple sacral neural foramina to the presacral space. The tissue involved sacral nervous roots (Figure 1) and the sciatic nerve (Figure 2). The

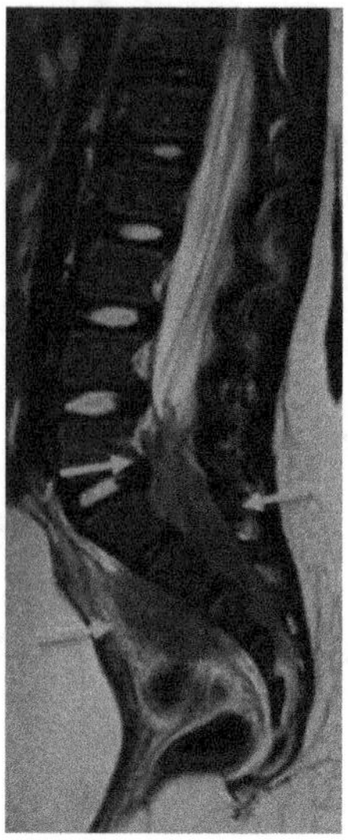

FIGURE 1: Sagittal T2-weighted MRI of the lumbosacral spine shows a large intracanalar epidural hypointense mass at L5 to S4, extending into the presacral space (blue arrows).

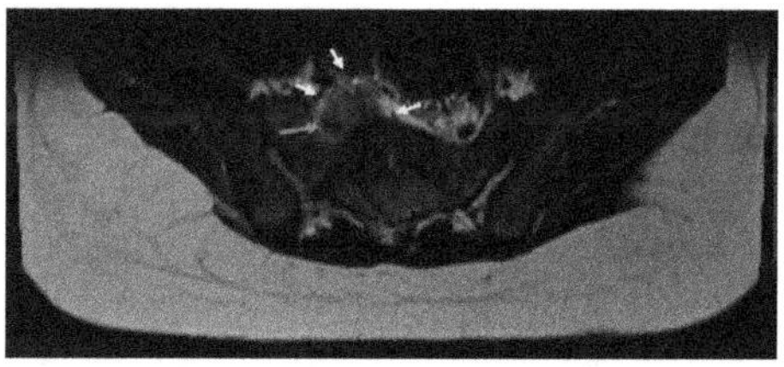

FIGURE 2: Axial T2-weighted MRI reveals anterior mass extension into the paraspinous soft tissues (yellow arrows), involving the sciatic nerve (blue arrow), which is thickened.

infiltrating mass was hypointense in T1- and T2-weighted images and enhanced after contrast (Figure 3). Based on the MRI findings, the authors suggested the diagnosis of chloroma. The chest X-ray was normal. In order to confirm the leukemic relapse, a bone marrow aspiration with biopsy and a minimal invasive biopsy of the sacral mass, guided by Computed Tomography, were performed. Bone marrow evaluation showed a hypercellular marrow with 2% myeloid blasts with fluorescent in situ hybridization (FISH) testing and was positive for the t(8;21) ETO/AML1 fusion. Histologic findings of the sacral mass revealed connective tissue without signs of invasion by previously diagnosed neoplasia. Flow cytometry could not verify the etiology of the mass, but ETO/AML1 translocation was confirmed by PCR in the biopsied sacral mass. The 2% of blasts in the bone marrow and the myeloid sarcoma as an epidural mass suggested the diagnosis of relapse combined with AML.

Following the institutional guidelines for relapsed AML, the patient started FLAG-IDA as a relapse protocol. Intrathecal chemotherapy was not performed in the first cycle due to the mass's large volume.

The patient was in remission by morphology and flow cytometry assessment after the first cycle of FLAG-IDA. Neurological assessment revealed normal and symmetric reflexes of the lower limbs, as well as symmetric and normal knee extension. At that time, the patient did not have pain in the right buttock or thigh. The MRI evaluation revealed a significant tumor mass volume reduction at that time (Figure 4).

Triple intrathecal therapy was performed at the beginning of the second FLAG-IDA cycle and there were no blasts detected in the cerebrospinal fluid. Following the second cycle, the patient experienced a four-month period of hematologic aplasia, which postponed the allogeneic stem-cell transplant (allo-HSCT). Meanwhile, she remained in remission but did not fully recover from the hematologic aplasia, while the platelets levels remained low. She started maintenance chemotherapy, in addition to intrathecal therapy (no blasts in the CNS fluid) as a bridge to allo-HSCT. At this point, the patient is waiting for allo-HSCT. The decision to undergo radiotherapy has been postponed until further evaluation after the transplant, as there was no growth of the sacral mass during the prolonged bone marrow aplasia.

3. Discussion

In literature, MS is classified according to the predominant cell type (blastic, monoblastic, and myelomonocytic) [6]. MS can have different clinical presentations. MS can appear simultaneously with AML. The case in this paper presents this type of clinical manifestation. MS can appear with blast phase/transformation of a myeloproliferative neoplasm, also known as chronic myelomonocytic leukemia. MS may also be associated with a normal bone marrow biopsy and blood smear, without a history of myeloid neoplasia [7–9]. Lastly, extramedullary relapse of AML may also occur after a bone marrow transplant procedure [9]. Extramedullary relapse is less frequent in patients treated without allo-HSCT, compared to patients treated with allo-HSCT. Children rarely have extramedullary relapse without bone marrow involvement [10].

Haversian channels serve as a bridge for tumor cell migration from the bone marrow to extramedullary sites. Spinal cord involvement is infrequent [11] and the spine segments most often affected are the thoracic followed by the lumbar, sacral, and cervical segments [12]. 18% of patients have multiple noncontiguous areas of involvement [13]. Lesions that have intraspinal invasion [14], as in the case described, may cause cord compression or *cauda equina syndrome*. Those complications are rare [13].

AML reservoirs are usually bone marrow, the central nervous system, and the testes. The sacral spinal canal is a specialized AML reservoir [15] and the average age for sacral MS manifestation is 22 years, being more predominant in males than in females [13]. The risk factors for extramedullary relapse are advanced disease conditions at the time of HSCT, chromosomes 5q and 7q deletions and FLT-3 mutations, history of an extramedullary disease, and FAB classification M4 or M5 AML [10].

Langerhans cell histiocytosis X, lymphoma, metastatic tumors, and Ewing sarcoma/PNET are the differential diagnoses of MS [16]. Bone marrow aspiration, biopsy, peripheral

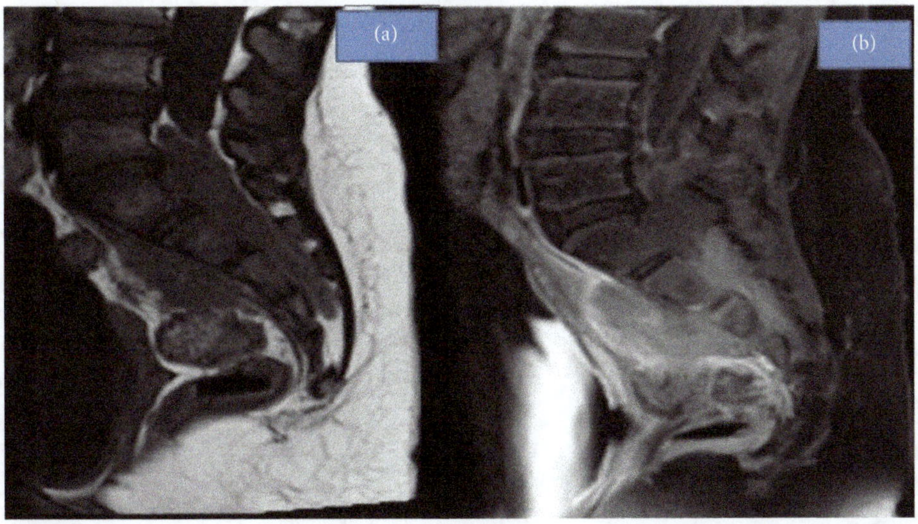

FIGURE 3: (a) Sagittal T1-weighted MRI shows a hypointense intracanalar and presacral infiltrating mass. (b) Postcontrast T1-weighted sagittal image with fat suppression shows heterogeneous enhancement of the mass and sacral vertebrae.

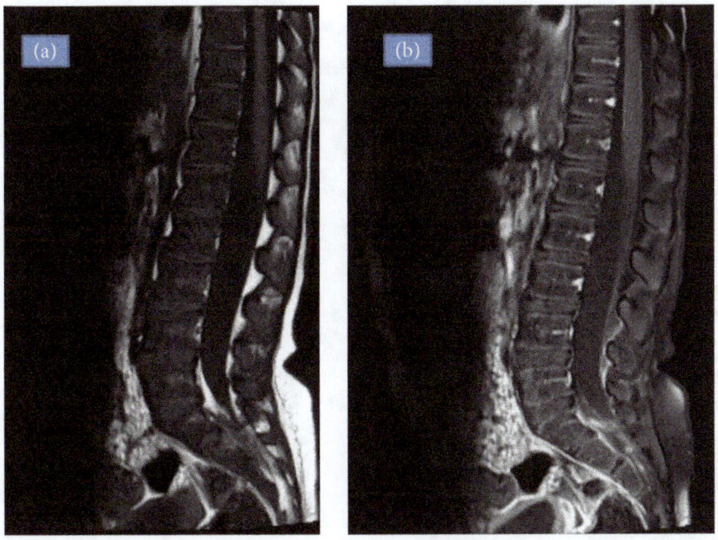

(a) (b)

FIGURE 4: Sagittal T1-weighted image (a) and sagittal postcontrast T1-weighted image with fat suppression (b) show a significant tumor mass volume reduction after treatment.

blood smears, and immunohistochemical detection are used to diagnose MS. The most suitable marker to identify MS is staining for myeloperoxidase. MS masses express lysozyme, Ki67, and myeloid/monocytoid antigens (CD13, CD14, CD33, CD64, CD68, and c-Kit (CD117)) [4].

MRI is the best imaging study to distinguish MS from other pathologies [4]. During MRI, MS commonly appears as a heterogeneous signal mass with isosignal or hypersignal intensity in T2-weighted images and with hyposignal or isosignal intensity in T1-weighted images, when compared to brain or muscle tissue [17]. After intravascular contrast, the MS masses usually present homogeneous enhancement [4]. In the case presented by the authors, the lesion was hypointense in T2-weighted images and hypointense in T1-weighted images and showed heterogeneous enhancement in postcontrast MRI images. The outcome of patients with systemic relapse is worse in comparison to the outcome of patients with isolated extramedullary relapse [10]. This is what occurred in this specific case.

Systemic chemotherapy using AML-like regimens should be initiated early, even in nonleukemic disease [9], with intrathecal chemotherapy as another option [13]. When the lesions are symptomatic or cause local organ dysfunction, surgery or/and radiotherapy might be carried out [9, 13]. In patients with complete remission, allo-HSCT can be performed [9]. There are no established treatment strategies for MS [4, 10]. None of the different specific treatments increase survival [13].

In this paper, the authors describe a rare case of leukemia relapse, presented as sacral MS in a girl with a progressive right-sided lumbosacral plexus neuropathy. The reader should bear in mind that sacral MS presents symptoms similar to other spinal lesions. MS should not be neglected and should be maintained under the differential diagnosis of spinal mass lesions. MRI, bone marrow aspiration, and pathological and histological staining can result in its correct diagnosis.

References

[1] J. H. Seok, J. Park, S. K. Kim, J. E. Choi, and C.-C. Kim, "Granulocytic sarcoma of the spine: MRI and clinical review," *American Journal of Roentgenology*, vol. 194, no. 2, pp. 485–489, 2010.

[2] E. Oliveira, J. Lavrador, J. Teixeira, A. Pignatelli, and S. Livraghi, "A purely extradural lumbar nerve root cavernoma mimicking acute myeloid leukemia recurrence: case report and literature review," *Surgical Neurology International*, vol. 7, supplement 38, pp. S908–S910, 2016.

[3] E. Ferri, C. Minotto, F. Ianniello, S. Cavaleri, E. Armato, and P. Capuzzo, "Maxillo-ethmoidal chloroma in acute myeloid leukaemia: case report," *Acta Otorhinolaryngologica Italica*, vol. 25, no. 3, pp. 195–199, 2005.

[4] S. Lama, S. Lui, Y. Xiao, H. Zhang, M. Karki, and Q. Gong, "Sacral myeloid sarcoma involving multiple metastases to the brain: A case report," *Experimental and Therapeutic Medicine*, vol. 9, no. 4, pp. 1429–1432, 2015.

[5] E. M. Valsamis and T. E. Glover, "Granulocytic sarcoma: A rare cause of sciatica," *BMJ Case Reports*, vol. 2017, 2017.

[6] S. A. Pileri, S. Ascani, M. C. Cox et al., "Myeloid sarcoma: clinico-pathologic, phenotypic and cytogenetic analysis of 92 adult patients," *Leukemia*, vol. 21, no. 2, pp. 340–350, 2007.

[7] F. Siraj, M. Kaur, V. Dalal, A. Khanna, and A. A. Khan, "Myeloid sarcoma: a report of four cases at unusual sites," *German Medical Science*, vol. 15, article Doc03, 2017.

[8] N. Orofino, D. Cattaneo, C. Bucelli et al., "An unusual type of myeloid sarcoma localization following myelofibrosis: A case report and literature review," *Leukemia Research Reports*, vol. 8, pp. 7–10, 2017.

[9] L. M. Almond, M. Charalampakis, S. J. Ford, D. Gourevitch, and A. Desai, "Myeloid sarcoma: presentation, diagnosis, and treatment," *Clinical Lymphoma, Myeloma & Leukemia*, vol. 17, no. 5, pp. 263–267, 2017.

[10] M. Samborska, K. Derwich, J. Skalska-Sadowska, P. Kurzawa, and J. Wachowiak, "Myeloid sarcoma in children—diagnostic and therapeutic difficulties," *Contemporary Oncology*, vol. 20, no. 6, pp. 444–448, 2016.

[11] H. Mostafavi, P. J. Lennarson, and V. C. Traynelis, "Granulocytic sarcoma of the spine," *Neurosurgery*, vol. 46, no. 1, pp. 78–84, 2000.

[12] D. M. Landis and D. M. Aboulafia, "Granulocytic sarcoma: An unusual complication of aleukemic myeloid leukemia causing spinal cord compression. A case report and literature review," *Leukemia & Lymphoma*, vol. 44, no. 10, pp. 1753–1760, 2003.

[13] M. L. Siker, J. Bovi, and B. Alexander, "Spinal cord tumors," in *Clinical Radiation Oncology*, pp. 521–540.e5, Elsevier, 2016.

[14] M. B. Dhakar, P. Bansal, and A. C. Tselis, "Sacral spine myeloid sarcoma," *The Neurohospitalist*, vol. 6, no. 2, pp. 87-88, 2015.

[15] S. M. McCarty and D. J. Kuo, "Persistent sacral chloroma in refractory acute myelogenous leukaemia," *BMJ Case Reports*, vol. 2017, 2017.

[16] T. Inoue, T. Takahashi, H. Shimizu et al., "Spinal granulocytic sarcoma manifesting as radiculopathy in a nonleukemic patient," *Neurologia Medico-Chirurgica*, vol. 48, no. 3, pp. 131–136, 2008.

[17] M. H. Pui, B. D. Fletcher, and J. W. Langston, "Granulocytic sarcoma in childhood leukemia: imaging features," *Radiology*, vol. 190, no. 3, pp. 698–702, 1994.

37

Urethral Duplication with a Cystic Phallic Urethra Associated with a Uterus Didelphys, Partial Agenesis of the Tibia, and an Equinovarus Foot

Edwige Kafando[1] **Boniface Moifo**[1,2] **Landry Mbouche,**[3] **Derek Ndangoh,**[1] **Evelyn Mah,**[1,4] **and Faustin Mouafo Tambo**[1,3]

[1]*Faculty of Medicine and Biomedical Sciences, University of Yaounde I, Yaounde, Cameroon*
[2]*Department of Radiology, Yaounde Gynaeco-Obstetric and Pediatric Hospital, Yaounde, Cameroon*
[3]*Department of Pediatric Surgery, Yaounde Gynaeco-Obstetric and Pediatric Hospital, Yaounde, Cameroon*
[4]*Department of Neonatology, Yaounde Gynaeco-Obstetric and Pediatric Hospital, Yaounde, Cameroon*

Correspondence should be addressed to Edwige Kafando; evikaf2001@yahoo.fr

Academic Editor: Vincent Low

Urethral duplication is a rare congenital malformation, especially in females. It may be associated with complex urogenital malformations, but the association with a cystic phallic urethra and a uterus didelphys is exceptional. We report a case of a newborn with urethral duplication, with the accessory urethra exteriorized by a large cyst, associated with a uterus didelphys and bone malformations. We discuss the clinical, radiographic, and therapeutic aspects as well as a literature review.

1. Introduction

Urethral duplications are among the rarest congenital malformations of the urinary tract, with about 500 cases described in the literature in 2008 [1]. They are defined by the existence of 2 urethras, with several reported anatomical variants, associated or not with genital malformations. They are encountered most often in males and are of exceptional occurrence in females [2]. To the best of our knowledge, no case having cystic phallic urethra with uterus didelphys has been described in literature. We, therefore, report clinical and radiological features of this case along with brief treatment.

2. Observation

A 2-day-old female newborn was referred to us for malformation assessment. A perineal cyst, a left equinovarus foot, and a single umbilical artery were demonstrated during third trimester obstetric ultrasound (Figure 1). Her mother is a 17-year-old primiparous lady whose pregnancy had been well monitored and without any particular incident. The delivery was done by Caesarean section. Physical examination of the newborn confirmed the presence of a cystic mass attached to the vulva, with an orifice in the anterosuperior part that occasionally emitted urine, with the mass emptying and gradually filling with the urine (Figure 2). Below the cyst was another orifice, through which the urine flowed more regularly. The anus was normal.

On ultrasound, this vulvar mass presented with thick walls and an anechoic content. Examination of the urinary tract revealed normal kidneys and a normally located bladder, behind which two uterine hemimatrices suggestive of a uterus didelphys were visualized (Figure 3).

In order to investigate the relationship between the cyst and the bladder, a retrograde urethrocystography was performed with simultaneous opacification of the two urine evacuation orifices. An X-ray of the left lower limb was performed to assess the deformity of the foot and leg. The analysis of the bony structures revealed a fusion of the last two sacral vertebrae with coccygeal agenesis and pubic diastasis and partial agenesis of the distal half of the left tibia with an equinovarus distortion of the foot (Figure 4). Opacification

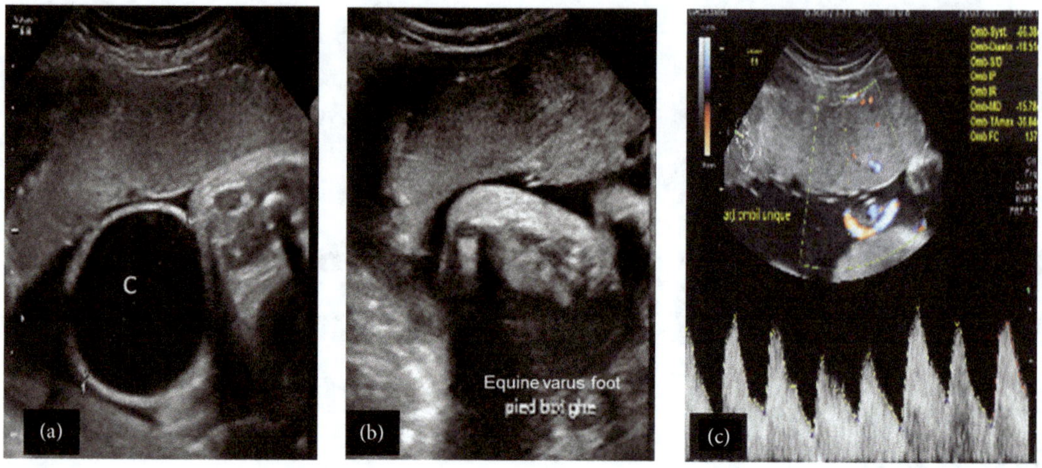

(a) (b) (c)

FIGURE 1: Morphological anomalies seen at antenatal ultrasound. (a) Cystic perineal mass (C), (b) equinovarus left foot, and (c) umbilical cord with a single artery.

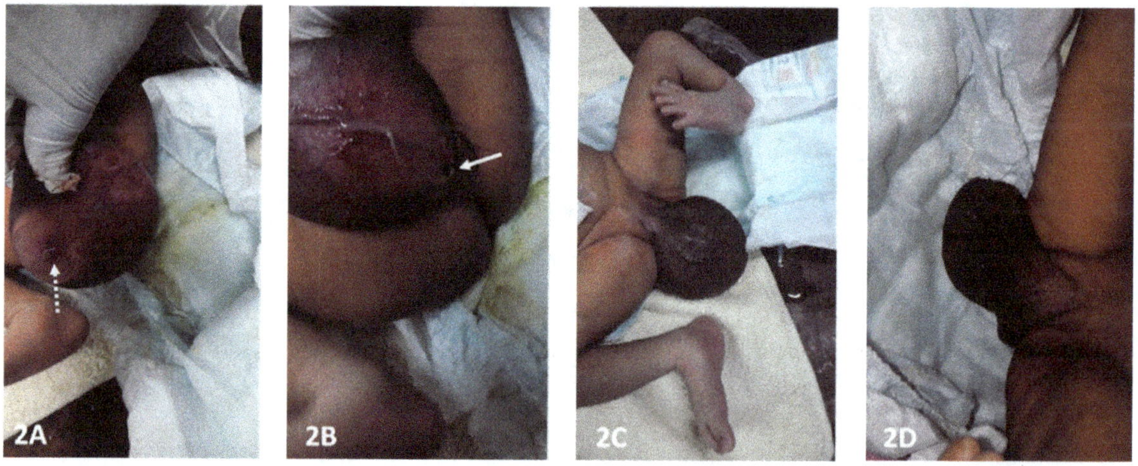

(a) (b) (c) (d)

FIGURE 2: Postnatal photographs of the newborn on day 2 of life. (a) Cystic vulvar mass with an orifice at the anterior superior part of the mass (broken arrow) emitting urine intermittently. (b) Below the cyst was another orifice (full arrow) emitting urine more regularly. (c) Equinovarus left foot. (d) Emptying of the mass after voiding.

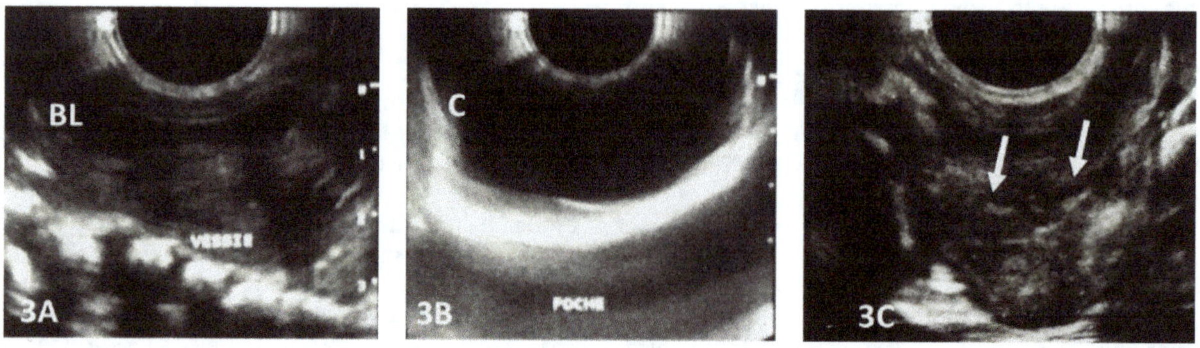

(a) (b) (c)

FIGURE 3: Postnatal pelvic and perineal ultrasound of the baby. (a-b) Suprapubic cross sections showing bladder (BL) and transperineal view showing cystic mass (C). (c) Uterus didelphys with the endometrial echogenic lines of the two hemiuteri (arrows).

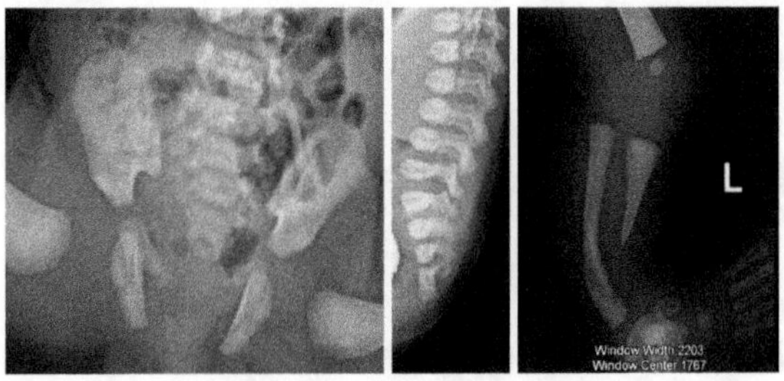

FIGURE 4: Radiographs centered on the anomalies of the bony structures (frontal view of the pelvis, lateral views of the lumbosacral spine and the left leg): VACTERL. Pubic diastasis, fusion of the last sacral vertebrae with agenesis of the coccyx, agenesis of the distal half of the tibia with fibular curvature, and an equinovarus deformation of the left foot.

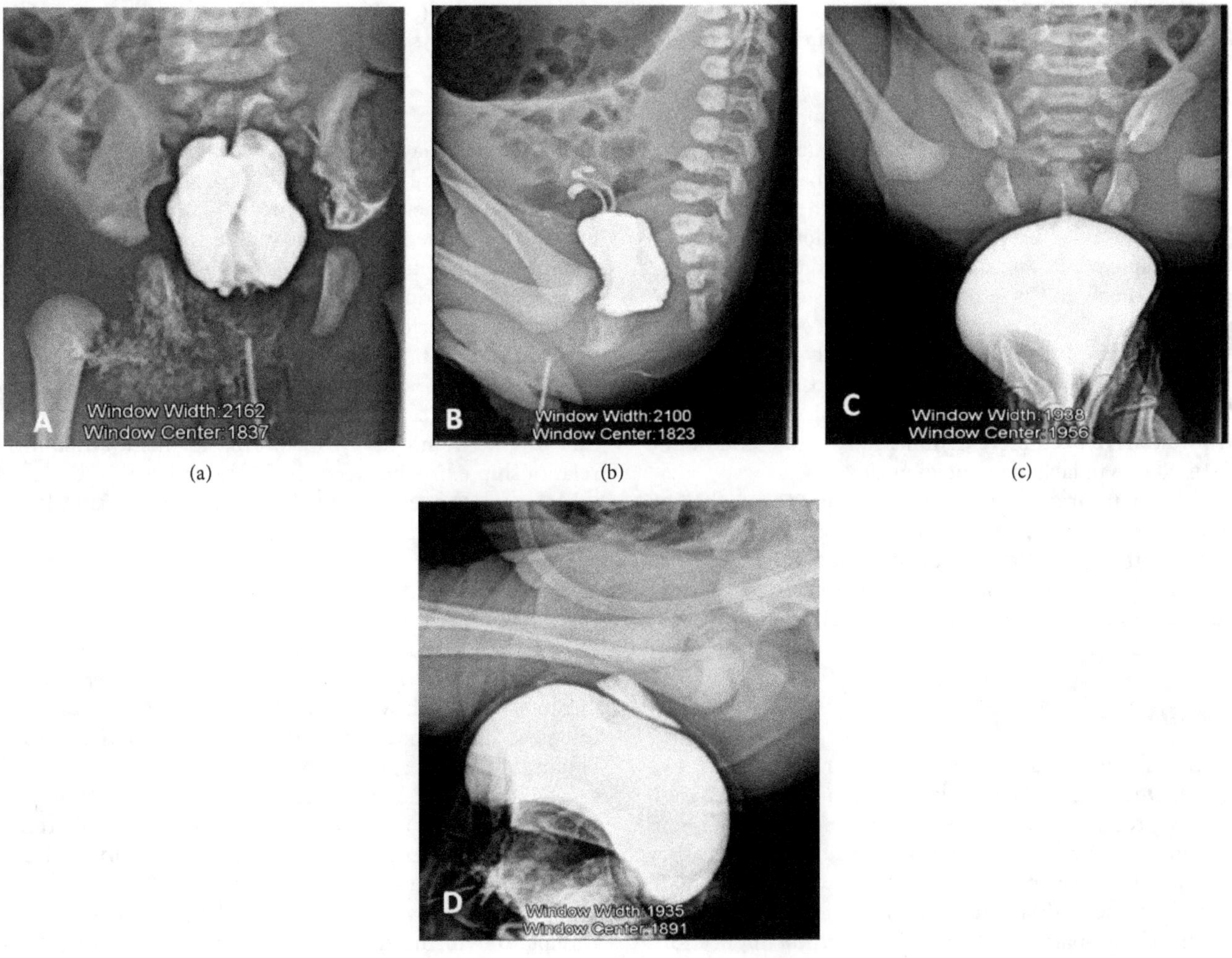

(a) (b) (c) (d)

FIGURE 5: Opacification with iodine-based contrast media. (a) and (b) Through the orifice below the cyst: evidence of two hemiuteri and tubes suggestive of a uterus didelphys. (c) and (d) Through the anterosuperior orifice: opacification of the vulvar cyst and of the phallic accessory urethra with the onset of bladder filling on the lateral view.

through the orifice below the cyst initially led to the filling of two oblong cavities, each continuous by a filamentous and tortuous structure suggestive of the tubal morphology, with the left being opacified right up to the distal portions and peritoneal spillage of the contrast medium, thus confirming the uterus didelphys (Figures 5(a) and 5(b)). During the evacuation of the contrast medium, there was reflux into the cystic mass with elimination through the two orifices, which made it possible to affirm the existence of a urogenital sinus thus explaining the communication between the urinary and genital tracts. The contrast medium injected through the orifice on the cyst completely molded the walls of the mass,

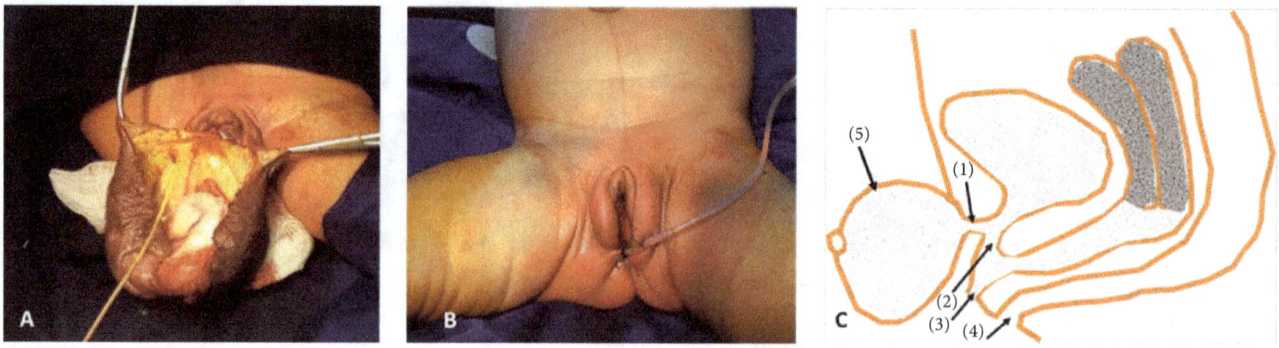

(a) (b) (c)

FIGURE 6: (a-b) Intraoperative view: resection of the cyst and phallic accessory urethra. (c) Illustrative diagram of urethral duplicity: (1) accessory phallic urethra, (2) main urethra, (3) urogenital sinus, (4) anus, and (5) clitoral cyst.

which were regular and thin. Pressure maneuvers revealed a short urethral pathway to the bladder that was partially opacified (Figures 5(c) and 5(d)). With these images, we suggested a complex urogenital malformation associating a uterus didelphys and a urethral duplicity: the main urethra communicating with the vagina by the persistence of the urogenital sinus opening externally via the orifice below the cyst; the accessory phallic urethra opens externally to the vulva via a voluminous cyst with an orifice at its anterosuperior surface and emitting urine intermittently. A complementary pelvic MRI would have been more demonstrative but could not be performed due to lack of financial means.

A multistep surgical management was proposed, the first consisting of an excision of the phallic accessory urethra with resection of the cyst and a vaginoplasty, thus allowing a complete separation of the urinary tract of the genital structures (Figures 6(a) and 6(b)): the repair of the malformations of the left lower limb having been deferred.

3. Discussion

Anatomically, urethral duplication is characterized by two urethras. One urethra is usually normal and the other is an accessory urethra. It may be either frontal or sagittal, and depending on whether the external orifice of the accessory urethra opens above or below the external orifice of the main urethra (the one with a markedly stronger urine flow), this distinguishes epispadic and hypospadic urethral duplications [1]. The male urethral duplication is divided into three types according to Effman's classification [3]. In girls, a classification of 5 types has been proposed [4]:

(i) Type I: double urethra and double bladder

(ii) Type II: double urethra with single bladder

(iii) Type III: accessory urethra posterior to the normal channel

(iv) Type IV: double proximal urethra and single distal urethra

(v) Type V: single proximal urethra and duplicated distal urethra.

Other authors have described two varieties: a duplication in the horizontal plane with 2 parallel channels and a duplication in the sagittal plane, with a posterior functional main channel opening into the vagina and a phallic accessory channel [2, 5]. Our findings were suggestive of the latter and were confirmed during the surgery (Figure 6(c)).

Various theories have been proposed for development of urethral duplication, but no single theory explains all the various types of anomalies [1]. The most widely accepted theory for the cause of complete urethral duplication is that of Patten and Barry. According to them, an abnormal relationship exists between the lateral anlagen of the genital tubercle and the ventral end of the cloacal membrane. [1, 4, 6]. The opening of the urethra in the vagina corresponds to a defect of the urethrovaginal septum which may be total, allowing a direct communication of the bladder with the vagina, or more frequently partial [2].

Urethral duplication can be observed in a context of complex urogenital malformations [2]. Until a certain age of intrauterine life, the development of the urinary tract is fully integrated with that of the genital tract in both males and females. In females, the cranial part of the pelvic portion of the final urogenital sinus remains narrow, constituting the very short female urethra. The pelvic part gradually reduces in depth and is incorporated into the phallic portion, leading to the urethral and vaginal orifices which open into the vestibule. The lower and horizontal part (phallic portion) widens and forms the vestibule, limited inferiorly by the urogenital membrane which breaks during the 7th week of embryonic life (Figure 7) [7]. This closeness during embryonic development thus explains the frequent association of urinary and genital malformations. This is the case in our observation where there is an association of urethral duplication by persistence of the phallic urethra with cystic exteriorization to the vulva, the urogenital sinus, and the uterus didelphys.

Besides endoscopy, the main work-up examinations include a voiding cystography showing the main channel as well as retrograde opacification from the accessory canal [2, 5]. In our case, voiding radiographs revealing the two ureters simultaneously were not obtained, but the two-stage

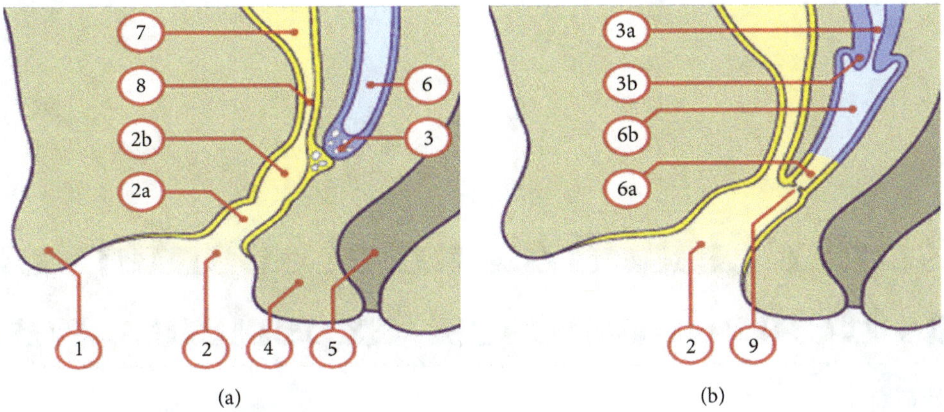

FIGURE 7: (a-b) Diagram of the urogenital sinus (UGS) at about 12 weeks and 9 months (source: http://www.embryology.ch/francais/ugenital/genitinterne06.html). (a) Urogenital sinus (UGS) at about 12 weeks: (1) genital tubercle, (2) vestibule, (2a) urogenital sinus (UGS) phallic portion, (2b) UGS pelvic portion, (3) vaginal epithelial blade, (4) perineum, (5) rectum, (6) uterovaginal canal, (7) bladder, and (8) urethra. (b) Definitive vestibule, uterus, and vagina at about the 9th month: (2) definitive vestibule, (3a) uterus (body), (3b) uterus (cervix), (6a) lower 1/4 of the vagina (endoblast), (6b) upper 3/4 of the vagina (mesoblast), and (9) hymen.

opacification of each urethral orifice made it possible to visualize the urethral pathways and their orifices. The plain films also revealed a pubic symphysis disjunction, which is often associated and must be systematically verified [1].

Ultrasound of the urinary tract can demonstrate the exact length of each urethra, looking for stenosis, diverticulations, and anomalies of the periurethral soft tissues as well as associated malformations such as bladder, ureteral duplication, or renal agenesis [1]. It has the advantage of being nonirradiating but it is an operator-dependent examination. In our case, it confirmed the existence of an intrapelvic bladder, which eliminated the hypothesis of a cystocele which could be mistaken for the vulvar cyst, and the existence of upper urinary tract malformations.

MRI provides a more accurate malformation assessment for the evaluation of urethral duplication by precisely demonstrating the sizes, shapes, and positions of both urethras as well as the existence of other genitourinary anomalies [1, 4]. But it is not always available or in our context.

Antenatal morphological ultrasound demonstrates once again its importance, having made it possible in our observation to demonstrate the vulvar cyst, the equinovarus foot, and the single umbilical artery. The family was quickly oriented towards a hospital structure adapted to the management of this kind of condition. An elective Caesarean section was performed and the newborn was treated early, the surgical act consisting of an excision of the cystic accessory phallic urethra with urogenital sinus septation and vaginoplasty. There were no postoperative complications.

Our patient presented with other bone abnormalities associated with the left foot equinovarus deformity; these included sacrococcygeal malformations and partial agenesis of the left tibia. These malformations can be integrated within the framework of a VACTERL and must trigger the verification of other malformations including cardiovascular and tracheoesophageal malformations.

4. Conclusion

Urethral duplication is a rare malformation especially in girls. The diagnosis of the anatomical form relies mainly in our context on voiding and retrograde cystography. Associated anomalies, in particular urogenital, should be systematically verified.

References

[1] I. Diabaté, C. Zé Ondo, B. Ouédraogo, M. Thiam, and G. Bazolo, "Epispadiac urethral duplication: Diagnosis and management. A case report," *African Journal of Urology*, vol. 22, no. 4, pp. 231–234, 2016.

[2] J. F. Lapray, *Imagerie de la vessie et de la dynamique pelvienne de la femme. Anomalies congénitales de l'urètre*, chapter 5, Masson, 1999.

[3] E. L. Effmann, R. L. Lebowitz, and A. H. Colodny, "Duplication of the urethra," *Radiology*, vol. 119, no. 1, pp. 179–185, 1976.

[4] S. Bhadury, U. Parashari, R. Singh, and N. Kohli, "MRI in congenital duplication of urethra," *Indian Journal of Radiology and Imaging*, vol. 19, no. 3, pp. 232–234, 2009.

[5] O. Helenon, K. Hamida, M. Augusti, M. Souissi, G. Ramella, and J. F. Moreau, "Radiologie de l'urètre pathologique. EMC," *Radiologie et Imagerie Medicale: Génito-urinaire - Gynéco-obstétricale - Mammaire*, 1992.

[6] S. Solanki, M. N. Babu, V. Jadhav, Gowrishankar, and S. Ramesh, "Female urethral duplication: Rare anomaly with unusual presentation," *Journal of Surgical Technique and Case Report*, vol. 7, no. 1, pp. 1–3, 2015.

[7] http://www.embryology.ch/francais/ugenital/genitinterne06.html.

38

Endovascular Embolization of Spontaneous Iliopsoas Hematoma: First Experience with Squidperi

Pierluca Torcia,[1] Silvia Squarza,[1] Umberto G. Rossi,[1,2] Paolo Rigamonti,[1] Lorenzo Carlo Pescatori,[3] Giovanni Damiani,[1] and Maurizio Cariati[1]

[1]*ASST Santi Paolo and Carlo, San Carlo Borromeo Hospital, Department of Diagnostic Science, Radiology and Interventional Radiology Unit, Via Pio II 3, 20153 Milano, Italy*
[2]*Department of Diagnostic Imaging, Interventional Radiology Unit, Galliera Hospital, Mura delle Cappuccine 14, 16128 Genova, Italy*
[3]*Postgraduation School in Radiodiagnostics, Università degli Studi di Milano, Via Festa del Perdono 7, 20122 Milano, Italy*

Correspondence should be addressed to Silvia Squarza; silvia.squarza@yahoo.it

Academic Editor: Roberto Iezzi

A 79-year-old man, suffering from atrial fibrillation and on anticoagulation therapy, was admitted at the emergency department of our institution because of a worsening respiratory insufficiency. After a diagnostic work-up, he was found to suffer from pneumonia, and antibiotic therapy was settled. He was kept under observation for his pulmonary conditions but, within a week, he developed a spontaneous iliopsoas hematoma, due to a sudden dysregulation of anticoagulation therapy subsequent to new in-hospital treatments. An endovascular approach was attempted and the bleeding vessels were embolized with a new liquid agent, named Squidperi (Emboflu, Switzerland). Complete exclusion of the diseased vessels was obtained and no complications occurred after the procedure. We conclude that Squidperi can be considered as an option for treatment of spontaneous iliopsoas hematomas.

1. Introduction

The incidence of spontaneous iliopsoas hematoma is 0.1% in general population and 0.6% in elderly patients receiving anticoagulant therapies or affected by coagulopathies [1].

As typically it is not considered a life threatening condition, a nonoperative approach should be attempted at first. In fact, a correction of the International Normalized Ratio (INR) can be sufficient to let the bleeding stop. More radical handling (i.e., endovascular or surgical therapies) should be taken into consideration when dealing with continuous and/or consistent bleeding, leading to hemodynamic instability [2].

At present, when an invasive treatment is needed, percutaneous management by selective embolization of the bleeding vessels is considered as gold standard [3].

Herein, we describe a case of spontaneous iliopsoas hematoma treated with Squidperi (Emboflu, Switzerland), a new formulation available for embolization procedures.

2. Case Report

A 79-year-old man was admitted at the emergency department of our institution because of a worsening respiratory insufficiency. After a first evaluation he was found to suffer from lobar right pneumonia, so he was hospitalized to receive proper antibiotic treatment and supportive medical care. At the time of admission, he was on oral anticoagulation therapy because of a persistent atrial fibrillation. After a week of treatment, his haemoglobin (Hb) level decreased by 1.5 g/dl (having 10 g/dl at admission). He did not report other symptoms and his blood tests were otherwise consistent with the previous ones obtained during hospitalization. Because of his pulmonary condition, a bronchial artery haemorrhage was suspected, so he underwent urgent Multidetector Computed Tomography (MD-CT).

A thoracic-abdominal CT with triphase technique was performed and it demonstrated a left iliopsoas hematoma with three active points of contrast extravasation

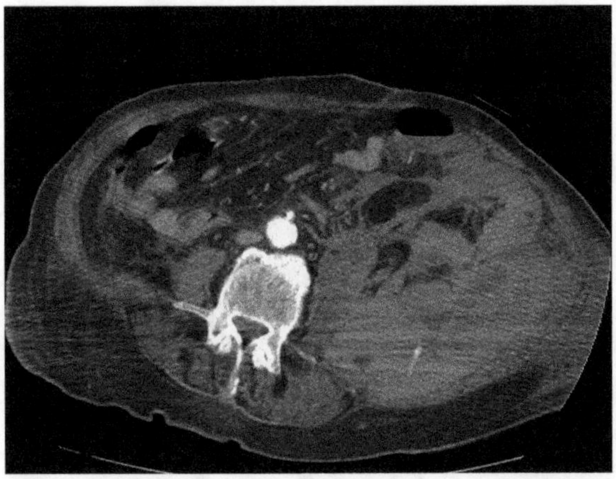

(a) MD-CT axial view in arterial phase demonstrates the presence of a haematoma into the left iliopsoas with a cranial spot of active bleeding

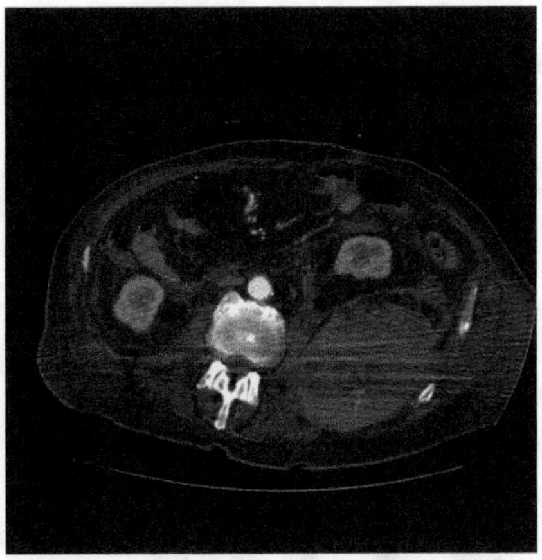

(b) MD-CT axial view in arterial phase demonstrates the presence of a haematoma into the left iliopsoas with a middle second spot of active bleeding

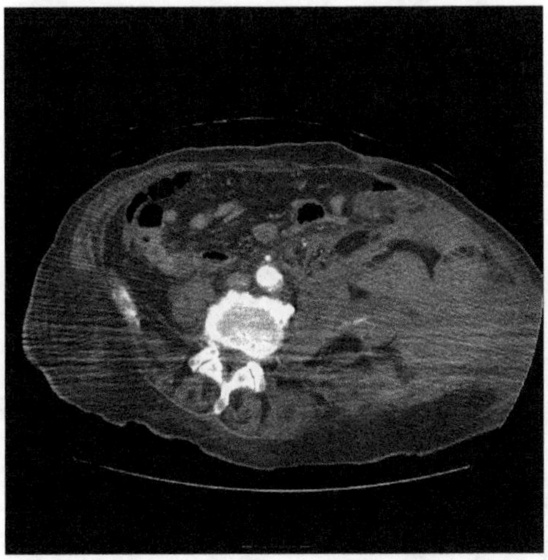

(c) MD-CT axial view in arterial phase demonstrates the presence of a haematoma into the left iliopsoas with a third caudal spot of active bleeding

FIGURE 1

(Figures 1(a)–1(c)). No active bleeding was detected at pulmonary level.

After multidisciplinary agreement, the patient underwent urgent Digital Subtraction Angiography (DSA) that confirmed the three points of bleeding described on CT, that is, gluteal artery, iliolumbar artery, and lumbar arteries (Figures 2(a) and 2(b)). DSA also demonstrated a site of active bleeding from circumflex iliac artery (Figure 3(a)). A coaxial superselective catheterization was performed for all these arteries with a Terumo Progreat microcatheter 2.7-Fr (Terumo, Tokyo, Japan) and then all the bleeding spots were embolized using the liquid embolic agent Squidperi 18 (Figures 3(a) and 3(b)). The final DSA control confirmed the complete embolization of all the diseased vessels and absence of active residual bleeding (Figure 4). The postoperative course was uneventful. Patient was discharged 3 days later, after completion of medical therapy for his pneumonia.

3. Discussion

Spontaneous iliopsoas hematoma is commonly found in elderly patients on anticoagulant therapies. As perfect compliance to anticoagulation treatments is not easy to obtain, patients' INR can be easily found over the therapeutic range for a number of reasons, and this is the main risk factor for spontaneous bleeding [2]. Likewise, several treatments can react with the anticoagulation drugs, leading to a sudden alteration of INR, like in the case presented.

Anyhow, spontaneous retroperitoneal bleeding is rare and detection can be difficult. In a typical setting, patients may report acute low back pain, but it can be underestimated (both by the patient and the clinician) and referred to spinal neuromuscular problems. However, when the pain is associated with decreasing Hb values and peripheral neurologic symptoms (due to compression by the increasing hematoma), the clinician should suspect a retroperitoneal bleeding [2].

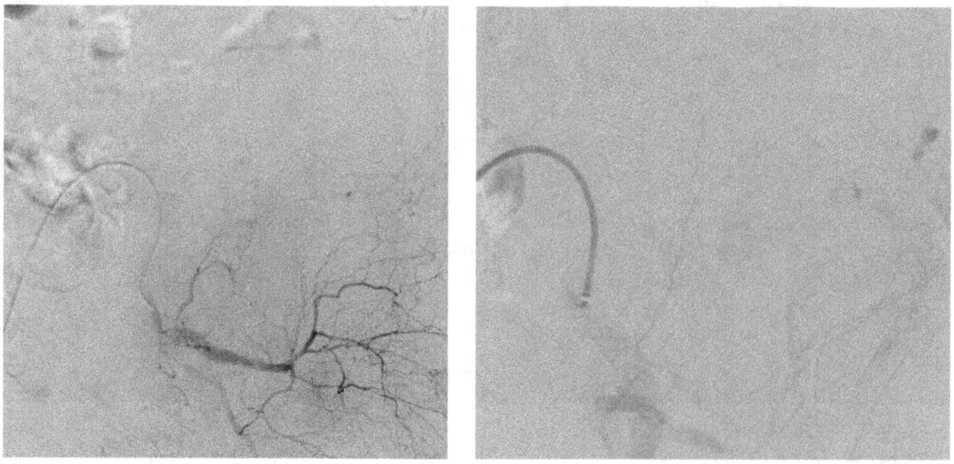

(a) Selective left internal iliac angiography confirmed multiple spots of active bleeding from distal collaterals

(b) Selective left internal iliac angiography confirmed multiple spots of active bleeding from distal collaterals

FIGURE 2

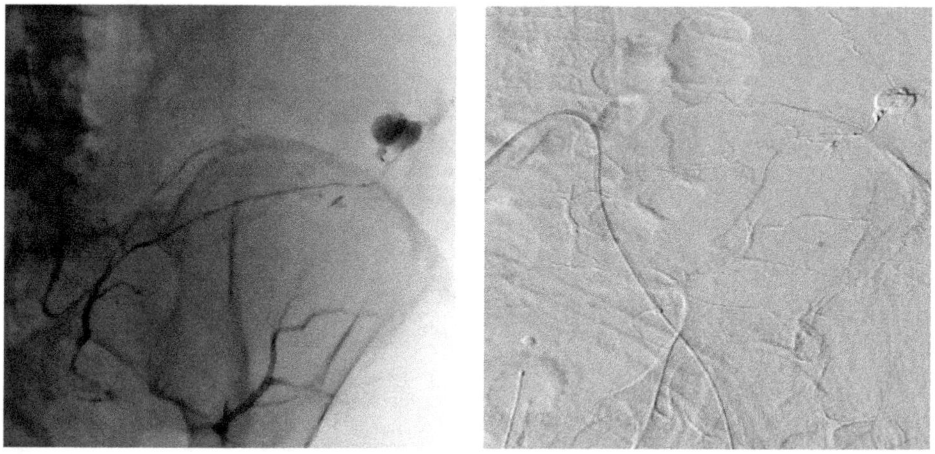

(a) Superselective catheterism and embolization with Squidperi of hematoma's arterial afferences

(b) Superselective catheterism of femoral artery demonstrates extravasation from circumflex iliac artery

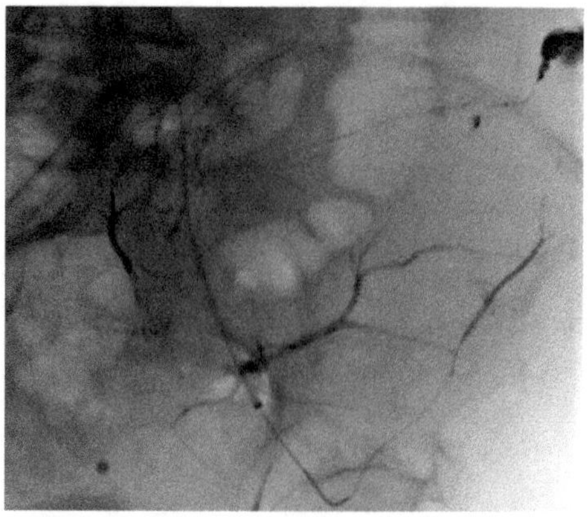

(c) Superselective catheterism and embolization with Squid 18 of the circumflex iliac artery

FIGURE 3

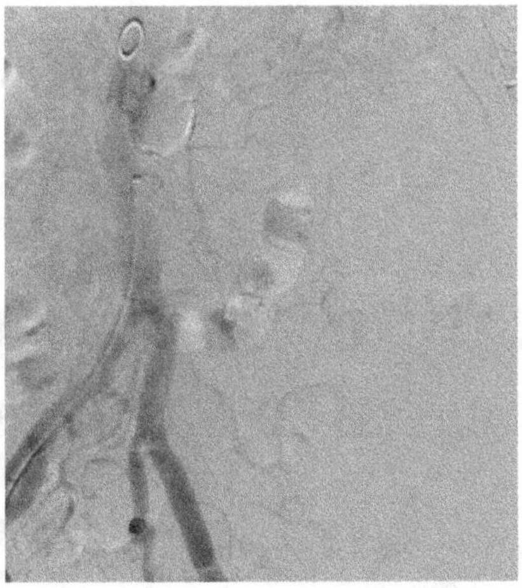

FIGURE 4: Final angiographic control demonstrates the complete exclusion of hematoma.

A triphase multislice CT angiography is considered the gold standard for diagnosis, as it allows detection of site and extension of hematoma as well as the evidence of active bleeding presenting as a blush of contrast media in arterial CT phase, that is, an indication for immediate treatment [4].

As stated, different approaches can be proposed when dealing with an iliopsoas hematoma and, at present, there is no general agreement about the best treatment options [3]. In our clinical practice, when a patient is found with a retroperitoneal hematoma but without signs of active bleeding or hemodynamic instability, a medical treatment is firstly proposed. Conversely, in case of blood loss and active arterial bleeding detected by CT scan, endovascular treatment is the first choice. Venous bleeding presents no indications to be treated with endovascular approach and, in case of patient's clinical instability, surgical approach is the only choice of treatment.

Angiography has multiple advantages in this cases as, thanks to high resolution images and to injection of intra-arterial contrast media, it allows confirming the diagnosis obtained with CT scan and searching for other bleeding points that can be missed with other diagnostic modalities. This particular role was demonstrated also in our case. Moreover, once the bleeding vessels are detected, they can be selectively embolized, saving surrounding tissue [5].

Because all of these reasons, surgery should be proposed only after endovascular failure, or when other surgical conditions occur or in case of significant compressive neurological symptoms [6].

After treatment, CT angiography has to be repeated after treatment only in case of unexpected clinical or hemodynamical instability to evaluate the presence of new bleeding; it can also play a role in recognizing complications such as pseudoaneurysms during the follow-up.

To our knowledge, there are no previous reports regarding the embolization of a spontaneous iliopsoas hematoma with Squidperi. It is a nonadhesive liquid embolic agent made with EVOH (ethylene vinyl alcohol) copolymer dissolved in DMSO (dimethylsulfoxide), and suspended in a micronized tantalum powder. First experiences were reported by Akmangit et al. who extensively used Squidperi to treat arteriovenous malformations, arteriovenous fistula, aneurysms, and tumors [7]. Shortly after, Erbahceci Salik et al. reported the use of Squidperi to embolize a pelvic arteriovenous malformation [8]. Recently our group described the successful use of Squid for the management of a spontaneous rectus sheat hematoma [9].

Two forms of the agent are available, with decreasing viscosity: Squidperi 12 and Squidperi 18.

The biggest advantages in using the Squidperi are the high homogeneity of suspension and its stability over time, which allows an easily controlled and prolonged injection. Squidperi presents also a homogenic radiopacity that improves the assessment of vascular architecture

The main limitation of Squidperi is the time needed to prepare the formulation (about 15–20 minutes), mainly in emergency cases. However, if the preparation starts before the superselective cannulation of the bleeding vessels, it can be efficiently delivered without losing precious time.

In conclusion, due to the good intraprocedural result obtained with this embolic agent, it can be considered for treatment of spontaneous iliopsoas hematomas, although further studies are needed to state the outcome of patients on long-term basis.

References

[1] X. Estivill Pallejà, P. Domingo, J. Fontcuberta, and J. Félez, "Spontaneous retroperitoneal hemorrhage during oral anticoagulant therapy," *JAMA Internal Medicine*, vol. 145, no. 8, pp. 1531–1534, 1985.

[2] J. Tsai, P. Yang, H. Lin, and C. Chang, "Spontaneous Iliopsoas Hematoma," *The Journal of Emergency Medicine*, vol. 51, no. 3, pp. e53–e54, 2016.

[3] Y. C. Chan, J. P. Morales, J. F. Reidy, and P. R. Taylor, "Management of spontaneous and iatrogenic retroperitoneal haemorrhage: conservative management, endovascular intervention or open surgery?" *International Journal of Clinical Practice*, vol. 62, no. 10, pp. 1604–1613, 2008.

[4] M. Scialpi, M. Scaglione, G. Angelelli et al., "Emergencies in the retroperitoneum: Assessment of spread of disease by helical CT," *European Journal of Radiology*, vol. 50, no. 1, pp. 74–83, 2004.

[5] J.-M. Isokangas and J. M. Perälä, "Endovascular embolization of spontaneous retroperitoneal hemorrhage secondary to anticoagulant treatment," *CardioVascular and Interventional Radiology*, vol. 27, no. 6, pp. 607–611, 2004.

[6] K. L. Sunga, M. F. Bellolio, R. M. Gilmore, and D. Cabrera, "Spontaneous retroperitoneal hematoma: Etiology, characteristics, management, and outcome," *The Journal of Emergency Medicine*, vol. 43, no. 2, pp. e157–e161, 2012.

[7] I. Akmangit, E. Daglioglu, T. Kaya et al., "Preliminary experience with Squid: A new liquid embolizing agent for AVM, AV fistulas and tumors," *Turkish Neurosurgery*, vol. 24, no. 4, pp. 565–570, 2014.

[8] A. Erbahceci Salik, F. Islim, A. Akgul, and B. E. Cil, "Concomitant transarterial and transvenous embolization of a pelvic arteriovenous malformation using a new liquid embolic agent, squid-12 and detachable coils," *Case Reports in Vascular Medicine*, vol. 2014, Article ID 972870, 5 pages, 2014.

39

Detection of Myofascial Herniation on Dynamic Sonography and Magnetic Resonance Imaging

Sanjay M. Khaladkar, Sushen Kumar Kondapavuluri, Anubhav Kamal, Raghav Kalra, and Vigyat Kamal

Department of Radio-Diagnosis, Dr. D. Y. Patil Medical College, Pimpri, Pune 411018, India

Correspondence should be addressed to Sanjay M. Khaladkar; drsanjaymkhaladkar@gmail.com

Academic Editor: Salah D. Qanadli

Muscle hernia is an uncommon cause of leg swelling. It can be detected in the early stages only if there is a high index of suspicion. It is common in lower extremity compared to the upper extremity. Tibialis anterior muscle in the leg is commonly involved. Dynamic sonography and magnetic resonance imaging (MRI) are the mainstay in their diagnosis, which demonstrate a facial defect with herniation of muscle fibers. We report a case of 23-year-old male patient who presented with a painless swelling in the anterolateral aspect of the left upper leg. Dynamic sonography done with high-resolution probe demonstrated a defect in fascia overlying tibialis anterior with herniation of outer muscle fibers which increased during dorsiflexion and reduced in the supine position at rest. MRI of the left leg confirmed the findings.

1. Introduction

Muscle hernia is also called myofascial herniation. Muscle herniation of the lower extremity is a rare entity and is often asymptomatic. Symptomatic muscle hernias commonly occur in the leg and cause chronic leg pain due to nerve involvement. The focal fascial defect with resultant muscle herniation into subcutaneous fat presents clinically as a soft tissue mass. Clinicians must remember to consider myofascial herniation in the differential diagnosis of chronic leg pain or neuropathy. We present a case of tibialis anterior muscle herniation due to overlying fascial defect presenting as a palpable mass detected on dynamic sonography and MRI.

2. Case Report

A 23-year-old male presented with painless swelling in the anterolateral aspect of the left upper leg for 1-year duration. The swelling was prominent in standing position and reduced in lying down position at rest. There was no history of trauma. On local examination, a diffuse swelling appeared in the anterolateral aspect of the left upper leg in standing position which accentuated dorsiflexion of the foot and reduced in the supine position. It was nontender. Overlying skin temperature and color were normal. Local ultrasonography (USG) done with a high-resolution linear probe (frequency: 7 to 12 MHz) in standing position showed intact echogenic fascia overlying tibialis anterior superior to site of swelling (Figure 1(a)) and a defect of size 9.9 mm in echogenic fascia in the anteroposterior direction overlying the tibialis anterior in upper third of leg, extending superoinferiorly over a length of approximately 5.5 cm at site of swelling. There was herniation of the outer fibers of tibialis anterior muscle through this defect (Figures 1(b) and 1(c)). Muscle hernia showed reduction in lying down position (Figure 1(d)). Limited MRI (static) of the left leg was performed at rest for confirmation of USG findings by taking coronal T1 and T2 sequences (Figures 2(a) and 2(b)) followed by axial PD fat saturated sequence (Figures 3(a) and 3(b)) after placing a marker at the site of diffuse swelling. MRI confirmed a fascial defect overlying tibialis anterior measuring 1.2 cm in width extending superoinferiorly over a length of 5.5 cm with resultant muscle herniation and outward bulge of tibialis anterior. Outer fibers of tibialis anterior revealed subtle hyperintense signal on PD fat saturated sequence suggestive of muscle edema (Figure 3(c)). The patient was referred to

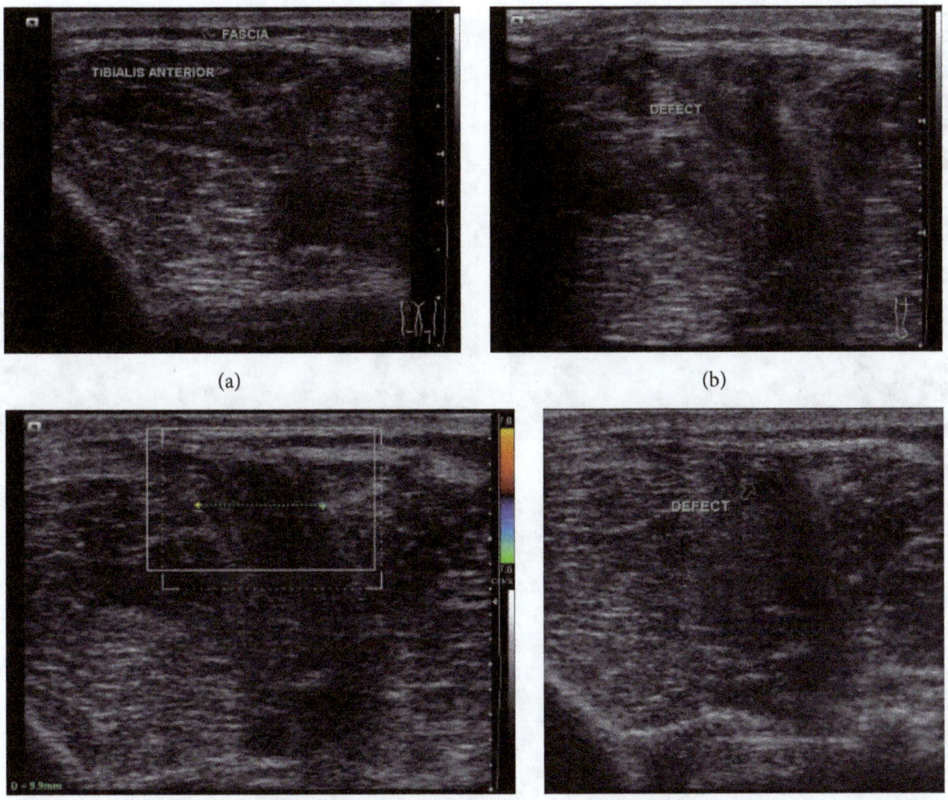

(a) (b) (c) (d)

FIGURE 1: (a) Longitudinal section on the anterolateral aspect of left upper leg superior to the site of muscle hernia showing intact echogenic fascia with underlying tibialis anterior muscle. (b) Transverse section on the anterolateral aspect of left upper leg in standing position showing a defect in echogenic fascia (marked by arrow) with an increase in herniation of underlying tibialis anterior muscle through the defect. (c) Transverse section on the anterolateral aspect of left upper leg in standing position showing the defect of size 9.9 mm in echogenic fascia with herniation of underlying tibialis anterior muscle through the defect. (d) Longitudinal section on the anterolateral aspect of left upper leg at rest at the site of muscle hernia showing a defect in echogenic fascia with herniation of underlying tibialis anterior muscle through the defect (marked by arrow).

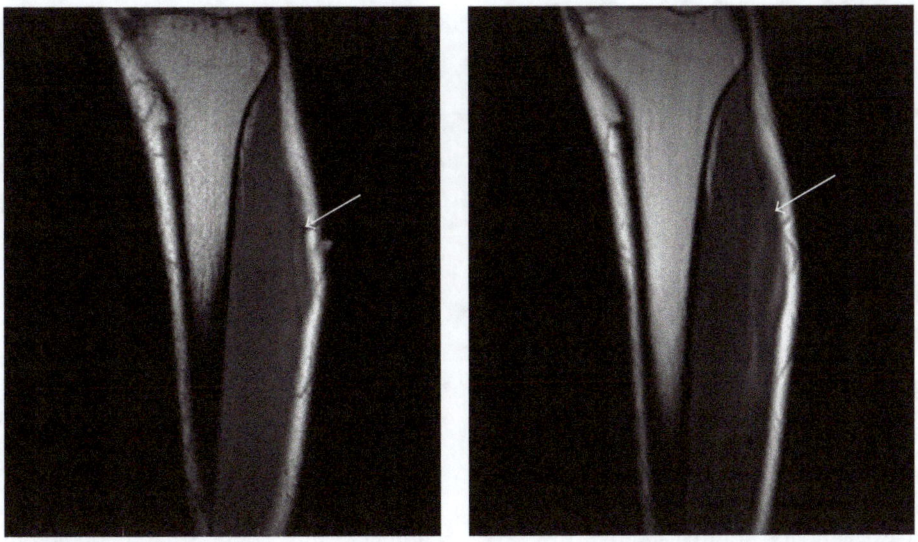

(a) (b)

FIGURE 2: (a) Coronal section of left leg T1-weighted sequence showing defect at the level of the marker (marked by arrow) with outward bulging of underlying tibialis anterior through the defect. (b) Coronal section of left leg T2-weighted sequence outward bulging of tibialis anterior due to muscle herniation through the defect (marked by arrow).

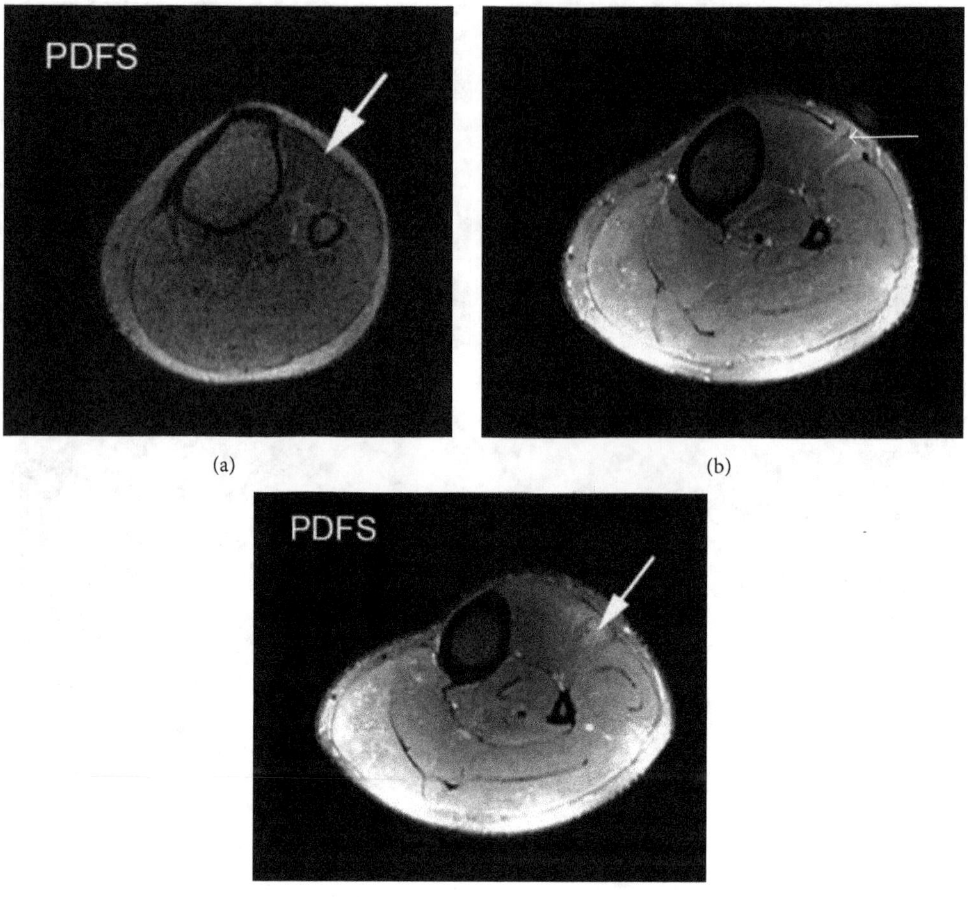

FIGURE 3: (a) Axial section of left upper leg PDFS sequence showing intact fascia overlying tibialis anterior muscle (marked by arrow). (b) Axial section of left upper leg PDFS sequence showing a defect in the fascia (marked by arrow) overlying tibialis anterior muscle at the level of the marker with resultant herniation of underlying muscle fibers. (c) Axial section of left upper leg PDFS sequence inferior to the level of defect showing intact fascia with a diffuse hyperintense signal in underlying tibialis anterior muscle due to muscle edema (marked by arrow).

the orthopedic department for repair of myofascial defect which he refused.

3. Discussion

Ihde provided original investigation and ground work on lower extremity muscle hernias [1]. Largest contribution is due to the combined efforts of military surgeons who observed muscle hernias in actively training military recruits; otherwise it occurs as sporadic cases. The majority of the earlier work of leg hernias is found in French medical literature which is based on military experience [1, 2]. Ihde in 1929 reported a series of 12 patients with hernias of leg and acknowledged the earlier description by Richet in 1853 and first actual definition provided in 1861 by Mourlon as "the displacement of muscle beyond its ruptured aponeurosis" [2]. Muscle hernias are caused by a focal defect in the fascial sheath. It is classified by Ihde [1] as constitutional (congenital) and traumatic (acquired). Congenital causes may be due to general weakness in muscular fascia (mesodermal insufficiency) or occur at sites of perforating nerves and vessels. Acquired cases are secondary to trauma as seen in penetrating trauma, direct trauma causing close fracture with fascial tear, and indirect trauma (force applied to contracted muscle causing fascial rupture) [3]. Increase in intracompartmental pressure seen in muscle hypertrophy or chronic exertional compartment syndrome (CECS) potentiates herniation [4]. Regular cardiovascular exercise and physical activity cause muscle hypertrophy with a 20% increase in muscle volume. CECS is a reversible form of abnormally increased intramuscular pressure during physical exertion or exercise secondary to noncompliance of osteofascial tissue to exercise-induced increase in muscle volume [4]. The true incidence of a leg hernia is not known, as most are asymptomatic and remain undiagnosed and are not brought to the attention of the physician. About 200 cases of muscle hernias are described in the literature [5]. Military soldier, athletes, mountain climbers, and skiers are the demographic population at highest risk who are prone to CECS. Fascial defects are found in 15–50% of patients undergoing surgery, even with normal preoperative examination [6].

The anterolateral tibial compartment is the commonest site due to superficial and tight fascial compartment [5].

A high index of suspicion and awareness of a muscle hernia helps in its early diagnosis. In the leg, tibialis anterior is the most commonly involved muscle and most reported in the literature. The fascia of tibialis anterior is more vulnerable to trauma as it is the weakest fascial point in the lower extremity [3]. Other muscles involved are peroneus longus, peroneus brevis, extensor digitorum longus, gastrocnemius, and flexor digitorum longus. Multiple hernias within the same muscle and bilateral symmetrical involvement may also be seen in the thigh. Iatrogenically induced hernia, involving rectus femoris and vastus lateralis, can occur as a complication following an anterolateral thigh perforator flap and after fascia lata harvest for cruciate ligament repair. The lower incidence of a muscle hernia in a peroneal compartment is due to a relatively large subcutaneous surface area aligning for increase compliance.

On clinical examination, muscle hernia may present as a palpable bulge, soft tissue mass, or subcutaneous nodule. It may be solitary, multiple, or bilateral. It is usually reducible on lying down. It may be irreducible when there is strangulated muscle. The patient may complain of pain, discomfort, weakness, cramping, or neuropathy. It worsens with standing and physical activity. On examination, local tenderness and decreased sensation may occur if there is associated nerve involvement. Herniation of tibialis anterior is pronounced with resisting dorsiflexion of the foot. If reducible, the fascial defect may be appreciated. A muscle hernia is commonly seen in adolescence and young adults who present with swelling which appears or enlarges on standing erect or when affected muscle is contracted. The swelling reduces when the patient is supine or muscle is relaxed. Differential diagnosis of muscle hernias are varicosities, angiomas, arteriovenous malformation, lipomas, ruptured muscle (a pseudohernia), and soft tissue tumors [3]. Dynamic sonography and MRI are diagnostic in detecting a myofascial defect. Dynamic sonography detects muscle bulge through the fascial defect on muscle contraction and reduces on relaxation. Sonography is advantageous as it is real time, muscle herniation is detected during dynamic examination, and nature of the lesion can be shown to the patient which helps in reassurance. The examination is done in standing position or by contracting the muscle. Marking of overlying skin is done as the mass may be difficult to be felt. High-frequency probe (more than 7.5 MHz) is used after liberal application of coupling gel. Gain and focus are set to optimize near field. The transducer is applied lightly as heavy pressure can efface a hernia [7].

Normal muscle is covered by thin echogenic fascia. In mild cases, fascia is thinned out with no demonstrable defect. There is a mild muscle bulge with an elevation of the overlying fascia. In overt cases, the margins of the defect are clearly defined with outward bulge and herniation of muscle through the defect. The herniated muscle and adjoining nonherniated muscle are less echogenic than normal muscle due to anisotropy or atrophy caused by low-grade repetitive trauma. Frank's hernia gives mushroom-like appearance causing convex superficial contour with herniated muscle overlapping the fascial defect. Spoke-like appearance caused by normal echogenic fibroadipose septae is seen as they are pinched through the fascial defect as they radiate from the center of the defect in the fascia. In a few cases, a prominent arterial pulsation can be identified on contour or power Doppler supporting the theory of muscle herniation at sites of weakness where vessels penetrate the fascia. USG is relatively easy and of low cost. 3D dynamic USG with surface rendering improves visualization of focal planes and the muscular protrusion and is superior to traditional 2-dimensional ultrasonography [7].

Though expensive, MRI confirms muscle herniation in equivocal USG findings. It better visualizes musculofascial demarcation and allows quantification of fascial splitting and muscle herniation. Dynamic ultrasonography and MRI incorporate fast imaging with forced muscular movements (dorsiflexion and plantar flexion at the ankle) and enable better visualization and pinpointing of the hernia and fascial defect. The defect is in the deep layer of the deep fascia. It may thin or elevate the superficial layer of deep fascia which is overlying the muscle [8–10]. Treatment of tibialis anterior herniation is controversial. Asymptomatic hernias require no specific treatment and rupture reassurance. Mildly symptomatic hernias often respond to conservative treatment with restriction of exercise and use of elastic support. The surgical option is the direct closure of the defect. However, it causes an increase in intracompartmental pressure accentuated in the postoperative period by edema causing recurrence. The fascial opening can be repaired with a patch of fascia lata or periosteal graft. However, this may be a cause of compartment syndrome and need an additional donor. Hence, recommended treatment is longitudinal fasciotomy which prevents the development of compartment syndrome [11].

4. Conclusion

A muscle hernia is an uncommon cause of swelling in the lower extremity which may cause chronic leg pain and neuropathy. It is common in lower extremity compared to the upper extremity. Tibialis anterior is commonly involved. Dynamic sonography and MRI are the investigations of choice in their detection.

Abbreviations

MRI: Magnetic resonance imaging
CECS: Chronic exertional compartment syndrome
USG: Ultrasonography.

References

[1] H. Ihde, "On muscular hernia of the leg," *Acta Chirurgica Scandinavica*, vol. 65, pp. 97–120, 1929.

[2] "Choux De la cure radicale des hernies musculaires," *Revue de Chirurgie*, vol. 485, 1983.

[3] J. T. Nguyen, J. L. Nguyen, M. J. Wheatley, and T. A. Nguyen, "Muscle hernias of the leg: a case report and comprehensive

review of the literature," *The Canadian Journal of Plastic Surgery*, vol. 21, no. 4, pp. 243–247, 2013.

[4] A. G. Schubert, "Exertional compartment syndrome: review of the literature and proposed rehabilitation guidelines following surgical release," *International Journal of Sports Physical Therapy*, vol. 6, no. 2, pp. 126–141, 2011.

[5] N. K. Rho, W. S. Kim, Y. J. Kim, K. H. Yoo, B. J. Kim, and M. N. Kim, "The use of dynamic ultrasonography for the confirmation of lower leg muscle herniation," *Annals of Dermatology*, vol. 20, no. 4, pp. 190–192, 2008.

[6] F. M. Azar, "Sports medicine," in *Campbell's Operative Orthopaedics*, S. T. Canale and J. H. Beaty, Eds., vol. 3, Mosby/Elsevier, Philadelphia, Pa, USA, 12th edition, 2012.

[7] I. Beggs, "Sonography of muscle hernias," *American Journal of Roentgenology*, vol. 180, no. 2, pp. 395–399, 2003.

[8] J. M. Mellado and L. Perez Del Palomar, "Muscle hernias of the lower leg: MRI findings," *Skeletal Radiology*, vol. 28, no. 8, pp. 465–469, 1999.

[9] S. Tyson and N. Subhas, "Radiologic case study. Gastrocnemius fascial defect and muscle herniation," *Orthopedics*, vol. 33, no. 11, pp. 785–854, 2010.

[10] S. E. Yochim, J. Jose, and P. D. Clifford, "Muscle herniation of the extremity," *The American Journal of Orthopedics*, vol. 39, no. 2, pp. 95–96, 2010.

[11] A. K. Dawar, R. Dawar, K. Gawri, and V. Gupta, "Tibialis anterior muscle hernia: a rare cause of leg pain," *Journal of Case Reports*, vol. 2, pp. 42–44, 2012.

40

Internal Jugular Vein Thrombosis in Isolated Tuberculous Cervical Lymphadenopathy

Sanjay Khaladkar, Avadhesh Chauhan, Arijit Ghosh, Kunaal Jain, and Surbhi Chauhan

Department of Radio-Diagnosis, Dr. D. Y. Patil Medical College and Research Center, Pimpri, Pune, India

Correspondence should be addressed to Sanjay Khaladkar; drsanjaymkhaladkar@gmail.com

Academic Editor: Vincent Low

Tuberculosis is a common infectious disease with a high prevalence in developing countries and presents a major public health issue. Internal jugular vein (IJV) thrombosis is a rare complication in tuberculous cervical lymphadenopathy. We report a case of 26-year male patient with a history of low-grade evening rise in fever, dry cough, loss of appetite, and loss of weight with swelling in lower neck on right side. Ultrasonography (USG) neck showed well-defined hypoechoic lymph nodes posterior to right IJV and common carotid artery in the lower neck at level IV and in the right supraclavicular region showing central necrotic areas with adjoining IJV thrombosis. The association between tuberculosis and deep vein thrombosis is rare. Awareness of IJV thrombosis in isolated cervical lymphadenopathy needs high diagnostic suspicion and prompt treatment to avoid fatal complication. Our case is rare as there was isolated tuberculous cervical lymphadenopathy with adjoining IJV thrombosis. Both USG and computed tomography (CT) are accurate and reliable radiological investigations for detecting IJV thrombosis along with cervical lymph nodes. They are useful in assessing surrounding soft tissue and fat planes and knowing the size and extent of cervical lymphadenopathy. USG is inexpensive and readily available for monitoring response to treatment.

1. Introduction

IJV thrombosis is a rare condition. It is usually associated with central venous catheterization, trauma, neck surgery, coagulation disorders, hypercoagulation states, endocrine alteration, local infection or malignancy, occult malignancy, neck massage, deep neck infection, and intravenous drug abuse [1, 2]. Tuberculous cervical lymphadenopathy with IJV thrombosis is extremely rare complication of isolated tuberculous cervical lymphadenopathy [3].

2. Case Report

A 26-year male patient that presented with swelling in the right supraclavicular region since 1.5 months was referred by surgeon to ultrasound department for evaluation of neck swelling. There was a history of low-grade evening rise in fever, dry cough, loss of appetite, and loss of weight.

USG neck showed well-defined hypoechoic lymph nodes measuring approx. 12×10 mm, 9×8 mm posterior to right IJV and common carotid artery (CCA) in the lower neck at level IV (Figures 1(a) and 1(b)). Lymph node measuring approx. 31×14 mm was noticed in the right supraclavicular region showing central hypoechoic areas due to necrosis showing multiple medium level internal echoes. A linear hypoechoic lesion of size approx. 20×5 mm was noted extending from this lymph node medially towards right lateral wall of internal jugular vein (Figure 1(c)). Echogenic fat plane noted between the lesion and right lateral wall of IJV was obscured with evidence of IJV invasion (Figures 2(a) and 2(b)). A medium level echogenic thrombus of size approx. 11(L) $\times$ 7(AP) $\times$ 8(T) mm was noted in adjoining right IJV in lower neck suggestive of IJV thrombosis (Figures 3(a) and 3(b)). Rest of the right IJV appeared normal with a normal flow on color Doppler. Contrast enhanced CT scan (CECT) of neck showed multiple lymph nodes at level IV on the right side and in the right supraclavicular region showing peripheral rim enhancement with central caseation necrosis (Figures 4, 5, and 6). A persistent filling defect was noted in

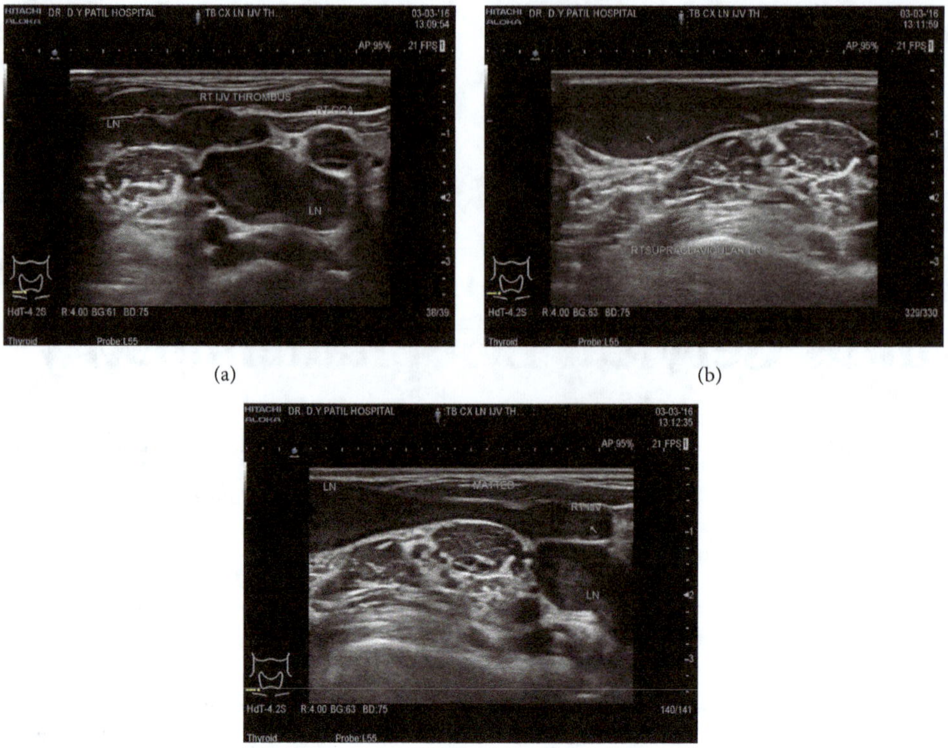

(a) (b)

(c)

FIGURE 1: USG neck showing well-defined hypoechoic lymph nodes posterior to right CCA and IJV and in the right supraclavicular region at level IV with echogenic thrombus in right IJV.

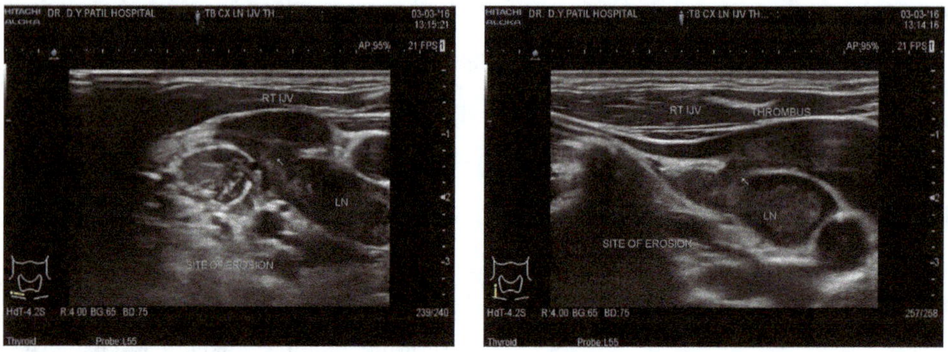

(a) (b)

FIGURE 2: Cervical lymph node at level IV eroding through posterior and the right lateral wall of IJV with medium level echogenic IJV thrombus.

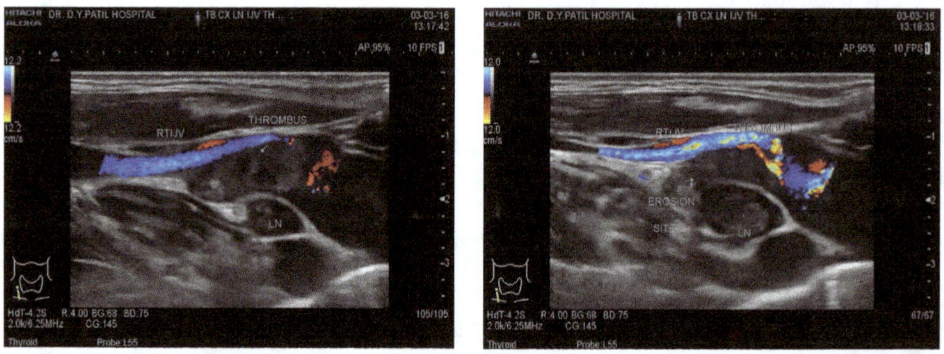

(a) (b)

FIGURE 3: Color Doppler study showing IJV thrombus seen as filling defect.

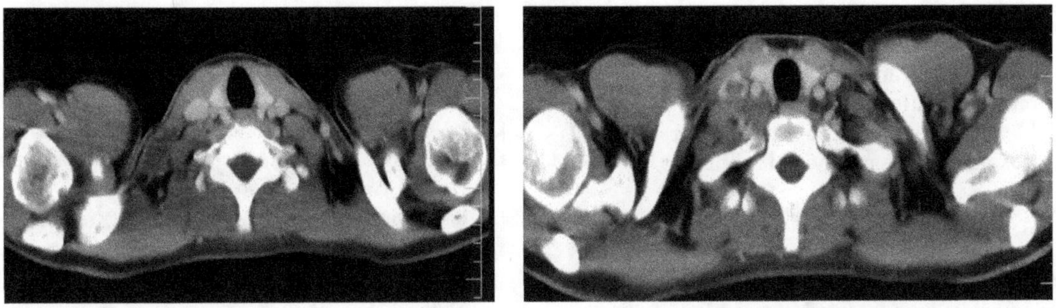

(a) (b)

FIGURE 4: Axial CECT neck showing well-defined hypodense lymph node in the right supraclavicular region and posterior to right CCA and IJV at level IV showing peripheral rim enhancement with central caseation necrosis eroding through the posterior wall of right IJV with filling defect in contrast filled IJV lumen suggestive of thrombus.

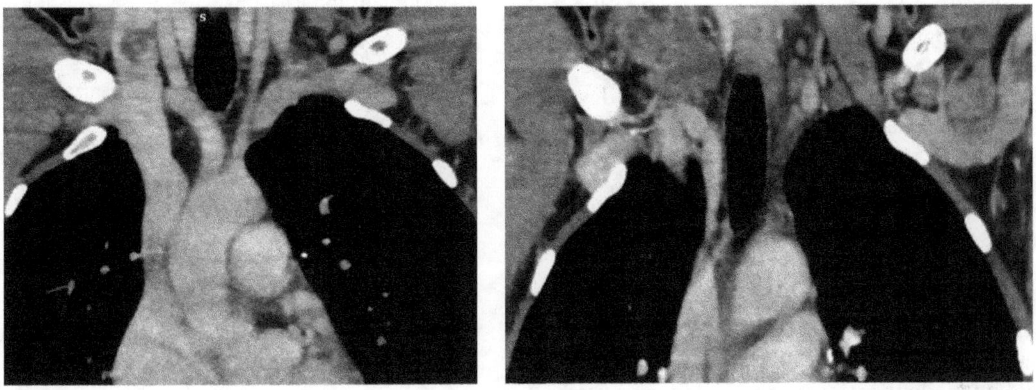

(a) (b)

FIGURE 5: Coronal CECT neck showing right IJV thrombus and matted lymph nodes posterior to right CCA and IJV.

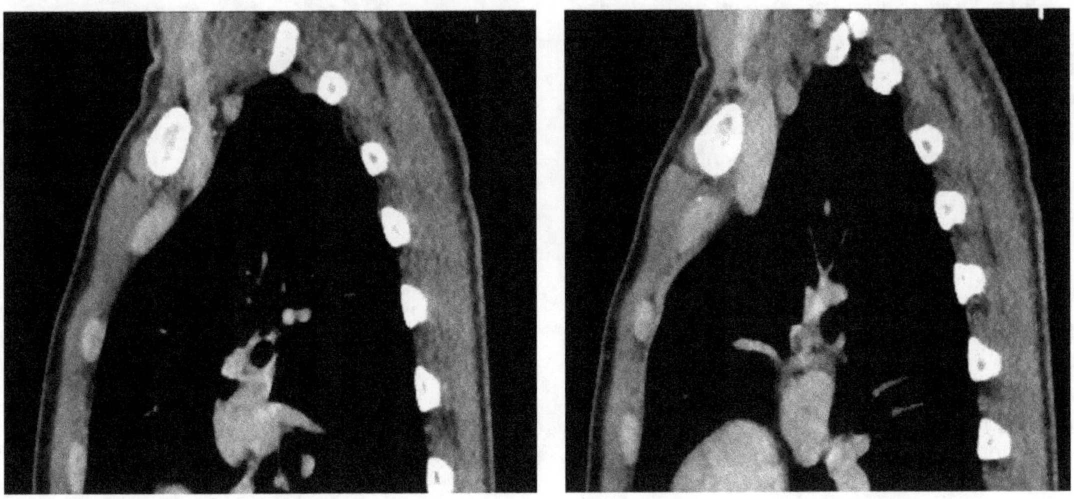

(a) (b)

FIGURE 6: Sagittal CECT neck showing matted lymph nodes posterior to right IJV eroding through the posterior wall of right IJV with IJV thrombus.

right IJV in lower neck suggestive of IJV thrombosis (Figures 4, 5, and 6). Fine needle aspiration cytology (FNAC) of right supraclavicular swelling done after ultrasound and CECT neck revealed necrotizing granulomatous inflammation suggestive of tuberculosis. Patient was put on antituberculous treatment (ATT) along with anticoagulants after diagnosis since last one week and has been advised follow-up.

3. Discussion

Venous thrombosis results from disturbance of pathophysiological mechanisms in Virchow's triad of endothelial damage, stasis, and hypercoagulable state [1]. Complication of IJV thrombosis is septic emboli, intracranial venous sinus thrombosis, raised intracranial pressure, pulmonary embolism, facial edema, and loss of vision [1]. IJV thrombosis is uncommon and possibly life threatening complication. Early diagnosis is must for appropriate management, to prevent potentially fatal complication due to IJV thrombosis [1].

The associations between inflammation, hypercoagulable state, and hemostatic changes are established [4, 5]. Elevated plasma fibrinogen, impaired fibrinolysis with decreased level of antithrombin III, and reactive thrombocytosis favor development of DVT in pulmonary tuberculosis [6]. Thrombosis can also occur due to compression of the vein by lymph nodes in ganglionar form of TB as thrombosis can occur in the absence of any hemostatic abnormality [7]. Tuberculosis can cause thrombosis by various mechanisms like transitory hypercoagulable state, venous compression, and local invasion [4, 5, 7]. IJV thrombosis can occur from intracranial IJV to the junction of IJV with subclavian vein with the formation of brachiocephalic vein.

Tuberculous lymphadenopathy can cause extensive vessel wall damage with endothelial damage predisposing to thrombosis [3].

IJV thrombosis in our case is likely to be due to venous compression, local invasion with resultant endothelial damage, and transitory hypercoagulable state.

Both USG and CT are accurate and reliable radiological investigations for detecting IJV thrombosis, along with cervical lymph nodes. They are useful in assessing surrounding soft tissue and fat planes, and knowing the size and extent of cervical lymphadenopathy. USG is inexpensive and readily available for monitoring response to treatment. Both USG and CT scan show number and extent of cervical lymph nodes, central caseation necrosis, matted lymph nodes, IJV invasion, and IJV thrombus. Doppler and contrast enhanced CT scan shows patency of remaining IJV lumen. Early detection of IJV thrombosis is must to avoid complications like raised intracranial pressure, cerebral venous sinus thrombosis, pulmonary embolism, and septic emboli.

ATT should be immediately started in addition to anticoagulant therapy. The optimum duration of anticoagulation in IJV thrombosis is not yet standardized [3].

4. Conclusion

Tuberculous cervical lymphadenopathy is a rare cause of IJV thrombosis. Early detection with USG and/or CT is essential for timely treatment and to avoid further complications.

References

[1] R. Erkoç, K. Uzun, K. Yuca et al., "Internal jugular vein thrombosis two different etiologies," *European Journal of General Medicine*, vol. 2, no. 3, pp. 123–128, 2005.

[2] K. Chowdhury, J. Bloom, M. J. Black, and K. Al-Noury, "Spontaneous and nonspontaneous internal jugular vein thrombosis," *Head & Neck*, vol. 12, no. 2, pp. 168–173, 1990.

[3] K. Gowrinath, M. I. Nizamiz, B. E. Kumar, P. Suneetha, and V. H. Kishor, "Unusual complication of cervical tuberculous lymphadenopathy," *Indian Journal of Tuberculosis*, vol. 58, no. 1, pp. 35–37, 2011.

[4] R. Naithani, N. Agrawal, and V. P. Choudhary, "Deep venous thrombosis associated with tuberculosis," *Blood Coagulation and Fibrinolysis*, vol. 18, no. 4, pp. 377–380, 2007.

[5] O. Turken, E. Kunter, M. Sezer et al., "Hemostatic changes in active pulmonary tuberculosis," *International Journal of Tuberculosis and Lung Disease*, vol. 6, no. 10, pp. 927–932, 2002.

[6] S. C. Robson, N. W. White, I. Aronson, R. Woollgar, H. Goodman, and P. Jacobs, "Acute-phase response and the hypercoagulable state in pulmonary tuberculosis," *British Journal of Haematology*, vol. 93, no. 4, pp. 943–949, 1996.

[7] I. M. Goncalves, D. C. Alves, A. Carvalho, M. D. C. Brito, F. Calvario, and R. Duarte, "Tuberculosis and venous thromboembolism: a case series," *Cases Journal*, vol. 2, no. 12, article 9333, 2009.

41

Isolation of Left Common Carotid Artery with Its Origin Proximal to Patent Ductus Arteriosus Presenting in Adult Age

Anagha R. Joshi, Saurabh Joshi, Kiran Kale, Rahul Jain, and Jernail Singh Bava

Department of Radiology, Lokmanya Tilak Municipal Medical College and General Hospital, Sion West, Mumbai, Maharashtra 400022, India

Correspondence should be addressed to Kiran Kale; drkirankale@gmail.com

Academic Editor: Atsushi Komemushi

Anomalies of aortic arch are a common occurrence. Such anomalies of right sided aortic arch with its various branching patterns are of clinical importance. Rarer anomalies include isolation (deficient connection) of either left subclavian artery or left common carotid artery; that is, they do not have their origin from aorta or its major branches. We present a case of an 18-year-old male who presented with gradual onset pulsatile swelling with bruit in neck on left side and was evaluated by CT brain and neck angiography. CT angiography revealed right sided aortic arch with aberrant left subclavian artery and isolated left common carotid artery. Very few cases of such an anomaly have been documented in the literature but none in an adult.

1. Introduction

Anomalies of aortic arch are a common occurrence. Few of such anomalies are right sided aortic arch with its various branching patterns, double aortic arch or left sided arch with aberrant right subclavian artery with or without formation of a vascular ring and variants in branching patterns of aortic arch. Edwards' hypothetical double aortic arch explains aortic arch abnormalities by selective regression of various parts of either arch [1].

Right sided aortic arch can have mirror branching which is associated with congenital cardiac defects in 98% of the cases. Another variant is right sided aortic arch with aberrant left subclavian artery. Rare anomalies include isolation of either left subclavian artery, left common carotid artery, or innominate artery; that is, they do not have their origin from aorta or its major branches [2]. Isolation of left common carotid artery is the rarest of the three. We report a case of an isolated left common carotid artery in an 18-year-old patient with right sided aortic arch and aberrant left subclavian artery.

2. Case Report

An 18-year-old previously asymptomatic male came with complaints of swelling in the left side of neck which was gradual in onset and slowly increasing in size and no other major complaints. Patient did not have any neurological symptoms at present or in the past and had normal development. On examination, the swelling was found to be pulsatile with audible bruit over it.

CT brain and neck angiography was advised in view of suspicion of a cervical AV malformation.

CT angiography revealed right sided aortic arch (Figures 1(a) and 1(b)). Right common carotid artery and right subclavian artery were seen originating as the first and second branches of arch, respectively. Aberrant origin of left subclavian artery noted coursing posterior to oesophagus with mild dilatation was seen at the origin of left subclavian artery s/o diverticulum of Kommerell (Figure 1(b)). Left common carotid artery was not seen originating from arch of aorta. It was seen originating from right side of main pulmonary artery before its bifurcation (Figure 2).

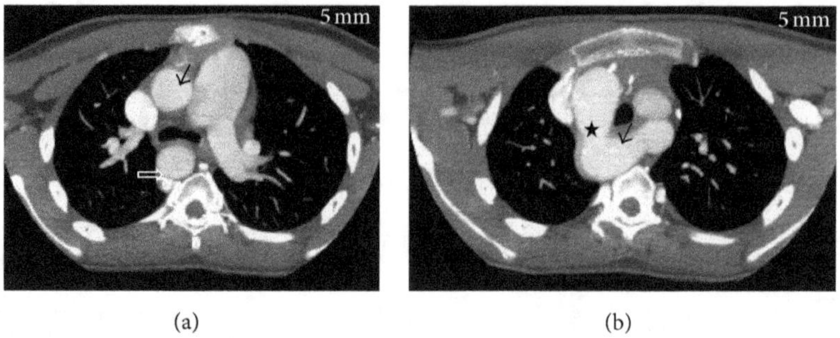

Figure 1: Axial MIP images at the level of ascending aorta and aortic arch showing right sided aortic arch and aberrant origin of left subclavian artery. (a) Ascending aorta (black arrow), descending aorta (open arrow), (b) aortic arch (star) and aberrant origin of left subclavian artery with diverticulum of Kommerell (black arrow).

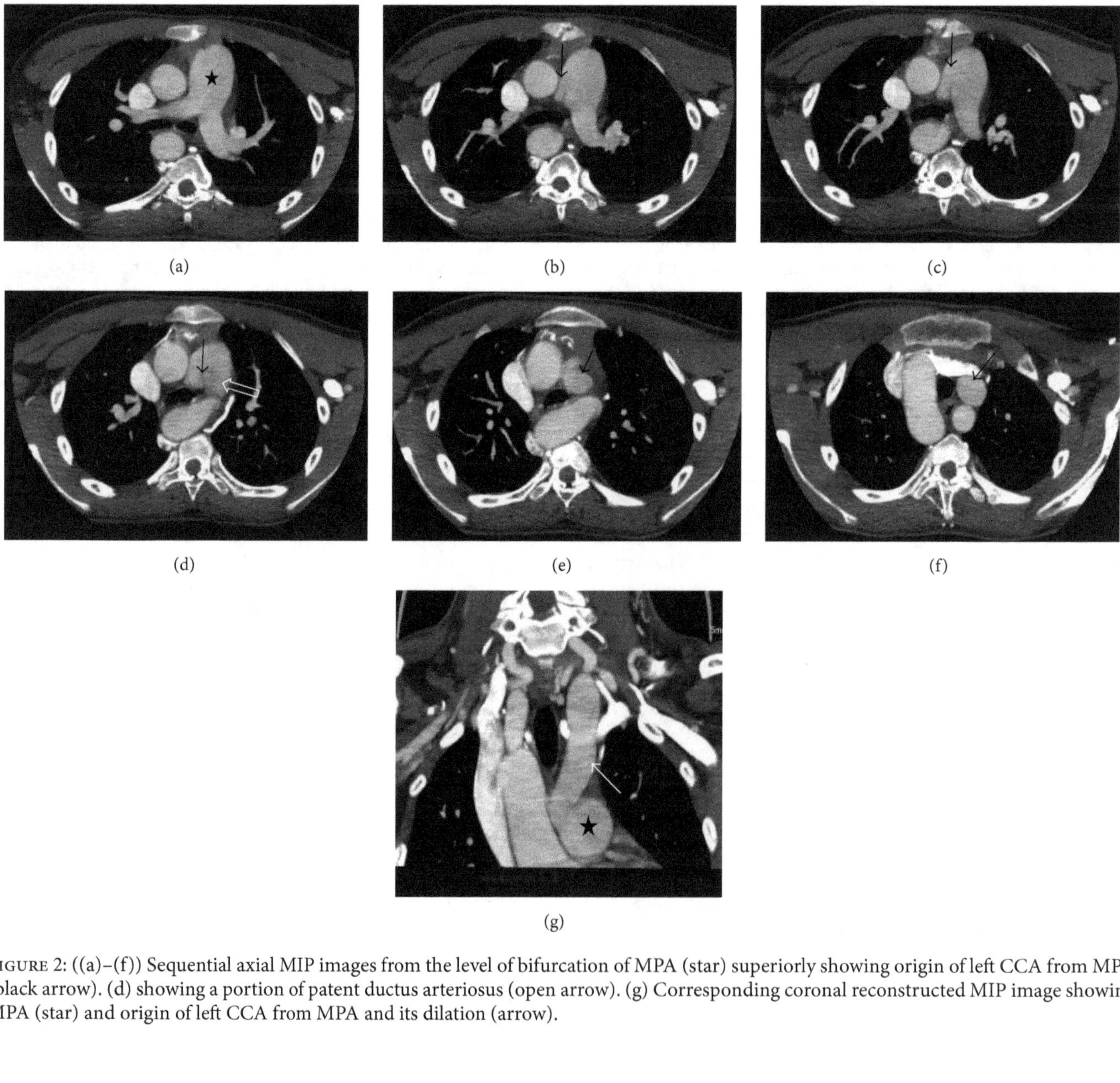

Figure 2: ((a)–(f)) Sequential axial MIP images from the level of bifurcation of MPA (star) superiorly showing origin of left CCA from MPA (black arrow). (d) showing a portion of patent ductus arteriosus (open arrow). (g) Corresponding coronal reconstructed MIP image showing MPA (star) and origin of left CCA from MPA and its dilation (arrow).

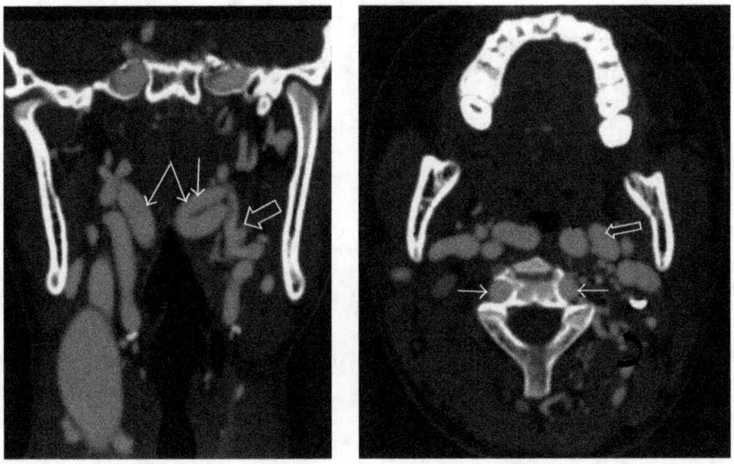

(a) (b)

Figure 3: (a) Coronal MIP image showing dilatation and tortuosity of left ICA (single white arrow) and ECA (open arrow) and kissing carotids (white arrows). (b) Axial MIP image at the level of bifurcation of CCA showing dilated left ICA (black arrow), ECA (open arrow) with multiple inter and intramuscular arterial collaterals on left side of neck (curved arrow), and prominent vertebral arteries (white arrows).

A small connection was also seen between the main pulmonary artery and left common carotid artery apart from its origin. This could represent a portion of patent ductus arteriosus (Figure 2(d)).

Left common carotid artery showed moderate dilatation in the cervical region, measuring 3 cm before bifurcation.

Left internal carotid artery, left external carotid artery, and main branches of external carotid artery were found to be tortuous and dilated with multiple arterial inter- and intramuscular collaterals on left side of neck. Incidental finding noted was kissing carotids (bilateral internal carotid arteries) due to its medial course (Figures 3(a) and 3(b)).

Bilateral vertebral arteries were prominent in cervical region (Figure 3(b)).

There is no evidence of dilatation of main pulmonary artery or right atrium.

3. Discussion

Aortic arch anomalies have been classically explained by Edward's hypothetical double aortic arch and regression of its parts on right or left side leading to various combinations. Right sided aortic arch with aberrant left subclavian artery can be explained on the basis of regression in left arch involving dorsal segment between left common carotid artery and left subclavian arteries with regression of right ductus arteriosus. In such cases, left common carotid artery is seen as the first branch of the arch followed by right common carotid artery and right subclavian artery, respectively. However, as left common carotid artery was isolated in our case, right common carotid artery was seen as the first branch followed by right subclavian artery and aberrant left subclavian artery.

Only eight cases of isolated left common carotid artery have been documented in the literature [2–8] till now. None of these cases were reported in adults.

According to Männer et al. [2], isolation of any aortic arch artery is explained not only by the regression of arch proximal and distal segments to it, but also by "deficient regression" that is persistence of ductus arteriosus. Presence of ductus arteriosus explains the communication with the pulmonary artery whereas regression of both proximal and distal segments explains the noncommunication to the arch.

Though this explains the basic anomaly in our patient, there remains an issue about a small connection that is seen separate from the origin of left common carotid artery from pulmonary artery. Similar cases have been reported before by Fouilloux et al. and Kaushik et al. [4, 5]. According to Männer [3] and Kaushik et al. [5], these cannot be explained based only on the Edward's hypothetical double arch model. Both of these authors have proposed malseptation of truncoaortic sac as a possible mechanism, that is, a disturbance in the septation of the truncoaortic sac secondary to abnormal migration of neural crest cells. In our case, presence of the small connection can only be explained by the same malseptation concept.

Fouilloux et al. [4] proposed two alternative hypotheses to explain the embryology of their case. (a) The initial segment of the isolated LCCA may represent a patent left ductus arteriosus at an abnormal position, while the fibrous band may represent the atretic left aortic arch segment between the LCCA and the left subclavian artery. (b) The fibrous band may represent the remnant of the left ductus arteriosus.

Importance of the detection and description of this anomaly is twofold. This finding, although rare, is always associated with other structural heart defects and aberrant left subclavian artery. Thus, when contemplating surgical corrections, it will play a major role in decision making. Secondly, with low pressure pulmonary circulation, a component of left to right shunting also develops. This is seen in our case as multiple collateral channels in the territory of left common carotid artery.

Such a case has not been described in an adult before. Therefore, our case should serve as an indicator of progression of cases diagnosed in infancy and childhood.

4. Conclusion

Our case is unique in the sense that it is the first case reported in an adult along with possible presence of a small connection being explained only by malseptation of truncoaortic sac along with regression of segments and persistence of ductus arteriosus. Therefore, our case should serve as indicator of progression of cases diagnosed in infancy and childhood.

References

[1] J. E. Edwards, "Anomalies of the derivatives of the aortic arch system," *The Medical Clinics of North America*, vol. 32, pp. 925–949, 1948.

[2] J. Männer, W. Seidl, and G. Steding, "The formal pathogenesis of isolated common carotid or innominate arteries: the concept of malseptation of the aortic sac," *Anatomy and Embryology*, vol. 196, no. 6, pp. 435–445, 1997.

[3] J. Manner, "Isolated left common carotid artery arising from the main pulmonary artery: where is the ductus arteriosus? An embryologist's view," *World Journal for Pediatric and Congenital Hearth Surgery*, vol. 4, no. 4, pp. 460–461, 2013.

[4] V. Fouilloux, C. Gran, and B. Kreitmann, "Isolated left common carotid artery connected to the pulmonary artery: where was the arterial duct?" *World Journal for Pediatric and Congenital Hearth Surgery*, vol. 4, no. 2, pp. 229–232, 2013.

[5] N. Kaushik, Z. Saba, H. Rosenfeld et al., "An isolated left common carotid artery from the main pulmonary artery: possible malseptation of the truncoaortic sac," *Pediatric Cardiology*, vol. 26, no. 5, pp. 707–709, 2005.

[6] S.-F. Huang and M.-H. Wu, "Left common carotid artery arising from the pulmonary artery in a patient with DiGeorge syndrome," *Heart*, vol. 76, no. 1, pp. 82–83, 1996.

[7] G. Oppido, C. P. Napoleone, D. Gabbieri et al., "Left common carotid artery isolation in a newborn with tetralogy of fallot and digeorge syndrome," *Circulation*, vol. 111, no. 1, pp. e4–e5, 2005.

[8] K. Ghalili, H. J. Issenberg, N. J. Freeman, and R. F. Brodman, "Isolated left carotid artery in CHARGE association: diagnosis and repair," *The Annals of Thoracic Surgery*, vol. 50, no. 1, pp. 130–132, 1990.

42

Imaging Manifestations of a Subependymal Giant Cell Astrocytoma in Tuberous Sclerosis

Joseph R. Stein and Daniel A. Reidman

The Regional Medical Center, 3000 St. Matthews Road, Orangeburg, SC 29118, USA

Correspondence should be addressed to Joseph R. Stein; jstein@carolinas.vcom.edu

Academic Editor: Amit Agrawal

Tuberous sclerosis is a rare genetic disorder resulting in benign tumor growth in various organs including the brain, heart, skin, eyes, kidney, and lung as well as systemic manifestations including seizures, cognitive impairment, and dermatologic abnormalities. This report shows the radiological findings and differentiation between a subependymal nodule and subependymal giant cell astrocytoma in a patient with tuberous sclerosis presenting with new onset seizures.

1. Introduction

Tuberous sclerosis complex (TSC) is an autosomal dominant genetic disorder resulting from mutations in the TSC1 gene or the TSC2 gene [1]. The disease is characterized by benign hamartoma development in several organs, including the brain, heart, skin, eyes, kidney, lung, and liver. The disease has an estimated prevalence between 1/6800 and 1/15000 [2–4]. Clinical manifestations of TSC seem to have an age-related expression pattern, as some manifestations are typically identifiable at birth while others develop later at different ages. Some patients may have a milder form of the disease and can remain undiagnosed while others can be debilitated by the disease from birth. Since the diagnosis of TS cannot be made based on a single clinical manifestation, careful attention to physical exam findings and radiologic abnormalities is vital for correct diagnosis. In this presentation, clinical and radiological findings of subependymal giant cell astrocytoma and cortical tubers leading to new onset seizures will be discussed.

2. Case Summary

A 26-year-old female with history of hypertension and dialysis-dependent ESRD with a GFR of 5 was admitted after having a seizure at work. Significant family history includes a father with tuberous sclerosis and brother with tuberous sclerosis and seizures. The patient stated she was at work the night before admission when she "felt hot" and started "shaking." She described 1-2-second duration and serial, generalized myoclonic twitching lasting roughly 5 minutes prior to reported loss of consciousness. During EMS stabilization and transfer another generalized tonic-clonic convulsion occurred accompanied by postictal lethargy and confusion. The patient denied any prior history of seizures, cognitive impairment, or frequent headaches.

On examination vital signs revealed the patient to be tachycardic (164 beats per minute) and hypertensive (249 mmHg/153 mmHg). Neurological examination was normal. Several facial and body hyperpigmented fibrous plaques and a posterior lumbar Shagreen patch were noted.

3. Imaging Findings

A nonenhanced head computed tomography was performed to exclude ischemia or hemorrhage. This revealed a rounded, heterogeneous, soft tissue mass with central calcifications opposing the ependymal surface in the ventral body of the right lateral ventricle measuring approximately 12 mm × 18 m. No accompanying hydrocephalus or local neoplastic extension was evident.

Subsequent contrast enhanced brain MRI demonstrated a 23 mm × 23 mm × 18 mm round, well-circumscribed mass in the right lateral ventricle and roof of the third ventricle. The mass was heterogeneous with several internal signal

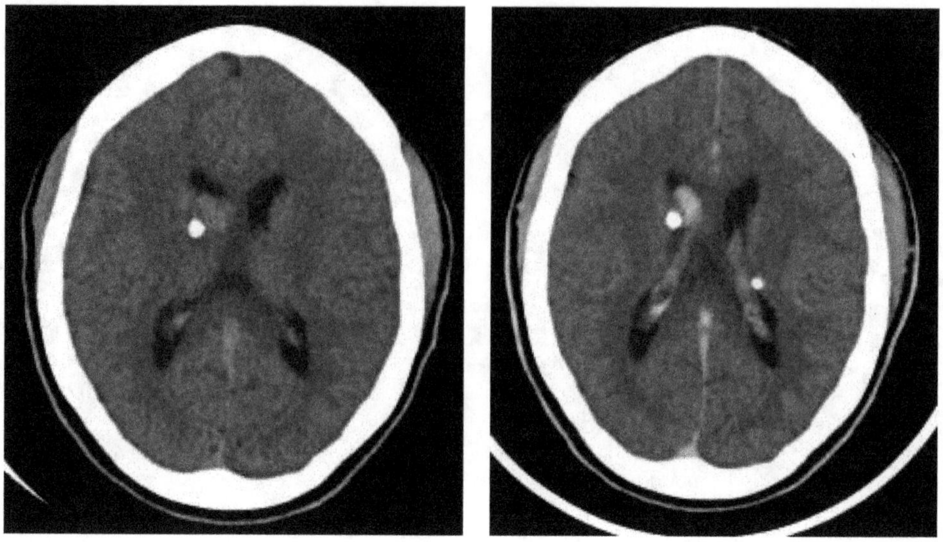

(a) (b)

Figure 1: Axial noncontrast CT demonstrating a 12 × 18 mm partially calcified, enhancing soft tissue mass in the anterior body of the right lateral ventricle (a). Axial CT with contrast showing SEGA enhancement but no enhancement of tubers (b).

voids. There was mild mass effect (4 mm septum pellucidum leftward shift), with adjacent white matter mild edema and gliosis. Scattered cortical based T2 and FLAIR hyperintensities were seen throughout both cerebral hemispheres, suggestive of cortical tubers.

Prior renal ultrasound and abdominal CT were obtained which demonstrated chronic cystic renal atrophy/chronic medical renal disease (Figures 4 and 5).

4. Discussion

The majority of TSC patients present with neurologic symptoms, with approximately 90% of affected individuals experiencing seizures and roughly half experiencing cognitive impairment, autism, or other behavioral disorders [5]. Epilepsy is seen in 70% to 90% of patients, most commonly presenting in the first year of life [6]. Autism spectrum disorder, intellectual disability, and other neurodevelopmental and psychiatric disorders associated with TSC also lead to a significant disability. Renal manifestations are the second most common finding associated with TS, with angiomyolipomas (AMLs) occurring in 80% and renal cystic disease in 50% of the patients [7]. Pulmonary involvement, specifically lymphangioleiomyomatosis (LAM), is the third most common cause of TSC associated morbidity, occurring in approximately 35% of reproductive age female TS patients [8, 9]. Cardiac rhabdomyoma can be found in 50%–65% of patients with TS [10]. Other features of TS include retinal nodular hamartomas, dental pits, gingival fibromas, rectal polyps, and bone cysts.

The main structural brain lesions include cortical tubers, subependymal nodules (SENs), and subependymal giant cell astrocytomas (SEGAs) [1, 5]. Cortical tubers develop prenatally and are seen in 90% of patients (Figure 1) [11]. Cortical tubers are a collection of giant cells, dysmorphic neurons, and gliosis that destroy the normal six-layer cortical structure [11]. There is a positive correlation between the number of cortical tubers and cognitive impairment and seizure control difficulty [12]. Magnetic resonance is the modality of choice for detecting cortical tubers. Increased signal intensity on T2-weighted images and decreased signal intensity on T1-weighted ones are demonstrated in almost all patients with the exception being infants and neonates where T1-weighted images show enhancement due to the similar relaxation time of T1 and the unmyelinated brain [13]. Only 10% of cortical tubers will be enhanced after administration of contrast material [13]. The patient in this case showed the typical findings of T2 and FLAIR hyperintensities in multiple areas suggesting cortical tubers, the likely etiology of her seizures (Figures 2 and 3).

Subependymal nodules are collections of abnormal, swollen glial cells and giant cells which cannot be differentiated as normal neural tissue. They have a tendency to calcify and can progress into subependymal giant cell astrocytomas, which are histologically indistinguishable from SENs but distinguishable based on their larger size, higher growth rate, and potential for mass effect compared to the relatively static course of SENs [14, 15]. The radiographic appearance of SENs on unenhanced CT will show small calcified foci along the wall of the lateral and third ventricle [13] (Figure 1). MR imaging will demonstrate hyperintensity on T1-weighted imaging and isointense or hyperintense T2 signal [13]. This variability is likely due to the extent of calcifications. SEGAs are slow growing tumors and most commonly manifest in the first two decades of life. Occurring in 1.7–26% of patients with TS, they consist of proliferative astrocytes and giant cells [11]. The most common location of SEGAs is the foramen of Monroe, leading to obstructive hydrocephalus and manifesting with signs and symptoms of increased intracranial pressure, but most are asymptomatic.

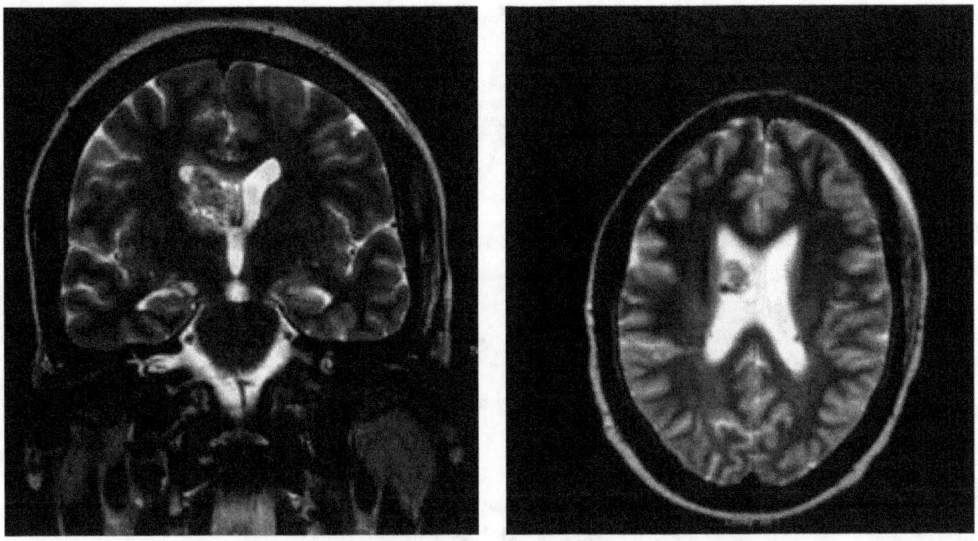

(a) (b)

FIGURE 2: T2 weighted coronal (a) and axial (b) MRI showing 23 × 23 × 18 m lobulated mass in the right lateral ventricle and roof of the third ventricle which is isointense to grey matter and has small signal voids in keeping with calcifications.

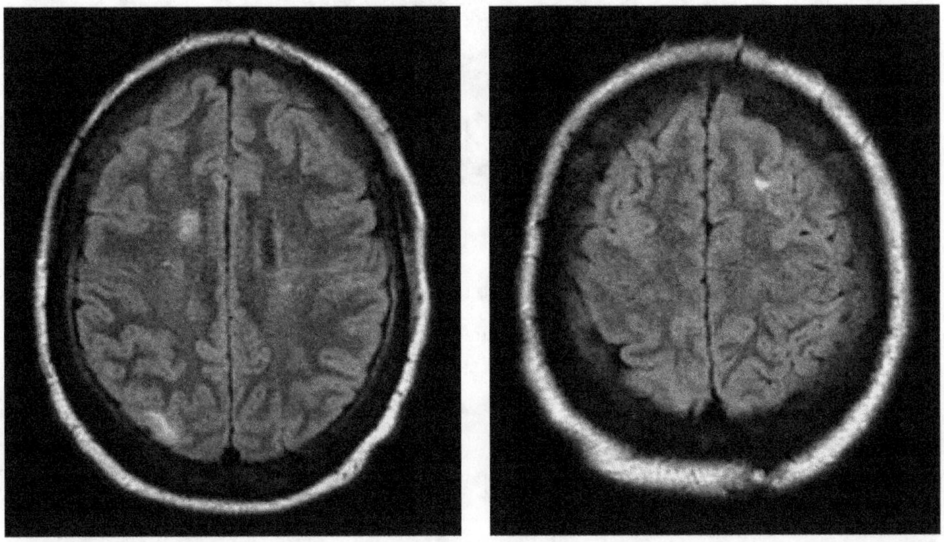

(a) (b)

FIGURE 3: T2 FLAIR axial MRI showing subcortical areas of mixed signal mass in the right occipital cortex (a) and left frontal cortex (b), suggestive of cortical tubers.

Intermediate cells have been identified in SENs and SEGAs suggesting that SENs can transform into SEGAs [16]. Serial imaging can monitor growth of subependymal nodules and potential for transformation into SEGAs [16]. Compared to SENs, SEGAs demonstrate more intense enhancement on CT and are larger tumors (>1 cm) [17] (Figure 1). Suspicion for transformation should be considered if lesions measure 5 mm or greater in diameter, are incompletely calcified, and demonstrate enhancement [18]. There is also a reported increased frequency of malignant transformation in masses approximating the foramen of Monroe [18]. SEGAs show heterogenous enhancement on MR imaging, demonstrating T1 isointense and hypointense signal and T2/FLAIR isointense and hyperintense signal [19] (Figures 2 and 3). The imaging findings of this patient are suggestive of a subependymal giant cell astrocytoma versus a subependymal nodule based on its incomplete calcification, enhancement with gadolinium, and size (>1 cm). Surgical resection remains the recommended treatment for symptomatic SEGAs [20]. Surgery also remains the standard treatment for SEGAs demonstrating serial growth on neuroimaging, but experts indicate that some patients may benefit more from medical

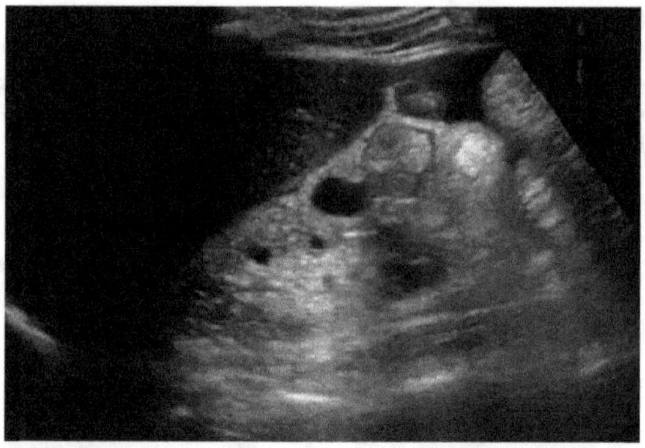

FIGURE 4: Renal US long R kidney demonstrating atrophy and cysts.

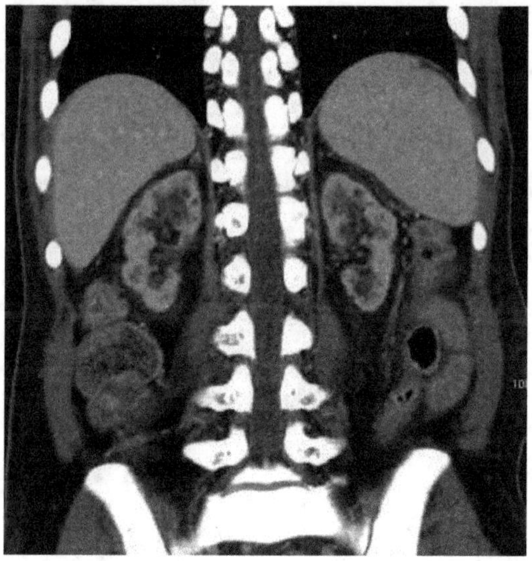

FIGURE 5: CT abdomen chronic cystic renal atrophy/chronic medical renal disease.

treatment depending on the size of the lesion [20]. Our patient's SEGA warranted neurosurgical consult given the above noted findings.

Generally speaking, tumors greater than 3 cm carry significant risk for complications and should be medically managed. Surgical intervention of SEGA > 3 cm carries a 67% risk of surgery-related complications and surgery on tumors > 4 cm was associated with a 73% risk of complications [21, 22]. Bilateral SEGAs, regardless their size, were associated with 67% risk of complications after surgery. No complications were observed in patients undergoing surgery for SEGAs < 2 cm. The 23 mm SEGA in our patient would likely benefit from surgical intervention and accordingly a neurosurgical consult was recommended. In the event in which surgical intervention is declined, serial monitoring of tumor growth in this patient would be based on clinical judgment. It is recommended that SEGAs are monitored serially with MRI every 1–3 years in patients younger than 25 as these tumors usually grow in children and adolescents but do not have a tendency to grow in adulthood [21, 22].

5. Conclusion

This case of a new onset seizure illustrated CNS manifestations of tuberous sclerosis. The patient presented with a new onset seizure and was found to have multiple cortical tubers and subependymal giant cell astrocytoma on brain imaging. The cortical tubers were the likely etiology of her seizure and the patient was placed on Keppra but more concerning was the astrocytoma mass in the body of the right lateral ventricle. The proximity to the right foramen of Monroe, its incomplete calcification, enhancement on MRI, and large size (>1 cm) make SEGA the likely diagnosis. A neurosurgery consult was recommended off-site, but surgery was not performed because of the patient's comorbidities and symptoms attributed to cortical tubers rather than symptomatic SEGA.

References

[1] P. Curatolo, R. Bombardieri, and S. Jozwiak, "Tuberous sclerosis," *The Lancet*, vol. 372, no. 9639, pp. 657–668, 2008.

[2] J. R. Sampson, S. J. Scahill, J. B. P. Stephenson, L. Mann, and J. M. Connor, "Genetic aspects of tuberous sclerosis in the west of Scotland," *Journal of Medical Genetics*, vol. 26, no. 1, pp. 28–31, 1989.

[3] F. J. K. O'Callaghan, A. W. Shiell, J. P. Osborne, and C. N. Martyn, "Prevalence of tuberous sclerosis estimated by capture-recapture analysis," *The Lancet*, vol. 351, no. 9114, p. 1490, 1998.

[4] J. R. W. Yates, "Tuberous sclerosis," *European Journal of Human Genetics*, vol. 14, no. 10, pp. 1065–1073, 2006.

[5] P. Curatolo and B. L. Maria, "Tuberous sclerosis," in *Handbook of Clinical Neurology*, vol. 111, chapter 38, pp. 323–331, Elsevier, 2013.

[6] C. J. Chu-Shore, P. Major, S. Camposano, D. Muzykewicz, and E. A. Thiele, "The natural history of epilepsy in tuberous sclerosis complex," *Epilepsia*, vol. 51, no. 7, pp. 1236–1241, 2010.

[7] P. Prather and P. J. de Vries, "Behavioral and cognitive aspects of tuberous sclerosis complex," *Journal of Child Neurology*, vol. 19, no. 9, pp. 666–674, 2004.

[8] D. N. Franz, J. J. Bissler, and F. X. McCormack, "Tuberous sclerosis complex: neurological, renal and pulmonary manifestations," *Neuropediatrics*, vol. 41, no. 5, pp. 199–208, 2010.

[9] C. J. Cudzilo, R. D. Szczesniak, A. S. Brody et al., "Lymphangioleiomyomatosis screening in women with tuberous sclerosis," *Chest*, vol. 144, no. 2, pp. 578–585, 2013.

[10] E. G. Muhler, V. Turniski-Harder, W. Engelhardt, and G. von Bernuth, "Cardiac involvement in tuberous sclerosis," *British Heart Journal*, vol. 72, no. 6, pp. 584–590, 1994.

[11] P. Van Tassel, J. K. Curé, and K. R. Holden, "Cystlike white matter lesions in tuberous sclerosis," *American Journal of Neuroradiology*, vol. 18, no. 7, pp. 1367–1373, 1997.

[12] R. S. Kandt, "Tuberous sclerosis complex and neurofibromatosis type 1: the two most common neurocutaneous diseases," *Neurologic Clinics*, vol. 21, no. 4, pp. 983–1004, 2003.

[13] J. C. Evans and J. Curtis, "The radiological appearances of tuberous sclerosis," *British Journal of Radiology*, vol. 73, no. 865, pp. 91–98, 2000.

[14] V. Moran and F. O'Keeffe, "Giant cell astrocytoma in tuberous sclerosis: computed tomographic findings," *Clinical Radiology*, vol. 37, no. 6, pp. 543–545, 1986.

[15] S. K. McMurdo Jr., S. G. Moore, M. Brant-Zawadzki et al., "MR imaging of intracranial tuberous sclerosis," *American Journal of Roentgenology*, vol. 148, pp. 791–796, 1987.

[16] K. Morimoto and H. Mogami, "Sequential CT study of subependymal giant-cell astrocytoma associated with tuberous sclerosis. Case report," *Journal of Neurosurgery*, vol. 65, no. 6, pp. 874–877, 1986.

[17] A. Nezu, K. Uetake, Y. Nomura, and M. Segawa, "Roles of a subependymal nodule of tuberous sclerosis on pathophysiology of epilepsy," *Japanese Journal of Psychiatry and Neurology*, vol. 45, no. 2, pp. 372–377, 1991.

[18] H.-D. Rott, B. Lemcke, M. Zenker, W. Huk, J. Horst, and K. Mayer, "Cyst-like cerebral lesions in tuberous sclerosis," *American Journal of Medical Genetics*, vol. 111, no. 4, pp. 435–439, 2002.

[19] Y. Baron and A. J. Barkovich, "MR imaging of tuberous sclerosis in neonates and young infants," *American Journal of Neuroradiology*, vol. 20, no. 5, pp. 907–916, 1999.

[20] M. Berhouma, "Management of subependymal giant cell tumors in tuberous sclerosis complex: the neurosurgeon's perspective," *World Journal of Pediatrics*, vol. 6, no. 2, pp. 103–110, 2010.

[21] K. Kotulska, J. Borkowska, M. Roszkowski et al., "Surgical treatment of subependymal giant cell astrocytoma in tuberous sclerosis complex patients," *Pediatric Neurology*, vol. 50, no. 4, pp. 307–312, 2014.

[22] J. Roth, E. S. Roach, U. Bartels et al., "Subependymal giant cell astrocytoma: diagnosis, screening, and treatment. Recommendations from the International Tuberous sclerosis Complex Consensus Conference 2012," *Pediatric Neurology*, vol. 49, no. 6, pp. 439–444, 2013.

43

Cardiac Magnetic Resonance for Evaluating Catheter Related FDG Avidity

Daniel Jeong, Kenneth L. Gage, Claudia G. Berman, and Jaime L. Montilla-Soler

Department of Radiology, H. Lee Moffitt Cancer Center, Tampa, FL 33612, USA

Correspondence should be addressed to Daniel Jeong; daniel.jeong@moffitt.org

Academic Editor: Atsushi Komemushi

A 53-year-old female with a history of metastatic left arm melanoma presented for F(18) fluorodeoxyglucose (FDG) positron emission tomography/computed tomography (PET/CT) which showed a moderately FDG avid focus at her port catheter tip near the cavoatrial junction. Although catheter tip related FDG avidity has previously been suggested to be bland thrombus or infection, melanoma can metastasize to unusual locations including the superior vena cava. In addition, the patient had an elevated risk of anticoagulation due to a history of hemorrhagic brain metastases. Therefore, confirmatory cardiac magnetic resonance (CMR) was obtained and findings were consistent with bland catheter-related thrombus.

1. Introduction

Cancer patients who receive PET/CT exams often have indwelling central catheters and ports. Rare reports have suggested catheter related FDG activity related to bland thrombus or infection [1, 2]. Bhargava et al. reported a series where 3 out of 4 patients with elevated FDG activity at the distal end of a central catheter were related to bland thrombus and 1 had clinical infection [2]. Each of the 4 FDG injections in this series was through a peripheral vein separate from the catheter [2]. Siösteen et al. presented a case of FDG activity at a catheter tip related to bland thrombus with the FDG injection occurring through the same catheter due to poor vascular access [1]. When FDG activity occurs at the superficial injection site of the port or port cavity, this is typically related to infection [3]. In addition, confirmatory diagnostic imaging of catheter tip related FDG avidity has not been previously presented in the literature.

2. Case Presentation

A 53-year-old female with a remote history of melanoma of the left arm had recurrence to the chest wall and brain. She presented for routine restaging positron emission tomography/computed tomography (PET/CT) (Figures 1(a) and 2(a)–2(c)) which showed an F(18) fluorodeoxyglucose (FDG) avid focus in the lower superior vena cava (SVC) just above the cavoatrial junction adjacent to the catheter tip of her right chest wall port. Maximum standard uptake value (SUV max) was 8.8. Due to poor vascular access, the patient's port was utilized to administer the FDG dose of 11.9 mCi for the exam. The patient had no clinical signs of catheter related infection. Figures 1(a) and 1(b) show the FDG avid focus on coronal fused PET/CT and the port catheter on frontal chest radiograph, respectively. Although catheter-related thrombus was initially suspected, the patient had a recent history of hemorrhagic brain metastases with an increased risk for anticoagulation. In addition, the SUV max of 8.8 was relatively higher than previous reports of bland thrombus. Cardiac magnetic resonance (CMR) was recommended for imaging confirmation. CMR demonstrated a hypointense lesion along the medial superior vena cava wall just above the catheter tip. The lesion demonstrated hypointense T1- and iso- to hypointense T2-weighted signal (Figures 1(c) and 3(a)–3(d)). No appreciable enhancement was noted on postcontrast (gadobutrol, 0.15 mmol/kg) or delayed gadolinium images. CMR findings were consistent with bland catheter-related thrombus.

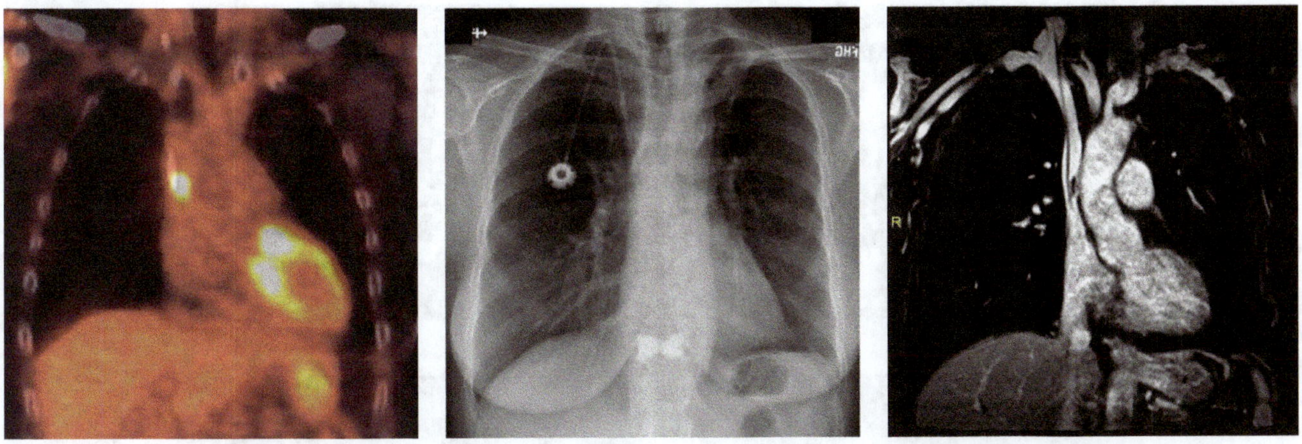

(a) (b) (c)

FIGURE 1: PET/CT, radiograph, and MR correlation. (a) Coronal reformatted PET/CT fusion image shows a moderately hypermetabolic focus at the approximate location of the catheter tip. SUV max was 8.8. (b) PA chest radiograph demonstrates a right chest wall port with its catheter tip at the cavoatrial junction. (c) Coronal T1 MR venous phase postcontrast image demonstrates a linear hypoenhancing structure along the medial lower SVC wall abutting the distal catheter. This finding was compatible with catheter related bland thrombus.

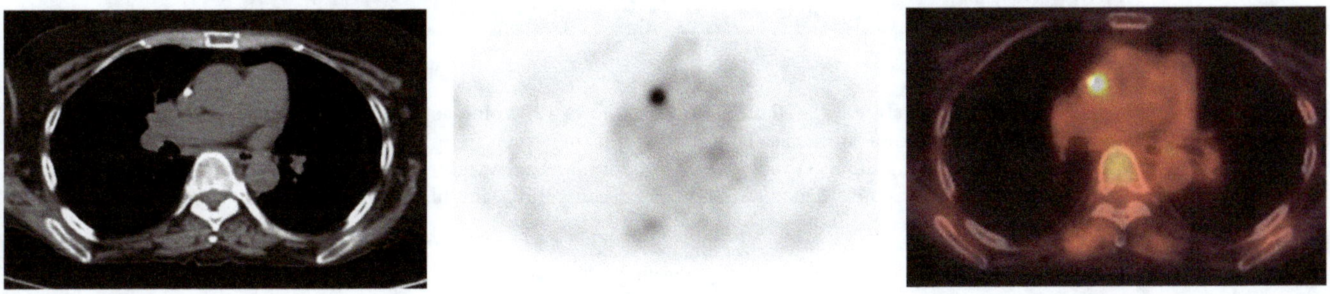

(a) (b) (c)

FIGURE 2: FDG PET/CT exam. Axial CT (a), PET (b), and (c) fused images from PET/CT exam demonstrate moderately hypermetabolic focus correlating with the catheter tip on CT.

3. Discussion

In higher risk cases such as ours, it can be clinically relevant to fully exclude tumor thrombus prior to initiating anticoagulation therapy. Ghattas et al. reported a case of melanoma of the left axilla with intravascular metastasis to the lower SVC which was also hypermetabolic on PET/CT, but with no central catheter present [4]. Bland non-catheter-related thrombus often has a lower SUV max compared to tumor thrombus. In general, SUV max greater than 3.35–3.63, contiguous intravascular spread from larger tumor, and location in the IVC have all been associated with tumor rather than bland thrombus [5–7].

Some authors suggest that an inflammatory process surrounding chronic bland thrombus is responsible for associated FDG avidity [1, 2, 5]. When FDG activity occurs at the tip of the catheter that was used for the injection, physical FDG trapping becomes another possibility [1]. Patients with long term indwelling central catheters can develop sleeve thrombus or an associated fibrin sheath that could theoretically cause physical trapping of FDG [1, 8]. In our case, the central port catheter with FDG activity finding at the tip was utilized for the FDG injection due to otherwise poor vascular access. Therefore physical bland thrombus/sheath related FDG trapping or associated inflammation are plausible explanations for FDG activity in our case.

CMR provides a unique diagnostic tool for evaluating a hypermetabolic cavoatrial junction mass. Cine balanced steady state free precession (BSSFP) images allow cardiac gated evaluation of thrombus which presents as a hypointense structure surrounded by normal bright blood signal. Acute thrombus can present with intermediate to hyperintense T1- and T2-weighted signal [9, 10]. Subacute thrombus appears hyperintense on T1-weighted images with hypointensity on T2-weighted images [9]. Chronic thrombus appears hypointense on T1- and T2-weighted images [9]. Thrombus presents as a filling defect on postcontrast sequences compatible with its avascular nature.

While lesions in the lower SVC may be imaged on postcontrast MR angiogram, T1-weighted sequences, or even CT angiography (CTA) without cardiac gating, lesions within the atrial cavity are subject to artifact from cardiac motion.

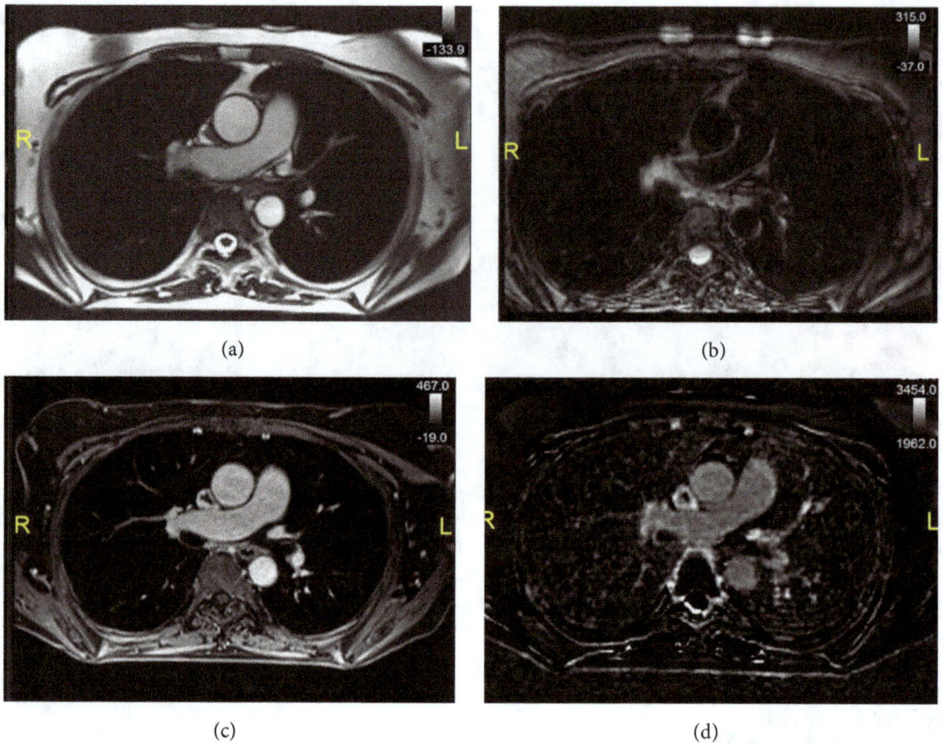

FIGURE 3: Cardiac magnetic resonance evaluation. (a) Axial SSFP image shows a hypointense structure conforming to the medial lower SVC wall. (b) Axial T2 SPAIR MR image shows isointense T2 signal within the structure. (c) Axial T1 postcontrast image demonstrates a well-defined intravascular filling defect along the SVC wall. (d) Late gadolinium enhancement phase sensitive inversion recovery image demonstrates hypoenhancement of the intravascular structure. Findings are compatible with bland thrombus.

Therefore cine and cardiac gated images provide a significant advantage in evaluating catheter related lesions which can often be located within the right atrium. Compared to CTA, real time gated perfusion imaging in CMR allows better detection of subtle enhancement with added benefit of temporal resolution of the enhancement. In addition, T2-weighted and late gadolinium enhanced imaging further increase specificity in mass evaluation compared to CTA.

Melanoma metastases demonstrate intrinsically hyperintense T1-weighted signal similar to that expected with subacute thrombus. Therefore, postcontrast imaging becomes a more important sequence to distinguish bland versus melanoma tumor thrombus. In our case, low T1- and T2-weighted signal without postcontrast enhancement were compatible with chronic bland thrombus. While Rinuncini et al. used CMR to diagnose a hypometabolic left ventricle mass as chronic bland thrombus, our case is the first to apply CMR to confirm bland thrombus at the cavoatrial junction associated with catheter tip FDG avidity [11]. Additionally, the emergence of PET/MR scanners will offer more clinical avenues for which PET can be obtained in similar cases. In this case, PET/MR would have provided seamless integration of the MR data needed to confidently diagnose the FDG avid focus as bland thrombus.

In conclusion, CMR is an excellent tool to further evaluate intravascular FDG avidity in the SVC, heart, and other major surrounding vessels. FDG avidity at the tip of a central catheter has classically been reported as bland. However, in cases where anticoagulation therapy has elevated risks and for primary tumors known to have unusual metastases such as melanoma, CMR should be the recommended next diagnostic exam.

References

[1] A.-K. Siösteen, F. Celsing, and H. Jacobsson, "FDG uptake in a catheter-related thrombus simulating relapse of lymphoma," *Clinical Nuclear Medicine*, vol. 30, no. 5, pp. 338–339, 2005.

[2] P. Bhargava, R. Kumar, H. Zhuang, M. Charron, and A. Alavi, "Catheter-related focal FDG activity on whole body PET imaging," *Clinical Nuclear Medicine*, vol. 29, no. 4, pp. 238–242, 2004.

[3] M. H. Miceli, L. B. J. Jackson, R. C. Walker, G. Talamo, B. Barlogie, and E. J. Anaissie, "Diagnosis of infection of implantable central venous catheters by [18F]fluorodeoxyglucose positron emission tomography," *Nuclear Medicine Communications*, vol. 25, no. 8, pp. 813–818, 2004.

[4] S. Ghattas, J. Howle, W. Wang, R. Kefford, and S. Gruenewald, "Intravascular metastatic melanoma: a difficult diagnosis," *The Australasian Journal of Dermatology*, vol. 54, no. 2, pp. 141–143, 2013.

[5] M. Ravina, S. Hess, M. S. Chauhan, M. J. Jacob, and A. Alavi, "Tumor thrombus: ancillary findings on FDG PET/CT in an oncologic population," *Clinical Nuclear Medicine*, vol. 39, no. 9, pp. 767–771, 2014.

[6] P. Sharma, R. Kumar, S. Jeph et al., "18F-FDG PET-CT in the diagnosis of tumor thrombus: can it be differentiated from benign thrombus?" *Nuclear Medicine Communications*, vol. 32, no. 9, pp. 782–788, 2011.

[7] S. Hu, J. Zhang, C. Cheng, Q. Liu, G. Sun, and C. Zuo, "The role of ^{18}F-FDG PET/CT in differentiating malignant from benign portal vein thrombosis," *Abdominal Imaging*, vol. 39, no. 6, pp. 1221–1227, 2014.

[8] M. Monreal and E. Davant, "Thrombotic complications of central venous catheters in cancer patients," *Acta Haematologica*, vol. 106, no. 1-2, pp. 69–72, 2001.

[9] P. J. Sparrow, J. B. Kurian, T. R. Jones, and M. U. Sivananthan, "MR imaging of cardiac tumors," *Radiographics*, vol. 25, no. 5, pp. 1255–1276, 2005.

[10] M. Motwani, A. Kidambi, B. A. Herzog, A. Uddin, J. P. Greenwood, and S. Plein, "MR imaging of cardiac tumors and masses: a review of methods and clinical applications," *Radiology*, vol. 268, no. 1, pp. 26–43, 2013.

[11] M. Rinuncini, M. Zuin, F. Scaranello et al., "Differentiation of cardiac thrombus from cardiac tumor combining cardiac MRI and 18F-FDG-PET/CT Imaging," *International Journal of Cardiology*, vol. 212, pp. 94–96, 2016.

44

Tailgut Cyst and Perineal Hydatid Cyst: A Case Report with Multimodality Imaging Findings

Ibtisam Musallam Aljohani,[1] Khalefa Ali Alghofaily,[2] Sebastian R. McWilliams,[3] and Mnahi Bin Saeedan[4]

[1] *Ministry of National Guard, Health Affairs, King Abdulaziz Medical City, Medical Imaging Department, Riyadh, Saudi Arabia*
[2] *College of Medicine, Medical Imaging Department, Al-Qassim University, Buraydah, Saudi Arabia*
[3] *Mallinckrodt Institute of Radiology, Washington University, St. Louis, MO, USA*
[4] *King Faisal Specialist Hospital & Research Center, Department of Radiology, P.O. Box 3354, Riyadh 1121, Saudi Arabia*

Correspondence should be addressed to Mnahi Bin Saeedan; mbinsaeedan@kfshrc.edu.sa

Academic Editor: Amit Agrawal

A tailgut cyst is a rare developmental lesion and usually is located in the retrorectal or presacral space. Extrahepatic hydatid disease has been reported in several locations including the pelvis and it often poses a diagnostic challenge. There are very few reported cases of primary perineal hydatid cysts. We present the multimodality imaging findings of a tailgut cyst and concurrent perineal hydatid disease in a 32-year-old male patient.

1. Introduction

A tailgut cyst is a rare congenital lesion. It has a female predilection and is usually asymptomatic and detected during middle age [1]. It is usually located in the presacral space and seen as a discrete and well-defined mass of variable attenuation on computed tomography (CT) depending on its contents. Cyst wall calcification may be seen. Rarely, a tailgut cyst may be complicated by infection or malignant transformation [2–4].

Hydatid disease is a zoonotic parasitic disease. *Echinococcus granulosus* and *Echinococcus multilocularis* are the two main infectious causative agents. Although liver and lung are the most commonly affected organs, hydatid cysts have the potential to affect any part of the human body. Primary extrahepatic hydatid cysts have been reported in different organs and anatomical locations and generally pose a diagnostic challenge [5, 6]. There are few reported cases of hydatid disease involving the perineal region [7–9]. We present the multimodality imaging findings of a retrorectal/presacral tailgut cyst with concomitant hydatid disease of the perineum.

2. Case Report

A 32-year-old male patient with a history of poliomyelitis in childhood complained of a progressively enlarging painless deep perianal mass for 1 year with a history of intermittent chronic constipation. The patient was referred to a tertiary healthcare center as a possible case of retroperitoneal sarcoma. Routine contrast enhanced CT showed a large (7.2 × 7.9 × 15.5 cm) multilocular, hypoattenuating, retrorectal cystic lesion. It displaced the rectum and rectosigmoid anteriorly and had no relation with the prostate, seminal vesicles, or adjacent major vessels. The CT also revealed a collection of smaller contiguous cysts in the left ischioanal fossa and the left perineal subcutaneous fat. This collection of cysts paralleled and was adjacent to the left puborectalis muscle and breached the left levator ani. No other lesion was found in the abdominal cavity. Atrophy of the right hemipelvis

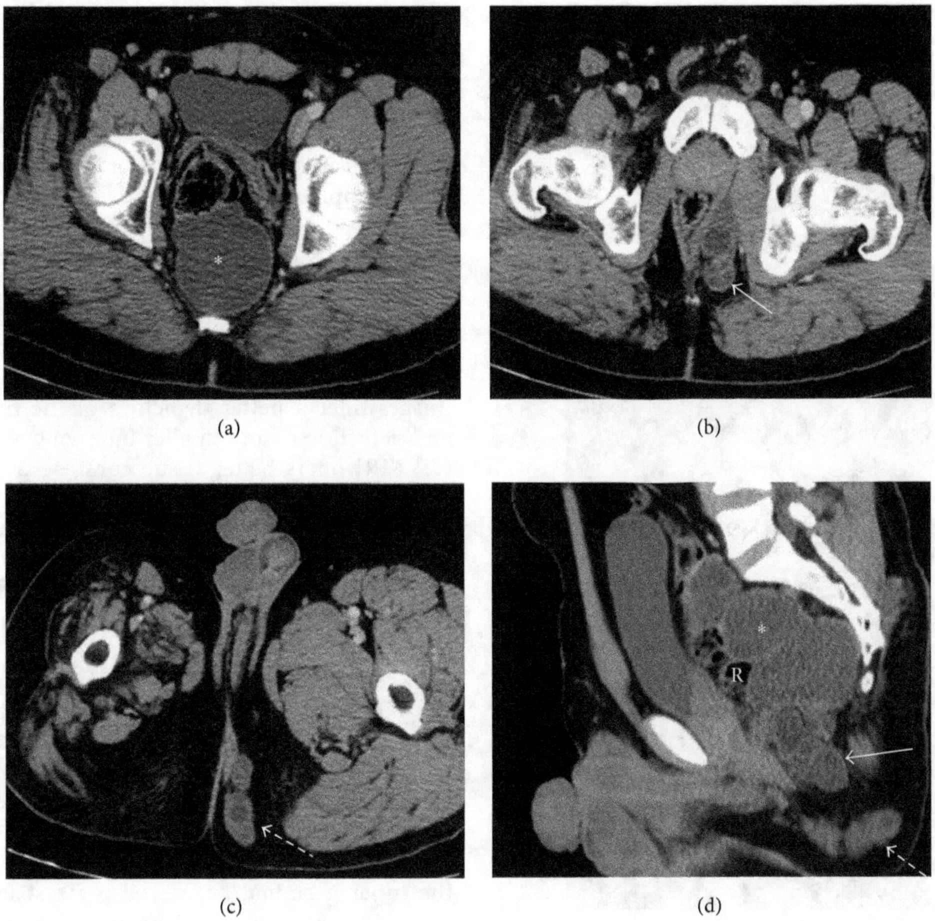

FIGURE 1: Multiple axial and sagittal contrast enhanced CT scan show a multilocular, hypoattenuating, retrorectal cystic lesion (asterisks) displacing the rectum (R) anteriorly. The left ischioanal fossa cystic lesion (solid arrow) shows enhancing wall and internal septations, breaching the left levator ani muscle and extending into the left perineal subcutaneous fat (dashed arrow). Atrophy of the right hemipelvis and proximal thigh muscles is noted and related to known poliomyelitis.

and proximal thigh muscles was related to the history of poliomyelitis (Figure 1). An ^{18}F-fluorodeoxyglucose (FDG) positron emission tomography (PET/CT) scan was performed and showed no abnormal uptake in these lesions; no regional lymphadenopathy or distant metastases were seen (Figure 2).

Pelvic magnetic resonance imaging (MRI) was performed. The retrorectal mass showed intermediate signal intensity on both T1 and T2 with multiple internal T1 hypointense foci and T2 hyperintense foci. The left ischioanal fossa collection of cysts showed low T1 and high T2 signal intensity with multiple internal cysts and T2 and T1 hypointense rim. There was thin peripheral enhancement with no enhancing mural solid component. There was no osseous involvement (Figure 3).

The patient underwent surgical resection. The histopathologic examination of the resected retrorectal cyst revealed a benign tailgut cyst. The resected left ischioanal and gluteal cystic lesions showed an outer histiocytic reaction to a hydatid cyst.

3. Discussion

The unique feature of this primary extrahepatic hydatid cyst is its very unusual location in the ischioanal fossa with extension to the left perianal and gluteal areas. While the hydatid cysts had increased signal on T2-weighted images, the tailgut cyst had intermediate signal, denoting proteinaceous or mucinous content. The presence of both a perineal hydatid cyst and tailgut cyst with differing signal characteristics on MRI in a contiguous location in one patient imposed a diagnostic challenge where the added information of MRI proved very useful. In fact, the interpreting radiologist suggested a developmental lesion such as a tailgut cyst and atypical hydatid disease. The differential diagnosis might include a myxoid tumor such as myxoid neurofibroma or aggressive angiomyxoma due to the presence of myxoid, proteinaceous, or mucinous contents. However, the lack of an enhancing solid component makes those diagnoses less likely.

A tailgut cyst is a rare developmental lesion that is a remnant of the embryonic tailgut. The tailgut is the most caudal

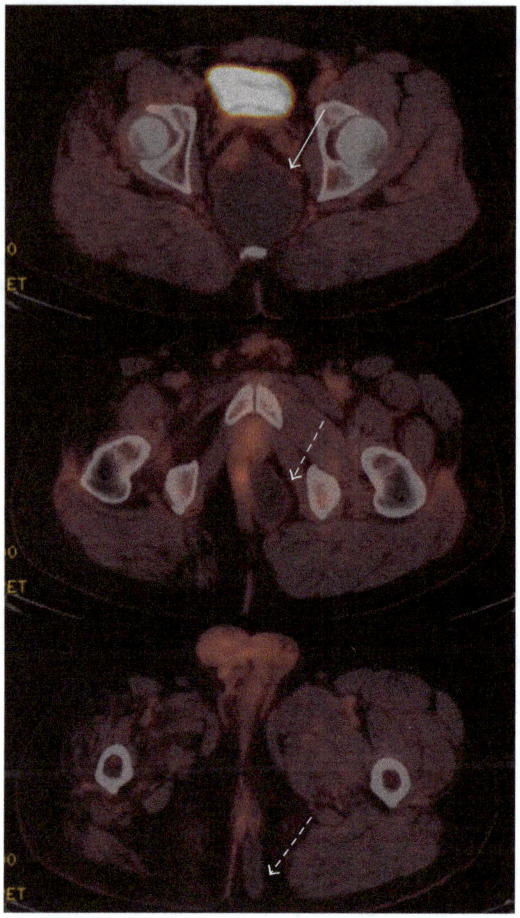

FIGURE 2: Fused FDG PET/CT images show no FDG uptake in the known retrorectal tailgut cyst (solid arrow) or the left ischioanal and perineal subcutaneous hydatid cysts (dashed arrows).

part of the hindgut that normally involutes during embryonic development. Tailgut cysts have a female predilection, are usually asymptomatic, and are often detected in middle age. They can be discovered at any age and may cause symptoms such as abdominal pain or constipation [1].

The imaging findings of tailgut cysts on CT and MRI have been described. Usually, CT shows a presacral, discrete, and well-marginated lesion of fluid or soft tissue attenuation depending on the cyst contents. Cyst wall calcifications may be seen and the rectum may be displaced if the lesion is large [2–4]. On MRI, tailgut cysts are usually hyperintense on T2-weighted images and hypointense on T1-weighted images. However, the presence of high protein content, mucinous materials, or internal hemorrhage may lead to high T1 signal intensity [4, 10, 11]. Malignant transformation of the tailgut cyst has been reported. Loss of discrete margins and involvement of contiguous structures can be detected on CT and might suggest the cyst is complicated by infection or malignant transformation [2]. Fibrous tissue within the cyst or malignant transformation may be seen as enhancing irregular wall thickening or a polypoid mass of intermediate signal intensity on both T1- and T2-weighted images [11, 12].

Because of the malignant potential of a tailgut cyst, to distinguish it from the other presacral cysts is essential. Differential diagnoses of a presacral cystic lesion might include rectal duplication cyst, dermoid cyst, epidermoid cyst, cystic lymphangioma, and anterior meningocele. These diagnoses are usually unilocular except for a tailgut cyst and cystic lymphangioma which are usually multicystic [13, 14]. Tailgut cysts have been reported as unilocular or multilocular cystic lesions on MRI [4, 10, 11]. Some suggest that a T2-weighted multilocular appearance with internal septa is a unique feature of a tailgut cyst [10, 14]. Another study observed the presence of small peripheral cysts within a large cyst [14]. Therefore, MRI and specifically T2-weighted MR images offer a better depiction of the multilocular nature and detection of any smaller internal cysts. As compared to CT, MRI offers better tissue contrast. Sagittal MRI can be used to assess the relationship of the presacral lesion with the rectum and osseous structures. Nevertheless, there is a considerable overlap in the imaging findings of presacral cystic lesions, and therefore histologic evaluation is essential to the establishment of a definitive diagnosis of tailgut cyst [10, 14].

Echinococcus granulosus and *Echinococcus multilocularis* are the two main infectious causative agents of hydatid disease. Dogs are usually the definitive hosts and sheep are the most common intermediate hosts. Humans are an intermediate host and may become infected after ingestion of food contaminated with *Echinococcus* eggs. Hydatid cysts have three components, the pericyst, middle laminated membrane, and the inner germinal layer. The pericyst is the surrounding host tissue inflammatory response. The scolex (the infectious parasite at the larval stage) arises from the inner endocyst [5, 6]. Although not highly sensitive or specific, serologic tests for the detection of *Echinococcus* antibody should be part of the work-up of any detected cystic lesion in an unusual location.

In humans, hydatid disease affects the liver, the lung, and other locations in approximately 75%, 15%, and 10% of cases, respectively [5, 6]. When occurring in unusual locations, most cases are secondary hydatid disease. Primary hydatid disease is considered when no other cysts are detected in the more common sites of occurrence. Primary pelvic hydatid disease has been reported with an incidence of 2%. It has be postulated that the hydatid scolex gains access to the pelvis by the lymphatic or haematogenous route [15, 16]. There are three reported cases of hydatid disease involving the perineal region [7–9]. However, one of the them was treated as perianal abscess with no preoperative imaging [9] and another one had a cyst centered in the retrorectal space with extension into the perineal and gluteal areas [8].

Hydatid disease has a variable imaging appearance. There is a standardized WHO classification of the hydatid cyst stages based on the Gharbi ultrasound classification [17, 18]. The hydatid cyst stages are a cyst with a visible cyst wall (stage 1), multiseptated, multivesicular cysts (stage 2), a cyst with a detached floating endocyst membrane (stage 3a), a unilocular cyst with solid or mucinous matrix and internal daughter cysts (stage 3b), a heterogeneous solid cyst with a degenerative internal canalicular structure (stage 4), and a

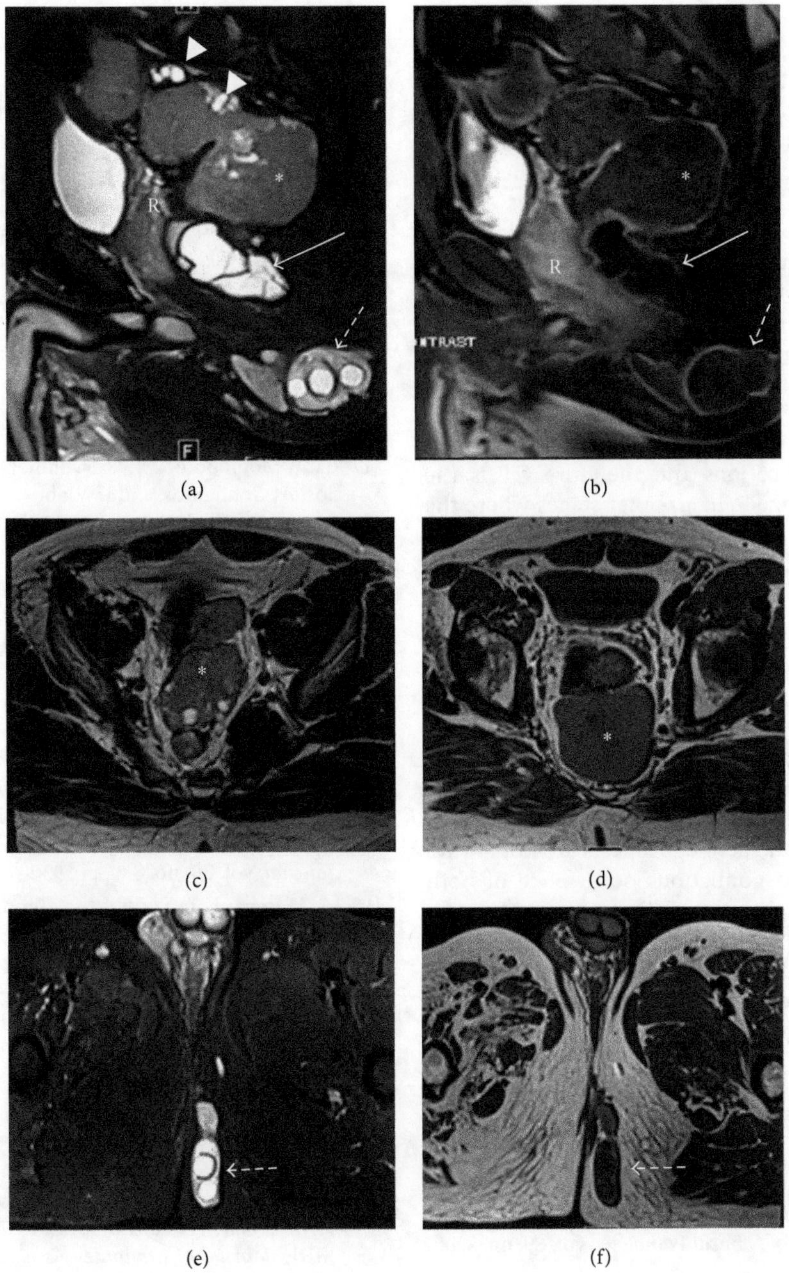

(a) (b) (c) (d) (e) (f)

FIGURE 3: (a) Sagittal T2-weighted MR image with fat saturation shows a predominantly intermediate T2 signal intensity presacral/retrorectal multilocular lesion (asterisk) with multiple internal T2 bright foci and smaller peripheral cysts (arrowheads). Note the anterior displacement of the rectum. The left ischioanal (solid arrow) and subcutaneous perineal hydatid cysts (dashed arrow) show high T2 signal intensity with dark internal septations and rims. (b) Sagittal T1-weighted postcontrast MR image shows peripheral rim enhancement of the retrorectal tailgut cyst (asterisks) as well as the ischioanal (solid arrow) and perineal subcutaneous hydatid cysts (dashed arrow). ((c) and (d)) Axial T2-weighted (c) and T1-weighted (d) MR images show the retrorectal lesion of intermediate signal intensity (asterisk) with peripheral small cyst. ((e) and (f)) Axial T2-weighted (e) and T1-weighted (f) MR images show the left subcutaneous perineal hydatid cysts (dashed arrow) of high T2 signal intensity and intermediately low T1 signal intensity with internal daughter cysts and a dark rim.

degenerated cyst with heavily calcified wall (stage 5) [17]. It is believed that the first two stages are active, the last two stages are inactive, and stage three is transitional. Treatment decisions are guided by imaging findings and therefore the adaptation of ultrasound-based classification of hydatid cyst into MR and CT imaging has been well described [19–21].

Stojkovic et al. compared the MR and CT imaging findings with ultrasound and concluded that the hydatid cyst matrix is the main defining feature of cyst stage. Also, the "double line sign" is diagnostic for hydatid stage 1. The cyst wall calcifications play some role in defining cyst stage 5 which may be challenging on MRI. Therefore when compared to ultrasound, MRI performs very well with WHO hydatid cyst stages 1, 2, 3, and 4. T2-weighted MR images provide the best sequence to detect cyst contents, that is, septa (stage 2) and daughter cysts (stage 3b) [21]. Singh and Gibikote concluded that T2-weighted MRI is also the best sequence to show the parent capsule and the detached germinal membrane. Both T2-weighted and T1-weighted images should be used to differentiate between the fluid signal intensity of the parent cyst and daughter cysts [22]. The rim sign is described as a low signal intensity rim that is suggestive of hydatid disease rather than other nonparasitic processes. It is more evident on T2-weighted MR images and represents the pericyst and the parasitic membranes. It has been described in hepatic and pulmonary hydatid disease but this sign lacks specificity [6, 23]. CT is superior to ultrasound and MRI in the detection of calcifications and therefore CT is the diagnostic standard for stage 5. In all other stages where the cyst matrix is an important classifying feature, CT performs moderately well compared to ultrasound [21].

4. Conclusion

While a tailgut cyst is a rare entity, it should be considered when there is a presacral multilocular mass. Hydatid disease may affect any part of the human body and often has non-specific imaging findings and serological tests are not always positive. The simultaneous contiguous occurrence of both diagnoses is rare. Attention to the unique imaging features of each cystic lesion facilitates the diagnosis. Clinicians and radiologists should entertain hydatid cysts in their differential diagnoses whenever they encounter cystic lesions especially if the patient is from an endemic area.

References

[1] B. M. Hjermstad and E. B. Helwig, "Tailgut cysts. Report of 53 cases," *American Journal of Clinical Pathology*, vol. 89, no. 2, pp. 139–147, 1988.

[2] A. R. Johnson, P. R. Ros, and B. M. Hjermstad, "Tailgut cyst: diagnosis with CT and sonography," *American Journal of Roentgenology*, vol. 147, no. 6, pp. 1309–1311, 1986.

[3] F. D. Ottery, R. A. Carlson, H. Gould, and J. L. Weese, "Retrorectal cyst-hamartomas: CT diagnosis," *Journal of Computer Assisted Tomography*, vol. 10, no. 2, pp. 260–263, 1986.

[4] G. Liessi, S. Cesari, M. Pavanello, and R. Butini, "Tailgut cysts: CT and MR findings," *Abdominal Imaging*, vol. 20, no. 3, pp. 256–258, 1995.

[5] I. Pedrosa, A. Saíz, J. Arrazola, J. Ferreirós, and C. S. Pedrosa, "Hydatid disease: radiologic and pathologic features and complications," *Radiographics*, vol. 20, no. 3, pp. 795–817, 2000.

[6] P. Polat, M. Kantarci, F. Alper, S. Suma, M. B. Koruyucu, and A. Okur, "Hydatid disease from head to toe," *Radiographics*, vol. 23, no. 2, pp. 475–494, 2003.

[7] A. J. Manouras, P. J. Tzardis, V. A. Katergiannakis, and N. S. Apostolidis, "Unusual primary locations of hydatid disease. Case report," *Acta Chirurgica Scandinavica*, vol. 155, no. 3, pp. 217–219, 1989.

[8] A. Baykan, S. Yildirim, H. M. Koksal, F. Celayir, and M. Oner, "Intrapelvic-perianal hydatid disease in an unusual location: report of a case," *Diseases of the Colon and Rectum*, vol. 47, no. 2, pp. 250–252, 2004.

[9] H. Soleimani, M. Seifi, and M. Shemshadi, "A primary hydatid cyst infestation as perianal abscess: a case report," *Journal of Isfahan Medical School*, vol. 29, pp. 491–494, 2011.

[10] M.-J. Kim, W. H. Kim, N. K. Kim et al., "Tailgut cyst: multilocular cystic appearance on MRI," *Journal of Computer Assisted Tomography*, vol. 21, no. 5, pp. 731–732, 1997.

[11] K.-E. Lim, W.-C. Hsu, and C.-R. Wang, "Tailgut Cyst with malignancy: MR imaging findings," *American Journal of Roentgenology*, vol. 170, no. 6, pp. 1488–1490, 1998.

[12] L. A. Moulopoulos, E. Karvouni, D. Kehagias, M. A. Dimopoulos, A. Gouliamos, and L. Vlahos, "MR imaging of complex tailgut cysts," *Clinical Radiology*, vol. 54, no. 2, pp. 118–122, 1999.

[13] H. Dahan, L. Arrivé, D. Wendum, H. D. Le Pointe, H. Djouhri, and J.-M. Tubiana, "Retrorectal developmental cysts in adults: clinical and radiologic-histopathologic review, differential diagnosis, and treatment," *Radiographics*, vol. 21, no. 3, pp. 575–584, 2001.

[14] D. M. Yang, C. H. Park, W. Jin et al., "Tailgut cyst: MRI evaluation," *American Journal of Roentgenology*, vol. 184, no. 5, pp. 1519–1523, 2005.

[15] V. Seenu, M. C. Misra, S. C. Tiwari, R. Jain, and C. Chandrashekhar, "Primary pelvic hydatid cyst presenting with obstructive uropathy and renal failure," *Postgraduate Medical Journal*, vol. 70, no. 830, pp. 930–932, 1994.

[16] A. Horchani, Y. Nouira, M. Chtourou, M. Kacem, and Z. Ben Safta, "Retrovesical hydatid disease: a clinical study of 27 cases," *European Urology*, vol. 40, no. 6, pp. 655–660, 2001.

[17] C. N. L. Macpherson, D. A. Vuitton, H. A. Gharbi et al., "International classification of ultrasound images in cystic echinococcosis for application in clinical and field epidemiological settings," *Acta Tropica*, vol. 85, no. 2, pp. 253–261, 2003.

[18] H. A. Gharbi, W. Hassine, M. W. Brauner, and K. Dupuch, "Ultrasound examination of the hydatic liver," *Radiology*, vol. 139, no. 2, pp. 459–463, 1981.

[19] P. Taourel, B. Marty-Ane, S. Charasset, M. Mattei, P. Devred, and J. M. Bruel, "Hydatid cyst of the liver: comparison of CT and MRI," *Journal of Computer Assisted Tomography*, vol. 17, no. 1, pp. 80–85, 1993.

[20] Z. Suwan, "Sonographic findings in hydatid disease of the liver: comparison with other imaging methods," *Annals of Tropical Medicine and Parasitology*, vol. 89, no. 3, pp. 261–269, 1995.

[21] M. Stojkovic, K. Rosenberger, H. U. Kauczor, T. Junghanss, and W. Hosch, "Diagnosing and staging of cystic echinococcosis: how do CT and MRI perform in comparison to ultrasound?" *PLoS Neglected Tropical Diseases*, vol. 6, no. 10, Article ID e1880, 2012.

[22] S. Singh and S. V. Gibikote, "Magnetic resonance imaging signal characteristics in hydatid cysts," *Australasian Radiology*, vol. 45, no. 2, pp. 128–133, 2001.

[23] S. A. Davolio Marani, G. C. Canossi, F. A. Nicoli, G. P. Alberti, S. G. Monni, and P. M. Casolo, "Hydatid disease: MR imaging study," *Radiology*, vol. 175, no. 3, pp. 701–706, 1990.

45

Tubular Carcinoma of the Breast: Advantages and Limitations of Breast Tomosynthesis

Filipa Vilaverde,[1] Ana Rocha,[2] and Alcinda Reis[1]

[1] *Serviço de Imagiologia, Centro Hospitalar de Entre o Douro e Vouga, Santa Maria da Feira, Portugal*
[2] *Servicio de Radiología, Hospital Povisa, Vigo, Spain*

Correspondence should be addressed to Filipa Vilaverde; filipavilaverde@gmail.com

Academic Editor: Roberto Grassi

Tubular carcinoma of the breast is a rare variant of invasive ductal carcinoma. We report a case of 42-year-old asymptomatic female with a histopathological proven multifocal tubular carcinoma, studied by mammography, Tomosynthesis, Ultrasound, and Magnetic Resonance. Herein, we discuss the advantages and limitations of Tomosynthesis, an emerging imaging technique, in this particular case.

1. Introduction

Mammography, the accepted technique for breast cancer screening, presents a global sensitivity of about 85%, reducing breast cancer deaths by 15 to 30% [1, 2]. Mammographic screening false negatives vary from 6 to 46% between series and are much more common in dense breasts. This is mainly related to the fact that a three-dimensional structure—the breast—is being studied with a two-dimensional image with subsequent tissue overlap [1, 3].

Digital Breast Tomosynthesis (DBT) is a new tool that can be expected to partially obviate this problem by reducing or eliminating tissue overlap. DBT technology enables the acquisition of a three-dimensional volume of thin-section data, and images are reconstructed in conventional orientations by using reconstruction algorithms similar to those used in computed tomography (CT). DBT is being progressively implemented in breast imaging clinics, as early clinical data have shown that it improves the accuracy of screening and diagnostic breast imaging, addressing some of the long-standing limitations of conventional mammography [4–6].

However, as with any new technique, several issues must be considered when implementing DBT into daily practice, and some limitations of the technique must be recognized.

This case illustrates some potential advantages and limitations of DBT.

2. Clinical Case

A 42-year-old asymptomatic female presented to our institution for routine screening breast study. The patient had family history of breast cancer (her mother at 45 years). Physical examination was normal.

Mammography showed an architectural distortion in the upper quadrants of the left breast, only clearly seen in the mediolateral oblique view (Figure 1). DBT—routinely performed at the patient's hospital—localized the lesion to the upper outer quadrant and further characterized it as a small irregular mass with long spicules (Figure 2). A targeted Ultrasound (US) showed a 10 mm solid nodule, with posterior acoustic shadowing (Figure 3). A tru-cut biopsy guided by US was performed, revealing a tubular carcinoma.

Breast Magnetic Resonance Imaging (MRI) was done to evaluate the local extension and showed, apart from this nodule, an additional one 8 mm in the upper inner quadrant, with the same imaging findings at MRI and US, and at a distance of 35 mm from the former (Figure 4). It was biopsied at second-look US, and the histologic diagnosis was also tubular carcinoma.

3. Discussion

Tubular carcinoma of the breast is a well-differentiated type of invasive ductal carcinoma that forms neoplastic tubules

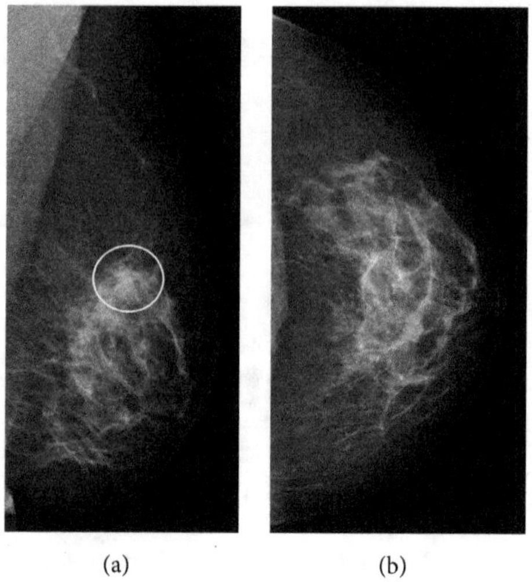

FIGURE 1: Left breast mammography, mediolateral oblique (a) and craniocaudal views (b). There is an architectural distortion in the upper quadrants of the left breast (white circle), not clearly seen in the craniocaudal view: Rocha A, Servicio de Radiologia, Hospital Povisa, Vigo, Spain.

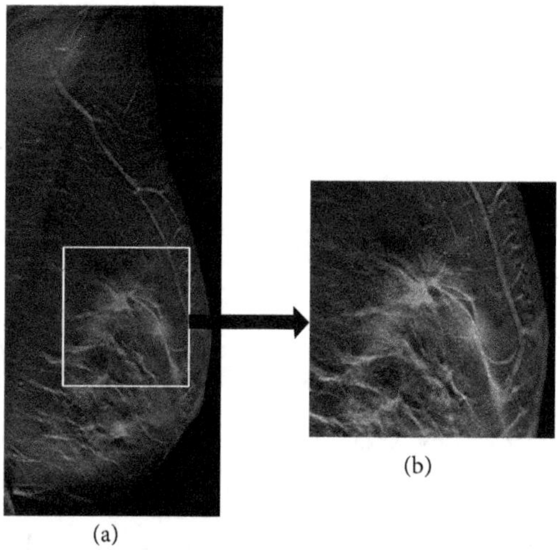

FIGURE 2: Left mediolateral oblique Tomosynthesis image section (a), with pathologic area close-up view (b). There was improved architectural distortion visualization further localized to the upper outer quadrant. Close-up view shows a small central mass with large spicules and focal retraction along the margin of the tissue: Rocha A, Servicio de Radiologia, Hospital Povisa, Vigo, Spain.

mimicking breast ductules and accounting for about 1% of all breast carcinomas [7]. It may contain other histologic elements, but an excess of 75% tubular elements is usually required for the diagnosis of tubular carcinoma [1]. Lesions are multifocal or multicentric in around 15% of cases [1]. Tubular carcinoma typically occurs in a younger population than the more common Invasive Ductal Carcinoma Not Otherwise Specified (IDC-NOS) [1]. The prognosis is excellent with survival of 97% at 10 years [8].

The lesion is usually very small (<1 cm) and nonpalpable, often first detected on screening mammography [8]. Some cases may be mammographically occult [9].

Tubular carcinoma presents on mammography as an architectural distortion or as an irregularly shaped mass with spiculated margins, with or without calcifications. The appearance mimics IDC-NOS. The spicules are often longer than the central mass [8, 9]. On US, the appearance also mimics IDC-NOS, manifesting as a hypoechoic solid mass with ill-defined margins and posterior acoustic shadowing. MRI shows characteristics of a malignant tumor, more commonly an irregular mass with a type 3 enhancement curve (rapid initial rise, followed by a drop-off with time/washout in the delayed phase) [8, 9]. Although DBT did not allow a specific diagnosis in this particular case, it was helpful for lesion localization seen on only one mammographic view, therefore obviating the need for additional projections. By scrolling through the image slices, a slider tool displays where the current image slice is positioned anatomically in a medial or lateral location on the mediolateral view and the superoinferior location on the craniocaudal view. Also, DBT improved diagnosis confidence in a malignant lesion, showing a central mass with large spicules, which was not featured on mammography. This is in accordance with known advantages of DBT: improved conspicuity and characterization of lesions due to reduced obscuration by overlapping breast tissue [5, 6]. Described false negatives of DBT are mainly related to areas of dense tissue without fat planes that blur tumor margins, particularly in the smaller ones [4]. Probably, an area of denser tissue was responsible for the inconspicuous second tumor.

Tubular carcinoma should be considered in the differential diagnosis of a small spiculated mass, especially if it has long spicules [10].

Our patient was submitted to partial mastectomy and the final diagnosis was compatible with multifocal tubular carcinoma with some foci of IDC-NOS, low grade.

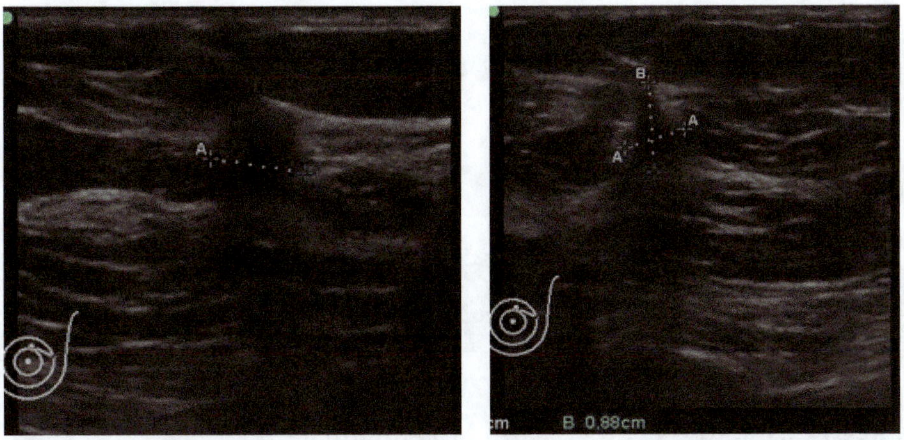

(a) (b)

FIGURE 3: Ultrasound, transverse (a) and longitudinal (b) sections. A 10 mm solid nodule was shown, with irregular and ill-defined margins, taller rather than wider shaped, with a hyperechoic rim and posterior acoustic shadowing: Rocha A, Servicio de Radiologia, Hospital Povisa, Vigo, Spain.

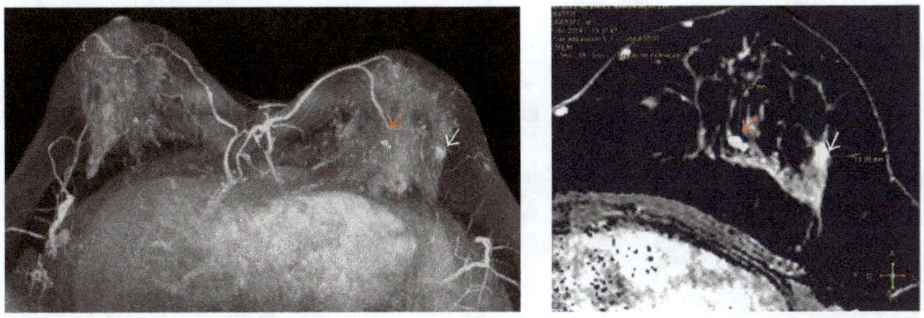

(a) (b)

FIGURE 4: Breast Magnetic Resonance T1-weighted images, after gadolinium administration and axial maximum intensity projection (MIP) reformations. In addition to the previously biopsied lesion in the upper outer quadrant, there was another nodule 35 mm apart, in the upper inner quadrant. It measured 8 mm and was also submitted to US-guided biopsy: Rocha A, Servicio de Radiologia, Hospital Povisa, Vigo, Spain.

4. Conclusion

DBT improves radiologist's diagnostic confidence allowing differentiation between fibroglandular tissue overlap and a true lesion, without the need of additional mammographic acquisitions. As tubular carcinoma frequently presents with an architectural distortion or as a small mass, it represents a potential tumor benefiting from DBT.

References

[1] Cardenosa, *Clinical Breast Imaging, A Patient Focused Teaching File*, Lippincott Williams & Wilkins, Philadelphia, Pa, USA, 2006.

[2] S. M. Moss, H. Cuckle, A. Evans, L. Johns, M. Waller, and L. Bobrow, "Effect of mammographic screening from age 40 years on breast cancer mortality at 10 years' follow-up: a randomised controlled trial," *The Lancet*, vol. 368, no. 9552, pp. 2053–2060, 2006.

[3] A. B. Miller, C. Wall, C. J. Baines, P. Sun, T. To, and S. A. Narod, "Twenty five year follow-up for breast cancer incidence and mortality of the Canadian National Breast Screening Study: randomised screening trial," *British Medical Journal*, vol. 348, article g366, 2014.

[4] M. P. Jeong, E. A. Franken Jr., M. Garg, L. L. Fajardo, and L. T. Niklason, "Breast tomosynthesis: present considerations and future applications," *RadioGraphics*, vol. 27, pp. S231–S240, 2007.

[5] H. R. Peppard, B. E. Nicholson, C. M. Rochman, J. K. Merchant, R. C. Mayo, and J. A. Harvey, "Digital breast tomosynthesis in the diagnostic setting: indications and clinical applications," *Radiographics*, vol. 35, no. 4, pp. 975–990, 2015.

[6] R. Gartner Roth, A. D. A. Maidment, S. P. Weinstein, S. Orel Roth, and E. F. Conant, "Digital breast tomosynthesis: lessons learned from early clinical implementation," *Radiographics* 34, no. 4, pp. E89–E102, 2014.

[7] D. Cyrlak, P. M. Carpenter, and N. B. Rawal, "Breast imaging case of the day," *Radiographics*, vol. 19, no. 1, pp. 245–247, 1999.

[8] J. A. Harvey, "Unusual breast cancers: useful clues to expanding the differential diagnosis," *Radiology*, vol. 242, no. 3, pp. 683–694, 2007.

46

Bilateral Congenital Agenesis of the Long Head of the Biceps Tendon: The Beginning

Francisco Rego Costa, Cátia Esteves, and Lina Melão

Department of Radiology, São João Hospital, Alameda Professor Hernâni Monteiro, 4200-319 Porto, Portugal

Correspondence should be addressed to Francisco Rego Costa; franciscoregocosta@gmail.com

Academic Editor: Toshihiro Akisue

The biceps brachii muscle is prone to variants but absence of the long head of the biceps (LHB) tendon is an exceptionally rare anomaly. This report concerns the fourth case of bilateral congenital absence of the LHB tendon and presents the ultrasonography (US) and magnetic resonance (MR) findings. Our case has the peculiarity of being the first in which bilateral LHB tendon agenesis is not associated with rotator cuff or labral tears.

1. Introduction

Absence of the long head of the biceps (LHB) tendon is a very unusual anomaly. We report the fourth case of bilateral congenital absence of the LHB tendon in the English literature. Ultrasonography (US) and magnetic resonance (MR) findings are exposed.

2. Case Report

A 29-year-old male, Muay Thai amateur fighter, presented with right anterior shoulder pain at rest that exacerbated with overhead activities. The pain was moderate for months but worsened in the last few weeks, specially after sports activity. He had no symptoms in the left shoulder.

Although the patient is a sportsman, there was no history of a significant lesion/traumatic event involving the upper limbs, including shoulder dislocation. He also denied orthopedic surgery to both shoulders.

The physical exam was almost unremarkable. The uppercut and Speed's tests were negative and the "Popeye" sign was absent. Digital pressure over the bicipital groove did not elicit pain. Although the rotatory stress test and the lateral decubitus load and shift test were negative, the anterior apprehension sign was doubtful. Also there was some limited range of motion when the patient tried to elevate the left arm with the forearm in supination. Overall, there was no clear evidence of biceps pathology or anterior instability.

On the ultrasonography of the painful and contralateral shoulder we were not able to demonstrate the LHB tendon in its groove (Figure 1), suggesting the presence of a tear or agenesis. There was no evidence of rotator cuff tears, bursitis, or effusion.

Magnetic resonance imaging of both shoulders revealed bilateral absence of the LHB tendon and shallow intertubercular sulci (Figures 2 and 3). There was no evidence of rotator cuff tears on the right side or labral tears bilaterally (Figures 4, 5, and 6). As the patient had no symptoms on the left side, only axial plane MR images were obtained, with the main purpose of proving bilateral agenesis. On these images there was no evidence of rotator cuff abnormalities (Figure 7).

3. Discussion

The biceps brachii muscle is one of the most diverse in the human body; however, congenital absence of the long head of the biceps tendon is a rare anomaly [1–7]. Frequently there are associated findings such as hypoplastic intertubercular groove [1–3] and shoulder instability [4–7]. Unilateral absence is associated with other skeletal and

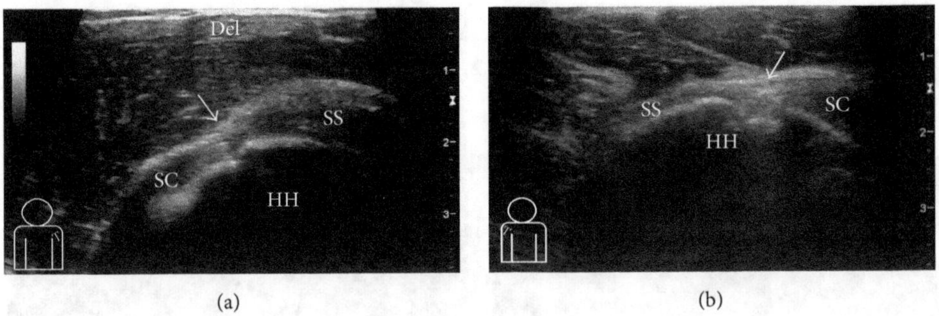

FIGURE 1: Ultrasound (US) images of both shoulders. (a) US parasagittal image of the left shoulder rotator interval. The long head of the biceps tendon is not identifiable in its normal position (white arrow). (b) US parasagittal image of the right shoulder rotator interval. The long head of the biceps tendon is not discernible in its normal position (white arrow). HH = humeral head; SS = supraspinatus tendon; SC = subscapularis tendon; Del = deltoid muscle.

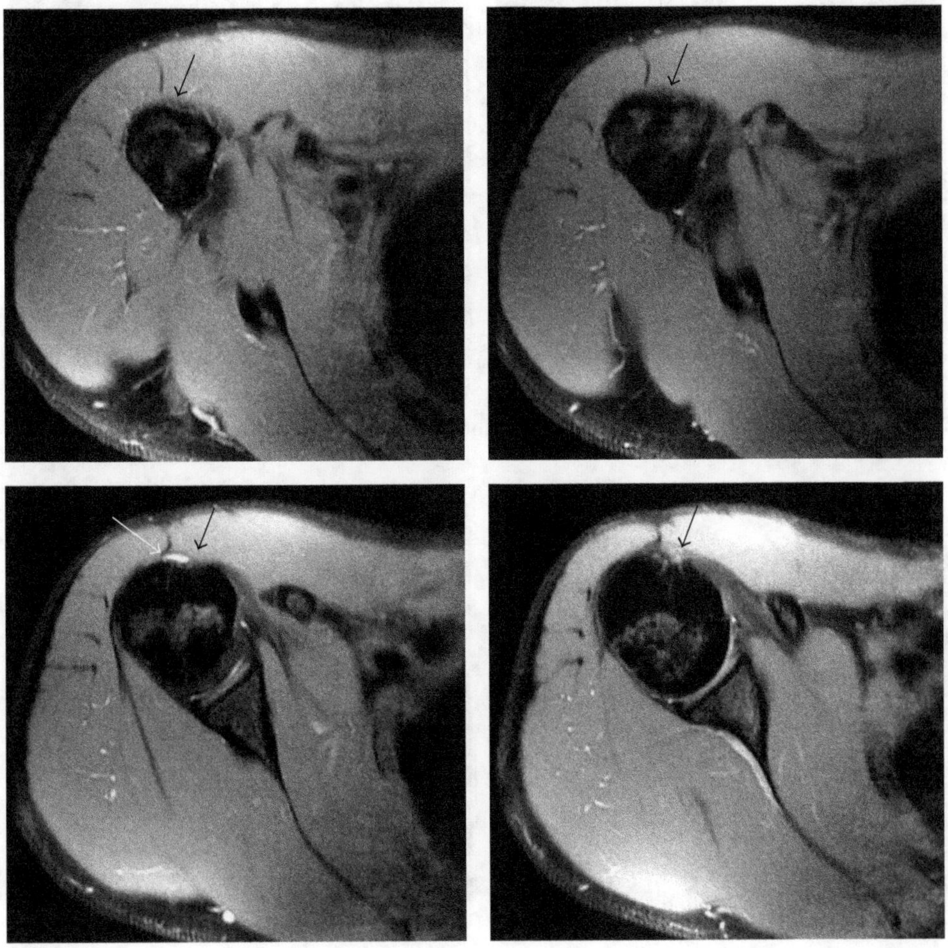

FIGURE 2: Axial DP FS SE MR sequential images of the right shoulder (TR = 2540; TE = 11.18; NEX = 2; EC = 1) demonstrating a shallow bicipital groove (black arrows) and absence of the long head of the biceps tendon. There is a small amount of fluid in the subacromial/subdeltoid bursa (white arrow), without pathologic significance.

nonskeletal congenital anomalies in 57% of cases [1, 4–6], including at least one case associated with VATER complex (vertebral defects, anal atresia, tracheoesophageal fistula with esophageal atresia, and radial and renal anomalies) [4]. Bilateral absence is extremely uncommon with only three prior reports in the English literature [1–3]. Solely one of these three cases presented with an additional skeletal abnormality (radial ray) [1].

In our case, the patient was healthy and physically active and no other congenital anomalies were evident. As in other reported cases, bilateral agenesis of the LHB tendon is most commonly diagnosed in a young adult patient complaining

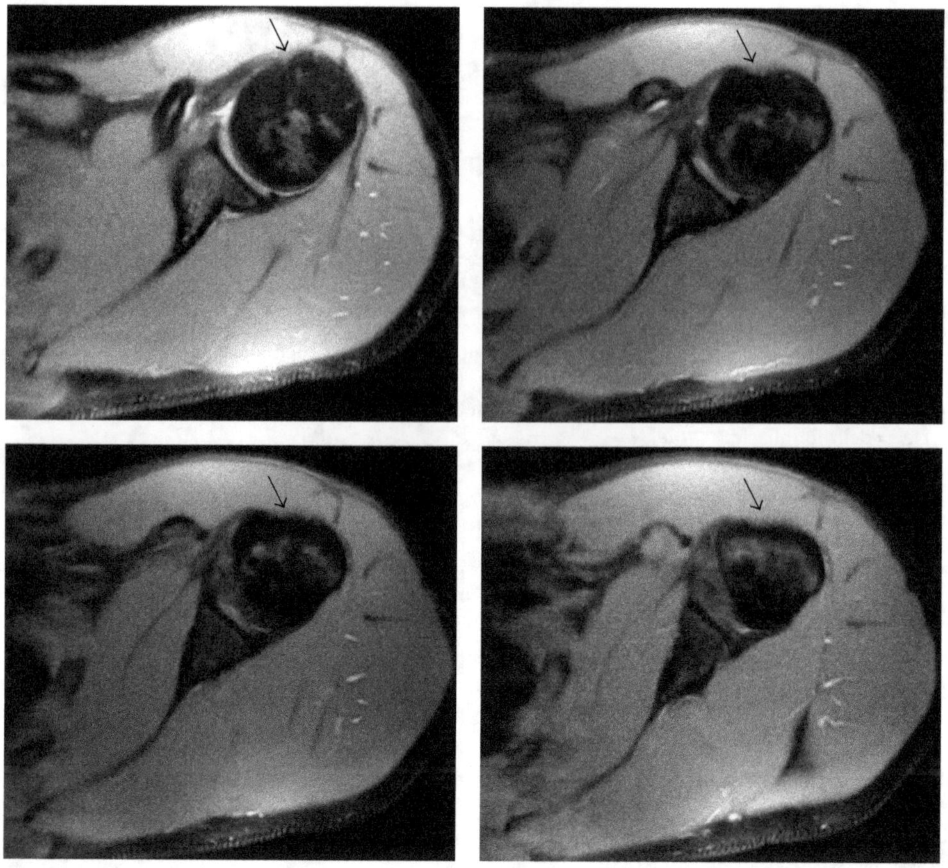

Figure 3: Axial DP FS SE MR sequential images of the left shoulder (TR = 2540; TE = 11.18; NEX = 2; EC = 1) showing a shallow bicipital groove (black arrows) and absence of the long head of the biceps tendon.

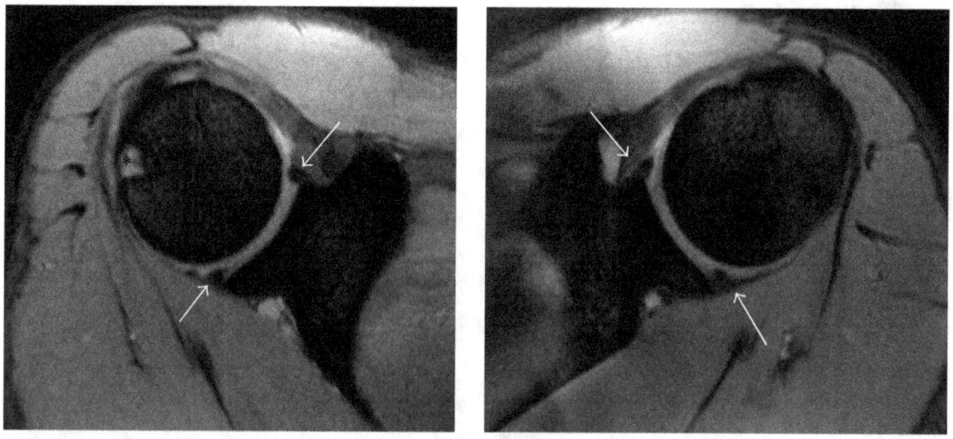

(a) (b)

Figure 4: Axial DP FS SE MR images of the right (a) and left (b) shoulder (TR = 475; TE = 13.43; NEX = 1; EC = 1) showing normal labrum morphology bilaterally, without evidence of tears (white arrows). In (a) there is a cyst beneath the lateral humeral head margin, without pathologic significance (asterisk).

of nonspecific shoulder pain [1–3]. Evidence of shallow intertubercular groove is the "rule," and our case is not an exception. The finding of a shallow groove is very helpful in the differential diagnosis, favoring agenesis over the much more common diagnosis of a biceps tear.

Our case is the first to describe bilateral absence of the LHB tendon not associated with rotator cuff or labral tears. No other significant abnormality was discernible in both shoulders. These findings support that agenesis of the LHB tendon can, by itself, be a source of symptoms and functional

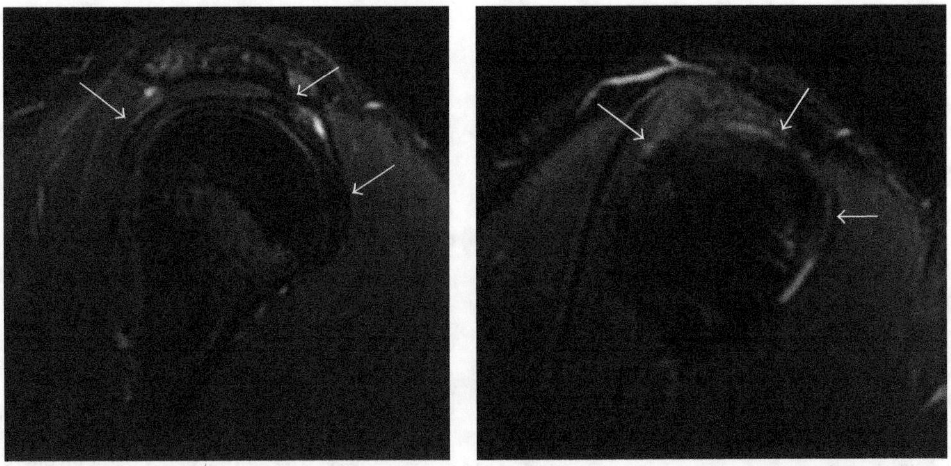

(a) (b)

FIGURE 5: Sagittal T2 FS SE MR images of the right shoulder (TR = 2600; TE = 63.9; NEX = 3; EC = 1) (a) and (b) demonstrating the rotator cuff tendons (white arrows) with normal thickness and hypointensity, without tears.

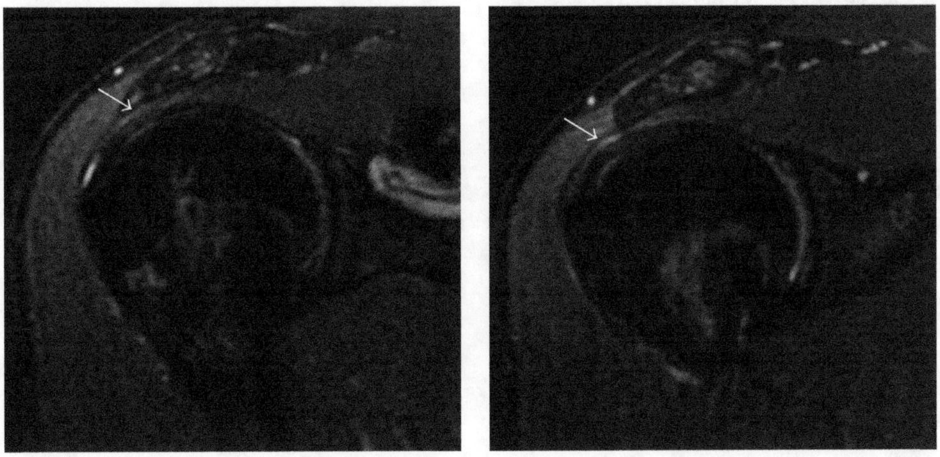

(a) (b)

FIGURE 6: Coronal T2 FS SE MR images of the right shoulder (TR = 3500; TE = 63.2; NEX = 2; EC = 1) (a) and (b) showing the normal supraspinatus tendon long axis (white arrows), without tears.

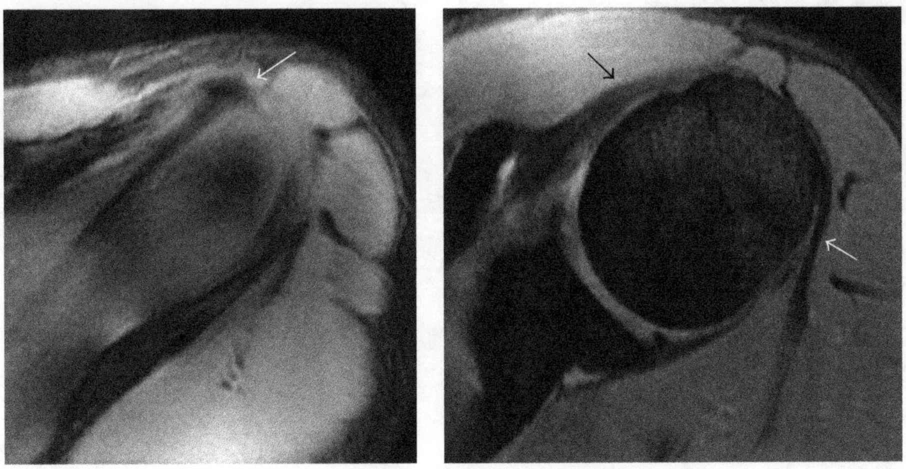

(a) (b)

FIGURE 7: Axial DP FS SE MR images of the left shoulder (TR = 475; TE = 13.4; NEX = 2; EC = 1). (a) The supraspinatus tendon is visible, without any discontinuity (white arrow). (b) The subscapularis tendon (black arrow) and the infraspinatus tendon (white arrow) show normal thickness and hypointensity, without tears.

deficit. Based on other cases described, which emphasized the role of the LHB tendon as a shoulder stabilizer [3, 8, 9], we believe that this case can represent the earliest stage of the shoulder disease process generated by the absence of the LHB tendon.

References

[1] C. Maldjian, C. Borrero, R. Adam, and D. Vyas, "Nature abhors a vacuum: bilateral prominent rotator cable in bilateral congenital absence of the long head of the biceps tendon," *Skeletal Radiology*, vol. 43, no. 1, pp. 75–78, 2014.

[2] M. C. Koplas, C. S. Winalski, W. H. Ulmer Jr., and M. Recht, "Bilateral congenital absence of the long head of the biceps tendon," *Skeletal Radiology*, vol. 38, no. 7, pp. 715–719, 2009.

[3] K. M. Kuhn, J. Carney, D. Solomon, and M. Provencher, "Bilateral absence of the long head of the biceps tendon," *Military Medicine*, vol. 174, no. 5, pp. 548–550, 2009.

[4] E. L. Smith, E. G. Matzkin, D. H. Kim, J. K. Harpstrite, and D. M. Kan, "Congenital absence of the long head of the biceps brachii tendon as a Vater association," *The American Journal of Orthopedics*, vol. 31, no. 8, pp. 452–454, 2002.

[5] J. C. Franco, T. P. Knapp, and B. R. Mandelbaum, "Congenital absence of the long head of the biceps tendon. A case report," *The Journal of Bone and Joint Surgery—American Volume*, vol. 87, no. 7, pp. 1584–1586, 2005.

[6] S. A. Sayeed, J. P. Shah, M. S. Collins, and D. L. Dahm, "Absence of the long head of the biceps tendon associated with glenoid dysplasia and posterior labral tear," *Clinical Anatomy*, vol. 21, no. 7, pp. 728–732, 2008.

[7] D. A. Glueck, S. D. Mair, and D. L. Johnson, "Shoulder instability with absence of the long head of the biceps tendon," *Arthroscopy*, vol. 19, no. 7, pp. 787–789, 2003.

[8] C. S. Neer II, "Impingement lesions," *Clinical Orthopaedics and Related Research*, vol. 173, pp. 70–77, 1983.

[9] E. Etoi, D. K. Kuechle, S. R. Newman, B. F. Morrey, and K. N. An, "Stabilizing function of the biceps in stable and unstable shoulders," *The Journal of Bone & Joint Surgery—British Volume*, vol. 75, no. 4, pp. 546–550, 1993.

47

Multifocal Head and Neck Neurofibromas with Osseous Abnormalities and Muscular Hypoplasia in a Child with Neurofibromatosis: Type I

Rachna Rath,[1] Sheetal Kaur,[2] Shadab Ali Baig,[3] Punyashlok Pati,[1] and Sonalisa Sahoo[1]

[1]*Department of Oral & Maxillofacial Pathology, SCB Government Dental College & Hospital, Cuttack 753007, India*
[2]*Department of Radio Diagnosis, Acharya Harihar Regional Cancer Centre, Cuttack 753007, India*
[3]*Department of Oral & Maxillofacial Surgery, SCB Government Dental College & Hospital, Cuttack 753007, India*

Correspondence should be addressed to Rachna Rath; drrachna.rath@gmail.com

Academic Editor: Amit Agrawal

Neurofibromatosis type 1 (NF1) is a clinically and genetically distinct disease involving both neuroectodermal and mesenchymal derivatives. Orofacial manifestations in NF1 have been documented before but occurrence of multifocal intraosseous (IO) and extraosseous (EO) neurofibromas is rare. The present case highlights the importance of imaging findings in the diagnosis and management of multifocal jaw, infratemporal, and parotid neurofibromas with muscular hypoplasia in an eight-year-old girl with NF1. Apart from orthopantomograms (OPG), three-dimensional computed tomography (3D CT) and cross-sectional reformations were valuable in delineating the extent of the lytic lesion and identifying additional bony deformities of the mandible. Magnetic resonance imaging (MRI) helped to identify the solid nature of the lesion and true extent of the soft tissue mass.

1. Introduction

NF1 or von Recklinghausen's disease is a neurocristopathy presenting with certain cutaneous, ophthalmologic, and skeletal manifestations [1]. Head and neck are a common location for NF; however other sites may be involved less frequently including nasal cavity, paranasal sinus, nasopharynx, orbit, larynx, maxilla, and mandible [2]. Intraoral involvement may be in the form of soft tissue neurofibromas, developmental defects, or dental abnormalities.

Neurofibroma (NF) extending to the maxilla and associated with multifocal lesions in the infratemporal fossa, temporomandibular joint, parotid, and external auditory canal is extremely rare. Only one such case has been stated in literature showing multifocal jaw and soft tissue tumors [3]. Management of IO neurofibroma varies depending on age of the patient, tumor location, size, extent, nature (simple or plexiform), presence of functional impairment, and the risk of malignant transformation [4]. It is in this context that advanced imaging tools like CT and MRI become increasingly important, as they aid in establishing the diagnosis, knowing the true extent of the tumor, identifying complications before they become clinically apparent, even in guiding the management as in this case of multifocal neurofibromas in an 8-year-old child with NF1.

2. Case Report

An 8-year-old girl referred to the Dental Department presented with right facial asymmetry due to a slow growing painless swelling of 6-month duration. There was periauricular soft tissue swelling and intraoral bony hard enlargement of right mandibular alveolar ridge (Figures 1(a) and 1(b)). A history of antibiotic administration and extraction of the deciduous canine and first and second molar under the assumption of odontogenic infection was elicited.

OPG showed the presence of a well demarcated radiolucency in the ramus and angle of the mandible. There was

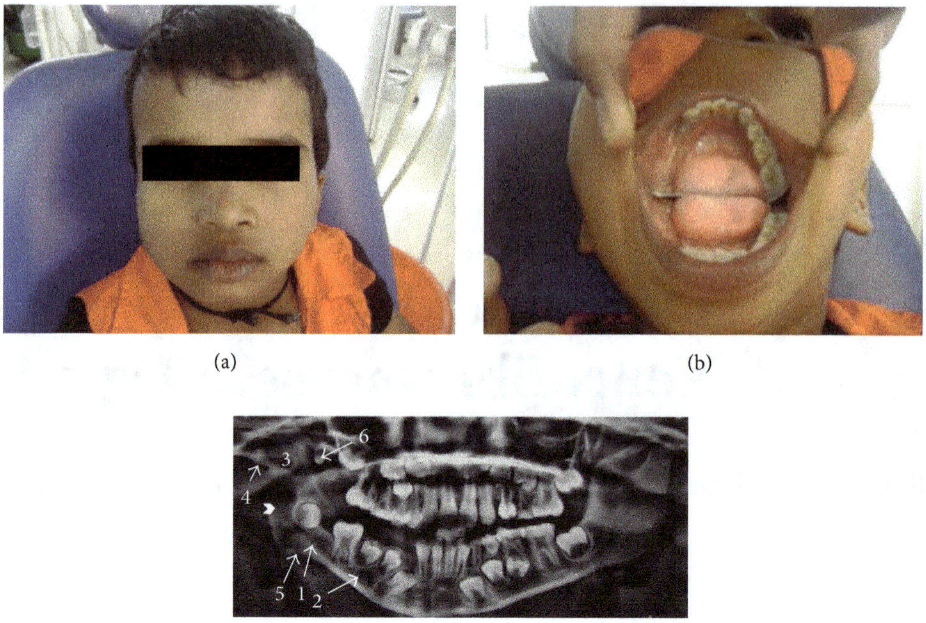

(a) (b) (c)

Figure 1: (a) Extraoral frontal view shows swelling on right side of face, (b) intraoral view shows alveolar enlargement and missing teeth on right side, (c) OPG shows intraosseous radiolucency (chevron) with impacted 46, enlarged mandibular canal (1), enlarged mental foramen (2), deep sigmoid notch (3), narrow condyle and pseudoelongation of condylar neck (4), notching of gonial angle (5), and supernumerary tooth in maxilla (6).

mandibular hypoplasia with narrow right condylar process, deepening of the right sigmoid notch, pseudoelongation of the ipsilateral condylar neck, thinner ramus and body, widened inferior alveolar canal, and enlarged mental foramen. Deep notching of gonial angle, narrowing of glenoid fossa, and presence of a supernumerary tooth in right maxillary third molar region were other findings (Figure 1(c)). An incision biopsy from the posterior mandibular lesion which microscopically revealed interlacing bundles of spindle shaped cells with wavy nuclei, delicate collagen fibres, plump fibroblasts, and a strong positive reaction with *S-100* (detection system, HRP polymer) confirmed the diagnosis of simple neurofibroma (Figures 2(a) and 2(b)).

Systemic examination revealed presence of multiple hyperpigmented macules, axillary freckling, and Lisch nodules (Figures 2(c), 2(d), and 2(e)). Patient had short height for her age and macrocephaly but no cutaneous neurofibromas. Examination revealed that her father and grandmother suffered from NF1 (Figure 2(f)). Based on family history and clinical and radiographic findings, NF1 was diagnosed.

As the patient was in an active growth period and had no alarming symptoms, conservative excision of the overlying tumor was done and the first molar was left in situ to erupt. Periodic OPGs revealed that the first molar erupted and the follicle of third molar appeared (Figures 3(a), 3(b), and 3(c)). However, the facial asymmetry and periauricular swelling were persistent. A 3D CT (bright speed 16 slice CT, GE Healthcare) of the mandible was done which revealed an irregular lytic lesion in the alveolar process of right side of mandible extending from lateral incisor to retromolar trigone (Figures 4(a) and 4(b)). An additional small bony defect was seen in the outer cortex of ramus of mandible. This apparent foramen was perhaps due to lytic erosion of the mandibular outer cortex (Figures 4(c) and 4(d)). There was associated lytic expansion of the alveolar margin of right maxilla at level of second molar and floor of right maxillary sinus. Presence of rudimentary supernumerary tooth was also confirmed. Right styloid process was rudimentary (2 mm) and right pterygopalatine fissure was widened (Figure 4(e)). There was persistent metopic suture in the frontal bone. There was also presence of sutural diastasis (12 mm defect of right occipitomastoid suture) (Figure 4(f)). MRI (Signa 1.5 T, Optima GE Healthcare) of the neck with mandible was performed with fat saturated postcontrast spin echo T1 weighted (T1W) and turbo spin echo T2 weighted (T2W) sequence to reevaluate the true extent of the lesion. The lesion had caused expansion of the lateral wall of the right maxillary sinus and alveolar margin of right maxilla and mandible extending from lateral incisor to retromolar area (Figure 5(a)). The lesion was isointense on T1W, hypointense on T2W with mild contrast enhancement on postgadolinium scans suggestive of fibrosis and residual tumor. Ill-defined increased T2W signal intensity and enhancement were seen in right TMJ, right temporal fossa, right infratemporal fossa, right parotid gland, right malar, and preauricular region of face indicating extraosseous infiltration (Figures 5(b) and 5(f)). Right external auditory meatus and canal were hypoplastic with thickened walls (Figures 5(c) and 5(d)).

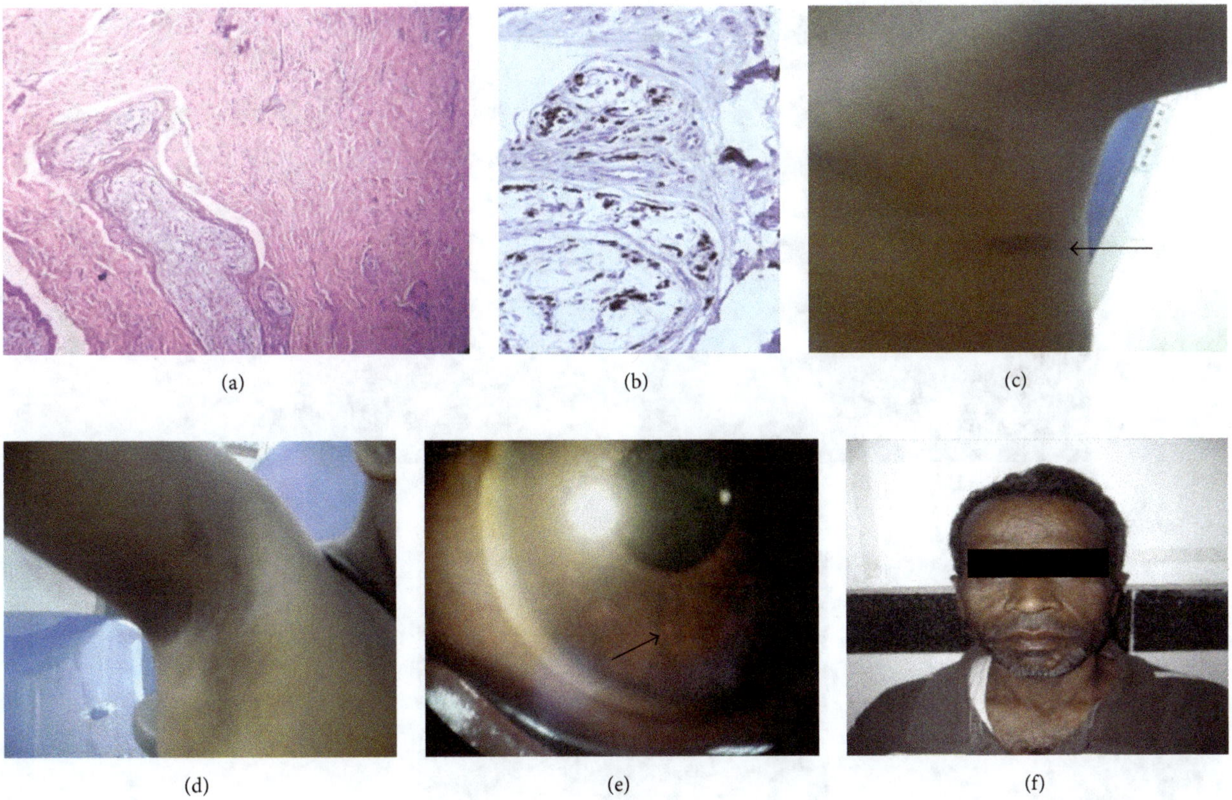

FIGURE 2: (a) Microsection showing bundles of wavy spindle cells with serpentine nuclei in fascicles (H&E, ×10x), (b) Strong S-100 positivity of tumor cells (×40x), (c) café au lait macule (arrow) in the back, (d) axillary freckle, (e) Lisch nodule (arrow) in slit lamp examination, and (f) father of patient with multiple cutaneous neurofibromas.

There was thinning and decreased bulk of right masticatory muscles suggesting *hypoplasia* (Figure 5(e)). Mucosal thickening and narrowing of right maxillary antrum and adenoid hypertrophy were associated findings. A repeat ENT evaluation was nonsubstantiative.

Due to lack of radiological evidence of malignant transformation or any functional impairment, patient has been put on a periodic follow-up till date and is being closely monitored.

3. Discussion

NF1 is a multisystem disorder that arises from mutation in the NF1 gene located on human chromosome 17q11.2 and encodes a protein neurofibromin [1, 2].

According to the National Institute of Health Consensus Development Conference, the diagnosis of NF1 is based on the presence of two or more of its seven diagnostic criteria [5]. Present case was confirmed as NF1 by presence of family history, numerous café au lait spots in the face and trunk, Lisch nodules, and axillary freckling under the arm.

Intraoral involvement includes the presence of neurofibromas usually affecting soft tissues like tongue, gingiva, palate, cheek, and floor of the mouth [2, 3]. Hypo- or hyperplasia of the maxilla, mandible, zygoma, and TMJ has all been reported [1–4]. Mandibular alterations may be unilateral or bilateral and include enlarged mandibular and mental foramen, widened inferior alveolar canal, branching of mandibular canal, hyperostosis, deepened sigmoid notch, elongated condylar neck, rarefied condylar and coronoid process, medial concavity in mandibular ramus, decreased or flat gonial angle, irregular inferior cortex, and cyst like lesions [1–4, 6]. Maxillary involvement may result in asymmetric maxillary sinuses, expansion of maxillary ridge, hemifacial hyperplasia, and so forth [7]. Neurofibromas of the gingivodentoalveolar complex particularly may cause displacement or impaction of the erupting permanent teeth [4]. Many of the above findings, multifocal neurofibromas in mandible and maxilla and musculoskeletal defects including *hypoplasia of the masticatory muscles* in the present case, were all revealed by CT and MRI. As a recently recognized function of neurofibromin in muscle formation, skeletal muscle deficiency might be a feature of NF1. In fact it is suggested that muscular weakness may contribute to the bone phenotype in NF1 [8]. In 90% children with NF1, NF presents with high frequency of hyperintense signal appearance on T2W and low signal intensity on TIW on MRI, as seen in present case. MRI with gadolinium enhancement is valuable as it offers superior soft tissue contrast and detailed imaging [9].

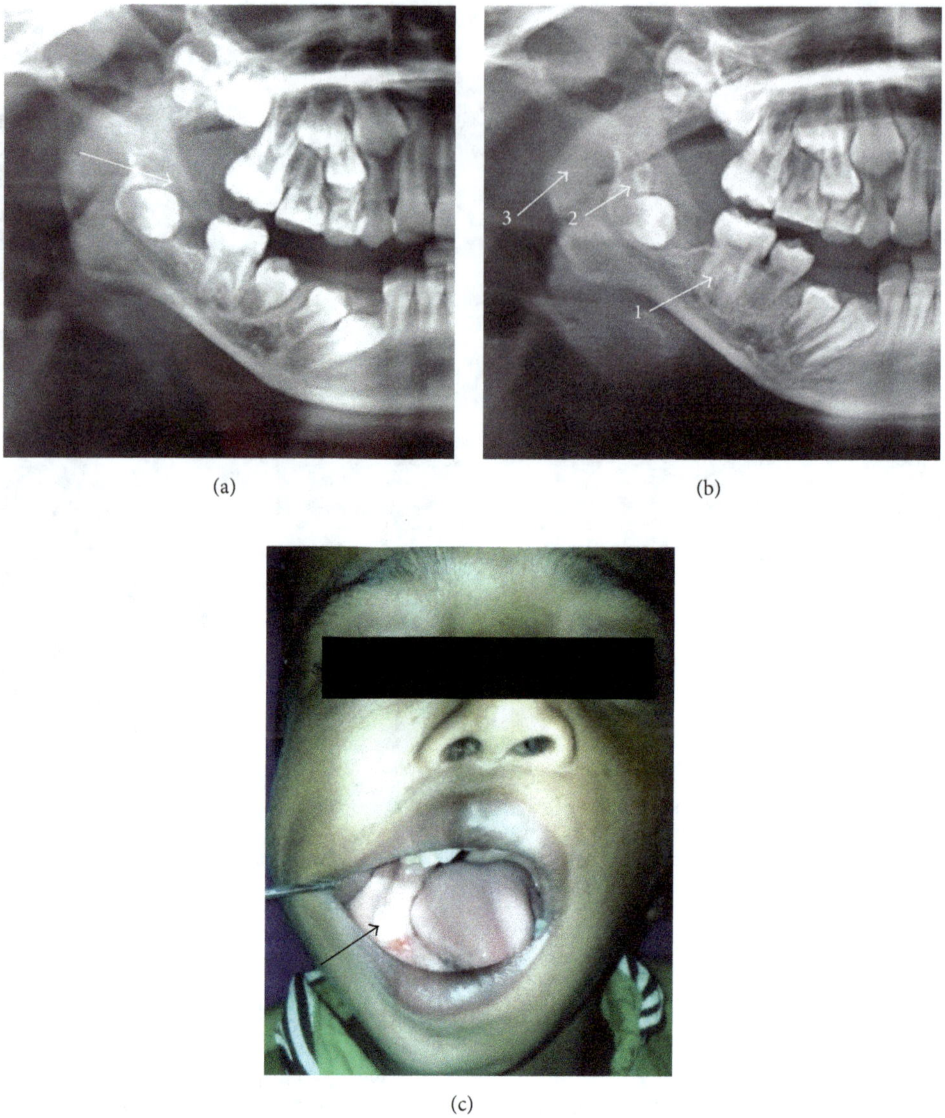

FIGURE 3: (a) One-year follow-up OPG shows reduced tumor size (arrow), (b) OPG after 1 year and 8 months shows erupted first molar (1), appearance of follicle of third molar (2) and presence of residual tumor (3), and (c) intraoral view after 1 year and 8 months shows fully erupted first molar (arrow).

Neurofibromas of head and neck may arise form cranial nerves like the trigeminal nerve (TGN), uncommonly the facial nerve, glossopharyngeal nerve, or upper cervical nerves [9, 10]. Location of the lesion dictates clinical symptoms and presentation. Upper cervical nerve involvement involves scalp, skull base, posterior auricular area, and so forth and causes massive expansion of these sites [9]. TGN root involvement in posterior fossa would present with intradural tumors, and the gasserian ganglion involvement in middle cranial fossa would present with extra dural mass apart from symptoms of continuous facial pain, facial paresthesia, numbness, and so forth. There would also be associated radiographic signs of erosion of petrous bone, displacement of carotid artery, and so on [11, 12]. Involvement of peripheral branches of TGN is more common. Upper TGN NF involves orbit, upper eyelid, and upper part of face, medial TGN tumor involves mid face and upper alveolus, and lower TGN involves jaws and lower alveolar region [9–11]. In our case due to multifocal involvement of the jaws, preauricular area, parotid, and TMJ and due to osteolytic enlargement of the mandibular canal, there is a possibility that the tumor has originated from medial and lower branches (inferior alveolar nerve) of TGN and facial nerve [10]. However, origin from TGN with extraosseous infiltration is more likely as facial nerve involvement was not identified on CT and MRI. In fact, hypoplastic right external auditory meatus and canal

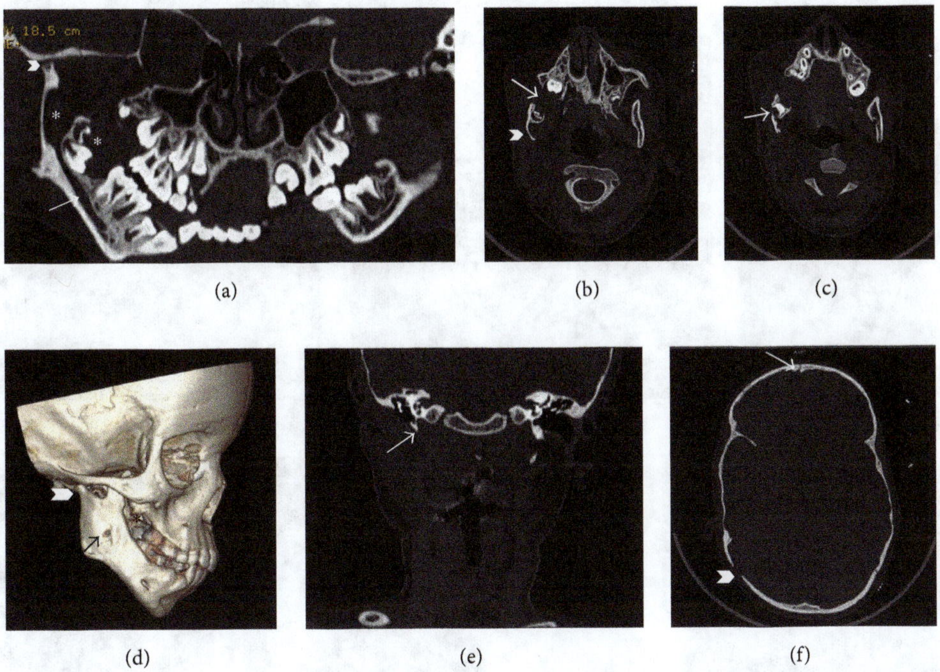

FIGURE 4: (a) *Panoramic dental scan* depicting enlarged inferior alveolar canal (arrow) with residual tumor mass (asterisk) and hypoplastic condylar process (chevron), (b) *axial CT* in bone window showing the residual mass in alveolar margins of maxilla and mandible (arrow) and concavity of mandibular ramus (chevron), (c) *axial CT scan* showing apparent foramen (arrow) due to lytic erosion of mandibular cortex, (d) *3D CT scan* image showing hypoplastic condylar process (chevron), apparent foramen (arrow), and tumor in maxillary alveolus (asterisk), (e) *coronal CT* image showing rudimentary styloid process of right side (arrow), and (f) *axial CT* image of sutural diastasis (chevron) and persistent metopic suture (arrow).

are attributed to developmental defects associated with NF1 [1].

D'Ambrosio et al. in a systematic clinicoradiographic study of 38 NF patients found head and neck manifestations in 92% of the subjects. They objectively defined the radiographic findings and highlighted the periodic monitoring of patients for oral and radiographic development [1]. Sigillo detected orofacial manifestations in all his paediatric cases of NF1 utilising OPG, CT, and MRI [6]. But only one other case of multifocal NF involving the mandible, maxilla, and orbit has been reported till date apart from the present one [3].

Plexiform NF is highly suggestive but not pathognomonic of NF1 [13]. Present case lacked the gross fusiform nerve expansion and "bag of worm" appearance as well as multiple fascicular arrangements of tortuous nerves histopathologically, which is characteristic of plexiform NF [9]. It was in fact a simple disseminated NF with multifocal involvement in the head and neck [4].

Management of NF1 requires periodic monitoring after baseline evaluation and carefully noticing the changes in consecutive visits to rule out onset of complications like malignant transformation that occurs in 6–29% of cases [1–4]. The indications of the latter feature are sudden increase in swelling, paresthesia, pain, and so forth. Radiographic findings of irregular widening of the canal, poorly circumscribed loss of jaw bone, and irregular loss of lamina dura around teeth raise the suspicion of malignancy in NF [4]. Also, plexiform NFs are associated with a higher rate of malignant transformation at 10–15% [9]. None of these alarming findings were present in our case to warrant surgery. In fact, age of patient at time of surgery influences the outcome. Tumors resected before 10 years of age recurred in 60% of cases compared to tumors resected after 10 years of age which showed a 30% recurrence [14]. So, it is prudent to delay surgery as long as possible in asymptomatic pediatric patients. Definitive management in our patient would need a combined surgical, orthodontic, and prosthodontic treatment which has to be delayed till the pubertal growth spurt has ended.

4. Conclusion

Periodic close surveillance is of utmost importance in management of a disease with unpredictable natural history and outcome as NF1. Present report of this rare case with multispectral radiological manifestations underlines the importance of imaging surveillance for the same.

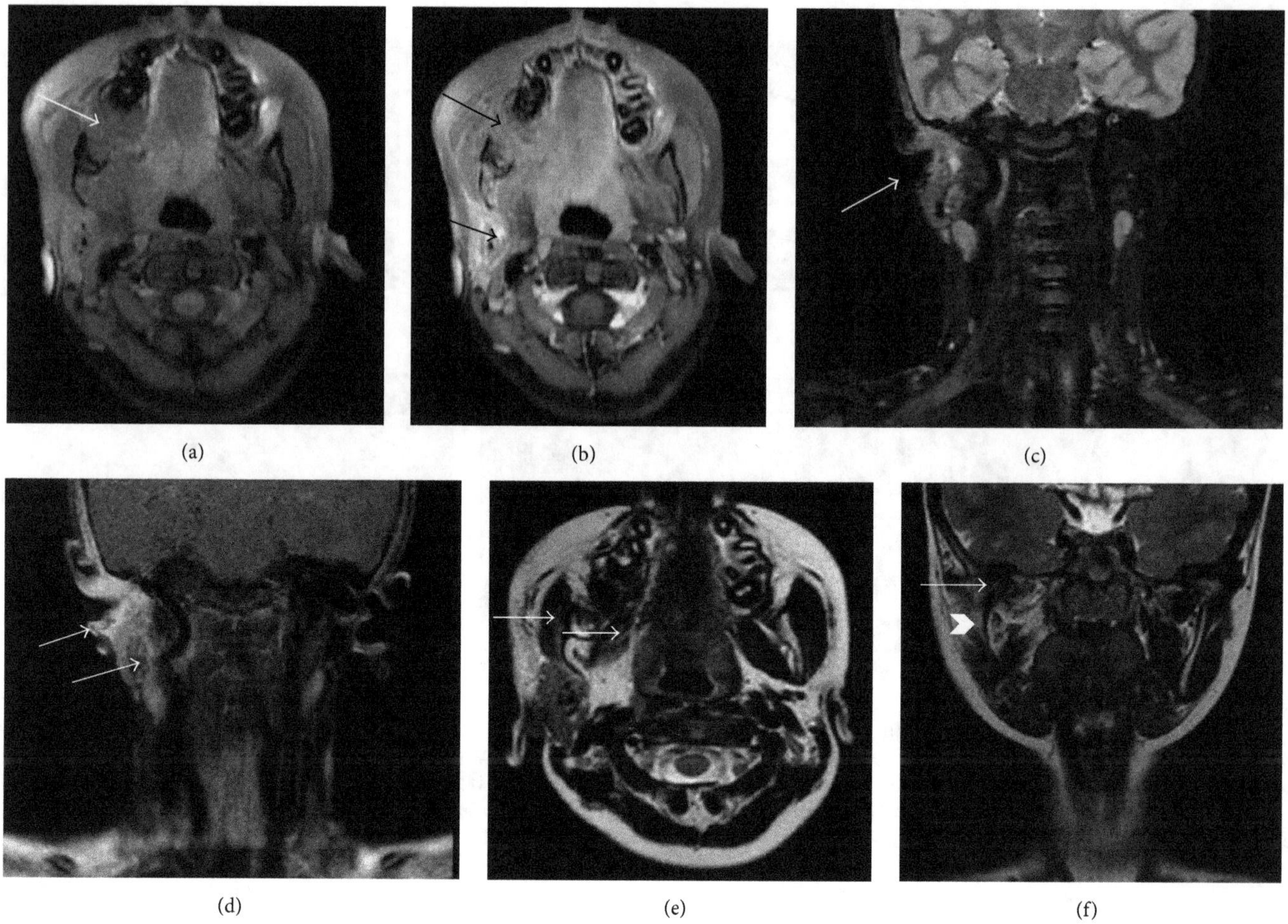

FIGURE 5: (a) *Precontrast T1W axial* image showing primary mass (arrow) in the alveolar process of maxilla and mandible with bony expansion, (b) *postcontrast T1W fat saturated axial* image showing enhancing intraosseous mass in maxilla and mandible, the parotid, and infratemporal fossa (arrows), (c) *coronal STIR* image showing narrow external auditory canal (arrow), (d) *coronal* postgadolinium image showing mass in infratemporal fossa, the parotid, and external auditory canal (arrows), (e) *axial T2W* image showing hypoplastic pterygoid and masseter muscles (arrows), and (f) *coronal T2W* image showing concave right mandibular ramus (chevron) and hypoplastic condyle with extension of mass into the TMJ (arrow).

References

[1] J. A. D'Ambrosio, R. P. Langlais, and R. S. Young, "Jaw and skull changes in neurofibromatosis," *Oral Surgery, Oral Medicine, Oral Pathology*, vol. 66, no. 3, pp. 391–396, 1988.

[2] S. D. Shapiro, K. Abramovitch, M. L. Van Dis et al., "Neurofibro matosis: oral and radiographic manifestations," *Oral Surgery, Oral Medicine, Oral Pathology*, vol. 58, no. 4, pp. 493–498, 1984.

[3] Z. Dalili and G. Adham, "Intraosseous neurofibroma and concurrent involvement of the mandible, maxilla and orbit: report of a case," *Iranian Journal of Radiology*, vol. 9, no. 1, pp. 236–240, 2012.

[4] N. Komerik, Z. Kirzioğlu, G. Ulu, and N. Kapucuoglu, "Neurofibroma of the mandible in a child with Neurofibromatosis Type 1," *Archives of Oral Sciences & Research*, vol. 1, no. 2, pp. 95–99, 2011.

[5] K. P. Boyd, B. R. Korf, and A. Theos, "Neurofibromatosis type 1," *Journal of the American Academy of Dermatology*, vol. 61, no. 1, pp. 1–14, 2009.

[6] R. Sigillo, H. Rivera, N. G. Nikitakis, and J. J. Sauk, "Neurofibromatosis type 1: a clinicopathological study of the orofacial manifestations in 6 pediatric patients," *Pediatric Dentistry*, vol. 24, no. 6, pp. 575–580, 2002.

[7] V. Visnapuu, S. Peltonen, T. Tammisalo, J. Peltonen, and R.-P. Happonen, "Radiographic findings in the jaws of patients with neurofibromatosis 1," *Journal of Oral and Maxillofacial Surgery*, vol. 70, no. 6, pp. 1351–1357, 2012.

[8] N. Kossler, S. Stricker, C. Rödelsperger et al., "Neurofibromin (Nf1) is required for skeletal muscle development," *Human Molecular Genetics*, vol. 20, no. 14, pp. 2697–2709, 2011.

[9] B. Y. Wang, D. Zagzag, and D. Nonaka, "Tumors of the nervous system," in *Surgical Pathology of the Head and Neck*, L. Barnes, Ed., pp. 669–773, Informa Healthcare, 2009.

[10] H. Papadopoulos, N. Zachariades, and A. P. Angelopoulos, "Neurofibroma of the mandible. Review of the literature and report of a case," *International Journal of Oral Surgery*, vol. 10, no. 4, pp. 293–297, 1981.

[11] W. G. Loutfy, D. E. Ryan, R. J. Toohill, and G. A. Meyer, "Trigeminal nerve neurofibroma: case report," *Journal of Oral and Maxillofacial Surgery*, vol. 48, no. 6, pp. 650–654, 1990.

[12] A. Gholkar, J. P. Stack, and I. Isherwood, "Case report: plexiform trigeminal neurofibroma," *Clinical Radiology*, vol. 39, no. 3, pp. 313–315, 1988.

[13] V. Lin, S. Daniel, and V. Forte, "Is a plexiform neurofibroma pathognomonic of neurofibromatosis type?" *Laryngoscope*, vol. 114, no. 8 I, pp. 1410–1414, 2004.

[14] M. T. Fadda, G. Verdino, M. C. Mustazza, D. Bartoli, and G. Iannetti, "Intra-parotid facial nerve multiple plexiform neurofibroma in patient with NF1," *International Journal of Pediatric Otorhinolaryngology*, vol. 72, no. 5, pp. 553–557, 2008.

48

CT and MR Unilateral Brain Features Secondary to Nonketotic Hyperglycemia Presenting as Hemichorea-Hemiballism

Víctor Manuel Suárez-Vega,[1] Carlos Sánchez Almaraz,[1] Ana Isabel Bernardo,[1] Ricardo Rodríguez-Díaz,[1] Ana Díez Barrio,[2] and Leticia Martín Gil[2]

[1]*Radiology Department, Hospital Infanta Elena, Valdemoro, 28342 Madrid, Spain*
[2]*Neurology Department, Hospital Infanta Elena, Valdemoro, 28342 Madrid, Spain*

Correspondence should be addressed to Víctor Manuel Suárez-Vega; vsuarezvega@gmail.com

Academic Editor: Atsushi Komemushi

Hemichorea-hemiballism is an unusual hyperkinetic movement disorder characterized by continuous involuntary movements of an entire limb or both limbs on one side of the body. The acute onset of this disorder occurs with an insult in contralateral basal ganglia. Ischemic events represent the most common cause. Nonketotic hyperglycemia comes in second place. Nonketotic hyperglycemic hemichorea-hemiballism (NHH) is a rare cause of unilateral brain abnormalities on imaging studies confined to basal ganglia (mainly putaminal region as well as caudate nucleus). Subtle hyperdensity in striatal region can be found on CT studies whereas brain MR imaging typically shows T1 hyperintensity and T2 hypointensity in the basal ganglia contralateral to the movements. Diagnosis is based on both glucose levels and neuroimaging findings. Elevated blood glucose and hemoglobin A1c levels occur with poorly controlled diabetes. In this case report, our aim is to present neuroimaging CT and MR unilateral findings in an elderly woman secondary to nonketotic hyperglycemia presenting as hemichorea-hemiballism.

1. Introduction

Hemichorea-hemiballism is an unusual hyperkinetic movement disorder characterized by continuous involuntary movements of an entire limb or both limbs on one side of the body. These movements are mostly irregular, variable in amplitude, and with no recognizable pattern [1].

Bedwell first described hemichorea-hemiballism associated with hyperglycemia in 1960. He reported the case of a 57-year-old woman with hemiballism that resolved as the blood glucose levels were normalized [2].

It was Yahikozawa et al. who first reported 3 diabetic patients with the unique combination of hemiballism and striatal hyperintensity on T1-weighted MRI as a new syndrome in 1994 [3].

NHH is most frequently reported in elderly patients, typically Asian, who have type II diabetes. The majority of cases published in the literature involve female patients [4]. Although this syndrome usually occurs in patients with previously known diabetes, it could also be an initial manifestation of diabetes [5].

2. Case Presentation

A 57-year-old female patient from East Europe was admitted in the emergency room of our institution with chest pain. Her serum glucose and hemoglobin A1c levels were 800 mg/dL and 15.9%, respectively. There were no ketones in the serum. Serum glucose was treated by insulin continuous perfusion and the patient was discharged.

A few hours later, she was readmitted presenting involuntary and violent movements on the left side of the body.

An unenhanced cranial CT was performed to rule out an ischemic event. Findings were initially misdiagnosed, reporting hypoattenuation of left basal ganglia instead of considering an abnormal increased attenuation on right basal

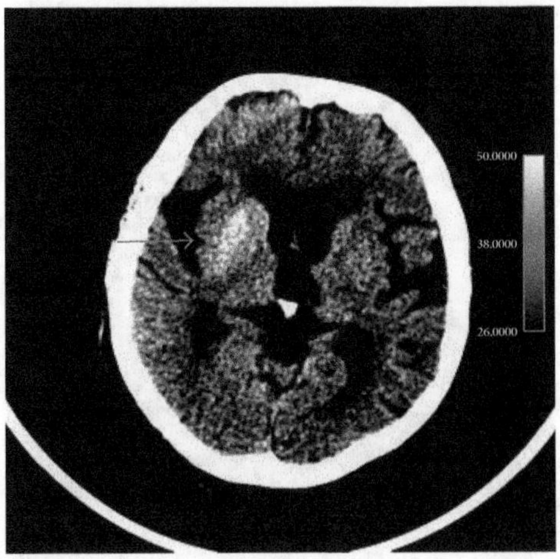

FIGURE 1: Findings: unenhanced axial brain CT depicts hyperdense striatum (caudate nucleus and putamen). This finding is better seen using narrow window width and higher center settings.

ganglia. Using narrow window width and slightly higher center settings better depicted this finding (Figure 1).

As correction of hyperglycemia did not lead to improvement of the involuntary movements, the patient was admitted in the Intensive Care Unit and an aggressive intravenous therapy was performed. Initially, risperidone up to 2 mg/dL and a continuous perfusion of clonazepam was administrated, with no response. Further treatment with tetrabenazine 25 mg twice a day was necessary for improvement of the movements in the next few days.

MR imaging of the brain was performed 2 days after the second admission showing right basal ganglia hyperintensity on T1-weighted sequences and fairly normal signal intensity on T2-weighted and FLAIR sequences (Figure 2). The apparent diffusion coefficients (ADCs) were slightly lower in right basal ganglia compared to those on the left side. ADC values were symmetrical on both basal ganglia (Figure 3).

One month later—movement disorders completely recovered—the patient was reimagined, depicting a striking increase on T1-weighted signal intensity, whereas the signal intensity of the rest of the sequences was within normal limits (Figure 4).

Both MR studies performed with one month difference did not show any abnormality within right striatum on T2 gradient echo sequences (Figure 5). However, a 10-month follow-up MR scan showed hypointensity within right striatum on susceptibility weighted images (SWI) (Figure 6).

Several follow-up MR studies have been performed with an elapsed time of 4 months and 10 months. Whereas the 4-month follow-up study still depicted right basal ganglia hyperintensity, the 10-month MR study finally confirmed a total regression of signal abnormalities, showing a normal appearance right striatum. No signs of striatum atrophy were shown (Figure 7).

3. Discussion

The underlying pathophysiology of imaging changes described in NHH is poorly understood.

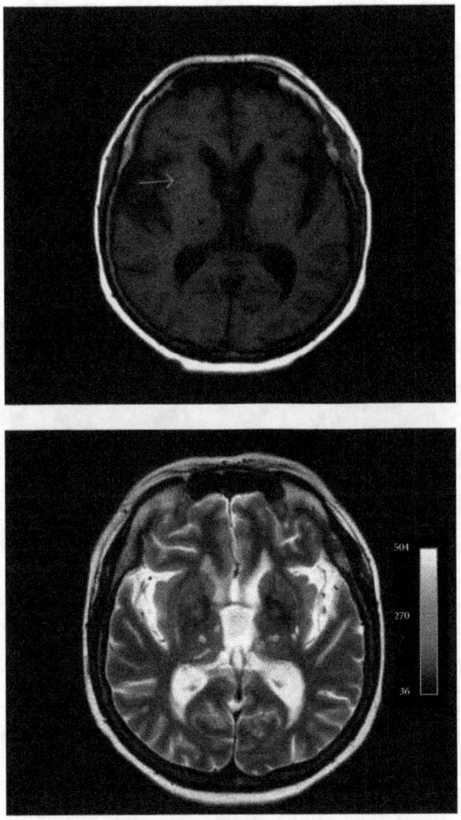

FIGURE 2: Axial T1-weighted sequence depicts right basal ganglia hyperintensity with unremarkable signal abnormality on axial T2-weighted.

Some mechanisms include blood hyperviscosity caused by hyperglycemia, leading to blood brain barrier disruption; increased sensitivity of dopaminergic receptors in postmenopausal period, remember female predominance; decreased gamma-aminobutyric acid (GABA) in striatum secondary to a nonketotic state.

In addition, acute infarct, petechial hemorrhage, myelinolysis, and calcium deposition have also been postulated [6, 7]. MR findings suggest that petechial hemorrhage is less plausible since if the high signal on T1 corresponds with methemoglobin it should also be high signal on T2. This is not reported in our case or in previous cases [7]. We could not find any alterations on T2 gradient echo images involving right striatum. However, the 10-month follow-up scan showed slightly hypointense signal within right striatum on SW images. To our knowledge, there is only one series of three cases describing SWI findings in NHH syndrome [8]. These authors explain T1 hyperintensity from the protein hydration layer inside the cytoplasm of swollen gemistocytes appearing after an acute cerebral injury. These astrocytes also express metallothionein with zinc, which is thought to be the cause of asymmetric hypointensity of the posterior putamen on SWI.

Other authors suggest that high T1 signal could be related to manganese accumulation on gemistocytes [9].

The differential diagnosis of conditions presenting with hemichorea includes ischemic or hemorrhagic stroke, vasculitis, central nervous system lupus, mass lesions,

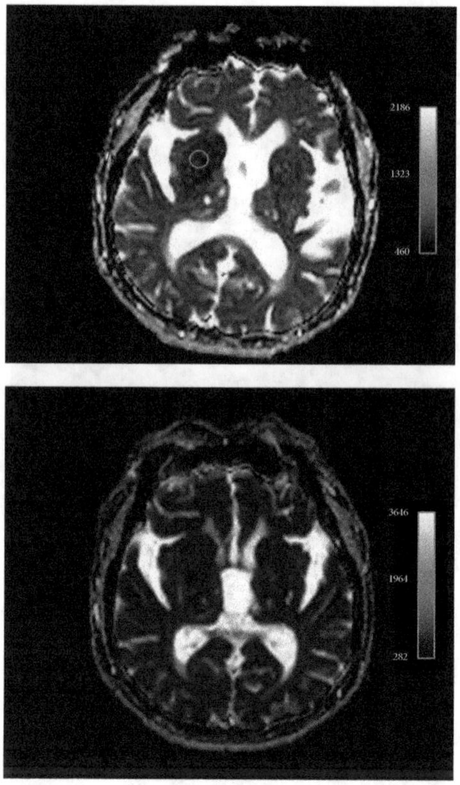

FIGURE 3: ADC map shows slight decreased apparent diffusion coefficient in right basal ganglia. Symmetrical normal ADC values one month later.

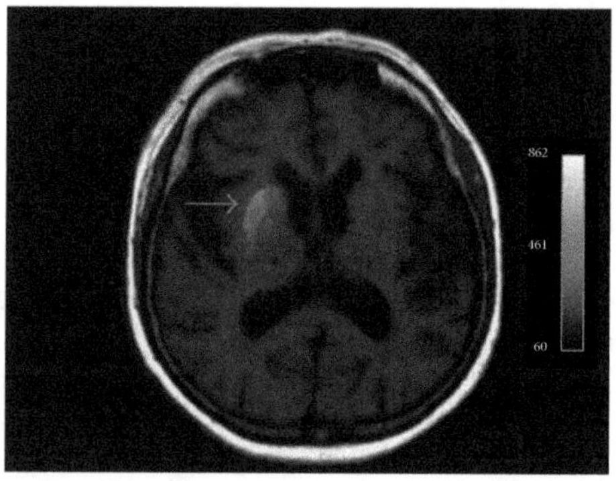

FIGURE 4: Striking increase of T1-weighted signal intensity within right striatum one month after the onset of symptoms. Patient was asymptomatic when this MR study was performed.

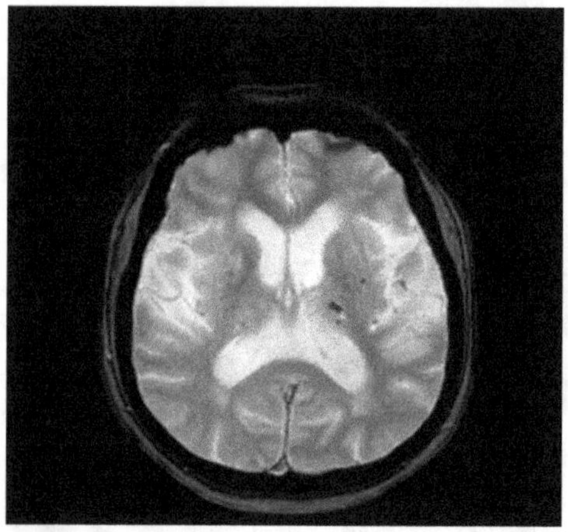

FIGURE 5: Axial T2 gradient echo sequence shows no signal abnormality within right striatum but some scattered blooming artifacts within left thalami consistent with petechial hemorrhages.

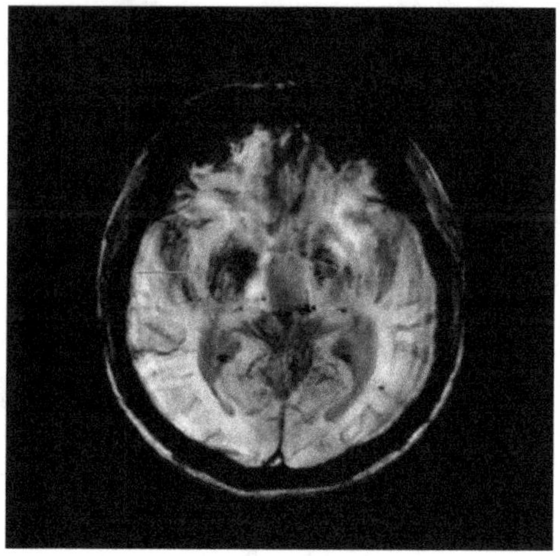

FIGURE 6: Axial minimum intensity projection of susceptibility weighted imaging at 10-month follow-up depicts slightly hypointense signal within right striatum.

multiple sclerosis, thyrotoxicosis, and drugs (such as neuroleptics or levodopa) [10].

However, clinical history and laboratory tests with striking increase of glucose levels make all these diagnoses unlikely.

Other causes to increased T1 signal in the basal ganglia are hypertensive hemorrhages, basal ganglia calcifications, Tay-Sachs disease, and tuberous sclerosis. A lenticulostriate isolated ischemic stroke can lead to a mismatch effect of false high signal on putaminal region.

Other metabolic or toxic disorders showing T1 signal increase include chronic hepatic encephalopathy, the most frequent, manganese toxicity during long-term parenteral nutrition, postcardiac arrest encephalopathy, hypoglycemic coma, hypothyroidism, neurofibromatosis, Fahr disease, Wilson disease, and carbon monoxide poisoning. In all these conditions a bilateral and symmetrical involvement is usually present [11].

Clinical course in patients with NHH is usually favorable and symptoms tend to resolve spontaneously within normalization of glucose levels. In addition, striatal high signal intensity may show resolution within a variable period of 2–11 months. In our case, T1 findings showed not only persistency but also increase of the signal whereas the other sequences partially resolved. We may emphasize that a period of 1 month separated both studies. Further follow-up studies confirmed resolution of findings in a period of 10 months, as reported previously in the literature.

One possible explanation could be acute putaminal dysfunction, secondary to hyperglycemic or hyperosmolar insult. This functional alteration could be associated with

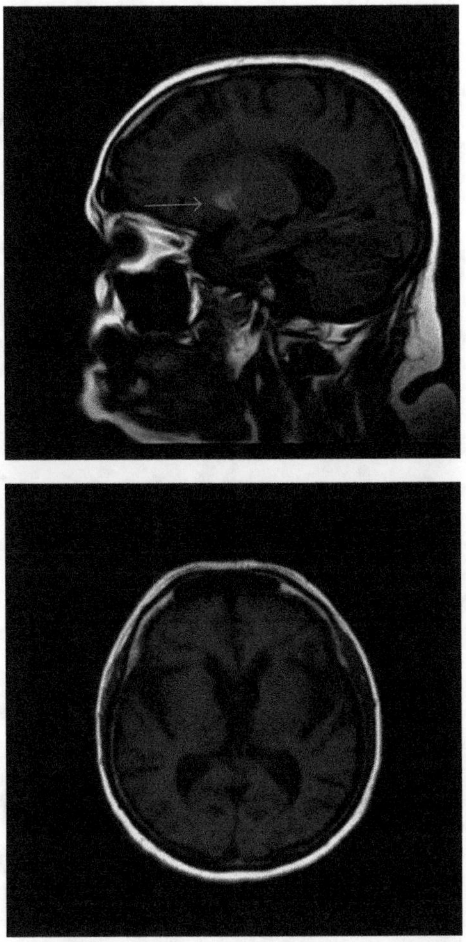

FIGURE 7: 4-month and 10-month follow-up MR studies. Sagittal T1 depicts persistent hyperintensity within right striatum (green arrow), whereas a 10-month follow-up MR shows complete regression of signal abnormalities.

some degree of Wallerian degeneration of the internal white matter of the putamen. Protein desiccation occurring in the course of Wallerian degeneration could explain the CT hyperattenuation and the MR and DW imaging patterns in the early phase, as well as the variable evolution of imaging features with time [12]. In our patient, no signs of atrophy affecting right striatum were found in follow-up studies after the disappearance of high intensity signals on T1 sequences. This might be explained by the early improvement in hemichorea-hemiballism, as suggested by the meta-analysis of Oh et al. [4].

In addition, we were not able to find an explanation for the increased signal on T1 sequences after one month onset. Some studies with larger number of cases report an increased T1 signal on follow-up MR scans compared to baseline CT images, with a posterior resolution of MR abnormalities [11].

4. Conclusion

NHH is a unique clinical-radiological entity with peculiar CT and MRI findings.

An early recognition is mandatory in order to establish the correct therapy (normalization of glucose levels) and avoid unnecessary treatments.

References

[1] R. B. Postuma and A. E. Lang, "Hemiballism: revisiting a classic disorder," *The Lancet Neurology*, vol. 2, no. 11, pp. 661–668, 2003.

[2] S. F. Bedwell, "Some observations on hemiballismus," *Neurology*, vol. 10, no. 6, pp. 619–622, 1960.

[3] H. Yahikozawa, N. Hanyu, K. Yamamoto et al., "Hemiballism with striatal hyperintensity on T1-weighted MRI in diabetic patients: a unique syndrome," *Journal of the Neurological Sciences*, vol. 124, no. 2, pp. 208–214, 1994.

[4] S.-H. Oh, K.-Y. Lee, J.-H. Im, and M.-S. Lee, "Chorea associated with non-ketotic hyperglycemia and hyperintensity basal ganglia lesion on T1-weighted brain MRI studya meta-analysis of 53 cases including four present cases," *Journal of the Neurological Sciences*, vol. 200, no. 1-2, pp. 57–62, 2002.

[5] J. J. Lin, G. Y. Lin, C. Shih, and W. C. Shen, "Presentation of striatal hyperintensity on T1-weighted MRI in patients with hemiballism-hemichorea caused by non-ketotic hyperglycemia: report of seven new cases and a review of literature," *Journal of Neurology*, vol. 248, no. 9, pp. 750–755, 2001.

[6] S. Ohara, S. Nakagawa, K. Tabata, and T. Hashimoto, "Hemiballism with hyperglycemia and striatal T1-MRI hyperintensity: an autopsy report," *Movement Disorders*, vol. 16, no. 3, pp. 521–525, 2001.

[7] D.-E. Shan, D. M. T. Ho, C. Chang, H.-C. Pan, and M. M. H. Teng, "Hemichorea-hemiballism: an explanation for MR signal changes," *American Journal of Neuroradiology*, vol. 19, no. 5, pp. 863–870, 1998.

[8] A. Cherian, B. Thomas, N. N. Baheti, T. Chemmanam, and C. Kesavadas, "Concepts and controversies in nonketotic hyperglycemia-induced hemichorea: further evidence from susceptibility-weighted MR imaging," *Journal of Magnetic Resonance Imaging*, vol. 29, no. 3, pp. 699–703, 2009.

[9] M. Fujioka, T. Taoka, Y. Matsuo et al., "Magnetic resonance imaging shows delayed ischemic striatal neurodegeneration," *Annals of Neurology*, vol. 54, no. 6, pp. 732–747, 2003.

[10] J. S. Hawley and W. J. Weiner, "Hemiballismus: current concepts and review," *Parkinsonism and Related Disorders*, vol. 18, no. 2, pp. 125–129, 2012.

[11] P.-H. Lai, R. D. Tien, M.-H. Chang et al., "Chorea-ballismus with nonketotic hyperglycemia in primary diabetes mellitus," *American Journal of Neuroradiology*, vol. 17, no. 6, pp. 1057–1064, 1996.

[12] M. Wintermark, N. J. Fischbein, P. Mukherjee, E. L. Yuh, and W. P. Dillon, "Unilateral putaminal CT, MR, and diffusion abnormalities secondary to nonketotic hyperglycemia in the setting of acute neurologic symptoms mimicking stroke," *American Journal of Neuroradiology*, vol. 25, no. 6, pp. 975–976, 2004.

New Insights about Pulmonary Epithelioid Hemangioendothelioma: Two Case Reports

Romeu Duarte Mesquita,[1] Marta Sousa,[1] Carmen Trinidad,[2] Eugénia Pinto,[3] and Iosu Antón Badiola[4]

[1]*Department of Radiology, Centro Hospitalar de Entre o Douro e Vouga, Santa Maria da Feira, Portugal*
[2]*Department of Radiology, Hospital Povisa, Vigo, Spain*
[3]*Department of Pathology, Centro Hospitalar de Lisboa Central, Lisboa, Portugal*
[4]*Department of Pathology, Hospital Povisa, Vigo, Spain*

Correspondence should be addressed to Romeu Duarte Mesquita; romeu.mesquita@gmail.com

Academic Editor: Suayib Yalcin

Pulmonary epithelioid hemangioendothelioma (PEH) is a rare neoplasm of vascular origin. There are three different major imaging patterns identified in thoracic manifestation of epithelioid hemangioendothelioma: (1) multiple pulmonary nodules; (2) multiple pulmonary reticulonodular opacities; and (3) diffuse infiltrative pleural thickening. Radiographically, presence of bilateral multiple nodules is the most common pattern of presentation. The diagnosis is made on the basis of histopathological findings and confirmed by positive immunohistochemistry staining. Although the prognostic factors for PEH have not yet been well established, a better prognosis is usually associated with the multinodular pattern. We report two different imagological presentations of this rare disease, based on two institutional experiences, along with a review of the relevant literature.

1. Introduction

Pulmonary epithelioid hemangioendothelioma (PEH) is a rare neoplasm of vascular origin. It is a low-to-intermediate grade malignant tumor, of borderline malignancy and a clinical course usually between hemangioma and angiosarcoma. Unfortunately, there is no clear definition of malignant PEH. The term "epithelioid hemangioendothelioma" was first introduced by Weiss et al. as a soft tissue vascular tumor of borderline malignancy [1].

However, the lesion was originally described in 1975 by Dail et al. as an "intravascular bronchoalveolar tumor," initially believed to be an aggressive form of the bronchoalveolar cell carcinoma [2].

Epithelioid hemangioendothelioma (EH) is classified as a vascular tumor because the neoplastic cells have characteristics in common with normal, nonneoplastic endothelial cells [3]. EH can behave in a locally aggressive fashion, with metastases being rare [4].

Corrin et al., using immunohistochemical techniques, demonstrated the presence of malignant cells deriving from a lineage capable of differentiation along endothelial lines [5]. Subsequently, Weldon-Linne et al., using electron microscopy, confirmed these results and revealed diffuse cytoplasmic staining of the tumor cells with a factor VIII-related antigen [6].

Histologic characteristics of EH include epithelioid cells with abundant eosinophilic cytoplasm in a fibromyxoid stroma, some of them with intracytoplasmic vacuoles, having a signet ring-like appearance. These features can, however, be also found in primary adenocarcinoma, mesothelioma, and large-cell lymphoma, so immunohistochemical analyses, especially those for the endothelial markers, are a mainstay [7–10].

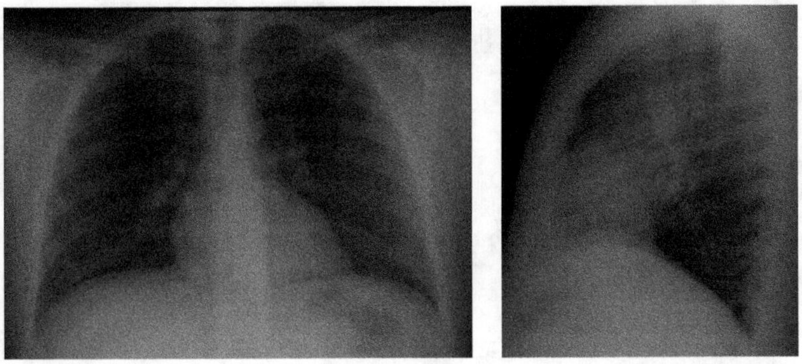

(a) (b)

FIGURE 1: Posteroanterior (a) and lateral (b) chest X-rays. The chest radiography showed a diffuse nodular pulmonary pattern in both lungs.

The 2015 WHO Classification of Tumors of the Lung, Pleura, Thymus and Heart [11] recently published, with numerous important changes from the 2004 WHO classification, has a significant change involving recognition of usefulness of *WWTR1-CAMTA1* fusions in diagnosis of pulmonary EH. The new information regarding this tumor is recognition of a translocation involving the *WWTR1* and *CAMTA1* genes and prognostic factors [12].

This update was based on the recent recognition that a recurrent t(1;3)(p36.3;q25) chromosomal translocation is characteristic of EH. Additionally, the genes involved in the EH translocation were identified, namely, WWTR1 (or TAZ) and CAMTA1, resulting in a transcription factor, WWTR1-CAMTA1 fusion protein. Also significant is the lack of CAMTA1 and WWTR1 rearrangements in *epithelioid hemangioma*, a benign vascular tumor that can be misdiagnosed as EH [13–17].

Tanas et al. [18] suggest that the *WWTR1/CAMTA1* gene fusion plays a pivot role in the tumor biology and can act as a transcription factor that ultimately may represent a therapeutic target for EH-specific drugs. Recently, Antonescu et al. [19, 20] report a novel subset of EH occurring in a specific group of young adults, where they found a distinct phenotype with YAP1-TFE3 fusions but similar morphologic features. Although further studies [21] confirm these results others question the utility of immunohistochemical YAP1-TFE3 fusion detection [7, 14].

Another hypothesis for the pathogenesis of this neoplasm, reported in the literature, mentions a possible causal relationship between chronic *Bartonella* infection and the development of this rare vascular tumor in immunocompetent patients [22].

Some authors also believe in a hormonal potential significance in this disease because the greater incidence is observed in women; also, hormone receptor expression has been reported in the literature [23, 24] and a recent case report describes recurrence of EH during pregnancy [25].

All these data highlight the current emerging development about the knowledge concerning biochemical and clinical behaviour of EH in general and PEH in particular and can lead to greater understanding of the molecular pathways in the tumor and great advances in potential therapies.

EH remains, however, a little-understood disease and one of the main reasons for that is the fact that the prevalence of EH is reported to be less than one in 1 million [26].

2. Case 1

A 35-year-old male, nonsmoker, without symptoms and with no prior history of lung diseases had a routine chest radiograph that showed alterations. His past medical history was not significant, without occupational exposures or family history of clinical relevance. The physical examination was unremarkable. Chest X-ray demonstrated the presence of a diffuse and bilateral micronodular infiltrate (Figure 1).

Serum levels of neoplastic markers and angiotensin converting enzyme were within normal values. The pulmonary function tests were also in the normal range. The bronchoscopy performed with bronchoalveolar lavage, brushing, and transbronchial biopsies were nondiagnostic. Chest high resolution (HR) computed tomography (CT) scan showed multiple, bilateral small pulmonary nodules (with diameters inferior to 10 mm) (Figure 2).

These nodules were present in all pulmonary lobes and adjacent to bronchioles and medium/small vessels. There were no enlarged lymph nodes, pleural effusion, or other relevant pulmonary changes. Abdominal and pelvic CT revealed no malignant lesions (Figure 3).

Radiological skeletal study also showed no bone involvement. Surgical lung biopsy was performed and histological examination of the nodules revealed epithelioid cells with eosinophilic cytoplasm and intracytoplasmic vacuolization. On immunohistochemical studies, the tumor cells were immunoreactive to CD34 and negative for cytokeratin (Figure 4).

Because the progression was slow, follow-up was suggested. In agreement with his decision, close follow-up with chest CT was planned.

He still has no symptoms and has survived for 48 months following the initial diagnosis.

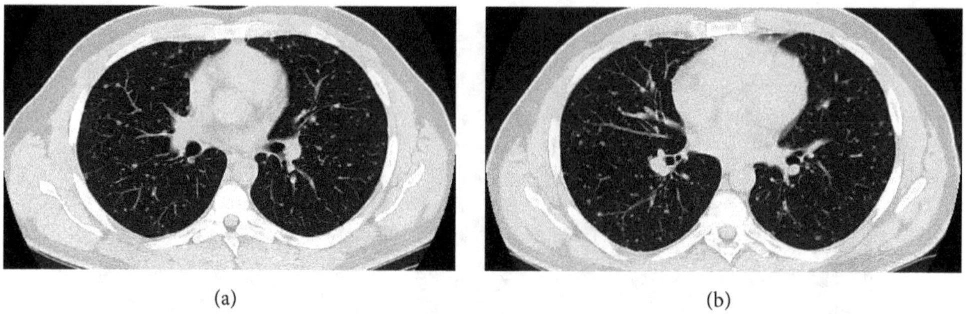

FIGURE 2: Chest CT (a and b). Multislice chest CT-images on lung window showed innumerable, well-defined, small, round, and noncalcified pulmonary nodular opacities, scattered in both lungs. These nodules were present in all pulmonary lobes and adjacent to bronchioles and medium/small vessels.

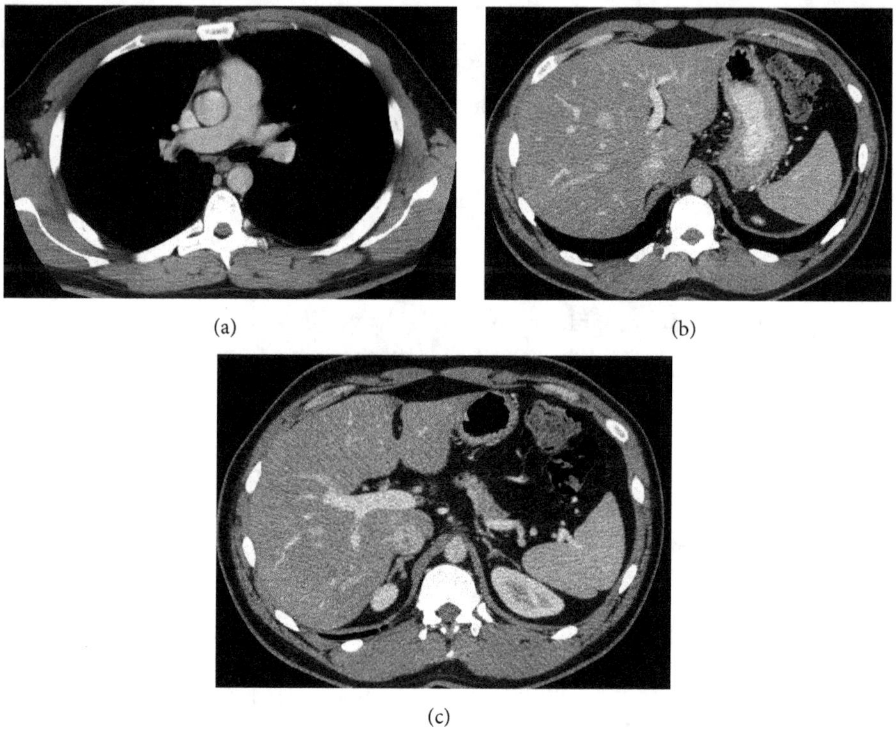

FIGURE 3: Contrast-enhanced multislice CT of the chest (a) on mediastinal window showed no thoracic lymphadenopathy. Multislice abdominopelvic CT scans (b and c) with intravenous contrast administration showed no significant findings, excluding focal liver or splenic lesions.

3. Case 2

A 67-year-old woman, nonsmoker, presented in the emergency department with a complaint of mild productive cough for 2 months with hematic sputum in the last 24 hours. She also reported progressive left-sided dorsal pain over 1-month duration. Her past medical history revealed a previous diagnosis of deep vein thrombosis in 2012. In a routine chest radiograph made 2 years previously, it was hard to depict any pulmonary pathology (Figure 5).

Her family history was unremarkable. There were no other specific abnormalities on physical examination. The laboratory findings were within normal range. Chest X-ray demonstrated the presence of a poorly defined opacity in the left lower lung and a blunt costophrenic angle in the left side (Figure 6).

Spirometry showed forced vital capacity (FVC) of 1.59 (69.1%), forced expiratory volume in 1 second (FEV1) of 1.16 (60.7%), FEV1/FVC of 76%, and diffusing capacity divided by the alveolar volume (DLCO/VA) of 103.3%. Extensive pulmonary workup for pulmonary nodules including bronchoscopy, bronchoalveolar lavage (BAL), and transbronchial lung biopsy was completed. Results were negative for infectious or rheumatologic processes. The transbronchial biopsy

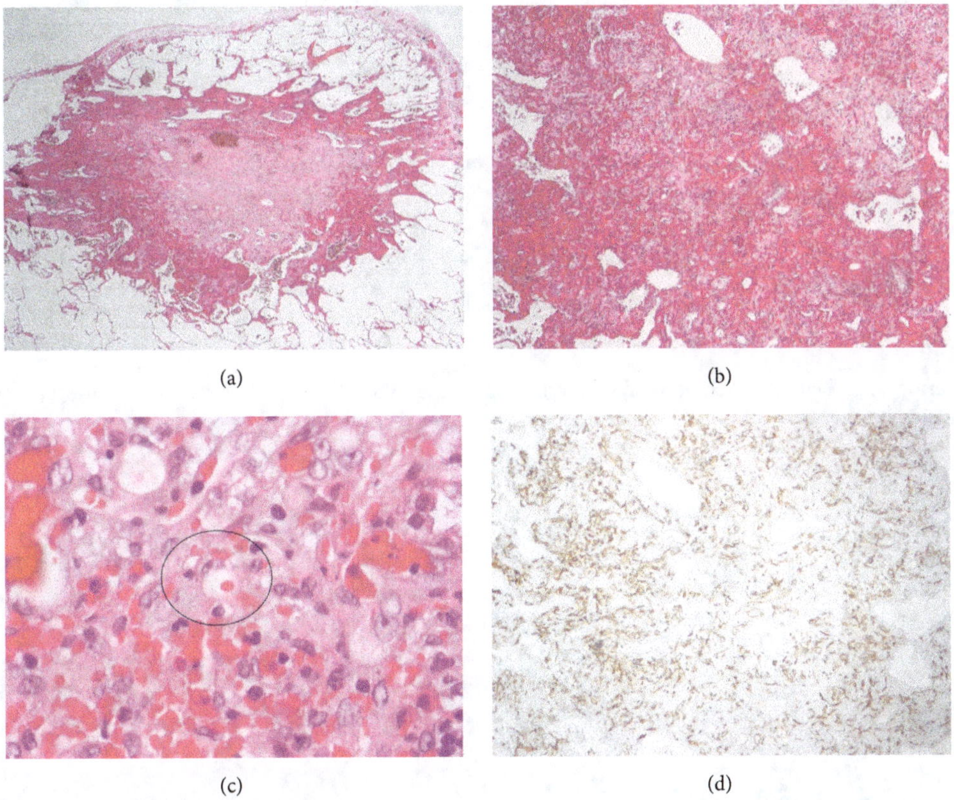

FIGURE 4: Histopathologic findings of hemangioendothelioma. (a) Low magnification of the specimen obtained from pulmonary wedge resection reveals a subpleural nodule that extends to adjacent alveoli, with vascular proliferation in the peripheral zone and areas of recent and old hemorrhage. (b) Neoplastic nodule showing tumor cells with an eosinophilic stroma at the periphery. The lesion contains blood filled spaces and respiratory epithelium "trapped" within the lesion is also shown. (c) Higher magnification of the tumor reveals vacuolation of some of the tumor cells, representing primitive angiogenesis. One of these epithelioid cells can be observed with intracytoplasmic lumen and an erythrocyte inside, indicating their vascular nature. (d) Immunostaining for CD34 revealed positivity of the neoplastic cells (brown colour), confirming the endothelial lineage of the tumor.

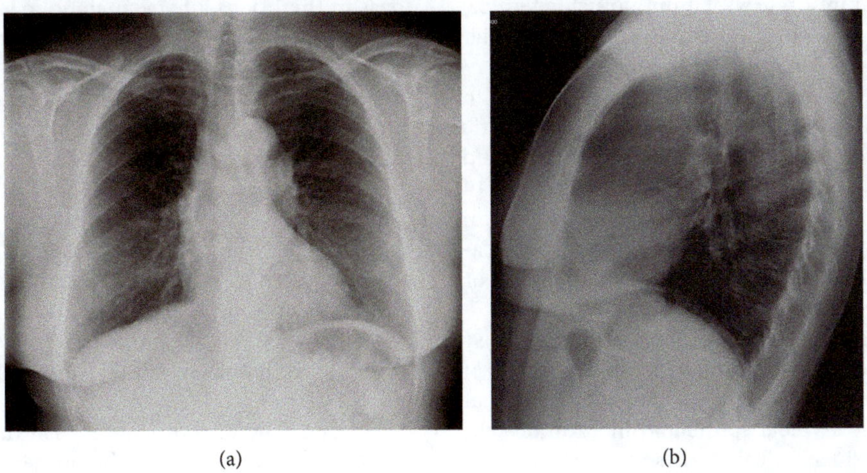

FIGURE 5: Posteroanterior (a) and lateral (b) chest X-rays. In a routine chest radiography 2 years before presentation in the ER it was difficult to detect the lesion in the left lower lung.

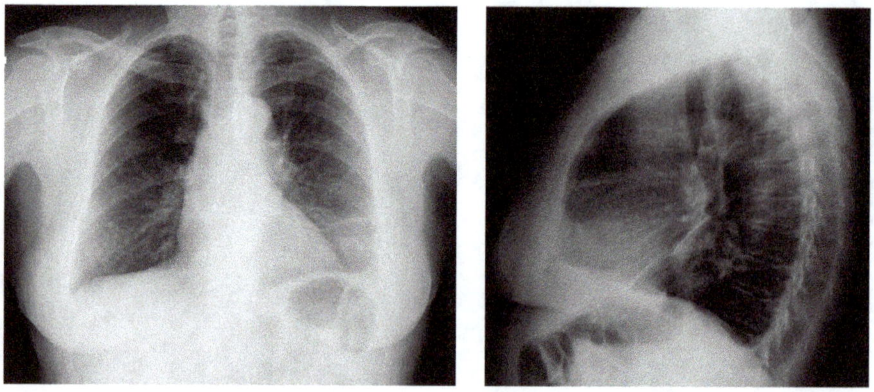

(a) (b)

Figure 6: Posteroanterior (a) and lateral (b) chest X-rays. The chest radiography showed a peripheral lesion in the left lower lung and a small volume of pleural effusion on the same side.

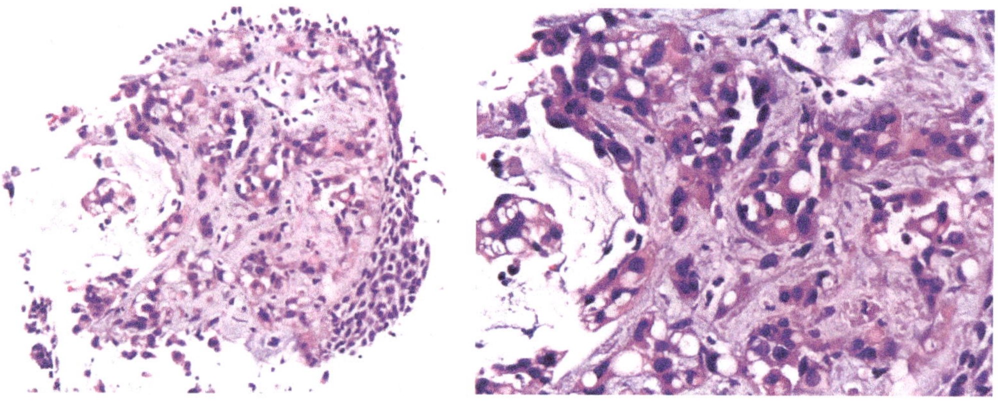

(a) (b)

Figure 7: Transbronchial biopsy of a pulmonary mass (H-E). (a) 10x. (b) 20x. Vascular proliferation and endothelial cells, frequently with citoplasmatic vacuolization, in a fibromyxoid stroma, with bronchial surface epithelial lining.

showed atypical cellular infiltrate with immunohistochemical expression very suggestive of proliferative lesion of vascular origin (Figure 7).

A chest CT scan revealed the presence of a lung mass in the parenchyma of the left inferior lobe (LIL), with necrotic component and in contact with the parietal pleura and diaphragmatic pleura, with associated partial atelectasis of the same lobe and coexisting multiple nodules scattered in both lungs (Figure 8); a single hilar ipsilateral lymphadenopathy was identified and no mediastinal lymphadenopathy or significant pleural effusion were present at presentation.

Patient underwent a first chest CT-guided lung biopsy that revealed intense fibrosis and focal changes suggestive of proliferative vascular lesion. She repeated the lung biopsy that showed the presence of atypical epithelioid-like tumor cells (Figure 9). Immunohistochemical studies were positive for CD31, CD34, and factor VIII. These results were consistent with the diagnosis of PEH.

She underwent a FDG PET/CT (not shown) that showed areas of increased uptake of FDG, including the pulmonary mass in the LIL as a hypermetabolic lesion and the left hilar lymphadenopathy. There was no abnormal FDG uptake in the small pulmonary nodules

One thoracic magnetic resonance (MR) with paramagnetic contrast, done two months later, demonstrated a left pleural effusion but did not show unequivocal abnormal pleural enhancement compatible with pleural metastases (Figure 10).

Three months later, under general anaesthesia, the surgeons performed a wedge resection by thoracotomy that also revealed multiple small pleural implants, both in visceral and in parietal pleural lesions, which were biopsied. Tumor specimens acquired showed pathological features of EH.

After a scheduled oncology visit the patient began treatment with six cycles of chemotherapy with carboplatin/paclitaxel, which changed to doxorubicin/cyclophosphamide.

Another chest CT, three months after the initial CT, showed rapid progression of the disease depicted by increase in number of the pulmonary nodules and the pleural lesions.

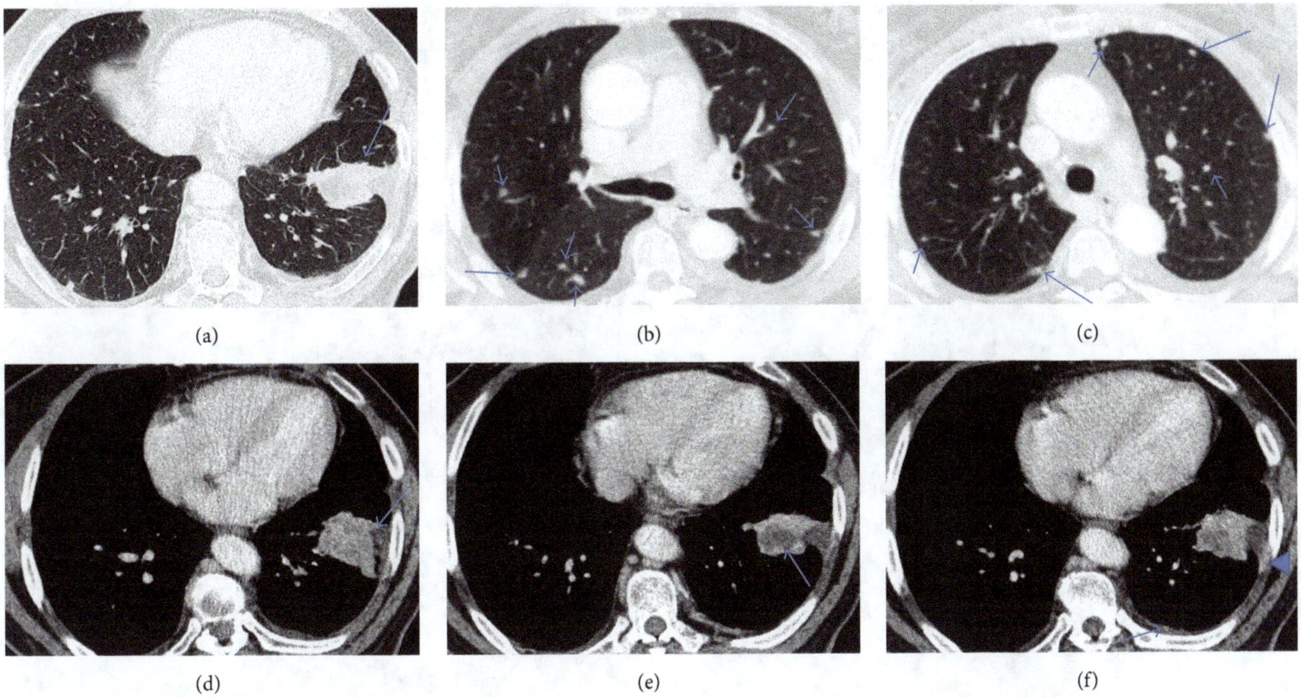

FIGURE 8: Chest CT. Multislice chest CT-images on lung window (a, b, and c) showed a lung mass with irregular borders (a); they also showed multiple small, round, and noncalcified pulmonary nodular opacities, scattered in both lungs (b and c). On mediastinal window (d, e, and f) it is possible to better identify the pleural invasion (d) and the necrotic areas in lesion (e), retrospectively, and valorization is hard when the exam was performed, and we can recognize areas of enhancement in the left pleura, more nodular (arrow) or linear (arrowhead) (f).

Also, showing increment in diameter, the splenic nodular lesions were compatible with metastases (Figure 11).

The patient returned to emergency department, seven months after the first visit, with progressive dyspnea.

A chest CT made at this time showed advance disease with a new lesion appearing in the contralateral pulmonary parenchymal and growth of the primary lesion in the left lung, illustrating the aggressive behaviour of the disease. The pulmonary nodules, however, did not show significant increment in size despite the completely different evolution seen in the lesion of the lower left lung (Figure 12).

Unlike this, the spleen showed an increase in number and size of the nodular lesions in his parenchyma. Although we did not have pathologic confirmation, because the patient did not have any other primary neoplastic lesion, these features reinforce the probable diagnosis of metastases from the PEH (Figure 13).

Upon her readmission, 2 weeks later, the patient succumbed to her condition due to respiratory failure.

4. Discussion

Using the International Hemangioendothioma, Epithelioid Hemangioendothelioma, and Related Vascular Disorders (HEARD) Registry, an Internet database with data of 206 patients, Lau et al. [15] found that the most commonly affected organs were liver and lung, and single organ involvement occurred in more than 60% of patients. The most common presentations were liver alone (21%), liver plus lung (18%), lung alone (12%), and bone alone (14%).

There is still no characteristic clinical or biological marker for PEH. PEH typically occurs among young patients and is more common in women than in men and many patients are asymptomatic at presentation, so it is often an incidental finding on imaging studies. Other possible symptoms can be minor or nonspecific pulmonary symptoms, such as chest pain, effort dyspnea, cough, and sputum [8, 14, 26–32]. There are sporadic reported cases of atypical symptoms related to unusual clinical course and/or extraordinary aggressiveness [33].

The prognosis is very variable, with survival ranging from less than one year up to 30 years [34]. Slow progression or growth for long periods and spontaneous regression may occur, especially in asymptomatic patients [27]. According to Lau et al. analysis, the 5-year overall survival is 73% [15]. The mortality for lung disease, with a minimum of follow-up of 4 years, was reported to be 65% [1].

The prognostic factors for PEH have not yet been well established. Pulmonary symptoms and, specially, pleural hemorrhagic effusions and hemoptysis are generally considered the worst prognostic factors [28]. Symptomatic patients and presence of pleural effusion were found to be independent predictors of survival. Other significant risk factors for PEH are male gender, presence of cough, chest pain, multiple unilateral nodules, metastases to more than one site, and lymph node metastases [26].

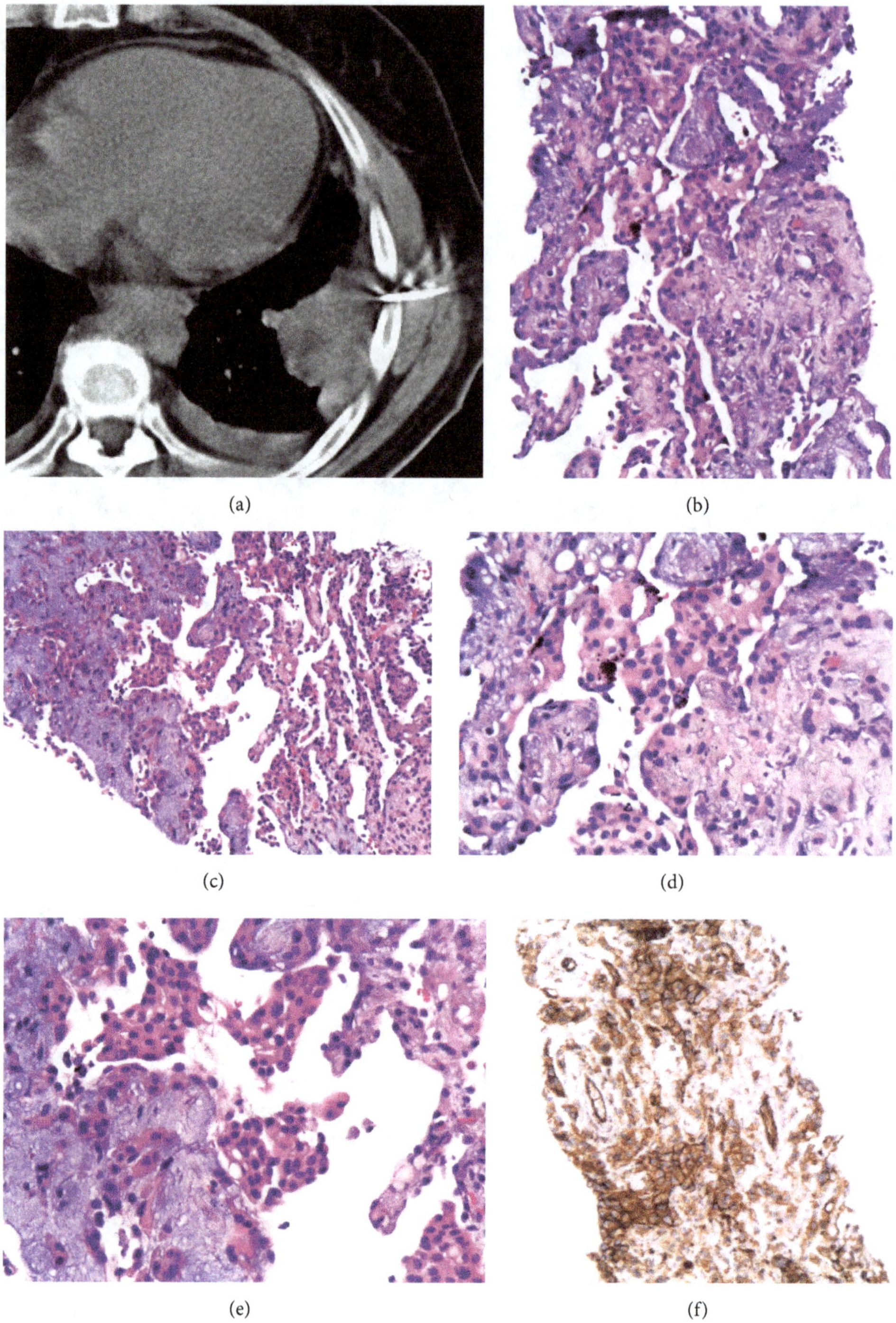

FIGURE 9: 20 G Tru-Cut biopsy of the lung mass (a). H-E (b–e) images show vascular proliferation with epithelioid cells in a fibromyxoid stroma and presence of haemosiderophages ((b, c) 10x; (d) 20x). Some of the epithelioid cells show vacuolation (e). Immunostaining for CD31 revealed positivity of the neoplastic cells (brown colour), confirming the endothelial lineage of the tumor.

Another study using cases from International HEARD Support Group found that although concurrent multiorgan involvement is common at the time of diagnosis, no specific organ or combination of organ involvement differentially affected survival, and there were no differences in patient's survival with single versus multiple organ involvement in their cohort [15]. They also confirmed that hemoptysis and pleural effusion or other signs of uncontained tumor growth have prognostic value and involve worse survival. These authors also categorized the patients into two different patterns of disease at presentation (A and B) based on presence or absence of lesions with discrete/defined borders, with

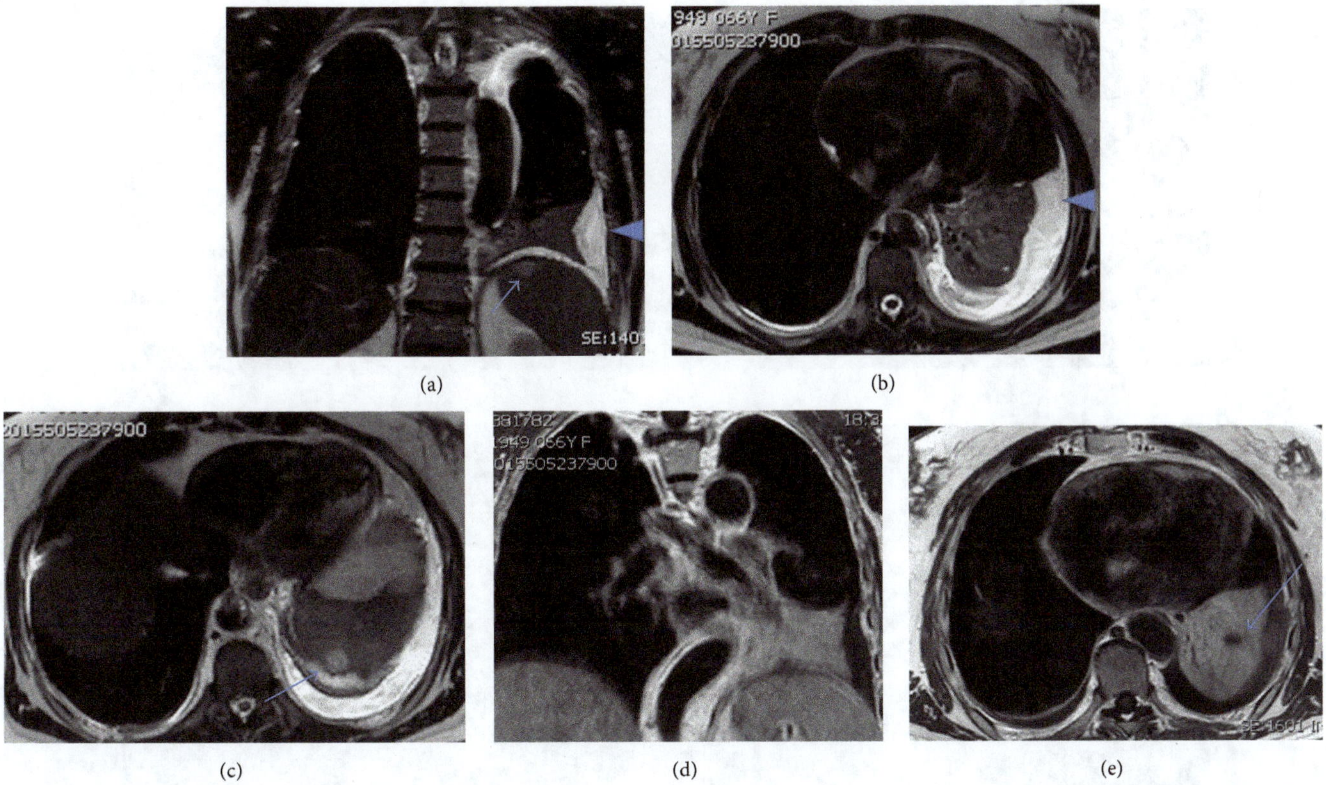

Figure 10: Thoracic MR images. Fluid sensitive sequences (a–c) show the presence of left pleural effusion (arrowhead) and also the nodular lesions in the spleen, which do not correspond to cysts (arrows). T1 weighted images with contrast (d and e) show the pulmonary mass and hypodense zones representing necrotic areas (arrow).

pattern B in the chest including pulmonary infiltrates, pleural effusion, extrapulmonary thoracic disease, and the symptom of hemoptysis and found a strong predictive prognostic value.

In terms of clinical features, it seems that the prognosis of PHE reflects primarily the vascular aggressiveness markers of hemorrhagic symptoms.

Although there are controversies regarding the multicentric or metastatic nature of EH, it can affect many organs simultaneously or sequentially, and lungs and liver are the two organs most frequently involved [15, 30, 35]. Although PEH is capable of producing regional and distant metastases, the metastases occur less frequently than in conventional angiosarcoma [26].

Dissemination of PEH can occur through blood vessels and lymphatics and within the pleural cavity [36]. Although rare, when the primary location is the lungs, distant metastases to the liver, skin, kidney, spleen, and retroperitoneum can occur and have been reported in the literature [2, 27, 28, 37–41]. Weiss et al. [1] reported that metastatic disease occurs in approximately 15% of patients with lesions affecting the lung.

Although it is unclear if the expression of CD44 has a major role in PEH invasiveness and metastases (because the number of patients tested is limited) Yi et al. [42] suggested the potential of intravascular invasion in a patient presenting with pulmonary thromboembolic disease and pulmonary hypertension.

Nevertheless, in patients with also hepatic involvement, knowledge of the CT manifestations in the liver may be helpful to narrow the differential diagnoses.

EH in the thorax can involve not just the lungs but also the pleurae and the mediastinum [14, 31, 43–45]. There are three major different patterns of CT findings identified in thoracic manifestation of EH [46–48]: (1) multiple pulmonary nodules; (2) multiple pulmonary reticulonodular opacities; and (3) diffuse infiltrative pleural thickening.

Radiographically, bilateral multiple nodular nodules are the most common presentation [27, 49]. The presence of multiple discrete pulmonary perivascular nodules with well- or ill-defined margins in both lungs on chest radiographs or CT is the characteristic finding. The nodules can range in size up to 3 cm, but most are less than 1 cm in diameter and are usually found in relation to small and medium-sized vessels and bronchi. This form of presentation may appear in many lung diseases and is easily mistaken for metastatic carcinoma, which is usually the initial radiologic interpretation [50]. However, little growth is shown on serial chest CT examinations [8, 50]. When this pattern is found the differential diagnosis list generally includes the following: pulmonary metastases, miliary granulomatous infection, sarcoidosis, silicosis, primary lung malignancy, and lymphangitic carcinomatosis.

There is a trend toward better prognosis for the multinodular pattern and the largest studies/reviews that assess

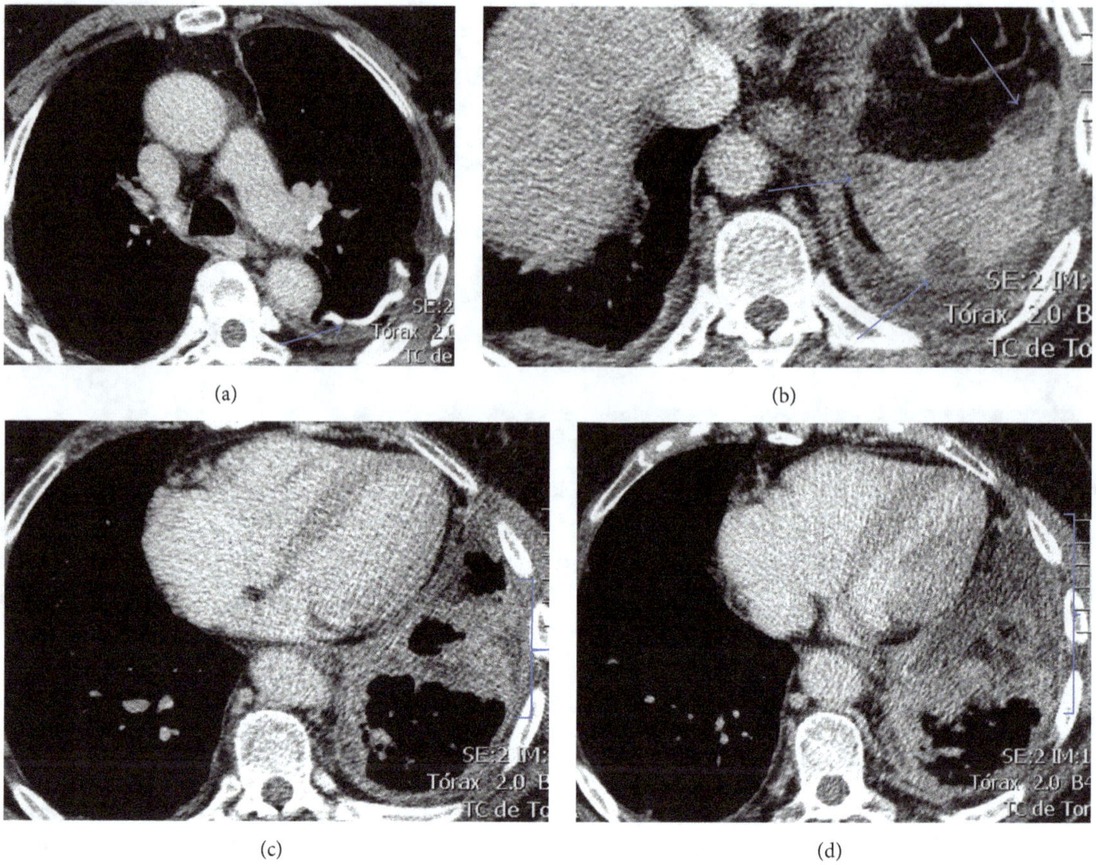

FIGURE 11: Chest CT. Multislice chest axial CT-images on mediastinal window show (a) signs of previous atypical wedge resection in the left lower lobe (arrow); (b) more nodular lesions in the spleen (arrows); (c and d) more pronounced and diffuse pleural invasion (brackets).

the relation between imaging features/different patterns and prognosis show that longer survival corresponds to the presence of multiple pulmonary nodules [26–28, 30, 32].

To the best of our knowledge, at least when the imaging pattern was specifically reported, all the cases that report complete/partial response or with spontaneous regression correspond to the multinodular pattern [1, 27, 34, 37, 51–61]

This issue is extremely important because, due to the heterogeneity of PEH, the specific imaging pattern from radiologic diagnosis may be a pivot step in the approach of the patient with PEH and ultimately can define the option about the treatment. Furthermore, perhaps the results about treatment efficacy cannot be compared when the lesions do not have homogeneous patterns.

Particularly interesting is the fact already described in other tumors not so distinct from PEH, like is the case of bronchioloalveolar carcinoma. In these tumors it is the clinical pattern and pathologic stage, and not the degree of invasion on histologic examination, that can predict survival [62].

Multiple pulmonary reticulonodular opacities represent, histopathologically, areas of infiltrating nodular proliferation of neoplastic cells within the lumina of small blood vessels and lymphatic vessels [26, 29, 47, 49]. In fact, in their study, Woo et al. [32] found a clinical significance in their similarity to pulmonary metastases in terms of prognosis, although just three patients had this pattern. This pattern may also suggest a more aggressive infiltrative growth into the lung interstitium, depicted histopathologically by infiltrative nodular proliferation of tumor cells within the vessel lumina [63, 64].

When the disease presents as diffuse infiltrative pleural thickening with associated pleural effusion, it can simulate malignant pleural mesothelioma or diffuse pleural carcinomatosis [16, 45, 65, 66].

An extra pattern can be added to the previous three identified ones, defined as parenchymal tumor with pleural invasion [32]. This pattern was previously described in some reports in the literature [27, 67–70] and Woo et al. described it in 4 patients. The major importance of this pattern relies on the fact that imaging features can greatly simulate the much more common primary non-small-cell lung tumor. Indeed, as was the case with all the four patients of Woo et al. study, also in one of our patients primary lung cancer with pleural seeding was the initial differential diagnosis.

Other unusual radiologic findings in sporadic cases are described in the literature, like irregular interstitial thickening and ground-glass opacities as the dominant feature, mimicking diffuse lung disease [63].

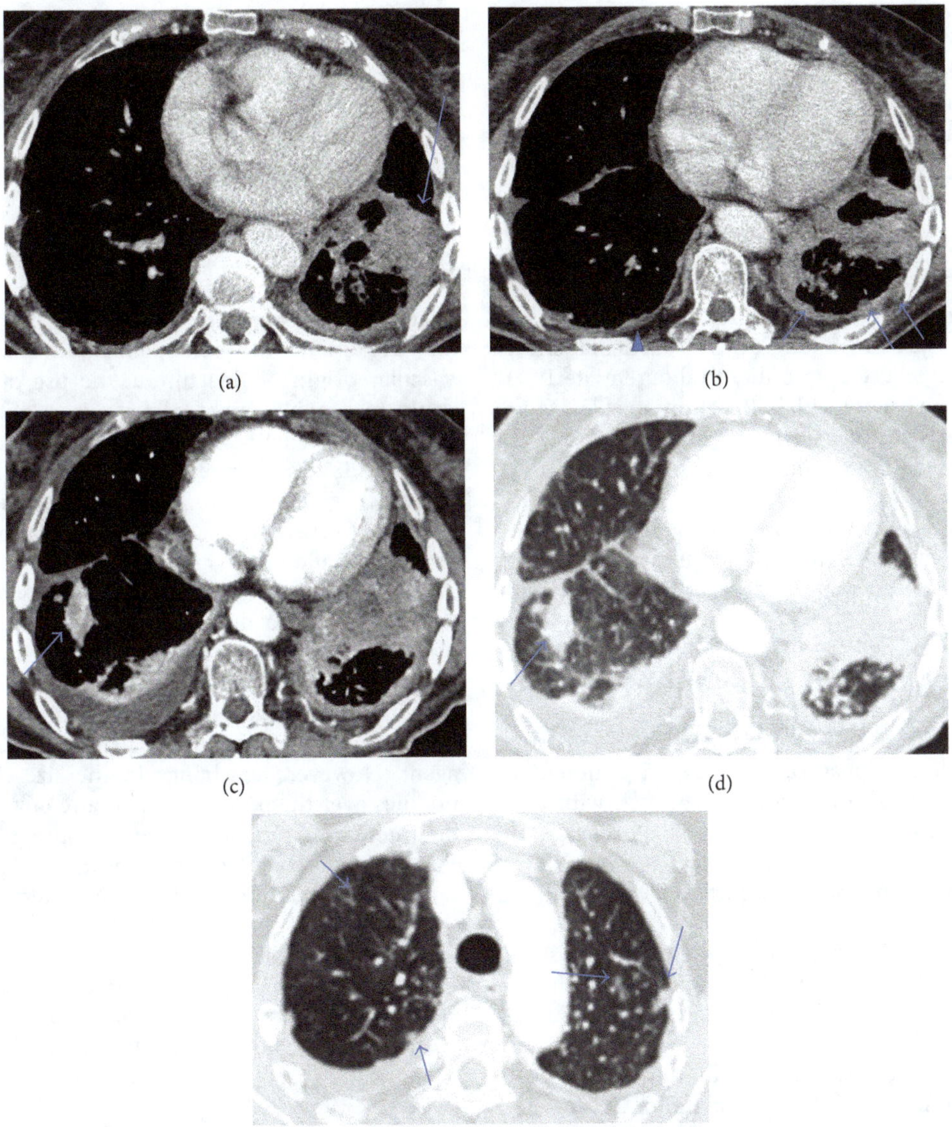

(a) (b) (c) (d) (e)

FIGURE 12: Chest CT. Multislice chest axial CT-images on mediastinal window (a, b, and c) show increase in size of the main lesion (a) and pleural metastases in the left side (arrows) and in contralateral side (arrowhead); a new lesion in the right lung is observed (arrow in (c)). Multislice chest axial CT-images on lung window (d and e) show the new contralateral lesion (arrow in (d)) and the parenchymal pulmonary nodules did not vary significantly in size from the previous studies (arrows in (e)).

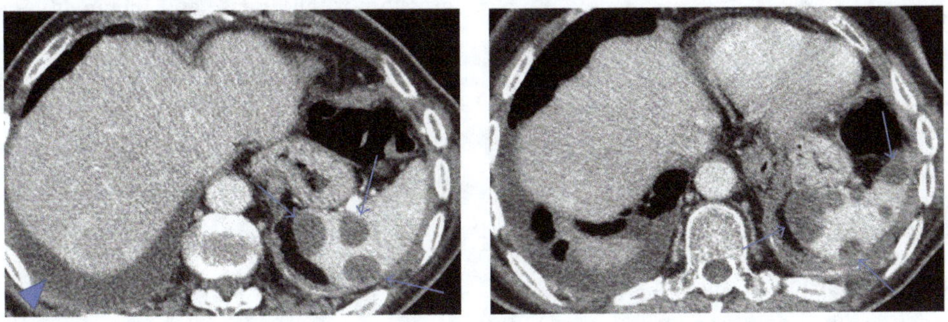

(a) (b)

FIGURE 13: Multislice chest CT. Axial images on mediastinal window at the pulmonary bases (a and b) show increase in size and number of the nodular spleen lesions (arrows). A pleural effusion in the right side is also apparent (arrowhead).

Although histologic calcifications are common, radiologic visible calcifications are rare. In long-standing cases or after treatment, extensive calcification of the nodules can be seen [67, 71].

PET/CT findings can demonstrate increased FDG-uptakes but usually are not a pivotal tool for the diagnosis, and a negative PET cannot exclude PEH [72, 73]. This false negative result is thought to be caused because of the small size of nodules, little FDG activity in the neoplasm, or low cellular density. Conversely, other studies show that FDG uptake may reflect the activation of PEH tumor cells, which is a sign of a poorer prognosis [74, 75]. One particular study demonstrated the PET/CT scan utility to differentiate PEH from amyloidosis in a patient with both conditions [73]. Most patients who underwent PET/CT in the study by Woo et al. [32] showed increased FDG uptake at the corresponding lung lesions on CT.

The most problematic pattern, undoubtedly, is the multinodular pattern where the lung nodules were 20 mm or less in diameter, decreasing the diagnostic accuracy and reliability of PET-CT.

Due to its rarity and heterogeneous mode of presentation, diagnosis of PEH can be really defiant. The diagnosis usually requires a lung biopsy, and histopathological samples are usually obtained from open-lung or thoracoscopic biopsy. Chest CT-guided lung biopsy can also be an option due to potential increased risk of bleeding associated with this vascular-like tumor or when the lesion is peripheral. A few reports report diagnosis made through bronchoscopy biopsies [8, 71, 76]. Fine needle aspiration can produce erroneous results [77].

The diagnosis is made on the basis of these histopathological features and confirmed by positive immunohistochemistry staining for vascular-endothelial markers, like CD31, CD34, and factor VIII [46].

Some histologic findings, like spindle tumor cells and fibrinous pleuritic lesion with extrapleural tumor cells proliferation, are linked to a worse prognosis [27, 28, 78]. Regarding correlation between the histopathological findings and prognosis Kitaichi et al. [27] found that fibrinofibrous pleuritic lesions with extrapleural proliferation of tumor cells and the presence of spindle tumor cells were the characteristics associated with worse prognosis. Interestingly, intravascular invasion and invasion of the visceral pleura by tumor cells without fibrinous pleuritis were observed in the two patients with spontaneous partial regression in their study.

In a more recent study, Anderson et al. [14], in 39 cases of EH with thoracic involvement, found that higher tumor grade and the presence of pleural involvement in lung and/or pleural tumors correlate with poor prognosis. They suggest that the reported criteria for classifying and grading malignant vascular tumors within soft tissue might be applicable to tumors in the thoracic cavity, including PEH.

There is no established standard treatment consensus for therapeutic regimens available, particularly owing to its borderline malignancy features and scarcity of cases [30, 79]. Spontaneous partial regressions are reported, particularly in asymptomatic patients, as we already reported [27]. Radiotherapy has proven to be ineffective for PEH because of the tumor's radiobiological characteristics, particularly the slow growth of tumor cells [37]. Surgery when tumor resection is feasible is usually considered the treatment of choice [80, 81]. However, a complete surgical resection is usually not feasible. Chemotherapy/immunostimulants in patients with disseminated disease and lung transplantation can also be an option [28, 58, 59, 61, 81–85]. Although there are a small number of reports about the effectiveness of chemotherapy, a general standard of chemotherapy is usually accepted for PEH [8]. Pinet et al. [82] reported a case of an aggressive form of pleural EH resulting in complete remission after treatment with carboplatin plus etoposide. Given the vascular origin of this tumor, the use of antiangiogenetic drugs reasonably might achieve good outcomes, including thalidomide, lenalidomide, and bevacizumab [61, 79, 84–86]. Ye et al. [58], in their review concerning chemotherapy and immunotherapy used in PEH, demonstrated a good partial response to chemotherapy with carboplatin, paclitaxel, bevacizumab, thalidomide, and α-interferon. In their study, these authors also described three patients with stabilization of the disease and a dramatic improvement in clinical status when treated with a combination regimen that included Endostar® or bevacizumab. This was the first report of the efficacy of Endostar, a recently introduced recombinant human endostatin, considered to be a valuable antiangiogenic agent. However, no change in the size of the pulmonary nodules over the period of chemotherapy was observed and treatment was unable to stop the progression of disease. Further studies of treatment are warranted to provide a better knowledge for different combination chemotherapies options to treat PEH.

Regular follow-up with no active therapy has been employed in asymptomatic patients, specifically in cases with diffuse lesions corresponding to multinodular pattern [2, 74, 87].

5. Conclusions

These two cases emphasise the large spectrum of presentation, clinical behaviour, and outcome of PHE.

Further investigations are essential to elucidate the progression of the disease and therapeutic options for patients with PEH.

Particularly, different imaging patterns of PHE need to be correlated with the recent molecular/genetic features identified, in order to confirm their prognostic value.

References

[1] S. W. Weiss, K. G. Ishak, D. H. Dail, D. E. Sweet, and F. M. Enzinger, "Epithelioid hemangioendothelioma and related lesions," *Semin Diagn Pathol*, vol. 3, no. 4, pp. 259–287, 1986, http://www.ncbi.nlm.nih.gov/pubmed/3303234.

[2] D. H. Dail, A. A. Liebow, J. T. Gmelich et al., "Intravascular, bronchiolar, and alveolar tumor of the lung (IVBAT): An analysis of twenty cases of a peculiar sclerosing endothelial tumor," *Cancer*, vol. 51, no. 3, pp. 452–464, 1983.

[3] de Albuquerque A. K. A. C., S. d. O. Romano, and A. L. A. Eisenberg, "Epithelioid hemangioendothelioma: 15 years at the National Cancer Institute. Literature review," *Brazilian Journal of Pathology and Laboratory Medicine*, vol. 49, no. 2, pp. 119–125, 2013, http://www.scielo.br/scielo.php?script=sci_arttext&pid=S1676-24442013000200007.

[4] C. D. M. Fletcher, J. A. Bridge, and M. F. Hogendoorn PCW, *WHO Classification of Tumours of Soft Tissue and Bone*, vol. 5, WHO/IARC Classification of Tumours, 4th edition, 2013, http://publications.iarc.fr/Book-And-Report-Series/Who-Iarc-Classification-Of-Tumours/Who-Classification-Of-Tumours-Of-Soft-Tissue-And-Bone-2013.

[5] B. Corrin, B. Manners, M. Millard, and L. Weaver, "Histogenesis of the so-called "intravascular bronchioloalveolar tumour"," *The Journal of Pathology*, vol. 128, no. 3, pp. 163–167, 1979.

[6] C. M. Weldon-Linne, T. A. Victor, M. L. Christ, and W. A. Fry, "Angiogenic nature of the "intravascular bronchioloalveolar tumor" of the lung: an electron microscopic study," *Archives of Pathology & Laboratory Medicine*, vol. 105, no. 4, pp. 174–179, 1981, http://www.ncbi.nlm.nih.gov/pubmed/6260056.

[7] U. Flucke, R. J. C. Vogels, N. de Saint Aubain Somerhausen et al., "Epithelioid Hemangioendothelioma: clinicopathologic, immunhistochemical, and molecular genetic analysis of 39 cases," *Diagnostic Pathology*, vol. 9, no. 1, p. 131, 2014.

[8] P. Cronin and D. Arenberg, "Pulmonary epithelioid hemangioendothelioma: an unusual case and a review of the literature," *Chest*, vol. 125, no. 2, pp. 789–792, 2004.

[9] M. Kim, J. Chang, H. Choi et al., "Pulmonary epithelioid hemangioendothelioma misdiagnosed as a benign nodule," *World Journal of Surgical Oncology*, vol. 13, no. 1, p. 107, 2015.

[10] R. Palfoldi, M. Radacs, and E. Csada, "Pulmonary epithelioid haemangioendothelioma studies in vitro and in vivo: new diagnostic and treatment methods," *In Vivo*, vol. 27, no. 2, pp. 221–225, 2013.

[11] W. D. Travis, E. Brambilla, A. P. Burke, and N. A. Marx A, *WHO Classification of Tumours of the Lung, Pleura, Thymus and Heart*, vol. 7, WHO/IARC Classification of Tumours, Accessed, 4th edition, 2015, http://publications.iarc.fr/Book-And-Report-Series/Who-Iarc-Classification-Of-Tumours/Who-Classification-Of-Tumours-Of-The-Lung-Pleura-Thymus-And-Heart-2015.

[12] W. D. Travis, E. Brambilla, A. G. Nicholson et al., "The 2015 World Health Organization Classification of Lung Tumors," *Journal of Thoracic Oncology*, vol. 10, no. 9, pp. 1243–1260, 2015.

[13] C. Errani, L. Zhang, Y. S. Sung et al., "A novel WWTR1-CAMTA1 gene fusion is a consistent abnormality in epithelioid hemangioendothelioma of different anatomic sites," *Genes Chromosomes and Cancer*, vol. 50, no. 8, pp. 644–653, 2011.

[14] T. Anderson, L. Zhang, M. Hameed, V. Rusch, W. D. Travis, and C. R. Antonescu, "Thoracic epithelioid malignant vascular tumors: a clinicopathologic study of 52 cases with emphasis on pathologic grading and molecular studies of WWTR1-CAMTA1 fusions," *The American Journal of Surgical Pathology*, vol. 39, no. 1, pp. 132–139, 2015.

[15] K. Lau, M. Massad, C. Pollak et al., "Clinical patterns and outcome in epithelioid hemangioendothelioma with or without pulmonary involvement: Insights from an internet registry in the study of a rare cancer," *Chest*, vol. 140, no. 5, pp. 1312–1318, 2011.

[16] S. Y. Ha, I. H. Choi, J. Han et al., "Pleural epithelioid hemangioendothelioma harboring CAMTA1 rearrangement," *Lung Cancer*, vol. 83, no. 3, pp. 411–415, 2014.

[17] M. R. Mendlick, M. Nelson, D. Pickering et al., "Translocation t(1;3)(p36.3;q25) is a nonrandom aberration in epithelioid hemangioendothelioma," *American Journal of Surgical Pathology*, vol. 25, no. 5, pp. 684–687, 2001.

[18] MR. Tanas, A. Sboner, AM. Oliveira et al., "Identification of a disease-defining gene fusion in epithelioid hemangioendothelioma," *Science Translational Medicine*, vol. 3, no. 98, p. 98ra82, 2011.

[19] C. R. Antonescu, F. Le Loarer, J.-M. Mosquera et al., "Novel YAP1-TFE3 fusion defines a distinct subset of epithelioid hemangioendothelioma," *Genes Chromosomes and Cancer*, vol. 52, no. 8, pp. 775–784, 2013.

[20] C. Antonescu, "Malignant vascular tumors—an update," *Modern Pathology*, vol. 27, S30–S38, 2014.

[21] N. R. Patel, A. A. Salim, H. Sayeed et al., "Molecular characterization of epithelioid haemangioendotheliomas identifies novel WWTR1-CAMTA1 fusion variants," *Histopathology*, vol. 67, no. 5, pp. 699–708, 2015.

[22] P. E. Mascarelli, J. R. Iredell, R. G. Maggi, G. Weinberg, and E. B. Breitschwerdt, "Bartonella species bacteremia in two patients with epithelioid hemangioendothelioma," *Journal of Clinical Microbiology*, vol. 49, no. 11, pp. 4006–4012, 2011.

[23] T. Haruki, T. Arai, H. Nakamura, K. Nosaka, K. Shomori, and H. Ito, "Pulmonary Epithelioid Hemangioendothelioma with PlGF Expression: Report of a Case," *Thoracic and Cardiovascular Surgeon*, vol. 59, no. 2, pp. 128–130, 2011.

[24] N. P. Ohori, S. A. Yousem, E. Sonmez-Alpan, and T. V. Colby, "Estrogen and progesterone receptors in lymphangioleiomyomatosis, epithelioid hemangioendothelioma, and sclerosing hemangioma of the lung," *American Journal of Clinical Pathology*, vol. 96, no. 4, pp. 529–535, 1991.

[25] M. Mcculloch, M. Russin, and A. Nachat, "Recurrence of epithelioid hemangioendothelioma during pregnancy: case report and systematic review," *The Permanente Journal*, vol. 20, no. 3, pp. 84–89, 2016.

[26] R. M. S. Amin, K. Hiroshima, T. Kokubo et al., "Risk factors and independent predictors of survival in patients with pulmonary epithelioid haemangioendothelioma. Review of the literature and a case report," *Respirology*, vol. 11, no. 6, pp. 818–825, 2006.

[27] M. Kitaichi, S. Nagai, K. Nishimura et al., "Pulmonary epithelioid haemangioendothelioma in 21 patients, including three with partial spontaneous regression," *European Respiratory Journal*, vol. 12, no. 1, pp. 89–96, 1998.

[28] P. Bagan, M. Hassan, F. L. P. Barthes et al., "Prognostic factors and surgical indications of pulmonary epithelioid hemangioendothelioma: a review of the literature," *The Annals of Thoracic Surgery*, vol. 82, no. 6, pp. 2010–2013, 2006.

[29] J. Shao and J. Zhang, "Clinicopathological characteristics of pulmonary epithelioid hemangioendothelioma: A report of four cases and review of the literature," *Oncology Letters*, vol. 8, no. 6, pp. 2517–2522, 2014.

[30] A. Sardaro, L. Bardoscia, M. F. Petruzzelli, and M. Portaluri, "Epithelioid hemangioendothelioma: an overview and update on a rare vascular tumor," *Oncol Rev*, vol. 8, no. 2, p. 259, 2014.

[31] J. Salijevska, R. Watson, A. Clifford, A. I. Ritchie, F. Mauri, and D. Adeboyeku, "Pleural epithelioid hemangioendothelioma: literature summary and novel case report," *Journal of Clinical Medicine Research*, vol. 7, no. 7, pp. 566–570, 2015.

[32] J. H. Woo, T. J. Kim, K. S. Lee, T. S. Kim, and B.-T. Kim, "Epithelioid hemangioendothelioma in the thorax: Clinicopathologic, CT, PET, and prognostic features," *Medicine (United States)*, vol. 95, no. 30, article no. 2010, 2016.

[33] S. Reich, H. Ringe, B. Uhlenberg, B. Fischer, and V. Varnholt, "Epithelioid hemangioendothelioma of the lung presenting with pneumonia and heart rhythm disturbances in a teenage girl," *Journal of Pediatric Hematology/Oncology*, vol. 32, no. 4, pp. 274–276, 2010.

[34] S. K. Teo, S. C. Chiang, and K. K. Tan, "Intravascular bronchioloalveolar tumour. A 20-year survival," *The Medical Journal of Australia*, vol. 142, no. 3, pp. 220–222, 1985, http://www.ncbi.nlm.nih.gov/pubmed/3969042.

[35] B. K. Bollinger, W. B. Laskin, and C. B. Knight, "Epithelioid hemangioendothelioma with multiple site involvement. Literature review and observations," *Cancer*, vol. 73, no. 3, pp. 610–615, 1994.

[36] J. F. Tomashefski, D. H. Dail, and Dail D. H., *Dail and Hammar's Pulmonary Pathology*, Springer, 2008.

[37] M. E. van Kasteren, A. A. van der Wurff, F. M. Palmen, A. Dolman, and J. F. Miseré, "Epithelioid haemangioendothelioma of the lung: clinical and pathological pitfalls," *The European Respiratory Journal*, vol. 8, no. 9, pp. 1616–1619, 1995, http://www.ncbi.nlm.nih.gov/pubmed/8575593.

[38] H. Yanagawa, Y. Hashimoto, H. Bando, Y. Takishita, and T. Nagano, "Intravascular bronchioloalveolar tumor with skin metastases," *Chest*, vol. 105, no. 6, pp. 1882–1884, 1994.

[39] S. R. Mehta, A. Das, N. Barnard, and A. Marcus, "Metastatic Pulmonary Epithelioid Hemangioendothelioma: A case report and review of the literature," *Respiratory Medicine Case Reports*, vol. 7, no. 1, pp. 17–20, 2012.

[40] H.-S. Ro, J. Y. Shin, S.-G. Roh, N.-H. Lee, K.-M. Yang, and W.-S. Moon, "A rare case of pulmonary epithelioid hemangioendothelioma presenting with skin metastasis," *Archives of Plastic Surgery*, vol. 43, no. 3, pp. 284–287, 2016.

[41] B. de Singly, E. Pommaret, F. Sailhan, and R. Coriat, "Colonic mestastasis of an epithelioid hemangioendothelioma: An unusual cause of periumbilical pain and weight loss," *Digestive and Liver Disease*, vol. 43, no. 5, p. e10, 2011.

[42] E. S. Yi, W. R. Auger, P. J. Friedman, T. A. Morris, and S. S. Shin, "Intravascular bronchioloalveolar tumor of the lung presenting as pulmonary thromboembolic disease and pulmonary hypertension," *Archives of Pathology & Laboratory Medicine*, vol. 119, no. 3, pp. 255–260, 1995, http://www.ncbi.nlm.nih.gov/pubmed/7534058.

[43] L. Yu, T. Gu, Z. Xiu, E. Shi, and X. Zhao, "Primary pleural epithelioid hemangioendothelioma compressing the myocardium," *Journal of Cardiac Surgery*, vol. 28, no. 3, pp. 266–268, 2013.

[44] S. Suster, C. A. Moran, and M. N. Koss, "Epithelioid hemangioendothelioma of the anterior mediastinum. Clinicopathologic, immunohistochemical, and ultrastructural analysis of 12 cases," *The American Journal of Surgical Pathology*, vol. 18, no. 9, pp. 871–881, 1994, http://www.ncbi.nlm.nih.gov/pubmed/8067508.

[45] D. Márquez-Medina, J. C. Samamé-Pérez-Vargas, N. Tuset-DerAbrain, A. Montero-Fernández, T. Taberner-Bonastre, and J. M. Porcel, "Pleural epithelioid hemangioendothelioma in an elderly patient. A case report and review of the literature," *Lung Cancer*, vol. 73, no. 1, pp. 116–119, 2011.

[46] E. Y. Kim, T. S. Kim, J. Han, J. Y. Choi, O. J. Kwon, and J. Kim, "Thoracic epithelioid hemangioendothelioma: Imaging and pathologic features," *Acta Radiologica*, vol. 52, no. 2, pp. 161–166, 2011.

[47] N. Sakamoto, S. Adachi, S. Monzawa et al., "High resolution CT findings of pulmonary epithelioid hemangioendothelioma: Unusual manifestations in 2 cases," *Journal of Thoracic Imaging*, vol. 20, no. 3, pp. 236–238, 2005.

[48] P. Luburich, M. C. Ayuso, C. Picado, J. Serra-Batlles, J. F. Ramirez, and M. Sole, "CT of pulmonary epithelioid hemangioendothelioma," *Journal of Computer Assisted Tomography*, vol. 18, no. 4, pp. 562–565, 1994, http://www.ncbi.nlm.nih.gov/pubmed/8040439.

[49] K. Liu, P. Xie, W. Peng, and Z. Zhou, "The computed tomographic findings of pulmonary epithelioid hemangioendothelioma," *Radiologia Medica*, vol. 119, no. 9, pp. 705–713, 2014.

[50] G. T. Noh, K. J. Lee, H. J. Sohn, K. H. Lee, W. S. Heo, and B. S. Koh, "Pulmonary epithelioid hemangioendothelioma misconceived as pulmonary metastasis of other malignancies," *Yeungnam University Journal of Medicine*, vol. 33, no. 1, pp. 72–75, 2016.

[51] M. J. Ledson, R. Convery, A. Carty, and C. C. Evans, "Epithelioid haemangioendothelioma," *Thorax*, vol. 54, no. 6, pp. 560-561, 1999.

[52] J. J. Erasmus, H. P. McAdams, and M. S. Carraway, "A 63-year-old woman with weight loss and multiple lung nodules," *Chest*, vol. 111, no. 1, pp. 236–238, 1997.

[53] C. Roudier-Pujol, O. Enjolras, J. Lacronique et al., "Multifocal epithelioid hemangioendothelioma with partial remission after interferon alfa-2a treatment," *Ann Dermatol Venereol*, vol. 121, no. 12, pp. 898–904, 1994, http://www.ncbi.nlm.nih.gov/pubmed/7632008.

[54] M. Miettinen, Y. Collan, P. Halttunen, T. Maamies, and P. Vilkko, "Intravascular bronchioloalveolar tumor," *Cancer*, vol. 60, no. 10, pp. 2471–2475, 1987.

[55] R. Rojas-Vigott, C. M. Castro, and S. R. Méndez, "P2.24: pulmonary-epithelioid hemangioendothelioma: a case report of spontaneous regression," *Journal of Thoracic Oncology*, vol. 11, S231-S232, no. 10, 2016.

[56] V. Semenisty, I. Naroditsky, Z. Keidar, and G. Bar-Sela, "Pazopanib for metastatic pulmonary epithelioid hemangioendothelioma-a suitable treatment option: Case report and review of anti-angiogenic treatment options," *BMC Cancer*, vol. 15, no. 1, article no. 402, 2015.

[57] S. Mirza, A. Glucksman, and J. McArdle, "Pulmonary epithelioid hemangioendothelioma: one cause of nodular parenchymal lung disease," *Chest*, vol. 148, no. 4, pp. 572A–572B, 2015.

[58] B. Ye, W. Li, J. Feng, J.-X. Shi, Y. Chen, and B.-H. Han, "Treatment of pulmonary epithelioid hemangioendothelioma with combination chemotherapy: Report of three cases and review of the literature," *Oncology Letters*, vol. 5, no. 5, pp. 1491–1496, 2013.

[59] E. Radzikowska, E. Szczepulska-Wójcik, M. Chabowski, K. Oniszh, R. Langfort, and K. Roszkowski, "Pulmonary epithelioid haemangioendothelioma—interferon 2-alpha treatment—case report," *Pneumonologia i Alergologia Polska*, vol. 76, no. 4, pp. 281–285, 2008, http://www.ncbi.nlm.nih.gov/pubmed/18785134.

[60] S. Saleiro, M. Barbosa, C. Souto Moura, J. Almeida, and S. Ferreira, "Epithelioid hemangioendothelioma - a rare pulmonary tumor," *Revista Portuguesa de Pneumologia*, vol. 14, no. 3, pp. 421–425, 2017, http://www.ncbi.nlm.nih.gov/pubmed/18528603.

[61] S. Gaur, A. Torabi, and T. J. O'Neill, "Activity of angiogenesis inhibitors in metastatic epithelioid hemangioendothelioma: a case report," *Cancer Biology & Medicine*, vol. 9, no. 2, pp. 133–136, 2012.

[62] M. I. Ebright, M. F. Zakowski, J. Martin et al., "Clinical pattern and pathologic stage but not histologic features predict outcome for bronchioloalveolar carcinoma," *Ann Thorac Surg*, vol. 74, no. 5, pp. 1640–1646-1647, 2002, http://www.ncbi.nlm.nih.gov/pubmed/12440623.

[63] G. Mukundan, B. A. Urban, F. B. Askin, and E. K. Fishman, "Pulmonary epithelioid hemangioendothelioma: Atypical radiologic findings of a rare tumor with pathologic correlation," *Journal of Computer Assisted Tomography*, vol. 24, no. 5, pp. 719-720, 2000.

[64] G. J. Ross, L. Violi, A. C. Friedman, P. R. Edmonds, and E. Unger, "Intravascular bronchioloalveolar tumor: CT and pathologic correlation," *Journal of Computer Assisted Tomography*, vol. 13, no. 2, pp. 240–243, http://www.ncbi.nlm.nih.gov/pubmed/2647795.

[65] A. Bahrami, T. C. Allen, and P. T. Cagle, "Pulmonary epithelioid hemangioendothelioma mimicking mesothelioma," *Pathology International*, vol. 58, no. 11, pp. 730–734, 2008.

[66] E. J. Crotty, H. P. McAdams, J. J. Erasmus, T. A. Sporn, and V. L. Roggli, "Epithelioid hemangioendothelioma of the pleura: Clinical and radiologic features," *American Journal of Roentgenology*, vol. 175, no. 6, pp. 1545–1549, 2000.

[67] X. Jinghong and C. Lirong, "Pulmonary epithelioid hemangioendothelioma accompanied by bilateral multiple calcified nodules in lung," *Diagnostic Pathology*, vol. 6, no. 1, article no. 21, 2011.

[68] R. P. Kumar, D. A. Smith, C. J. Hilton, and D. V. Parums, "A case of epithelioid haemangioendothelioma (EHE) of the lung with bronchial brushing cytology," *Cytopathology*, vol. 10, no. 2, pp. 132–136, 1999.

[69] J. H. Kim, E. B. Lee, S. Kim et al., "A case of hypertrophic osteoarthropathy associated with epithelioid hemangioendothelioma," *Journal of Korean Medical Science*, vol. 19, no. 3, pp. 484–486, 2004.

[70] K. Fagen, E. D. Silverman, and Cole R. L., "Detection of a pulmonary epithelioid hemangioendothelioma by FDG PET scan," *Clinical Nuclear Medicine*, vol. 29, no. 11, pp. 758-759, 2004, http://www.ncbi.nlm.nih.gov/pubmed/15483505.

[71] D. Rosengarten, M. R. Kramer, G. Amir, L. Fuks, and N. Berkman, "Pulmonary epithelioid hemangioendothelioma," *The Israel Medical Association Journal*, vol. 13, no. 11, pp. 676–679, 2011.

[72] R. Cazzuffi, N. Calia, F. Ravenna et al., "Primary pulmonary epithelioid hemangioendothelioma: a rare cause of pet-negative pulmonary nodules," *Case Reports in Medicine*, vol. 2011, Article ID 262674, 2011.

[73] L. Yi, D. Cheng, H. Shi et al., "Pulmonary epithelioid hemangioendothelioma coexisting with pulmonary nodular amyloidosis: Case discussion and review of the literature," *International Journal of Clinical and Experimental Medicine*, vol. 7, no. 7, pp. 1891–1897, 2014.

[74] K. Okamura, T. Ohshima, R. Nakano, H. Ouchi, K. Takayama, and Y. Nakanishi, "A case of pulmonary epithelioid hemangioendothelioma surviving 10 years without treatment," *Annals of Thoracic and Cardiovascular Surgery*, vol. 16, no. 6, pp. 432–435, 2010.

[75] S. Watanabe, F. Yano, T. Kita et al., "18F-FDG-PET/CT as an indicator for resection of pulmonary epithelioid hemangioendothelioma," *Annals of Nuclear Medicine*, vol. 22, no. 6, pp. 521–524, 2008.

[76] K. K. Sakata, M. B. Gotway, M. L. Smith et al., "Pulmonary epithelioid hemangioendothelioma diagnosed with endobronchial biopsies: A case report and literature review," *Journal of Bronchology and Interventional Pulmonology*, vol. 23, no. 2, pp. 168–173, 2016.

[77] H. S. Ryu, S.-S. Lee, H.-S. Choi, H. Baek, and J. S. Koh, "A case of pulmonary malignant epithelioid hemangioendothelioma misdiagnosed as adenocarcinoma by fine needle aspiration cytology," *Diagnostic Cytopathology*, vol. 39, no. 11, pp. 801–807, 2011.

[78] T. Schattenberg, R. Kam, M. Klopp et al., "Pulmonary epithelioid hemangioendothelioma: Report of three cases," *Surgery Today*, vol. 38, no. 9, pp. 844–849, 2008.

[79] L. B. Angela Sardaro, M. F. Petruzzelli, and B. D. Maurizio Portaluri, "Pulmonary epithelioid hemangioendothelioma: advances in treatment options despite a rare vascular tumor," *Chemother Open Access*, vol. 4, no. 3, pp. 2014-2015, 2014.

[80] K. Eguchi and M. Sawafuji, "Surgical management of a patient with bilateral multiple pulmonary epithelioid hemangioendothelioma: report of a case," *Surgery Today*, vol. 45, no. 7, pp. 904–906, 2014.

[81] Y. Mizuno, H. Iwata, K. Shirahashi, Y. Hirose, and H. Takemura, "Pulmonary epithelioid hemangioendothelioma," *General Thoracic and Cardiovascular Surgery*, vol. 59, no. 4, pp. 297–300, 2011.

[82] C. Pinet, A. Magnan, L. Garbe, M.-J. Payan, and D. Vervloet, "Aggressive form of pleural epithelioid haemangioendothelioma: Complete response after chemotherapy," *European Respiratory Journal*, vol. 14, no. 1, pp. 237-238, 1999.

[83] N. Desie, D. E. Van Raemdonck, L. J. Ceulemans et al., "Combined or serial liver and lung transplantation for epithelioid hemangioendothelioma: A case series," *American Journal of Transplantation*, vol. 15, no. 12, pp. 3247–3254, 2015.

[84] A. Mizota, K. Shitara, and T. Fukui, "Bevacizumab chemotherapy for pulmonary epithelioid hemangioendothelioma with severe dyspnea," *Journal of Thoracic Oncology*, vol. 6, no. 3, pp. 651-652, 2011.

[85] L. Belmont, L. Zemoura, and L. J. Couderc, "Pulmonary epithelioid haemangioendothelioma and bevacizumab," *Journal of Thoracic Oncology*, vol. 3, no. 5, pp. 557-558, 2008.

[86] Y. H. Kim, M. Mishima, and A. Miyagawa-Hayashino, "Treatment of pulmonary epithelioid hemangioendothelioma with bevacizumab," *Journal of Thoracic Oncology*, vol. 5, no. 7, pp. 1107-1108, 2010.

[87] A. Haro, G. Saitoh, S. Tamiya, and A. Nagashima, "Four-year natural clinical course of pulmonary epithelioid hemangioendothelioma without therapy," *Thoracic Cancer*, vol. 6, no. 4, pp. 544–547, 2015.

50

An Uncommon Case of Bilateral Breast Enlargement Diagnosed as Tumoral Pseudoangiomatous Stromal Hyperplasia: Imaging and Pathological Findings

Isabel Sollozo-Dupont,[1] Héctor Alejandro Domínguez-Hernández,[1] Cecilia Pavón-Hernández,[1] Yolanda Villaseñor-Navarro,[1] Robin Shaw-Dulin,[2] Victor Manuel Pérez-Sánchez,[3] Alejandro Javier España-Ferrufino,[3] Laura Marysol Álvarez-Guadarrama,[3] Fany Iris Porras-Reyes,[3] and M. Patricia Pérez-Badillo[1]

[1]*Department of Radiology and Imaging, Instituto Nacional de Cancerología (INCan), Mexico City, Mexico*
[2]*Department of Surgical Oncology, Instituto Nacional de Cancerología (INCan), Mexico City, Mexico*
[3]*Department of Surgical Pathology, Instituto Nacional de Cancerología (INCan), Mexico City, Mexico*

Correspondence should be addressed to M. Patricia Pérez-Badillo; mperezb@incan.edu.mx

Academic Editor: Soon Thye Lim

The incidence of reported pseudoangiomatous stromal hyperplasia (PASH), as well as the variability and severity of clinical presentations, is increasing in the literature. In parallel, several authors posit the need for an improved classification of PASH to avoid possible variables associated with this diagnosis. Here, we present a 25-year-old woman with PASH accompanied by severe bilateral and symmetrical breasts enlargement, highlighting an uncommon clinical presentation of PASH as much as the careful interdisciplinary review and correlation of histology and all available imaging studies to confirm the definitive diagnosis.

1. Introduction

Pseudoangiomatous stromal hyperplasia (PASH) is an uncommon nonneoplastic proliferation of the myofibroblastic cells in the mammary stroma [1, 2]. Clinically, PASH is frequently presented as a unilateral or bilateral focal microscopic changes. However, diffuse massive processes accompanied with masses are also reported [1, 3]. In the presence of masses, mammography typically shows well-defined masses with smooth borders [4, 5]. Meanwhile, sonographic appearances are a well-circumscribed hypoechoic or isoechoic oval masses, with enhanced through transmission [6].

To the diagnosis, core needle biopsy or vacuum-assisted biopsy is indicated in order to differentiate PASH from low-grade angiosarcoma, principally [2, 7, 8]. Histopathologic features of PASH have been clearly outlined by several authors who describe it as a complex pattern of interanastomosing empty slit-like spaces lined by spindle-shaped stromal cells that are positive for CD34, vimentin, actin, and calponin and negative for vascular markers such as factor VIII protein and CD31 [8–11]. After diagnosis, the prognosis of PASH is usually good although there are reports indicating recurrence rates ranging between 13 and 26% [12], by which the treatment of choice is generally a complete resection by wide excision [13].

From the original article by Vuitch et al. (1986) to the current literature, available data appear to be sufficient to provide an accurate diagnosis in any case of PASH. However, due to the variability in clinical features, the criteria for defining PASH, as well as the associated radiographic and pathological findings, are not well established [10, 14]. One of the points of confusion, for example, is whether PASH might be histopathologically defined as a diffuse process in the presence of masses [10]. This is important because discordance of histology and breast imaging presents a diagnostic situation that might require further evaluation, including repeating biopsy with a consequent delay in appropriate treatment [10, 13].

Here, we present a 25-year-old woman with an uncommon PASH characterized by several skin symptoms and multiple large masses, accompanied by a simultaneous and symmetrical breast enlargement. In addition, we enriched the present report discussing diagnostic criteria defining diffuse versus tumoral PASH since a discrepancy between histopathology and imaging is exposed. We suggest that this case is relevant to enrich the different clinical presentations of PASH, but also to reinforce the need for more definitive classification of PASH that helps with clinical management.

2. Case Report

A 25-year-old multiparous woman presented in November 2015 with eight months' history of bilateral breast enlargement. The chief complaint was painful and swollen breasts, accompanied by multiple palpable nodules and erythema. She reported use of birth control implant by two years at the age of 23 years, after her last pregnancy.

On clinical examination, the woman showed bilateral and symmetrical breast enlargement and a palpable mass of 4 cm diameter in the lower inner quadrant of the right breast, while no palpable lesions were found in the left breast. The breast skin was red and swelling, with peau d'orange appearance, whereas nipple areola complex was normal. Edema was also observed in both breasts (Figure 1). Notably, an axillary lymph node was palpable in the right axilla. At the interview, she stated no familiar or personal history of breast cancer.

Since inflammatory breast carcinoma was suspected, a bilateral mammography was initially recommended. Nevertheless, the diagnosis was not conclusive due to the extremely dense breast tissue. Then, a complementary ultrasound was performance, revealing heterogeneous breast echotexture with hypoechoic areas and multiple circumscribed solid masses in both breasts, ranging in diameter from 3 to 8 cm (Figures 2(a)–2(e)). In addition, ultrasound examination revealed two suspicious axillary right lymph nodes with increased cortical thickness. After imaging examination, this case was categorized as BI-RADS 4A.

To the pathologic diagnostic, fragments of the large mass from the right breast were obtained by percutaneous core needle biopsy. Also, a fine needle aspiration biopsy of the right axillary lymph node was performed. Pathologists reported breast parenchyma that was composed of ductal-lobular unit and breast stromal tissue containing a complex pattern of linear spaces lined by endothelial-like spindle cells. Those cells exhibited strong positivity for CD34, actin, and calponin (Figures 4(a)–4(d)) and negativity for estrogen and progesterone receptors. The diagnosis was benign breast lump with features of a diffuse PASH. Meanwhile, fine needle aspiration biopsy of right node reported lymphoid hyperplasia.

Due to the extension of the disease, the patient was subjected to a bilateral mastectomy with immediate reconstruction. A magnetic breast resonance was performed for surgical planning, confirming multiple bilateral circumscribed masses with avid and persistent enhancement after gadolinium administration, which is usually related to a benign etiology (Figures 3(a)–3(f)). After the referred surgery, and taking into account the imaging features of the lesion, the diagnosis was changed from diffuse PASH to tumoral PASH in a careful interdisciplinary review of the case.

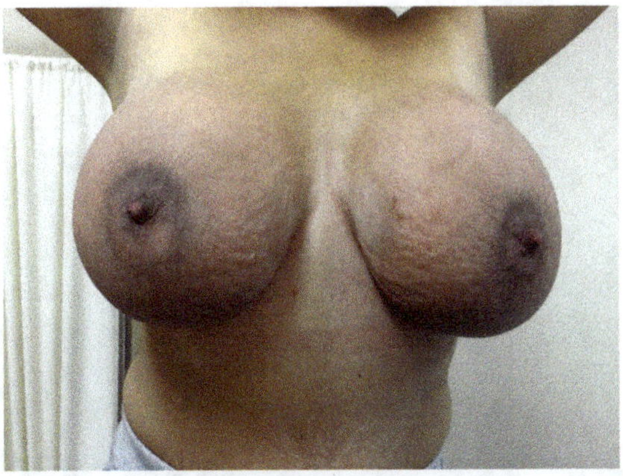

FIGURE 1: Clinical photograph of a 25-year-old woman presenting with symmetrical breast enlargement, thickened skin, and redness.

Currently, the patient is tumor-free on one-year follow-up with excellent cosmetic outcome and breast symmetry.

3. Discussion

PASH of the breast is a rare benign proliferation of mesenchymal stromal cells with irregular slit-like formations resembling angiomatous structures that are similar to vascular spaces. However, these slit-like spaces are not true vascular structures and lack red blood cells. In fact, these spaces are lined by myofibroblasts that are attenuated, lack atypia, and resemble endothelial cells [8, 10, 13, 15, 16]. Although PASH is frequently incidental microscopic findings, evidence shows that its spectrum might include sizeable or symptomatic masses [10, 13, 15, 16].

In the present report, we expose a case of a 25-year-old mastectomized woman by the presence of PASH that is unique for its radiographic and clinical presentation, for example, her bilateral and pronounced symmetrical breast enlargement, accompanied by multiple large masses comprising both breasts. Despite the fact that bilateral nodular cases of PASH are reported in the English medical literature, contrary to our patient, women of those cases have been mostly presented with more growth of one of the breasts causing significant asymmetry [1, 17–19]. Also, it is common to find cases coursing with unilateral processes, or with a unique round mass that resembles a fibroadenoma or a phyllodes tumor [9, 20–23].

Notably, at the clinical examination, the woman presented with painful breasts that were hyperemic and markedly enlarged. Additionally, she had skin changes such as erythema, thickening, edema, and "peau d'orange" appearance, all of which were accompanied with increased breast hardness. The extension and severity of those symptoms led

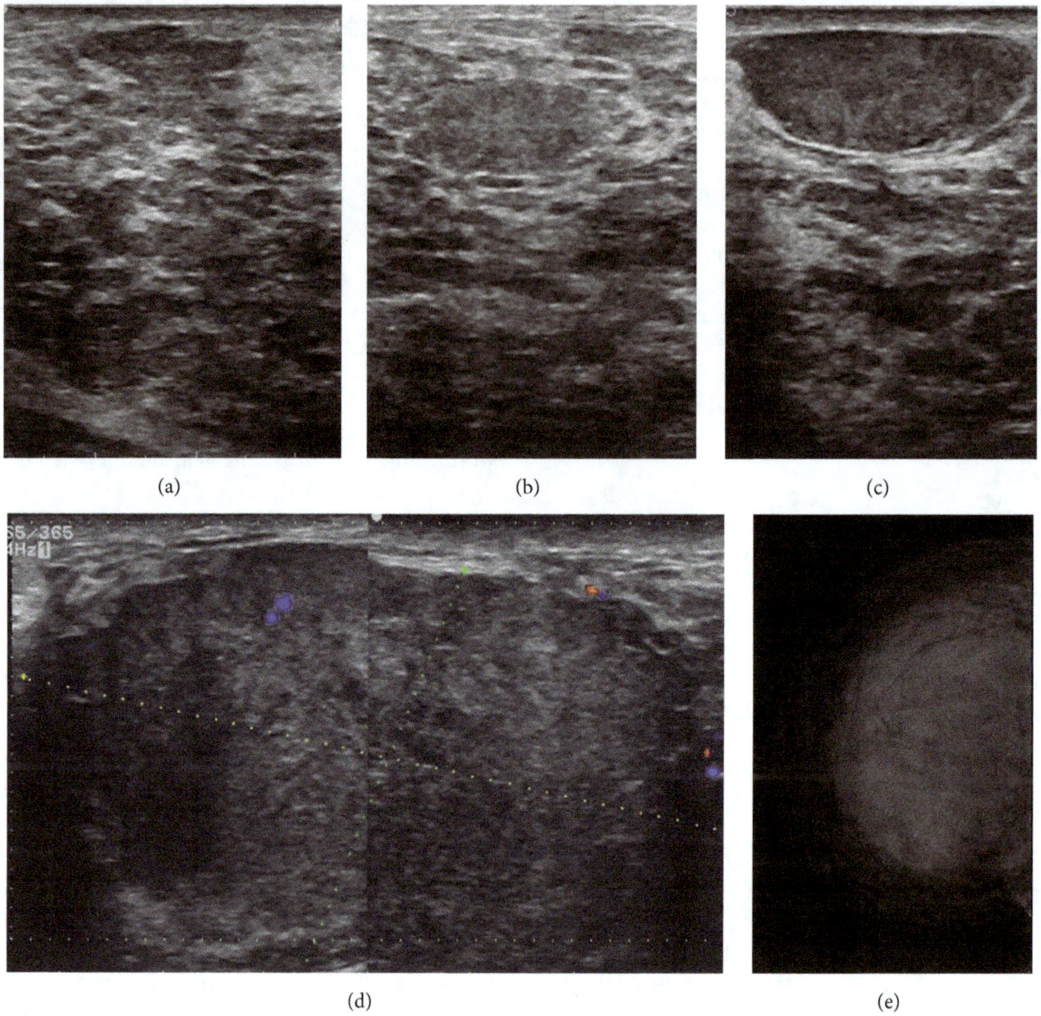

FIGURE 2: Sonographic and mammographic findings. Ultrasound of the left and right breasts showing different heterogeneous, hypoechoic, well circumscribe oval masses. Note the heterogeneous echogenicity of the breast parenchyma (a–c). Sonogram of the left breast demonstrating a hypoechoic well-circumscribed oval mass measuring 80 mm (longitudinal axis), with low flow vascularity detected by Doppler imaging (d). Craniocaudal (CC) breast mammogram of the right breast with increase in density, which decreased the sensitivity of mammography (e).

clinicians to suspect breast inflammatory carcinoma. Noteworthily, within the diagnostic possibilities, PASH was not suspected due to its relative rarity as a symptomatic disease. However, there is increasing evidence on aggressive forms of PASH, suggesting that this clinical presentation may be more common than expected [1, 16, 18, 19].

On the other hand, mammography has a limited use here because of the increased mammary density. Meanwhile, sonographic findings revealed benign-appearing, circumscribed oval hypoechoic masses ranging in size from 3 cm to 8 cm. In spite of the fact that many reports exhibit marked variability in tumoral PASH when it is evaluated through ultrasonography, this lesion is consistently defined as being oval and hypoechoic with no posterior acoustic shadowing, varying in size between 1 cm and 12 cm [3, 5, 24, 25], which concur with our breast imaging.

In addition, ultrasonographic features of PASH were corroborated by using magnetic resonance imaging (MRI), where circumscribed masses with isointense signal as that of the surrounding parenchyma on T1 weighted images were revealed. The enhancement was type 1, corroborating the benign etiology of the disease. Nonetheless, there are reports indicating that curves generated for dynamic contrast also can be of type II [24, 26]. Even though nonspecific markers of PASH were defined by using MRI, we consider that the present findings are important because of more recent reports describing mammographic and ultrasonographic features of PASH [16]. However, little is known about the MRI characteristics up to today [24, 26].

Multimodality imaging patterns of PASH presented here are suggestive but not conclusive. Thus, following BI-RADS criteria, the initial recommendation was core needle biopsy

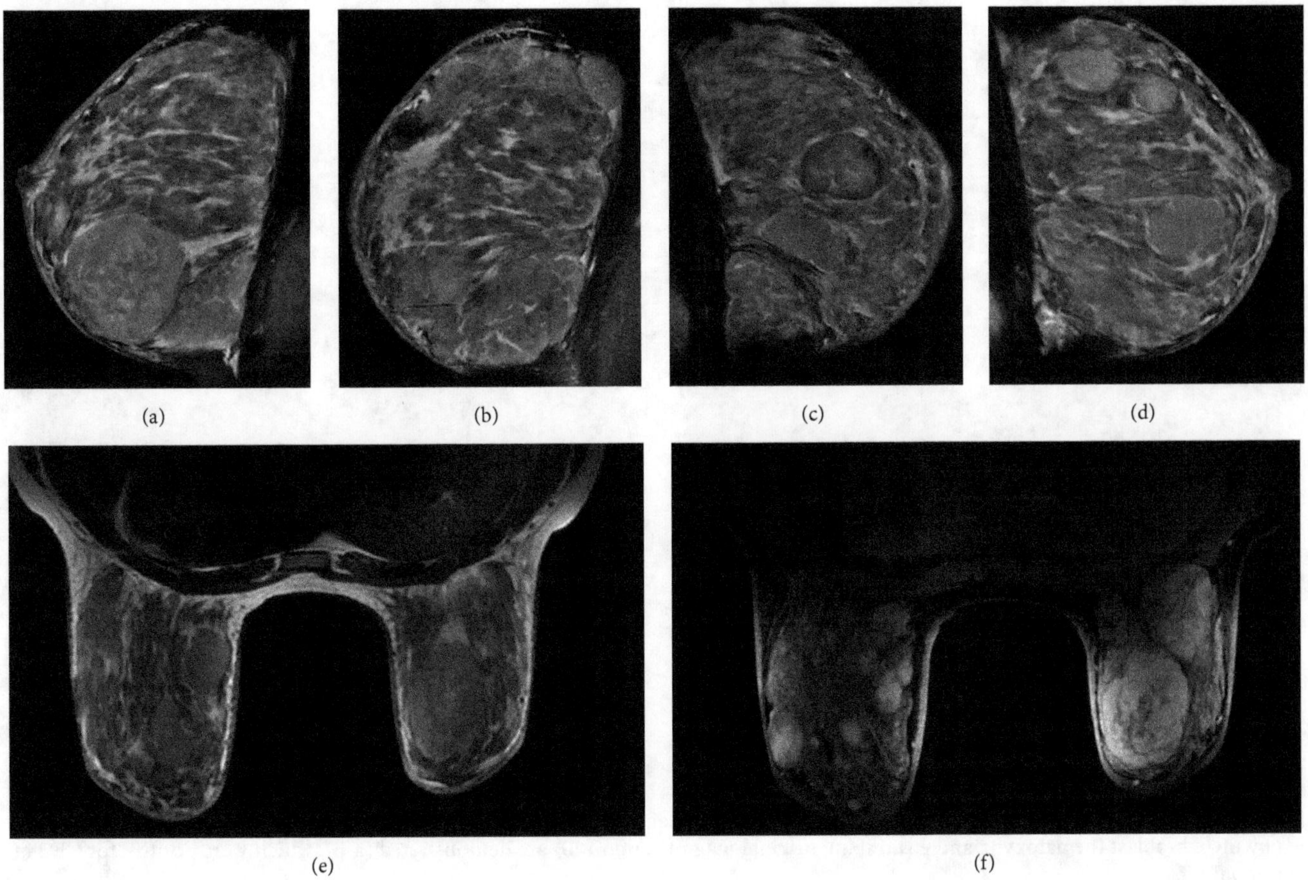

FIGURE 3: Magnetic resonance imaging findings. Right (a-b) and left (c-d) sagittal noncontrast fat suppressed T2-weighted image (T2W-FATSAT) showing extreme fibroglandular tissue and multifocal well-circumscribed masses, with internal linear reticular strands. Axial noncontrast fat suppressed T2-weighted image (T2W-FATSAT) (e) and axial contrast fat suppressed T1-weighted dynamic sequence after 6 minutes (T1WFATSAT+G) (f) demonstrating bilateral breast enlargement, with multiple circumscribed masses that present heterogeneous and persistent enhancement. Areas of nonmass enhancement with diffuse distribution also are observed in the inner and external quadrants of both breasts.

by which histopathological examination revealed a "diffuse PASH." Noteworthily, this diagnosis was originally focused on stromal changes and immunohistochemistry. However, following an interdisciplinary review of this case, the diagnosis changes from "diffuse" to "tumoral PASH," an aspect that was supported by imaging.

Undoubtedly, the aggressive form of stromal hyperplasia exposed here is not similar to what is reported in the literature. This is demonstrated by the quality of imaging and pathologic representation suggesting that this case might contribute to the differential diagnosis of a rapidly growing breast mass.

On the other hand, some authors assert that, under today's literature, it is no longer possible to obtain an assertive diagnosis of PASH due to inconsistences underlying its classification, an aspect that could be inadequate for the patient management after the initial biopsy [10]. One of the points of confusion, for which this report argues, is whether PASH could be pathologically defined as a diffuse process when it results in a mass lesion by imaging [10, 24, 27]. Although, with one case, the exposed confusion will never be resolved, according to previous reports [10], we consider that a diffuse PASH in the presence of masses is technically concordant with the diagnosis of "tumoral PASH."

Concerning etiology, the most prevalent theory is that of a hormone-dependent process on the basis of observations that PASH is most frequently seen in premenopausal women or in elderly women taking hormone-replacement therapy [2, 10]. Therefore, it is possible to suggest that the use of contraceptive in an altered hormonal milieu could modify the reactivity of myofibroblasts causing the masses-forming PASH in our patient [10, 11, 25, 27, 28]. Lastly, because of the extension of the disease and severity of the clinical presentation, the treatment of choice was bilateral subcutaneous mastectomy with immediate silicone implant reconstruction, producing a satisfactory cosmetic result.

In conclusion, we present a unique case of a PASH that demanded an aggressive treatment due to its extended presentation. With the apparent discrepancy present here, we attempt to emphasize that it is not enough to check only pathology, but also the sequence of actions underlying the diagnosis should be checked, including clinical findings and

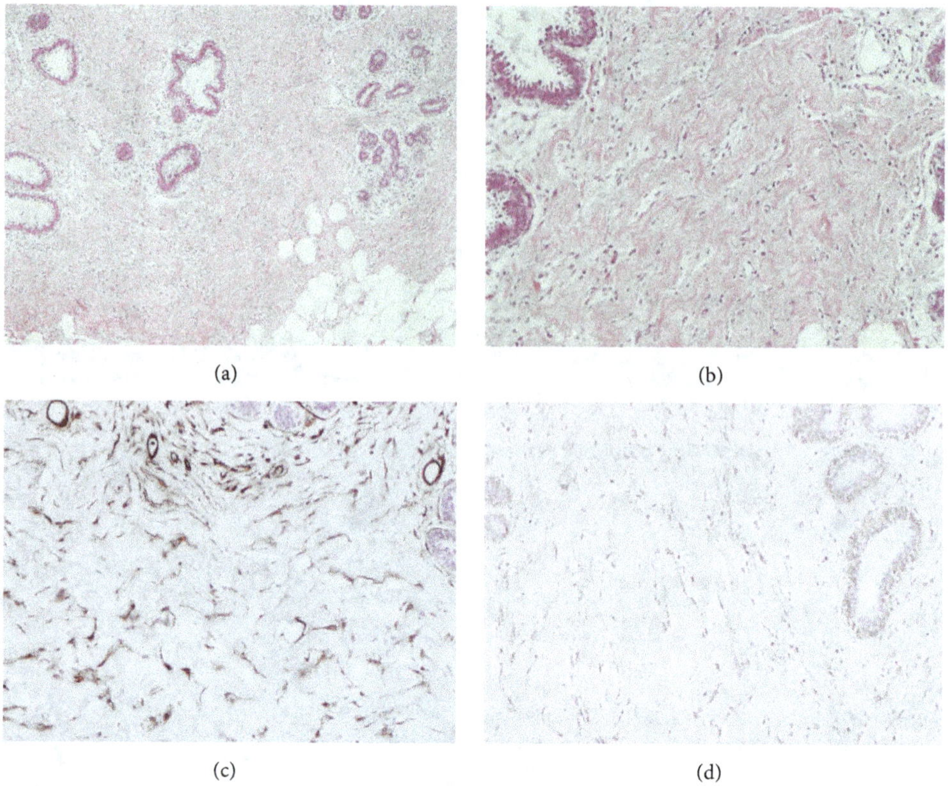

FIGURE 4: Photomicrograph shows high stromal cellularity of glandular tissue with intralobular and perilobular involvement. Slit-like spaces lined by myofibroblast (hematoxylin and eosin stain, original magnification ×10) are demonstrated (a-b), which were positive for CD34 (c) and calponin (d).

imaging modalities that may be needed to ensure correct diagnosis.

References

[1] A. Alikhassi, F. Ensani, R. Omranipour, and A. Abdollahi, "Bilateral Simultaneous Pseudoangiomatous Stromal Hyperplasia of the Breasts and Axillae: Imaging Findings with Pathological and Clinical Correlation," *Case Reports in Radiology*, vol. 2016, pp. 1–4, 2016.

[2] E. Bowman, G. Oprea, J. Okoli et al., "Pseudoangiomatous stromal hyperplasia (PASH) of the breast: a series of 24 patients," *The Breast Journal*, vol. 18, no. 3, pp. 242–247, 2012.

[3] S. S. Jaunoo, S. Thrush, and P. Dunn, "Pseudoangiomatous stromal hyperplasia (PASH): A brief review," *International Journal of Surgery*, vol. 9, no. 1, pp. 20–22, 2011.

[4] S. Pruthi, C. Reynolds, R. E. Johnson, and J. J. Gisvold, "Tamoxifen in the management of pseudoangiomatous stromal hyperplasia," *The Breast Journal*, vol. 7, no. 6, pp. 434–439, 2001.

[5] C. L. Mercado, S. A. Naidrich, D. Hamele-Bena, S. A. Fineberg, and S. S. Buchbinder, "Pseudoangiomatous stromal hyperplasia of the breast: sonographic features with histopathologic correlation," *The Breast Journal*, vol. 10, no. 5, pp. 427–432, 2004.

[6] G. C. Hargaden, E. D. Yeh, D. Georgian-Smith et al., "Analysis of the mammographic and sonographic features of pseudoangiomatous stromal hyperplasia," *American Journal of Roentgenology*, vol. 191, no. 2, pp. 359–363, 2008.

[7] Y. J. Choi, E. Y. Ko, and S. Kook, "Diagnosis of pseudoangiomatous stromal hyperplasia of the breast: Ultrasonography findings and different biopsy methods," *Yonsei Medical Journal*, vol. 49, no. 5, pp. 757–764, 2008.

[8] F. A. Tavassoli and J. Soares, "Myoepithelial lesions," in *in Pathology and Genetics Tumours of the Breast and Female Genital Organs. World Health Organization Classification of Tumours*, F. A. Tavassoli and P. Devilee, Eds., pp. 9–112, IARCPress, Lyon, France, 4th edition, 2003.

[9] C. M. Powell, M. L. Cranor, and P. P. Rosen, "Pseudoangiomatous stromal hyperplasia (PASH): a mammary stromal tumor with myofibroblastic differentiation," *The American Journal of Surgical Pathology*, vol. 19, no. 3, pp. 270–277, 1995.

[10] G. Rosa, A. Dawson, and J. J. Rowe, "Does Identifying Whether Pseudoangiomatous Stromal Hyperplasia (PASH) Is Focal or Diffuse on Core Biopsy Correlate With a PASH Nodule on Excision?" *International Journal of Surgical Pathology*, vol. 25, no. 4, pp. 292–297, 2016.

[11] C. Anderson, A. Ricci Jr., C. A. Pedersen, and R. W. Cartun, "Immunocytochemical analysis of estrogen and progesterone receptors in benign stromal lesions of the breast: evidence for hormonal etiology in pseudoangiomatous hyperplasia of mammary stroma," *The American Journal of Surgical Pathology*, vol. 15, no. 2, pp. 145–149, 1991.

[12] C. M. Gresik, C. Godellas, G. V. Aranha, P. Rajan, and M. Shoup, "Pseudoangiomatous stromal hyperplasia of the breast: A contemporary approach to its clinical and radiologic features and ideal management," *Surgery*, vol. 148, no. 4, pp. 752–758, 2010.

[13] A. Mizutou, K. Nakashima, and T. Moriya, "Large pseudoangiomatous stromal hyperplasia complicated with gynecomastia and lobular differentiation in a male breast," *SpringerPlus*, vol. 4, no. 1, article 282, 2015.

[14] A. Irshad, S. J. Ackerman, T. L. Pope, C. K. Moses, T. Rumboldt, and B. Panzegrau, "Rare breast lesions: correlation of imaging and histologic features with WHO classification," *RadioGraphics*, vol. 28, no. 5, pp. 1399–1414, 2008.

[15] P. Zúbor, K. Kajo, C. A. Dussan, N. Szunyogh, and J. Danko, "Rapidly growing nodular pseudoangiomatous stromal hyperplasia of the breast in an 18-year-old girl," *APMIS-Acta Pathologica, Microbiologica et Immunologica Scandinavica*, vol. 114, no. 5, pp. 389–392, 2006.

[16] A. C. Degnim, M. H. Frost, D. C. Radisky et al., "Pseudoangiomatous stromal hyperplasia and breast cancer risk," *Annals of Surgical Oncology*, vol. 17, no. 12, pp. 3269–3277, 2010.

[17] K. A. Singh, M. M. Lewis, R. L. Runge, and G. W. Carlson, "Pseudoangiomatous stromal hyperplasia. A case for bilateral mastectomy in a 12-year-old girl," *The Breast Journal*, vol. 13, no. 6, pp. 603–606, 2007.

[18] E. M. Ryu, I. Y. Whang, and E. D. Chang, "Rapidly growing bilateral pseudoangiomatous stromal hyperplasia of the breast," *Korean Journal of Radiology*, vol. 11, no. 3, pp. 355–358, 2010.

[19] I. Vasconcelos, C. M. Perez Fernandez, S. Günzel, and W. Schoenegg, "Multifocal Tumorous Pseudoangiomatous Stromal Hyperplasia Presenting as Asymmetric Bilateral Breast Enlargement," *Geburtshilfe und Frauenheilkunde*, vol. 75, no. 2, pp. 183–187, 2015.

[20] S. N. Prasad, D. Houserkova, I. Svach, N. Zlamalova, L. Kucerova, and K. Cwiertka, "Pseudoangiomatous stromal hyperplasia of breast: a case report," *Biomedical Papers*, vol. 152, no. 1, pp. 117–120, 2008.

[21] S. Kimura, A. Tanimoto, S. Shimajiri et al., "Unilateral gynecomastia and pseudoangiomatous stromal hyperplasia in neurofibromatosis: Case report and review of the literature," *Pathology-Research and Practice*, vol. 208, no. 5, pp. 318–322, 2012.

[22] T. L. Holloway and I. Jatoi, "Tumorous PASH presenting as rapid unilateral breast enlargement," *Mayo Clinic Proceedings*, vol. 88, no. 7, p. e75, 2013.

[23] S. G. Fine, A. T. Powell, and M. K. Murray, "Resection of giant pseudoangiomatous stromal hyperplasia: Expectant observation and avoidance of complex breast surgery," *International Journal of Surgery Case Reports*, vol. 15, article no. 1495, pp. 32–34, 2015.

[24] S. D. Raj, V. G. Sahani, B. E. Adrada et al., "Pseudoangiomatous Stromal Hyperplasia of the Breast: Multimodality Review With Pathologic Correlation," *Current Problems in Diagnostic Radiology*, vol. 46, no. 2, pp. 130–135, 2017.

[25] M. A. Cohen, E. A. Morris, P. P. Rosen, D. D. Dershaw, L. Liberman, and A. F. Abramson, "Pseudoangiomatous stromal hyperplasia: mammographic, sonographic, and clinical patterns," *Radiology*, vol. 198, no. 1, pp. 117–120, 1996.

[26] E. Solomou, P. Kraniotis, and G. Patriarcheas, "A case of a giant pseudoangiomatous stromal hyperplasia of the breast: magnetic resonance imaging findings," *Rare Tumors*, vol. 4, no. 2, p. 23, 2012.

[27] C. Y. Castro, G. J. Whitman, A. A. Sahin, and C. F. Wogan, "Pseudoangiomatous stromal hyperplasia of the breast," *American Journal of Clinical Oncology*, vol. 25, no. 2, pp. 213–216, 2002.

[28] R. K. Virk and A. Khan, "Pseudoangiomatous stromal hyperplasia: an overview," *Archives of Pathology & Laboratory Medicine*, vol. 134, no. 7, pp. 1070–1074, 2010.

Direct Intrahepatic Portosystemic Shunt in Budd-Chiari Syndrome: A Case Report

V. Chandra, E. Wajswol, M. Shahid, A. Kumar, and S. Contractor

Department of Radiology, Rutgers New Jersey Medical School, Newark, NJ, USA

Correspondence should be addressed to S. Contractor; contrasg@njms.rutgers.edu

A ademic Editor: Roberto Iezzi

Transjugular intrahepatic portosystemic shunt (TIPS) is an alternative interventional procedure used to manage refractory Budd-Chiari syndrome (BCS) when conservative medical therapy has failed. However, TIPS is not always technically successful because of hepatic vein thrombosis and inability to catheterize the hepatic veins. In these situations, direct intrahepatic portosystemic shunt (DIPS) with access to the portal vein from the IVC has been shown to be a viable alternative that may ameliorate portal hypertension in these patients. Typically, DIPS involves the use of transabdominal ultrasound to target the portal vein. Herein a case in which a 39-year-old female underwent DIPS without the use of ultrasound guidance is presented. Instead, a hepatic venogram generated using collateral circulation was used to opacify and guide access to the portal vein.

1. Introduction

Budd-Chiari syndrome (BCS) is associated with occlusion of hepatic venous outflow by thrombosis or structural compression at the level of the main hepatic vein or the extrahepatic segment of the inferior vena cava [1]. Initial management of BCS is usually medical (nonoperative/noninterventional), with the most common intervention for BCS nonresponsive to medical management being transjugular intrahepatic portosystemic shunt (TIPS). However, this is not always technically successful because of hepatic vein thrombosis and inability to catheterize the hepatic veins. In these situations, direct intrahepatic portosystemic shunt (DIPS) with access to the portal vein from the IVC is a viable alternative that may ameliorate portal hypertension in these patients [2–5]. This procedure generally involves the use of transabdominal ultrasound or endovascular ultrasound to accurately identify and access the portal vein. If the portal vein can be identified by catheterizing the collateral vessels seen in BCS, the portal vein may be targeted from the IVC without the use of ultrasound. Herein is presented a case in which a 39-year-old female underwent DIPS after the portal vein was localized utilizing the opacified collateral circulation as a roadmap.

2. Clinical History

A 39-year-old Hispanic female with no significant past medical history presented to an outside hospital with complaints of nausea, vomiting, and abdominal pain. The patient's presentation and workup was consistent with decompensated liver cirrhosis. The patient was started on diuretics and underwent multiple paracentesis for ascites, as well as being treated for spontaneous bacterial peritonitis (SBP). Primary prophylaxis with propranolol was initiated after esophagogastroduodenoscopy (EGD) showed grade II esophageal varices and portal gastropathy. The patient was also found to have a large deep vein thrombosis (DVT) extending from the IVC to the right common and external iliac veins and was started on heparin drip for anticoagulation. Cirrhosis workup for chronic liver disease was negative, including viral and autoimmune etiologies. Polycythemia vera or other chronic myeloproliferative disorder was suspected given patients high peripheral red blood cell count (RBC 6.15/uL, Hemoglobin 16.0 g/dL, and Hematocrit 48.9%). Further workup, including Factor V Leiden, Factor II prothrombin gene mutation, antiphospholipid antibody syndrome, and JAK2 mutation, was negative and biopsy of the liver showed complete cirrhosis without marked steatosis. Despite receiving maximal

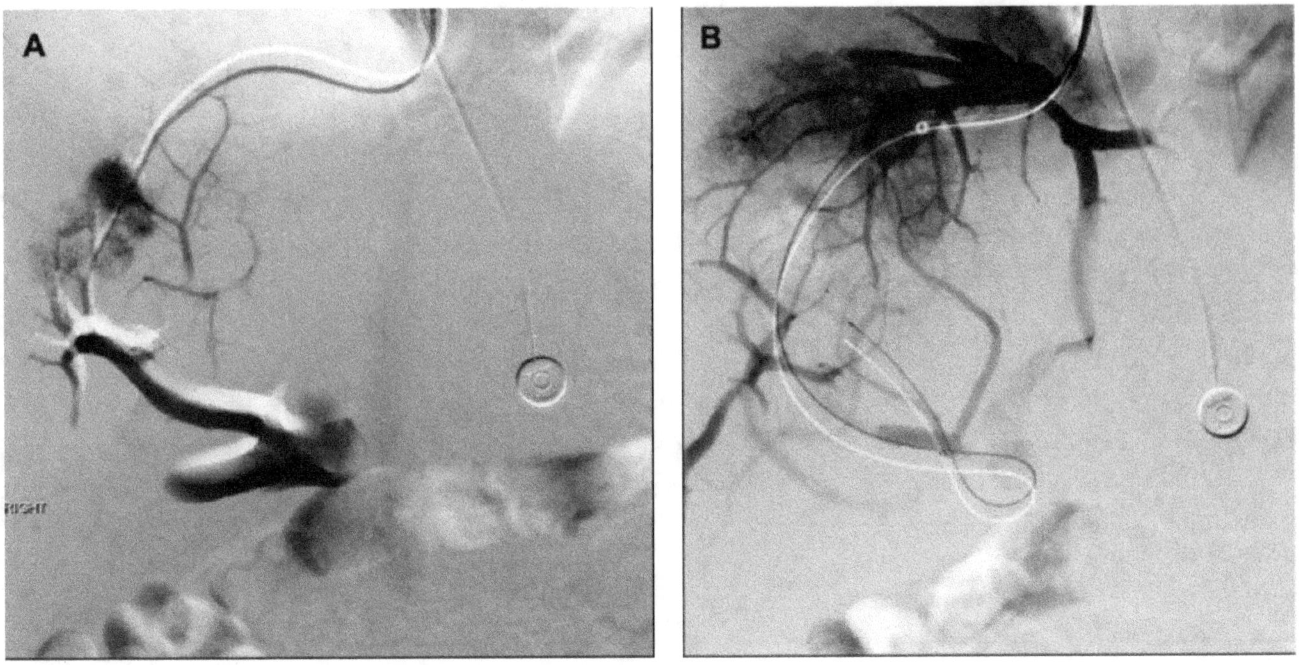

(a) (b)

Figure 1: (a) Initial venography of right hepatic venous system. Note parenchymal blush and opacification of the hepatic veins and portal venous system. (b) Venography following distal placement of the guidewire. Note the guidewire is now within the portal venous system. Parenchymal blush can be seen as well as opacification of the hepatic venous system and multiple collaterals leading, from the hepatic venous system to the portal system.

medical therapy, the patient continued to have significant ascites requiring multiple large-volume paracentesis. Given the refractory ascites and the presence of a DVT, Budd-Chiari syndrome was suspected and TIPS placement was attempted at the outside hospital. TIPS placement was abandoned after the hepatic veins could not be catheterized due to narrowing vs. occlusion.

The patient was transferred to this author's hepatology service for liver transplant workup and potential surgical shunt placement. On initial presentation the patient denied abdominal pain, nausea, vomiting, diarrhea, confusion, and weakness. The patient appeared jaundiced but in no acute distress, with scleral icterus noted on HEENT exam. On neurological exam, the patient was alert and oriented to person, place, and location, with no asterixis noted. Examination of the abdomen yielded distension, a positive fluid wave, and right upper quadrant tenderness to palpation. On presentation, the patient had a Child-Pugh Score of 7, model end-stage liver disease (MELD) score of 23, and a class I Rotterdam score of 1.04.

3. Imaging Review

Doppler ultrasound of the abdomen demonstrated hepatomegaly, hepatic parenchyma consistent with cirrhosis, a patent portal vein and IVC, significant ascites, and splenomegaly. Hepatopetal flow was noted in the main, right, and left portal veins. The hepatic vein could not be visualized. CT imaging displayed classic features of BCS, including heterogenous "starry sky" liver parenchyma, lack of visualization of the hepatic venous trunks, and an enlarged caudate lobe. CT imaging was also significant for changes consistent with portal hypertension. In view of this picture, TIPS was considered as a means of alleviating her portal hypertension.

4. Treatment Options/Results

Under ultrasound guidance, vascular access was obtained via the right internal jugular (RIJ) vein using a 5 Fr micropuncture kit. An Amplatz wire was passed into the IVC and a 12 Fr vascular sheath was then advanced over the wire into the IVC. A venogram was performed which demonstrated the site of inflow from the hepatic veins. Utilizing a hydrophilic Glidewire and 5 Fr Berenstein catheter, attempts were made to catheterize the right hepatic vein. Venogram at this point demonstrated outflow venous obstruction with reflux of contrast into the right portal vein (RPV), shown in Figure 1(a). Angiography following further distal advancement of the guidewire revealed the presence of the guidewire within the portal system, introduced without assistance from a needle (Figure 1(b)).

Attempts were made to catheterize the occluded hepatic veins; however, the sheath of the TIPS set could not be placed in the hepatic vein. The Glidewire was left within the portal system and the sheath was pulled back to level of the IVC. Using the Glidewire as a guide, serial balloon catheter dilations were performed without technical success.

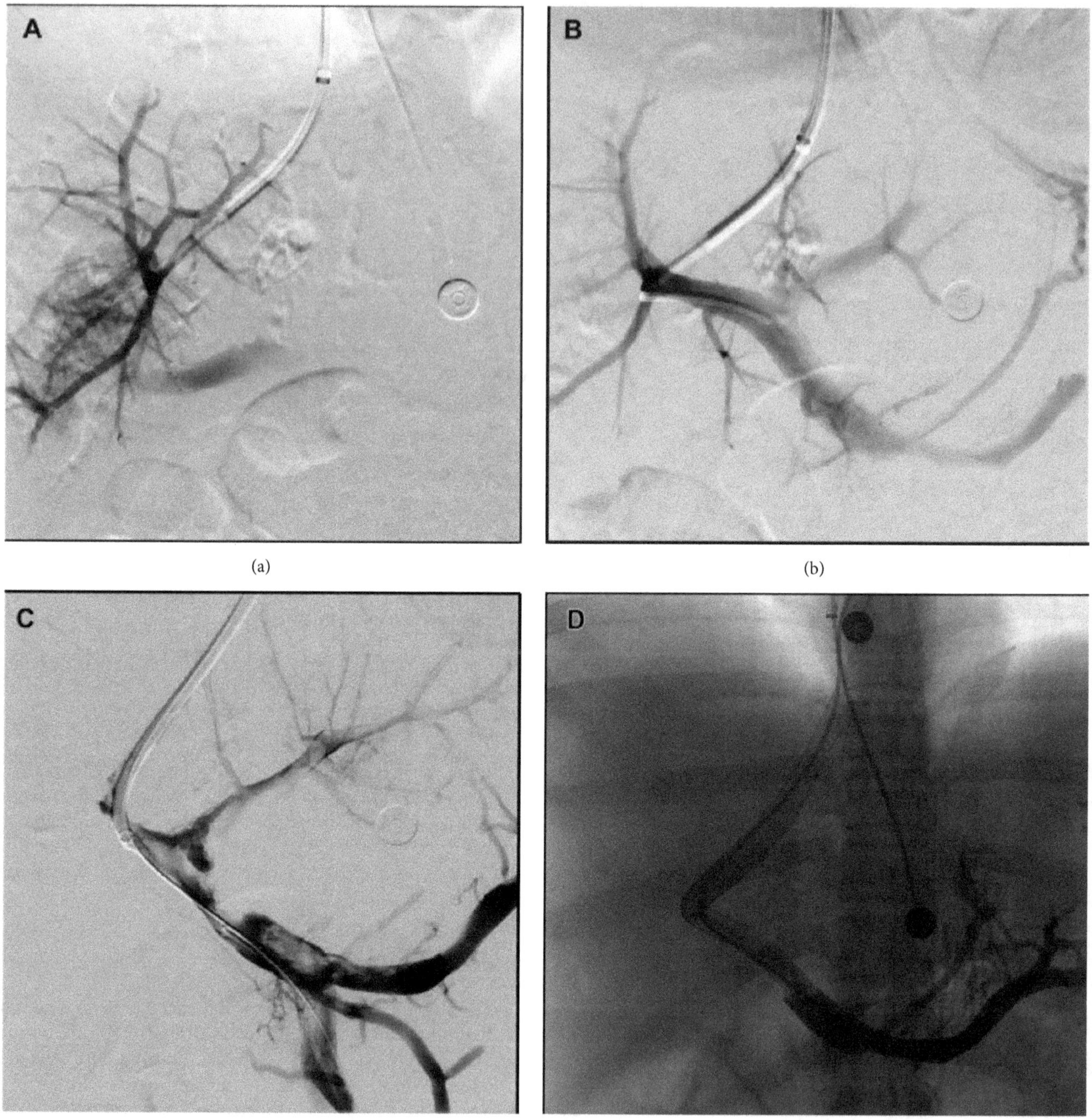

(a) (b) (c) (d)

FIGURE 2: (a) Portal venography after initial needle access through DIPS. (b) Portal venography after introduction of sheath into the portal venous system. Note the presence of gastric varices. (c) Portal venography prior to creation and stenting of the DIPS. Note portal venous thrombosis disseminated throughout. (d) Unsubtracted post-DIPS and stenting portal venography. Note the absence of thrombosis and patency of the DIPS with brisk flow of contrast.

At this point, a decision to perform a DIPS was made. An exaggerated curve of the outer cannula of the TIPS sheath was made. The liver was probed with the puncture needle from the IVC just below the previously identified origin of the hepatic vein. The cannula was then rotated counterclockwise and advanced through the liver parenchyma until a portal vein was successfully accessed (Figure 2(a)).

A hydrophilic wire and catheter were then passed into the portal vein and a portal venogram demonstrated hepatic flow with evidence of prominent esophageal and gastric varices (Figure 2(b)). An Amplatz wire was then passed into the RPV; the hepatic parenchymal tract was dilated using a 6 mm angioplasty balloon. A 10 Fr introducer sheath was then passed into the RPV and a 10 mm × 8 cm Viatorr covered stent

(W.L. Gore & Associates, Inc, Flagstaff, Arizona) and a second 10 mm × 98 mm Wallstent (Boston Scientific, Marlborough, Massachusetts) were placed spanning from the portal vein to the hepatic vein IVC junction. The stent was then dilated utilizing a 10 mm angioplasty balloon. Venograms prior to creation of DIPS and stenting demonstrated new partial thrombosis of the portal vein (Figure 2(c)). At this time, a 5 Fr Fogarty balloon catheter was used to sweep the thrombus and free flow in the portal vein was restored. Poststenting venogram demonstrated the absence of significant residual thrombus and excellent flow through the stented segment, with decompression of the previously visualized esophageal and gastric varices (Figure 2(d)). The patient tolerated the procedure well and with the exception of the aforementioned resolved intraprocedural thrombosis experienced no complications.

Ultrasound evaluation 2 weeks later revealed the main portal vein to have hepatopetal flow, with a flow velocity of 47.3 cm/s. The left portal vein was patent with hepatopetal flow, and the right portal vein was patent with bidirectional flow. Velocity was 92 cm/s within the proximal DIPS, 131 cm/s within the mid DIPS, and 127 cm/s within the distal DIPS.

5. Discussion

Budd-Chiari syndrome (BCS) is a group of disorders characterized by hepatic venous outflow occlusion, by either thrombosis or structural compression, leading to hepatovenous congestion, ischemic necrosis, and eventually cirrhosis [1]. While the progression of BCS can be fulminant, acute, or chronic, it is usually asymptomatic for a long period of time until progressing rapidly to liver cirrhosis and the development of portal hypertension [6]. If timely diagnosis and disease management are not initiated, there is a significant morbidity associated with BCS, with 1-year and 3-year untreated mortality exceeding 70% and 89%, respectively [7, 8]. The principal goal of treatment and disease management in BCS is to decrease hepatic congestion and thereby reduce the associated morbidity and mortality.

Since BCS is a pathophysiologic process that encompasses multiple etiologies, management in patients with BCS depends on clinical symptoms and anatomic considerations. The American Association for the Study of Liver Diseases recommends a stepwise approach in management of BCS, beginning with medical treatment prior to interventional approaches [9]. Since an underlying condition can be diagnosed in up to 80% of patients with BCS, appropriate medical management should be initiated promptly [10]. This most often involves anticoagulation to address the primary hypercoagulability disorder and prevent propagation of clot formation [11]. However, one study showed the use of anticoagulation alone to be successful in only 18% of patients and radiographically guided treatments were required to restore patency of the thrombosed hepatic veins [7].

Minimally invasive interventional treatment options include recanalization of hepatic veins with balloon angioplasty, hepatic vein stenting, and transjugular intrahepatic portosystemic shunt (TIPS). In China, balloon angioplasty, with or without stenting, is the most common interventional treatment employed in treating BCS and TIPS is rarely used [12, 13]. This success of balloon angioplasty in China is likely attributable to the etiology of BCS in the Asian population; BCS in the Asian population is usually associated with suprahepatic stenosis of the IVC and therefore TIPS is not therapeutic [14, 15]. This is in contrast to the pathophysiology of BCS in Western countries, as it includes typically hypercoagulable states that lead to hepatic vein occlusion [16]. Recanalization procedures in this population only provided a clinical benefit in 15% of patients [7]. Studies have also shown that placement of metal stents along with angioplasty is associated with decreased incidence of reocclusion and may in fact improve long-term survival [17–20].

Interventionalists are often conservative when considering the use of stent, as it can complicate liver transplantation should the patient require one. While angioplasty and stenting are attractive options, they seem to have a low applicability in the treatment of BCS patients in the western world, as they only prevent progression of treatment to TIPS and liver transplant in a third of patients [6, 21, 22]. Furthermore, it has been shown that among pediatric BCS patients success rates for angioplasty, hepatic vein stenting, and TIPS were 43%, 66%, and 72%, respectively [23]. A comprehensive study has not yet reported results in the adult population, and currently there are no randomized controlled trials comparing these interventional procedures.

TIPS has been shown to have a high technical success rate of 93%, with a 1- and 5-year transplant-free survival rate of 93% and 74%, respectively [24, 25]. While only 50% of patients who underwent recanalization procedures showed a clinical response, TIPS showed an increased response rate of 84% [7]. Moreover, TIPS is associated with less morbidity and mortality when compared to open surgical procedures [1, 26]. Despite the lack of RCTs, there exists some retrospective evidence suggesting that TIPS may improve survival in BCS patients who fail to respond to medical therapy [25, 27].

Despite these high success rates of TIPS among BCS patients, TIPS is sometimes not technically successful because of significant hepatic vein thrombosis and inability to catheterize the hepatic vein. In these situations, direct intrahepatic portosystemic shunt (DIPS) is a viable alternative technique that can ameliorate portal hypertension in these patients.

In DIPS, a portocaval shunt is created between the inferior vena cava and the portal vasculature through the enlarged caudate lobe. The most crucial and difficult part of this procedure is identifying and gaining access to the portal vein. To address this issue, Haskal et al. first described the gun-sight technique in 1996 as method of guiding access into the portal vein [2]. Boyvat et. al then modified this technique and used transabdominal ultrasound guidance to percutaneously insert a needle into a portal venous branch and subsequently directly into the IVC [3]. Over the next two years, this simultaneous approach was technically and clinically successful in 11 patients [28]. Use of intravascular sonographic-guided placement of DIPS has been described by Petersen and Binkert [4, 29], wherein ultrasound is used to transhepatically puncture the portal vein from the IVC. A disadvantage of this approach is that it requires special equipment (endovascular ultrasound) and is therefore more expensive. Transabdominal ultrasound guidance with simultaneous fluoroscopy has been used successfully for intrahepatic puncture directly from the IVC to a portal venous branch [5]. In all cases described above, ultrasound guidance (both transabdominal and endovascular) was used to locate and target the portal vein for access.

In the case presented herein, ultrasound guidance was not used to generate the DIPS. Rather, a wedged hepatic venogram through catheterization of a thrombosed hepatic vein opacified the portal vein and provided a road map to guide access to the portal vein. In this approach, there are several important variables to consider. First, understanding the pathophysiology of Budd-Chiari syndrome is crucial to the success of interventional treatments, especially in DIPS. Because primary BCS is most often chronic in nature, several collateral pathways develop, varying based on the level of thrombosis and the span of the obstructed segment. Hepatic vein obstructions cause increased pressure within the hepatic venous system, resulting in formation of collateral venous circulation. However, the sites of these collateral veins in BCS are different from the portosystemic collaterals secondary to portal hypertension [30]. Multiple subcapsular vessels develop to bypass thrombosed portions of the hepatic veins as well as connect open portions of hepatic veins directly to systemic veins [30, 31]. This has been described as the pathognomonic "spiderweb" pattern on hepatic venocavography [9]. This existence of collaterals plays an important role in the course of BCS and must be considered during interventional treatment of BCS, as they may enable identification of the portal circulation and serve as a guide for DIPS.

In patients with Budd-Chiari syndrome, direct intrahepatic portosystemic shunt (DIPS) is a viable alternative technique to TIPS that can ameliorate portal hypertension. While DIPS generally involves the use of transabdominal or endovascular ultrasound to target the portal vein, the collateral vessels in BCS can be used to create a roadmap to facilitate targeting the portal vein. Importantly, long-term anticoagulation is needed in these patients to prevent Budd-Chiari recurrence and DIPS occlusion.

References

[1] H. L. A. Janssen, J.-C. Garcia-Pagan, E. Elias, G. Mentha, A. Hadengue, and D.-C. Valla, "Budd-Chiari syndrome: a review by an expert panel," *Journal of Hepatology*, vol. 38, no. 3, pp. 364–371, 2003.

[2] Z. Haskal, R. Duszak Jr., and E. E. Furth, "Transjugular intrahepatic transcaval portosystemic shunt: The gun-sight approach," *Journal of Vascular and Interventional Radiology*, vol. 7, no. 1, pp. 139–142, 1996.

[3] F. Boyvat, C. Aytekin, A. Harman, and Y. Özin, "Transjugular intrahepatic portosystemic shunt creation in Budd-Chiari syndrome: Percutaneous ultrasound-guided direct simultaneous puncture of the portal vein and vena cava," *CardioVascular and Interventional Radiology*, vol. 29, no. 5, pp. 857–861, 2006.

[4] B. D. Petersen and T. W. I. Clark, "Direct Intrahepatic Portocaval Shunt," *Techniques in Vascular and Interventional Radiology*, vol. 11, no. 4, pp. 230–234, 2008.

[5] A. Hatzidakis, N. Galanakis, and E. Kehagias, "Ultrasound-guided direct intrahepatic portosystemic shunt in patients with BuddChiari syndrome: Short- and long-term results," *Interventional Medicine Applied Science*, vol. 9, no. 2, pp. 86–93, 2017.

[6] K. V. N. Menon, V. Shah, and P. S. Kamath, "The Budd—Chiari syndrome," *The New England Journal of Medicine*, vol. 350, no. 6, pp. 578–585, 2004.

[7] A. Plessier, A. Sibert, Y. Consigny et al., "Aiming at minimal invasiveness as a therapeutic strategy for Budd-Chiari syndrome," *Hepatology*, vol. 44, no. 5, pp. 1308–1316, 2006.

[8] A. S. Tavill, E. J. Wood, L. Kreel, E. A. Jones, M. Gregory, and S. Sherlock, "The Budd-Chiari Syndrome: Correlation Between Hepatic Scintigraphy and the Clinical, Radiological, and Pathological Findings in Nineteen Cases of Hepatic Venous Outflow Obstruction," *Gastroenterology*, vol. 68, no. 3, pp. 509–518, 1975.

[9] L. D. DeLeve, D.-C. Valla, and G. Garcia-Tsao, "Vascular disorders of the liver," *Hepatology*, vol. 49, no. 5, pp. 1729–1764, 2009.

[10] S. D. Murad, A. Plessier, M. Hernandez-Guerra et al., "Etiology, management, and outcome of the Budd-Chiari syndrome," *Annals of Internal Medicine*, vol. 151, no. 3, pp. 167–175, 2009.

[11] D.-C. Valla, "The diagnosis and management of the Budd-Chiari syndrome: Consensus and controversies," *Hepatology*, vol. 38, no. 4, pp. 793–803, 2003.

[12] W. Zhang, X. Qi, X. Zhang et al., "Budd-Chiari Syndrome in China: A Systematic Analysis of Epidemiological Features Based on the Chinese Literature Survey," *Gastroenterology Research and Practice*, vol. 2015, Article ID 738548, 8 pages, 2015.

[13] X. Yang, T. O. Cheng, and C. Chen, "Successful Treatment by Percutaneous Balloon Angioplasty of Budd-Chiari Syndrome Caused by Membranous Obstruction of Inferior Vena Cava: 8-Year Follow-Up Study," *Journal of the American College of Cardiology*, vol. 28, no. 7, pp. 1720–1724, 1996.

[14] J. H. Lim, J. H. Park, and Y. H. Auh, "Membranous obstruction of the inferior vena cava: Comparison of findings at sonography, CT, and venography," *American Journal of Roentgenology*, vol. 159, no. 3, pp. 515–520, 1992.

[15] A. H. Sonin, M. J. Mazer, and T. A. Powers, "Obstruction of the inferior vena cava: a multiple-modality demonstration of causes, manifestations, and collateral pathways.," *RadioGraphics*, vol. 12, no. 2, pp. 309–322, 1992.

[16] X. Qi, X. Guo, and D. Fan, "Difference in Budd-Chiari syndrome between the West and China," *Hepatology*, vol. 62, no. 2, p. 656, 2015.

[17] T. Wu, L. Wang, Q. Xiao et al., "Percutaneous balloon angioplasty of inferior vena cava in Budd-Chiari syndrome-R1," *International Journal of Cardiology*, vol. 83, no. 2, pp. 175–178, 2002.

[18] A. M. Witte, L. J. Kool, R. Veenendaal et al., "Hepatic vein stenting for Budd-Chiari syndrome," *The American Journal of Gastroenterology*, pp. 492–498, 1997.

[19] H. Xue, Y.-C. Li, P. Shakya, M. Palikhe, and R. K. Jha, "The role of intravascular intervention in the management of Budd-Chiari syndrome," *Digestive Diseases and Sciences*, vol. 55, no. 9, pp. 2659–2663, 2010.

[20] G. Han, X. Qi, W. Zhang et al., "Percutaneous recanalization for Budd-Chiari syndrome: an 11-year retrospective study on patency and survival in 177 Chinese patients from a single center," *Radiology*, vol. 266, no. 2, pp. 657–667, 2013.

[21] C. E. Eapen, D. Velissaris, M. Heydtmann, B. Gunson, S. Olliff, and E. Elias, "Favourable medium term outcome following hepatic vein recanalisation and/or transjugular intrahepatic portosystemic shunt for Budd Chiari syndrome," *Gut*, vol. 55, no. 6, pp. 878–884, 2006.

[22] S. Seijo, A. Plessier, J. Hoekstra et al., "Good long-term outcome of Budd-Chiari syndrome with a step-wise management," *Hepatology*, vol. 57, no. 5, pp. 1962–1968, 2013.

[23] V. K. Sharma, P. R. Ranade, S. Marar, F. Nabi, and A. Nagral, "Long-term clinical outcome of Budd-Chiari syndrome in children after radiological intervention," *European Journal of Gastroenterology & Hepatology*, vol. 28, no. 5, pp. 567–575, 2016.

[24] M. Rössle, M. Olschewski, V. Siegerstetter, E. Berger, K. Kurz, and D. Grandt, "The Budd-Chiari syndrome: Outcome after treatment with the transjugular intrahepatic portosystemic shunt," *Surgery*, vol. 135, no. 4, pp. 394–403, 2004.

[25] J. C. Garcia-Pagán, M. Heydtmann, S. Raffa et al., "TIPS for Budd-Chiari Syndrome: Long-Term Results and Prognostics Factors in 124 Patients," *Gastroenterology*, vol. 135, no. 3, pp. 808–815, 2008.

[26] P. Michl, M. Bilzer, T. Waggershauser et al., "Successful treatment of chronic Budd-Chiari syndrome with a transjugular intrahepatic portosystemic shunt," *Journal of Hepatology*, vol. 32, no. 3, pp. 516–520, 2000.

[27] A. Perelló, J. C. García-Pagán, R. Gilabert et al., "TIPS is a useful long-term derivative therapy for patients with Budd-Chiari syndrome uncontrolled by medical therapy," *Hepatology*, vol. 35, no. 1, pp. 132–139, 2002.

[28] F. Boyvat, A. Harman, U. Ozyer, C. Aytekin, and Z. Arat, "Percutaneous sonographic guidance for tips in Budd-Chiari syndrome: Direct simultaneous puncture of the portal vein and inferior vena cava," *American Journal of Roentgenology*, vol. 191, no. 2, pp. 560–564, 2008.

[29] B. Petersen and C. Binkert, "Intravascular ultrasound-guided direct intrahepatic portacaval shunt: Midterm follow-up," *Journal of Vascular and Interventional Radiology*, vol. 15, no. 9, pp. 927–938, 2004.

[30] O. K. Cho, J. H. Koo, Y. S. Kim, H. C. Rhim, B. H. Koh, and H. S. Seo, "Collateral pathways in Budd-Chiari syndrome: CT and venographic correlation," *American Journal of Roentgenology*, vol. 167, no. 5, pp. 1163–1167, 1996.

[31] A. Bozorgmanesh, D. A. Selvam, and J. G. Caridi, "Budd-Chiari syndrome: Hepatic venous web outflow obstruction treated by percutaneous placement of hepatic vein stent," *Seminars in Interventional Radiology*, vol. 24, no. 1, pp. 100–105, 2007.

52

Primary Osteosarcoma of the Breast Arising in an Intraductal Papilloma

Khalefa Ali Alghofaily,[1] Musab Hamoud Almushayqih,[2] Muhannad Faleh Alanazi,[3] Abdullah Abdulrahman Bin Salamah,[2] and Halldor Benediktsson[4]

[1]*Radiology Department, Al Qassim University, Buraydah, Saudi Arabia*
[2]*King Saud University and King Khalid University Hospital, Riyadh, Saudi Arabia*
[3]*Radiology Department, Al Jouf University, Al Jawf, Saudi Arabia*
[4]*King Faisal Specialist Hospital and Research Centre, Riyadh, Saudi Arabia*

Correspondence should be addressed to Musab Hamoud Almushayqih; mousab2@gmail.com

Academic Editor: Suayib Yalcin

Introduction. Primary osteosarcoma of the breast is extremely rare, and an osteosarcoma arising from an intraductal papilloma is exceptional. *Case Presentation.* A 72-year-old Saudi Arabian woman presented with a solid, bone-containing breast mass that was diagnosed as primary osteosarcoma of the breast on biopsy. She had a history of untreated intraductal papilloma. Treatment was completed with a modified mastectomy after excluding extramammary metastases. However, she subsequently developed multiple recurrent lesions at the same site. *Conclusion.* Primary osteogenic sarcomas of the breast are very rare. Although the main treatment is resection the optimal management remains uncertain and prognosis is poor.

1. Introduction

Breast cancer is the second leading cause of death in women, with invasive ductal carcinoma by far the commonest subtype. Breast sarcomas are rare neoplasms accounting for less than 1% of total breast malignancies [1]. Extraskeletal osteosarcomas have been reported throughout the body including the thyroid, kidneys, bladder, colon, testes, and penis [2]. At extraskeletal sites including the breast, osteosarcomas are thought to arise either as metaplastic differentiation of a preexisting benign or as malignant tumor or de novo from normal breast tissue. Here we present a case of osteogenic sarcoma arising in an intraductal papilloma of the breast.

2. Case Report

A 72-year-old Saudi Arabian woman had a small right breast opacity detected on a screening mammogram, which revealed right upper outer mid and posterior third regional clusters of microcalcifications with underlying increased density associated with partially marginated nodule (Figures 1(a) and 1(b)). The target ultrasound shows partially marginated hypoechoic mass with tubular extension from the lateral aspect and relatively soft in elastography (Figure 2). The lesion was asymptomatic and impalpable. Histological examination of a core biopsy revealed intraductal papilloma, and although follow-up was recommended unfortunately it was not performed.

Two years later she represented with a three-month history of a painless palpable lump in her right breast. On examination, a hard, mobile, well-circumscribed 5 cm mass occupying most of lower outer quadrant of the breast was detected. There was no nipple discharge or skin involvement and there were no palpable axillary lymph nodes. The contralateral breast, axilla, and nipple were normal. There was no history of breast trauma, radiotherapy, or hormonal therapy or a family history of breast cancer. Mammography revealed a heavily calcified, lobulated, hyperdense irregular mass in the outer mid breast. The lesion was adjacent

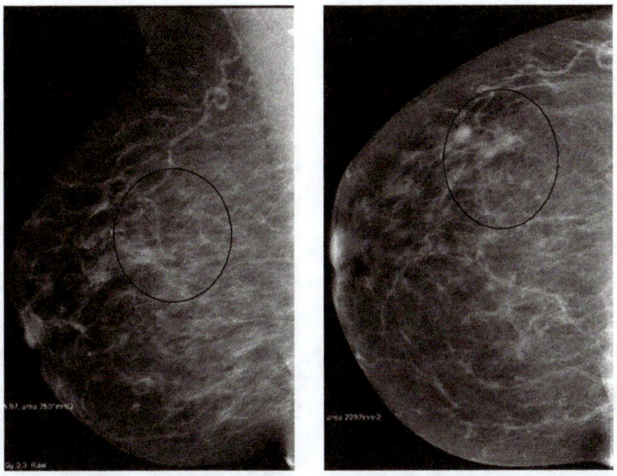

(a) (b)

FIGURE 1: MLO (a) and CC (b) mammogram views of the right breast revealed right upper outer mid and posterior third regional clusters of microcalcifications (circle) with underlying increased density associated with partially marginated nodule; the imaging appearance is suspicious.

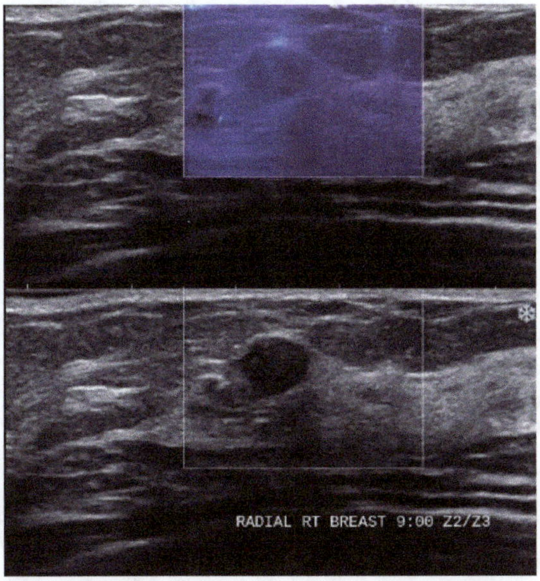

FIGURE 2: Target ultrasound corresponding to mammogram, there is partially marginated hypoechoic mass noted at 9 o'clock mid to posterior third of the right breast measuring 0.7 × 0.8 × 0.5 cm. This mass shows tubular extension from the lateral aspect and shows no internal vascularity. This mass appears relatively soft in elastography.

to a blood vessel, closely resembled bone, and measured 4.8 × 3.9 cm with minimal perilesional edema. The visualized axilla was unremarkable (Figures 3(a) and 3(b)).

Axial and coronal contrast-enhanced computerized tomography (CT) scans were ordered to better characterize the lesion and rule out metastasis. A heavily calcified right breast mass was noted in the axial plane measuring 3.2 × 5.8 cm with overlying skin thickening (Figures 4(a) and 4(b)).

The patient underwent diagnostic lumpectomy. On macroscopic examination, the mass measured 5.5 × 4.7 × 4.2 cm and was ill defined with a heterogeneous, tan, hard cut surface and extending to within 0.05 cm of the closest medial, deep, and superior margins. On histological and immunohistochemical examination, the lesion was negative CTK, CK5/6, CK7, CKLMW8/18, p63, and CK14. The lesion was diagnosed as a primary osteosarcoma of the breast.

She subsequently underwent a right modified radical mastectomy in which a 5 × 4 × 3 cm tan, firm mass in the lower outer quadrant was resected. The mass contained cystic spaces filled with blood but no further residual osteosarcoma was identified and the sentinel lymph node was negative. She did not receive any adjuvant chemotherapy but did receive close follow-up.

Three months after mastectomy she presented again with recurrent, multiple firm lumps in the outer lower quadrant of her right breast at the mastectomy site (Figure 5). She underwent reoperation, at which multiple, white masses were identified measuring 6 × 5.5 × 3.5 cm maximum with cystic walls underneath the previous scar. No tumor tissue was identified.

3. Discussion

Primary osteosarcoma of the breast (POB) is a very rare tumor, accounting for less than 1% of all breast malignancies [1]. The prognosis for patients with POB is poor, with a reported 5-year overall survival of only 38% [3].

The carcinogenetic pathway of primary osteosarcoma is poorly understood, but the leading hypotheses are that they either arise from totipotent mesenchymal cells in the breast stroma or from transformation of preexisting phyllodes tumors or fibroadenomas [3, 4]. There is a known association between a history of trauma or radiation exposure to the breast and POB [3], although neither of these factors were reported in this case.

On radiographic examination, mammary osteosarcomas usually show pathological bone formation in the breast tissue

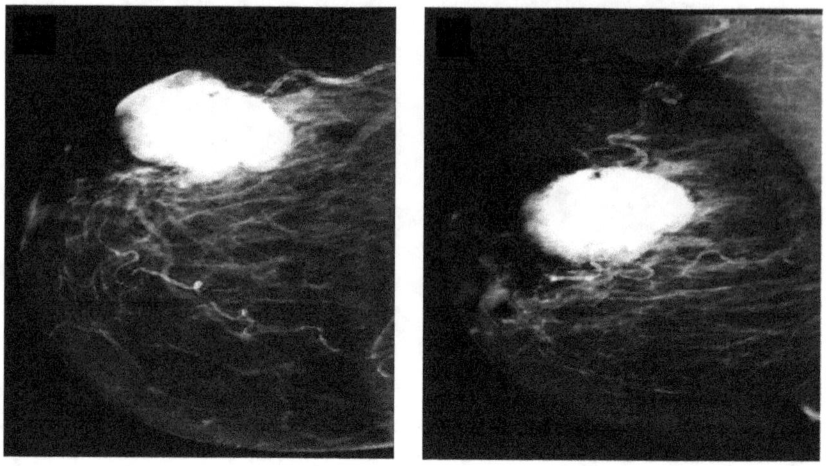

(a) (b)

FIGURE 3: MLO (a) and CC (b) mammogram views of the right breast revealed a heavily calcified lobulated mass in the outer mid breast measuring 4.8 × 3.9 cm adjacent to a blood vessel with minimal perilesional edema.

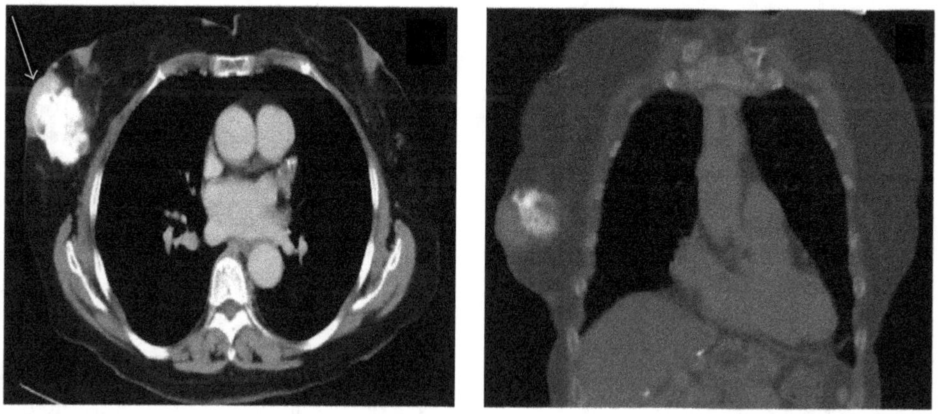

(a) (b)

FIGURE 4: Axial (a) and coronal (b) contrast-enhanced CT to characterize the lesion and rule out metastasis. A heavily calcified right breast mass was noted measuring about 3.2 × 5.8 cm with overlying skin thickening.

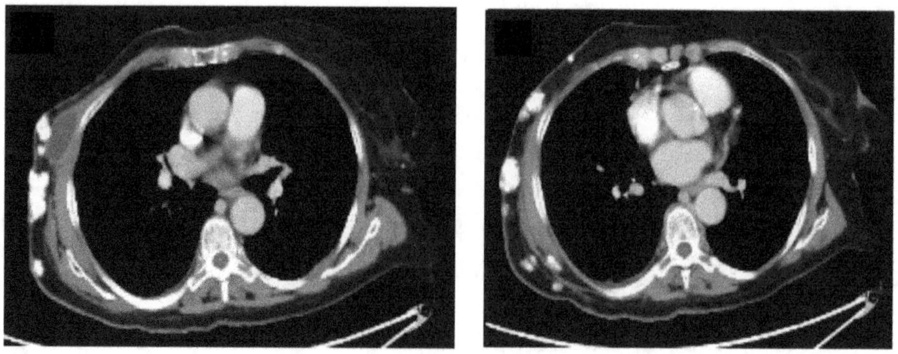

(a) (b)

FIGURE 5: Axial contrast-enhanced postoperative CT performed after three months demonstrates postoperative changes including seroma and multiple right chest wall subcutaneous calcified nodules compatible with metastasis.

as a result of intermembranous ossification but marrow is not present [5]. The management of POB is similar to that of other sarcomas. Surgery aims to remove the lesion in its entirety with clear margins, since margin status is a major risk factor for recurrence [2, 6]. Nevertheless, mammary osteosarcomas are biologically aggressive tumors characterized by early recurrence and hematogenous metastasis, frequently to the lungs [7]. Patients may require chemotherapy when tumors are large (>5 cm) and/or high-grade, with doxorubicin, cisplatin, methotrexate, and ifosfamide showing cytotoxic effects in osteosarcomas [8]. However, administration of chemotherapy must be balanced against side effects especially in older or unfit patients, such as in this case.

References

[1] M. Szajewski, W. J. Kruszewski, M. Ciesielski, U. Śmiałek-Kusowska, M. Czerepko, and J. Szefel, "Primary osteosarcoma of the breast: A case report," *Oncology Letters*, vol. 7, no. 6, pp. 1962–1964, 2014.

[2] A. M. Thomas and B. E. Nathan, "Primary osteosarcoma of the breast," *The British Journal of Radiology*, vol. 57, no. 680, pp. 762-763, 1984.

[3] S. A. Silver and F. A. Tavassoli, "Primary osteogenic sarcoma of the breast: A clinicopathologic analysis of 50 cases," *American Journal of Surgical Pathology*, vol. 22, no. 8, pp. 925–933, 1998.

[4] S. Remadi, I. Doussis-Anagnostopoulu, and W. Mac Gee, "Primary Osteosarcoma of the Breast," *Pathology - Research and Practice*, vol. 191, no. 5, pp. 471–474, 1995.

[5] V. Singhal, Chintamani, and J. Cosgrove, "Osteogenic sarcoma of the breast arising in a cystosarcoma phyllodes: a case report and review of the literature," *Journal of Medical Case Reports*, vol. 5, article 293, 2011.

[6] C. Adem, C. Reynolds, J. N. Ingle, and A. G. Nascimento, "Primary breast sarcoma: clinicopathologic series from the Mayo Clinic and review of the literature," *British Journal of Cancer*, vol. 91, no. 2, pp. 237–241, 2004.

[7] U. Kaiser, P. Barth, V. Duda, K.-H. Pflüger, and K. Havemann, "Primary osteosarcoma of the breast-case report and review of the literature," *Acta Oncologica*, vol. 33, no. 1, pp. 74–76, 1994.

[8] ESMO/European Sarcoma Network Working Group. Bone sarcomas: ESMO Clinical.

53

Mandibular Osteitis Leading to the Diagnosis of SAPHO Syndrome

Tomohiro Kikuchi,[1] Hiroyuki Fujii ,[1] Akifumi Fujita,[1] Tomoko Sugiyama,[2] and Hideharu Sugimoto[1]

[1] *Department of Radiology, Jichi Medical University, School of Medicine, 3311-1 Yakushiji, Shimotsuke, Tochigi 329-0498, Japan*
[2] *Department of Dentistry, Oral and Maxillofacial Surgery, Jichi Medical University, School of Medicine, 3311-1 Yakushiji, Shimotsuke, Tochigi 329-0498, Japan*

Correspondence should be addressed to Hiroyuki Fujii; hiroyuki.fujii@jichi.ac.jp

Academic Editor: Bruce J. Barron

Synovitis, acne, pustulosis, hyperostosis, and osteitis (SAPHO) syndrome is a disorder characterized by pustular skin lesions and osteoarticular lesions. Mandibular involvement of SAPHO syndrome is clinically rare, and it is difficult to reach a diagnosis of SAPHO syndrome from only mandibular manifestations. This report describes the case of a 26-year-old woman who presented with mandibular osteitis. Orthopantomogram and computed tomography showed sclerotic change of the right body of the mandible with periosteal reaction without odontogenic infection, which suggested the possibility of SAPHO syndrome. Detailed medical interview found that she had a history of palmoplantar pustulosis treated at a local dermatology clinic and additional bone scintigraphy showed diffuse increased uptake in the right mandible, as well as in the sternum and the sternocostoclavicular joints. She was eventually diagnosed as having SAPHO syndrome. We should consider SAPHO syndrome when we encounter a patient with mandibular osteitis of unknown etiology.

1. Introduction

Synovitis, acne, pustulosis, hyperostosis, and osteitis (SAPHO) syndrome is a disorder characterized by pustular skin lesions and osteoarticular lesions proposed in 1987 by Chamot et al. [1]. It is known to present at any age ranging from childhood to adulthood and is characterized by repeated episodes of remission and recurrence. SAPHO syndrome can be difficult to diagnose because of its variable clinical presentation, widespread distribution, and broad spectrum of imaging features [2]. Generally, combinations of osteoarticular and skin manifestations lead to its diagnosis.

Mandibular involvement of SAPHO syndrome is clinically rare and has been reported to comprise 10% of this entity [1]. It is often seen as recurrent mandibular osteitis demonstrating bone sclerosis, mainly involving the body of the mandible [3]. Because a mandibular lesion in SAPHO syndrome is often misdiagnosed as bacterial osteomyelitis, some affected patients received long-term antibiotic therapy combined with surgical procedures and it is rare that the mandibular lesion triggers the diagnosis of SAPHO syndrome [3, 4]. Herein, we report the case of a 26-year-old woman with mandibular osteitis leading to the diagnosis of SAPHO syndrome.

2. Case Report

A 26-year-old woman presented to a local dentist due to right mandible pain. She did not complain of any other manifestations, and she had no pertinent past medical history. She was diagnosed with periapical periodontitis, which is an infection of the dental pulp with an apical lesion, of the right lower first molar. She subsequently underwent a root canal therapy. However, she also complained of swelling of the right mandibular region. Since her symptoms had been worsening for 4 months, she was referred to our hospital for further examination and treatment. At our hospital, facial conditions

Table 1: Diagnostic criteria for SAPHO syndrome [11, 12].

Inclusion criteria
(i) Bone and/or joint involvement associated with palmoplantar pustulosis and psoriasis vulgaris, or hidradenitis suppurativa
(ii) Bone and/or joint involvement associated with severe acne
(iii) Isolated sterile hyperostosis/osteitis (adults)[a]
(iv) Chronic recurrent multifocal osteomyelitis (children)
(v) Bone and/or joint involvement associated with chronic bowel diseases
Exclusion criteria
(i) Infectious osteitis
(ii) Tumoral conditions of the bone
(iii) Noninflammatory condensing lesions of the bone

[a]With the exception of *Propionibacterium acnes*.

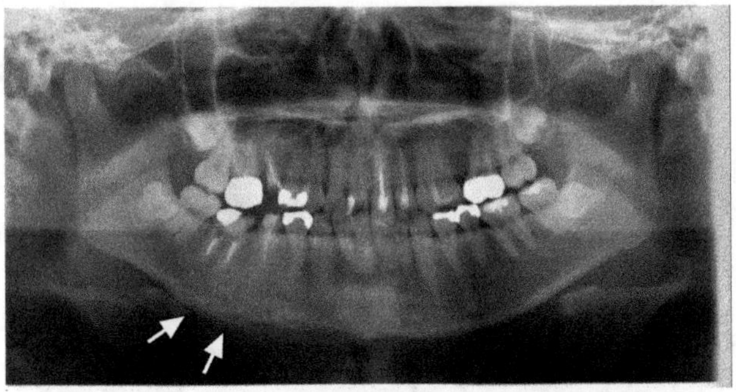

Figure 1: Orthopantomography. Sclerotic changes are seen in the right body of the mandible with periosteal reaction (arrows).

revealed right mandibular swelling and tenderness. Oral conditions showed no percussion and occlusal pain of teeth in the swelling region, and tooth mobility, gum swelling, and gum redness were not seen. Hence, there was no dental infection that could cause osteomyelitis/osteitis. Blood samples were unremarkable with no signs of inflammation.

Orthopantomogram showed sclerotic change at the right body of the mandible with periosteal reaction (Figure 1). Plain computed tomography (CT) showed sclerotic change at the right body of the mandible with periosteal reaction and spotted osteolysis was seen in the cortex of the mandible (Figure 2). On magnetic resonance imaging (MRI), the right body of the mandible showed low signal intensity on T1-weighted images and high signal intensity on short tau inversion recovery (STIR) images with perilesional soft tissue swelling (Figure 3). Bilateral palatine tonsils and reactive lymphadenopathy were also seen. These findings indicated active mandibular osteomyelitis/osteitis without odontogenic infection. At this time, the possibility of SAPHO syndrome was considered. Detailed medical interview found that she had a history of palmoplantar pustulosis (PPP) for about 1 year, which was treated at a local dermatology clinic. To investigate the presence of other osteoarticular involvement, technetium-99m hydroxymethylene diphosphonate (^{99m}Tc-HMDP) scintigraphy was performed, which demonstrated diffuse increased uptake at the right mandible, as well as in the sternum and the sternocostoclavicular joints (Figure 4). These characteristics of clinical and radiological manifestations led to the diagnosis of SAPHO syndrome.

Tonsillectomy was performed for PPP, and bone biopsy of the right mandible was simultaneously performed. Histopathological examination showed enlarged and sclerotic bone trabeculae with little inflammatory cell infiltration, which was compatible with SAPHO syndrome (Figure 5).

She was treated with salazosulfapyridine 1000 mg/day and nonsteroidal anti-inflammatory drugs as needed, and the pain resolved. Thus far, after a 5-month follow-up period, she has not experienced recurrence of pain.

3. Discussion

SAPHO syndrome affects individuals of any age, ranging from childhood to adulthood, and its prevalence has been estimated to be no greater than one in 10,000 in Caucasians and is rarer in Asians [5]. Most patients present with local inflammatory symptoms of pain, swelling, and limitation of movement at the site of active involvement without suppuration [6]. The pathogenesis of SAPHO syndrome remains unknown and several hypotheses, such as infectious, immunological, and genetic mechanisms, have been proposed. An infective cause is a widely accepted theory, and it is described as an autoinflammatory process triggered by low-virulence pathogens [7, 8]. *Propionibacterium acnes*, a member of normal flora of the skin and gastrointestinal tract, is occasionally identified from osteoarticular biopsy samples. However, in many instances, biopsy culture is negative and antibiotic therapy is generally ineffective [9]. SAPHO syndrome shares clinical and radiologic features with spondyloarthropathy (SpA), including sacroiliitis, enthesis, paravertebral ossifications, and ankylosis, and many times is associated with psoriasis and inflammatory bowel disease. However, its consideration as a variant of SpA is controversial [10]. Serum rheumatoid factor is usually absent, and human leukocyte antigen-B27 is positive in 4–18% of patients, which is less frequent compared to SpA [7].

The rationale for establishing SAPHO syndrome is that unusual bone involvement is the common denominator among the four skin diseases, such as PPP, acne, psoriasis vulgaris, and generalized pustular psoriasis, by either its radiologic appearance or pathologic features [13]. In 1994, Kahn et al. reported three diagnostic criteria that characterize SAPHO syndrome, which were modified in 2003 (see Table 1) [11, 12]. In many cases, combinations of osteoarticular and

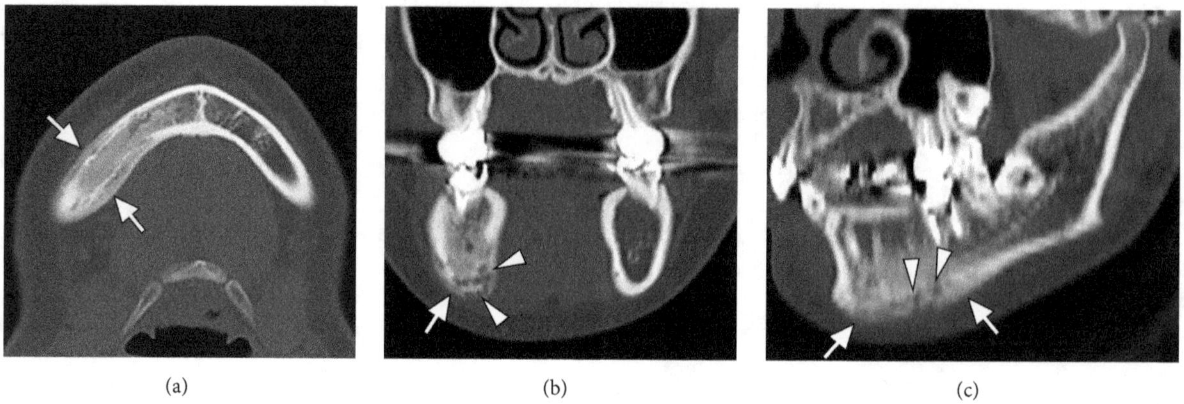

(a) (b) (c)

FIGURE 2: CT scan of the mandible. Axial (a) and coronal (b) and oblique sagittal reconstruction (c) plain CT images show sclerotic change and periosteal reaction in the right body of the mandible (arrows). Spotted osteolysis is also seen mainly in the cortical bone (arrowheads).

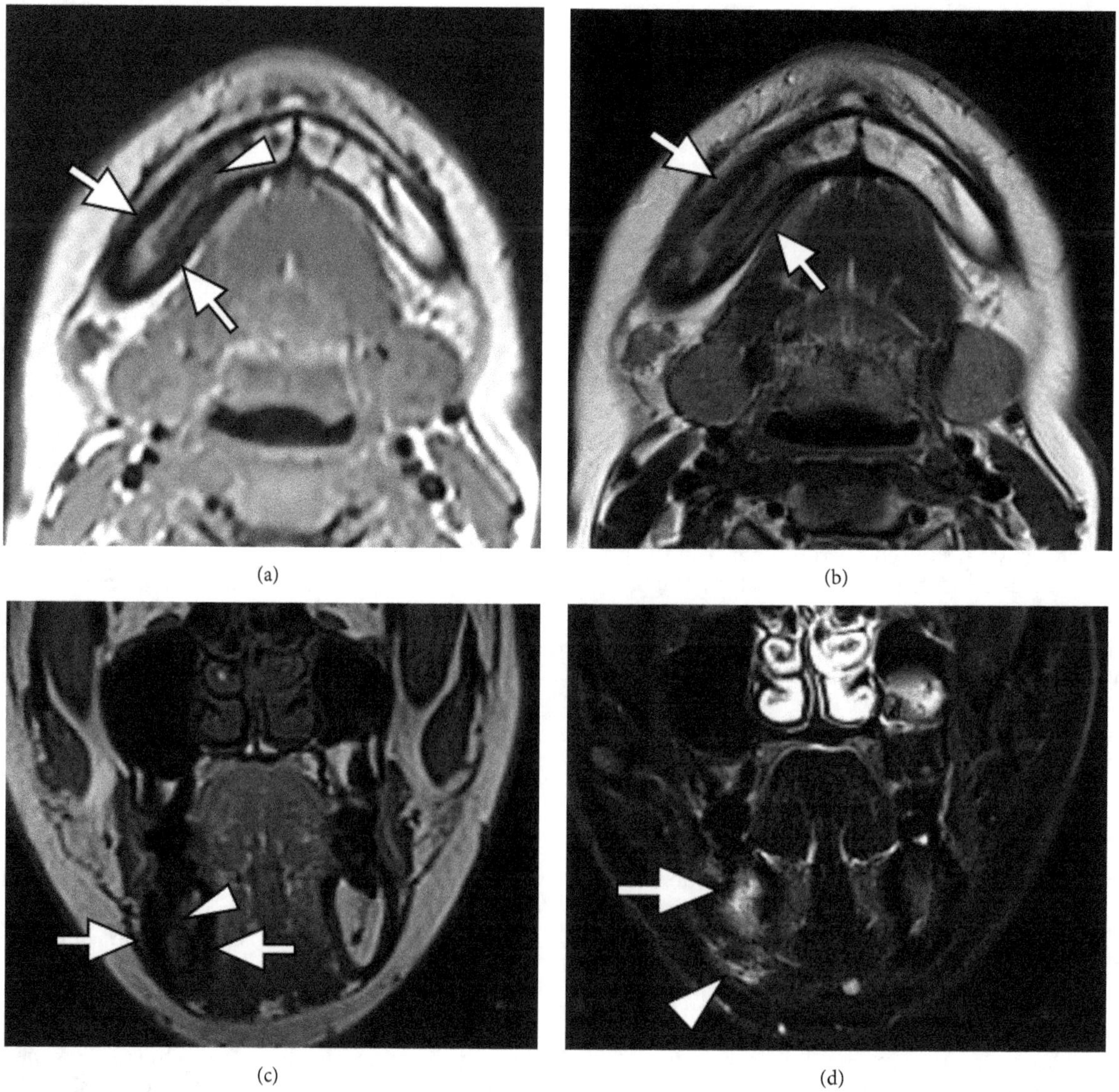

(a) (b) (c) (d)

FIGURE 3: MR imaging of the mandible. Axial (a) and coronal (c) T1-weighted images and axial T2-weighted image (b) show thickening of the right mandible (arrows) and decreased bone marrow fat signal (arrowheads). Coronal short tau inversion recovery image (d) shows high signal intensity in the right body of the mandible (arrow), with perilesional soft tissue swelling (arrowhead).

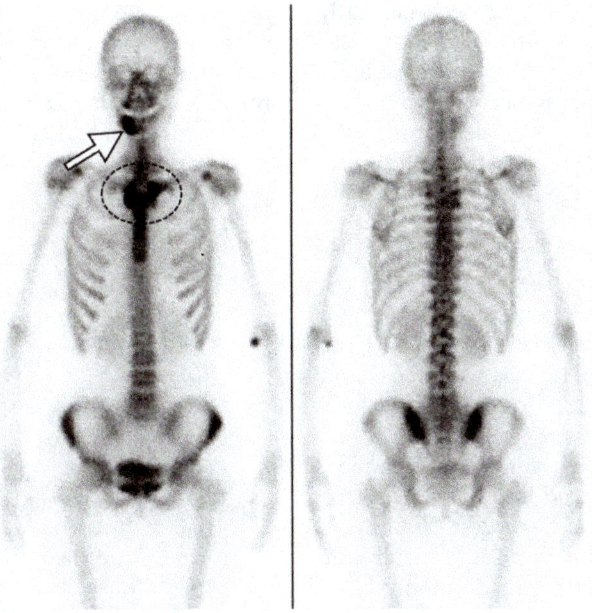

FIGURE 4: Bone scintigraphy. There is increased tracer uptake in the right mandible (arrow), sternum, and the sternocostoclavicular joints (dotted circle).

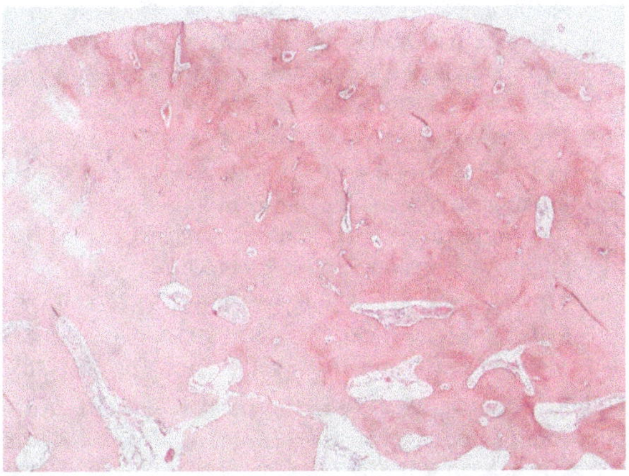

(a)

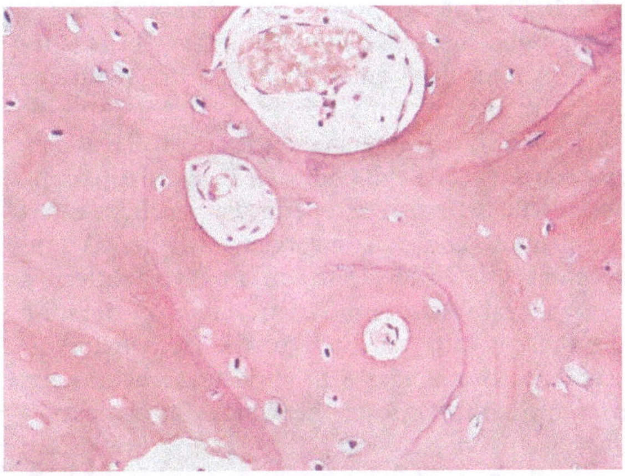

(b)

FIGURE 5: Histopathological findings of the mandible. Enlarged and sclerotic bone trabeculae with little inflammatory cell infiltration [hematoxylin-eosin staining; magnification: 100× (a), 400× (b)].

skin manifestations lead to the diagnosis of SAPHO syndrome. Our case showed PPP in addition to sterile osteitis of the mandible, and it met the diagnostic criteria.

The most common target site of osteoarticular lesions for SAPHO syndrome in adults is the anterior chest wall, in particular, the clavicles, sternum, and sternoclavicular joints, followed by the sacroiliac region and the spine [14]. Mandibular involvement is relatively rare and has been reported to comprise 10% of this entity [1, 3]. Bone lesions tend to be osteolytic in early stages and osteosclerotic at later stages [14]. Osteosclerotic manifestations include hyperostosis and osteitis, which are chronic inflammatory reactions involving both cortical and medullary bones.

On CT, hyperostosis appears as endosteal and periosteal reactions resulting in generalized cortical thickening and narrowing of the medullary canal. Osteitis appears as increased osteosclerosis involving the trabecular infrastructure of cancellous bone in response to the underlying inflammation [9, 15]. MRI provides better definition of the extent of the inflammatory process in relation to bone marrow edema and soft tissue swelling. Fat-suppressed T2-weighted or STIR images may show high signals on affected sites and are useful to differentiate active lesions from quiescent lesions. Erosions and osteosclerosis are not well depicted, which are well depicted on CT [15]. Bone scintigraphy shows increased tracer uptake in the affected region. In addition, bone scintigraphy is useful because it frequently reveals clinically silent lesions. High tracer uptake in the sternocostoclavicular region yields the so-called "bull's head sign," with the body of the sternum representing the upper skull and the inflamed sternoclavicular joint with the adjacent clavicles forming the horns [16]. A mandibular lesion also demonstrates the imaging findings described above. The mandibular lesion usually shows unilateral involvement at the body of the mandible [3, 17]. Although it is rare, extension to the temporomandibular joint evolves into ankylosis [18]. In the present case, the right body of the mandible showed sclerotic change with prominent periosteal reaction on CT and showed low signal intensity on T1-weighted images and high signal intensity on STIR images, which were compatible with reported imaging findings.

Some cases with imaging findings similar to mandibular involvement of SAPHO syndrome have been reported under various names, such as chronic recurrent multifocal osteomyelitis, diffuse sclerosing osteomyelitis, and juvenile mandibular chronic osteomyelitis (Garre's osteomyelitis), and some of these cases are considered to be included in SAPHO syndrome [14, 19]. The differential diagnosis for imaging findings of mandibular lesion may include suppurative osteomyelitis, fibrous dysplasia, Paget's disease, osseous neoplasms including osteoid osteoma, osteosarcoma, Ewing's sarcoma, lymphoma, metastases, and Langerhans' cell histiocytosis [14]. It is difficult to differentiate SAPHO syndrome from suppurative osteomyelitis because of its nonspecific findings, such as bone marrow edema and periosteal reaction. Suei et al. reported that SAPHO syndrome revealed osteosclerotic and osteolytic patterns, solid periosteal reaction, external bone resorption, and bone enlargement, whereas suppurative osteomyelitis demonstrated an osteolytic pattern, a lamellated periosteal reaction, and cortical bone perforation [15]. In the present case, the body of the right mandible showed osteosclerotic changes with periosteal reaction and osteolysis mainly in the cortical bone, which was compatible with findings of a previous report [17].

The key to diagnose SAPHO syndrome is to depict both osteoarticular and skin manifestations; however, only the single bone may be symptomatic at disease onset and the skin manifestation does not always occur at the same time [17, 20]. Thus, making a diagnosis of SAPHO syndrome with the mandibular lesion alone as an initial presentation is difficult. In addition, patients may regard skin lesions and mandibular pain/swelling as irrelevant and sometimes skin lesions are hidden. In our case, the medical history of PPP was concealed, and she did not complain of any symptoms except right mandibular pain and swelling when she was first referred to our hospital. We could consider the possibility of SAPHO syndrome from mandibular osteitis because there was no evidence of dental infection, which could cause osteomyelitis.

4. Conclusion

We experienced a case of SAPHO syndrome revealed by mandibular osteitis. Although it is difficult to diagnose SAPHO syndrome from only the presence of a mandibular lesion, we should consider the possibility of SAPHO syndrome when we encounter patients with mandibular osteitis of unknown etiology. Detailed medical interview and further imaging examination including bone scintigraphy can lead to the diagnosis of SAPHO syndrome.

References

[1] A. M. Chamot, C. L. Benhamou, and M. F. Kahn, "The syndrome acne-pustulosis-hyperostosis-osteitis (SAPHO). Results of a national investigation. 85 case-reports," *Revue du Rhumatisme et des Maladies Ostéo-Articulaires*, vol. 54, no. 3, pp. 187–196, 1987.

[2] M. Magrey and M. A. Khan, "New insights into synovitis, acne, pustulosis, hyperostosis, and osteitis (SAPHO) syndrome," *Current Rheumatology Reports*, vol. 11, no. 5, pp. 329–333, 2009.

[3] W. Zemann, M. Pau, M. Feichtinger, B. Ferra-Matschy, and H. Kaercher, "SAPHO syndrome with affection of the mandible: diagnosis, treatment, and review of literature," *Oral Surgery, Oral Medicine, Oral Pathology, Oral Radiology, and Endodontology*, vol. 111, no. 2, pp. 190–195, 2011.

[4] E. Karadag-Saygi, O. Hakan Gunduz, G. Gumrukcu, and G. Akyuz, "SAPHO syndrome: misdiagnosed and operated," *Acta Reumatólogica Portuguesa*, vol. 33, no. 4, pp. 460–463, 2008.

[5] S. Hukuda, M. Minami, T. Saito et al., "Spondyloarthropathies in Japan: nationwide questionnaire survey performed by the Japan ankylosing spondylitis society," *The Journal of Rheumatology*, vol. 28, no. 3, pp. 554–559, 2001.

[6] J. C. Roldán, H. Terheyden, A. Dunsche, W. U. Kampen, and J. O. Schroeder, "Acne with chronic recurrent multifocal osteomyelitis involving the mandible as part of the SAPHO syndrome: case report," *British Journal of Oral and Maxillofacial Surgery*, vol. 39, no. 2, pp. 141–144, 2001.

[7] M. T. Nguyen, A. Borchers, C. Selmi, S. M. Naguwa, G. Cheema, and M. E. Gershwin, "The SAPHO Syndrome," *Seminars in Arthritis and Rheumatism*, vol. 42, no. 3, pp. 254–265, 2012.

[8] F. Ciccarelli, M. De Martinis, and L. Ginaldi, "An update on autoinflammatory diseases," *Current Medicinal Chemistry*, vol. 21, no. 3, pp. 261–269, 2014.

[9] G. Hayem, A. Bouchaud-Chabot, K. Benali et al., "SAPHO syndrome: a long-term follow-up study of 120 cases," *Seminars in Arthritis and Rheumatism*, vol. 29, no. 3, pp. 159–171, 1999.

[10] S. Carneiro and P. D. Sampaio-Barros, "SAPHO Syndrome," *Rheumatic Disease Clinics of North America*, vol. 39, no. 2, pp. 401–418, 2013.

[11] M.-F. Kahn and M. A. Khan, "The SAPHO syndrome," *Best Practice & Research Clinical Rheumatology*, vol. 8, no. 2, pp. 333–362, 1994.

[12] I. Rukavina, "SAPHO syndrome: a review," *Journal of Children's Orthopaedics*, vol. 9, no. 1, pp. 19–27, 2015.

[13] H. Sugimoto, K. Tamura, and T. Fujii, "The SAPHO syndrome: defining the radiologic spectrum of diseases comprising the syndrome," *European Radiology*, vol. 8, no. 5, pp. 800–806, 1998.

[14] R. Depasquale, N. Kumar, R. K. Lalam et al., "SAPHO: what radiologists should know," *Clinical Radiology*, vol. 67, no. 3, pp. 195–206, 2012.

[15] J. W. S. Earwaker and A. Cotten, "SAPHO: Syndrome or concept? Imaging findings," *Skeletal Radiology*, vol. 32, no. 6, pp. 311–327, 2003.

[16] J. Freyschmidt and A. Sternberg, "The bullhead sign: scintigraphic pattern of sternocostoclavicular hyperostosis and pustulotic arthroosteitis," *European Radiology*, vol. 8, no. 5, pp. 807–812, 1998.

[17] Y. Suei, A. Taguchi, and K. Tanimoto, "Diagnostic points and possible origin of osteomylitis in synovitis, acne, pustulosis, hyperostosis and osteitis (SAPHO) syndrome: a radiographic study of 77 mandibular osteomyelitis cases," *Rheumatology*, vol. 42, no. 11, pp. 1398–1403, 2003.

[18] E. R. Utumi, M. A. Oliveira Sales, E. H. Shinohara et al., "SAPHO syndrome with temporomandibular joint ankylosis: clinical, radiological, histopathological, and therapeutical correlations," *Oral Surgery, Oral Medicine, Oral Pathology, Oral Radiology, and Endodontology*, vol. 105, no. 3, pp. e67–e72, 2008.

[19] Y. Suei, A. Taguchi, and K. Tanimoto, "Diagnosis and classification of mandibular osteomyelitis," *Oral Surgery, Oral Medicine, Oral Pathology, Oral Radiology, and Endodontology*, vol. 100, no. 2, pp. 207–214, 2005.

[20] S. Van Doornum, D. Barraclough, G. McColl, and I. Wicks, "Sapho: Rare or just not recognized?" *Seminars in Arthritis and Rheumatism*, vol. 30, no. 1, pp. 70–77, 2000.

54

Extraosseous Intradural Chondrosarcoma of the Cervical Spine: A Case Report

Elizabeth Presutto,[1] **Sejal Patel**,[1] **Joseph Fullmer**,[2] **and Sajeev Ezhapilli**[1]

[1]*Department of Radiology, SUNY Upstate Medical University, Room 3530, 750 East Adams Street, Syracuse, NY 13210, USA*
[2]*Department of Pathology, SUNY Upstate Medical University, 750 East Adams Street, Syracuse, NY, USA*

Correspondence should be addressed to Elizabeth Presutto; presutte@upstate.edu

Academic Editor: Ruben Dammers

Mesenchymal chondrosarcoma (MCS) is a malignant cancer of the cartilage that accounts for less than 1% of all chondrosarcomas and typically occurs within the bone. One-third of all mesenchymal chondrosarcomas are extraosseous soft tissue sarcomas, rendering this as an uncommon entity. We report a rare case of an extraosseous chondrosarcoma with the cervical spinal canal in a 21-year-old male. The purpose of this case report is to discuss the imaging characteristics of this pathology proven diagnosis.

1. Introduction

Extraosseous mesenchymal chondrosarcoma (MCS) is an aggressive, high-grade malignant tumor predominantly of the bone and also of the soft tissue that demonstrates a biphasic pattern of small cells with islands of atypical cartilage. It represents 1% or less of all chondrosarcomas, in which one-third are extraosseous [1]. Most cases of MCS originate in the head and neck region, followed by trunk and extremities. Craniofacial, spine, and ribs are most commonly affected [2]. MCS affects all ages, with a peak incidence in the second decade of life and a slight predilection for women. Overall survival rate is poor with a 10-year survival of less than 30% [3, 4].

Extramedullary, intradural location of MCS is exceedingly rare with a limited number of cases reported in the United States [5–7]. Herein, we report a case of extraosseous mesenchymal chondrosarcoma in a young male involving the cervical spinal canal.

2. Case Presentation

A 21-year-old white male presented to his primary care provider with a 3-month history of neck pain with stiffness, tingling, and paresthesias in his right arm at the C6–C8 dermatomal distribution. He also complained of loss of dexterity, loss of grip strength, and some gait instabilities. His exam was positive for Babinski's sign on the right and some vision loss. An initial brain magnetic resonance imaging (MRI) was normal. Contrast enhanced cervical spine MRI demonstrated an enhancing intradural extramedullary T1 isointense and T2 hypointense mass at the level of C2-C3, anterior to cervical spinal cord and resulting in severe spinal canal stenosis. There is mass effect with posterior displacement of the cord, cord compression, and cord edema (Figures 1(a) and 1(b)).

Subsequently, decompression with bilateral posterior cervical C2-C3 laminectomies and tumor resection was attempted by neurosurgery. However, full resection of the mass was not achieved after significant loss of motor signals was evoked. As a result, the patient only received posterior decompression at this level. The patient's postoperative course was uneventful and the patient was discharged with plan to attend occupational and physical rehabilitation. On pathology, gross section demonstrated fragments of tissue ranging from 0.1 to 0.4 cm. Microscopy revealed tightly packed small blue cells with greatly increased nuclear to cytoplasmic ratios and some areas of cartilage. Pathology was sent to an

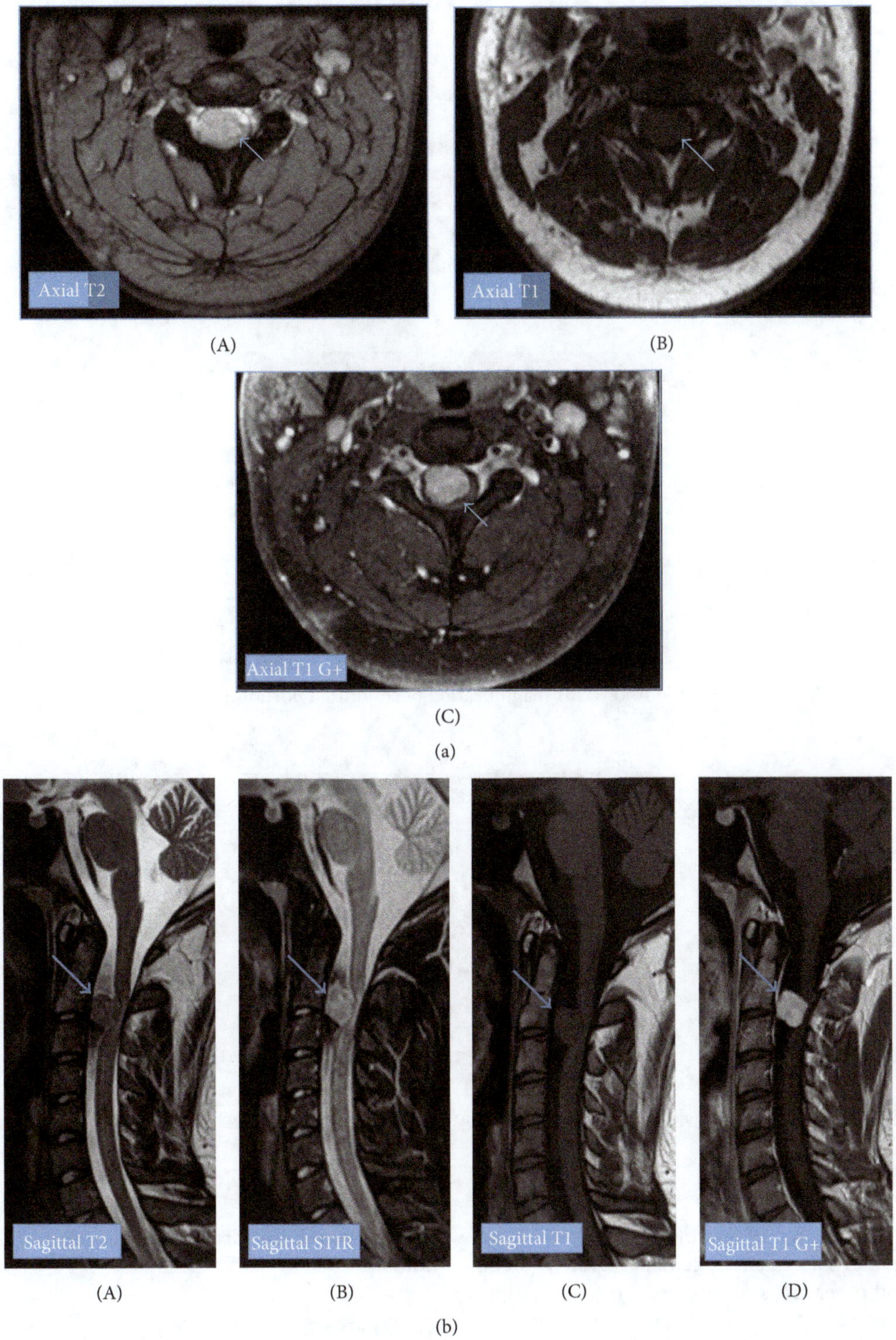

FIGURE 1: There is a slightly lobulated well-demarcated 1.4 × 1.7 × 1.2 cm intradural extramedullary mass lesion (blue arrow) in the spinal canal, anterior to the spinal cord at the level of C2-C3. There is mass effect with posterior displacement of the cord as well as cord edema. There is widening of the ventral subarachnoid space. It is homogeneously isointense on T1 and slightly heterogeneously hypointense on T2. Postcontrast imaging demonstrates avid diffusely homogenous enhancement.

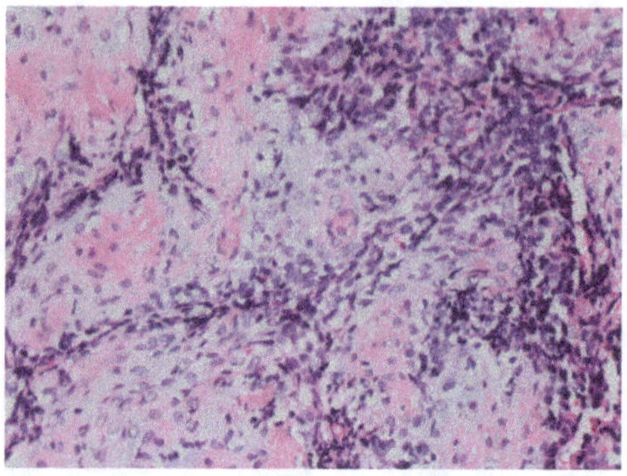

FIGURE 2: 10x magnification of chondroid and mesenchymal portions.

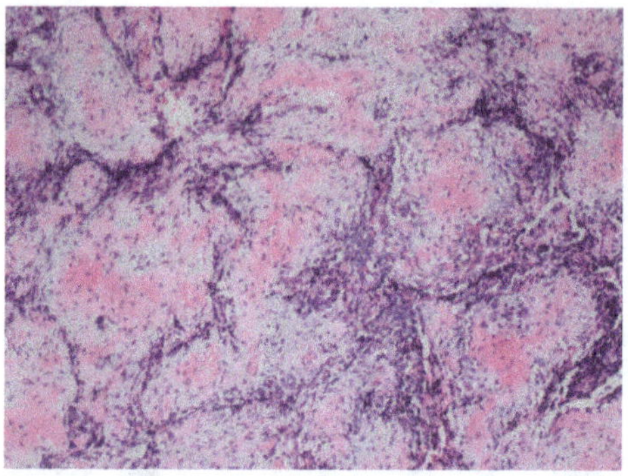

FIGURE 3: 10x magnification of chondroid portion.

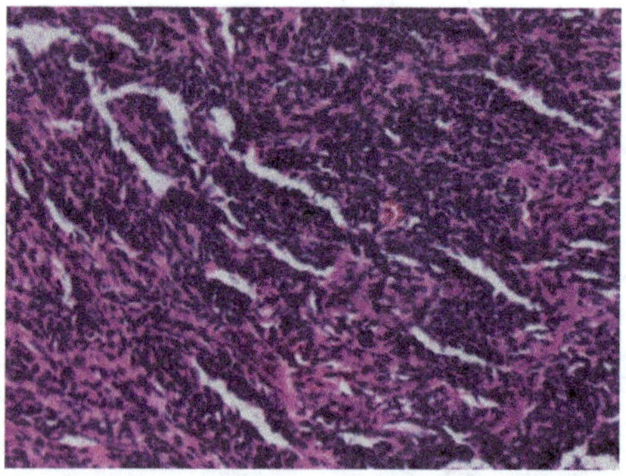

FIGURE 4: 20x magnification of mesenchymal portion.

outside institution for further evaluation. It was determined to show biphasic pattern with densely cellular regions of small anaplastic cells and other areas of chondroid differentiation, consistent with diagnosis of mesenchymal chondrosarcoma (Figures 2–4).

The patient subsequently underwent definitive radiotherapy followed by adjuvant chemotherapy with an Ewing sarcoma protocol for a total of one year. Nonenhanced CT (NECT) of cervical spine was performed at an outside institution for radiotherapy planning (Figures 5(a) and 5(b)). Most current follow-up at two years demonstrates stable findings on MRI with no new abnormalities. The patient has persistent weakness in the left arm but denies any new neurologic symptoms.

3. Discussion

Mesenchymal chondrosarcoma (MCS) is a rare malignant tumor that is classified as chondrosarcoma due to its focal appearance of cartilage with alternating undifferentiated stroma. The first two examples of MCS were described by Lichtenstein and Bernstein in 1959 [8]. Mesenchymal chondrosarcoma represents a rare subset of chondrosarcoma, only few of which are extraskeletal in nature [9]. Shapeero et al.

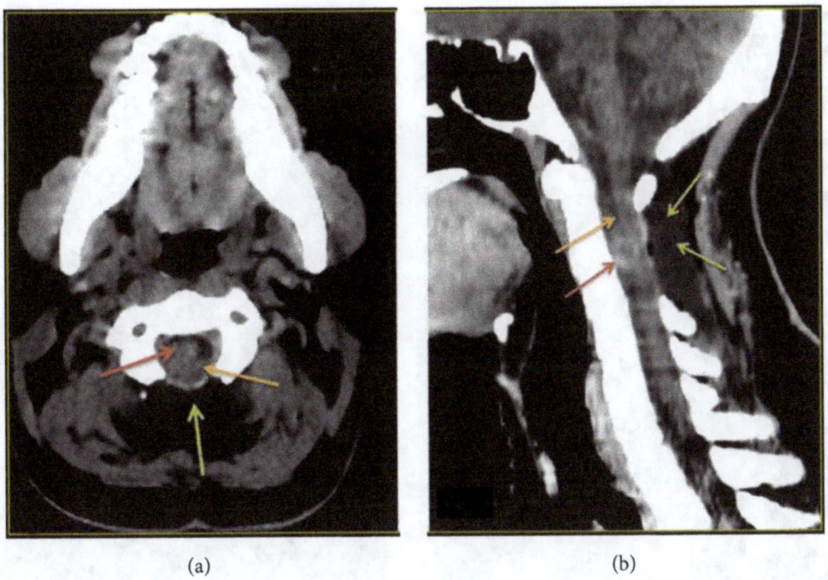

FIGURE 5: Axial NECT (Figure 5(a)) and sagittal NECT (Figure 5(b)) of cervical spine demonstrate surgical changes secondary to posterior spinal decompression (green arrows) at C2 and C3 levels, as well as a well-defined soft tissue density lesion (red arrows) anterior to cervical spinal cord (orange arrows) at C2-C3.

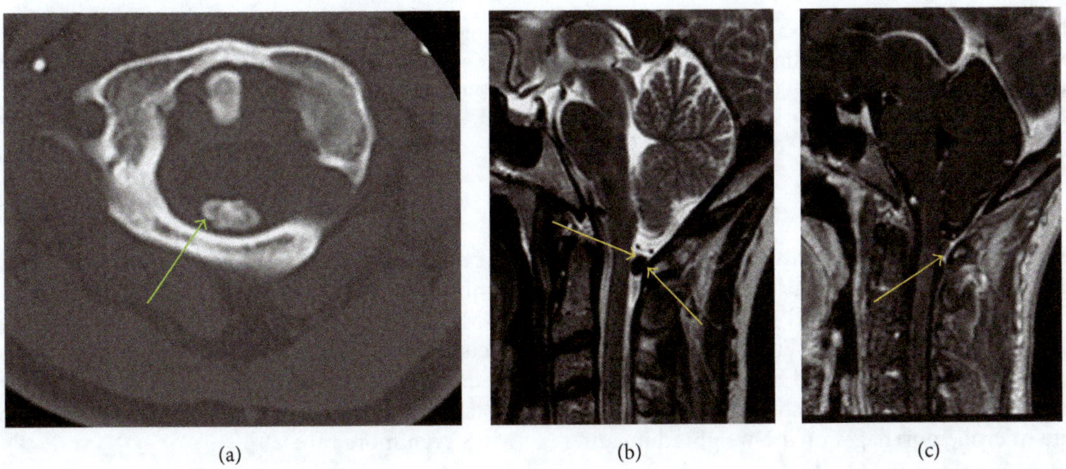

FIGURE 6: Axial NECT of cervical spine (Figure 6(a)) demonstrates a calcified well-marginated lesion (green arrow) within posterior aspect of central canal at C1 level. On sagittal T2WI (Figure 6(b)) and sagittal postgadolinium (Figure 6(c)) MR images, this extramedullary intradural lesion (orange arrows) is noted to be T2 hypointense and mildly rim enhancing, respectively, causing effacement of posterior thecal sac and abutment of cervical spinal cord at the level of posterior arch of C1. The imaging findings favor a calcified meningioma.

reported that only 7 of 224 cases of MCS were extraosseous in origin [10]. It tends to grow rapidly, predominantly affects teens and young adults, and usually involves bone and somatic soft tissue [4].

Given the extraosseous presentation of our case, MCS was not initially suggested. Extraskeletal MCS is exceedingly rare, representing about 0.33% of all chondrosarcomas [2]. Chondrosarcomas generally occur in the pelvis, shoulder, or proximal femur and present in the 4th or 5th decade of life [11]. Despite the mesenchymal type often in the head and neck region, the rarity of the disease and unlikeliness to occur in the soft tissue resulted in its nonconsideration made for initial differential diagnosis. Initial preoperative imaging differential diagnoses instead included meningioma and schwannoma. Meningioma typically presents on MRI as well-defined, extra-axial dural-based mass that is isointense to hypointense to gray matter on T1 demonstrating avid, homogenous contrast enhancement after gadolinium administration, similar to the imaging findings in our case (Figures 6 and 7) [12]. Given the symptoms of sensory loss and weakness, a peripheral nerve tumor such as schwannoma was also considered [12]. Classic enhancement patterns on MRI

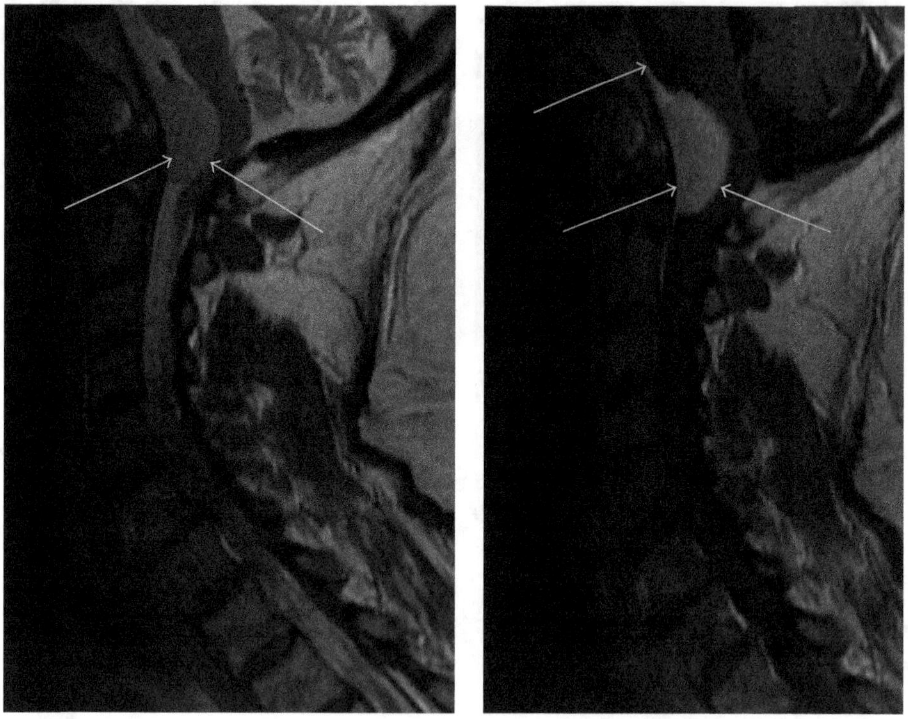

(a) (b)

FIGURE 7: Sagittal T2WI (Figure 7(a)) and sagittal postgadolinium images (Figure 7(b)) show a homogeneously enhancing T2 hyperintense dural-based lesion (green arrows) representing a meningioma, occupying the anterior aspect of foramen magnum. This lesion demonstrates a characteristic dural tail (blue arrow) on postgadolinium image. This lesion causes effacement of anterior subarachnoid space and exerts mass effect resulting in posterior displacement of the adjacent medulla and upper cervical spinal cord with impingement at the level of foramen magnum.

have been described for extracranial schwannomas. Characteristically, schwannomas present with findings such as the target sign, fascicular appearance, and hypointense rim on T2-weighted images (Figure 8) [13, 14]. Furthermore, vestibular schwannomas may be differentiated from a cerebellopontine angle meningioma by the predilection of schwannomas to demonstrate microhemorrhages on T2-weighted imaging [15].

MRI is the preferred imaging modality for intraspinal tumors, but there is no pathognomonic description for extraosseous MCS. Chondrosarcomas share similar findings with chordomas, making the differential diagnosis challenging [16]. On imaging, extraosseous MCS can present as calcified area of low intensity on both T1-weighted and T2-weighted MRI images, whereas the noncalcified areas present as low and high intensity on T1-weighted (T1WIs) and T2-weighted images (T2WIs), respectively. Therefore, the two components typically show clear demarcation on T2WIs and can be used in differentiation. However, Bae et al. reported a case of intraspinal MCS with no evidence of calcification, which elucidates the variation and difficulty in diagnosis by imaging. They described findings of isointensity to the spinal cord on T1WIs and high intensity or isointensity on T2WIs [16]. An additional study of imaging in 10 extraskeletal MSC patients found that, on gadolinium-enhanced MRI, MCS is expected to show heterogeneous enhancement in both calcified and uncalcified areas, although sensitivity and specificity of this finding are unknown [17]. Harsh IV and Wilson reviewed 16 MCS in the primary central nervous system, of which 5 occurred indurally. These tumors typically occur at an extramedullary, extradural site, but majority occur with dural attachment making this case of extramedullary, intradural MCS even more rare [18].

4. Management

Due to the rarity of the disease, no universal management protocol has been established. Total resection with wide margins is typically suggested and surgery has shown to be essential for a positive outcome. Adjunctive chemotherapy and/or radiotherapy may be considered; however, little evidence for their utility has been demonstrated so far. Careful, long-term follow-up and monitoring should last at least 10 years due to the tendency toward recurrence and metastasis in >70% of cases [9, 18].

5. Conclusion

Our case demonstrated an unusual and rare extraskeletal location of mesenchymal chondrosarcoma: extramedullary, intradural within the cervical spine. We suggest the importance of considering the diagnosis of mesenchymal

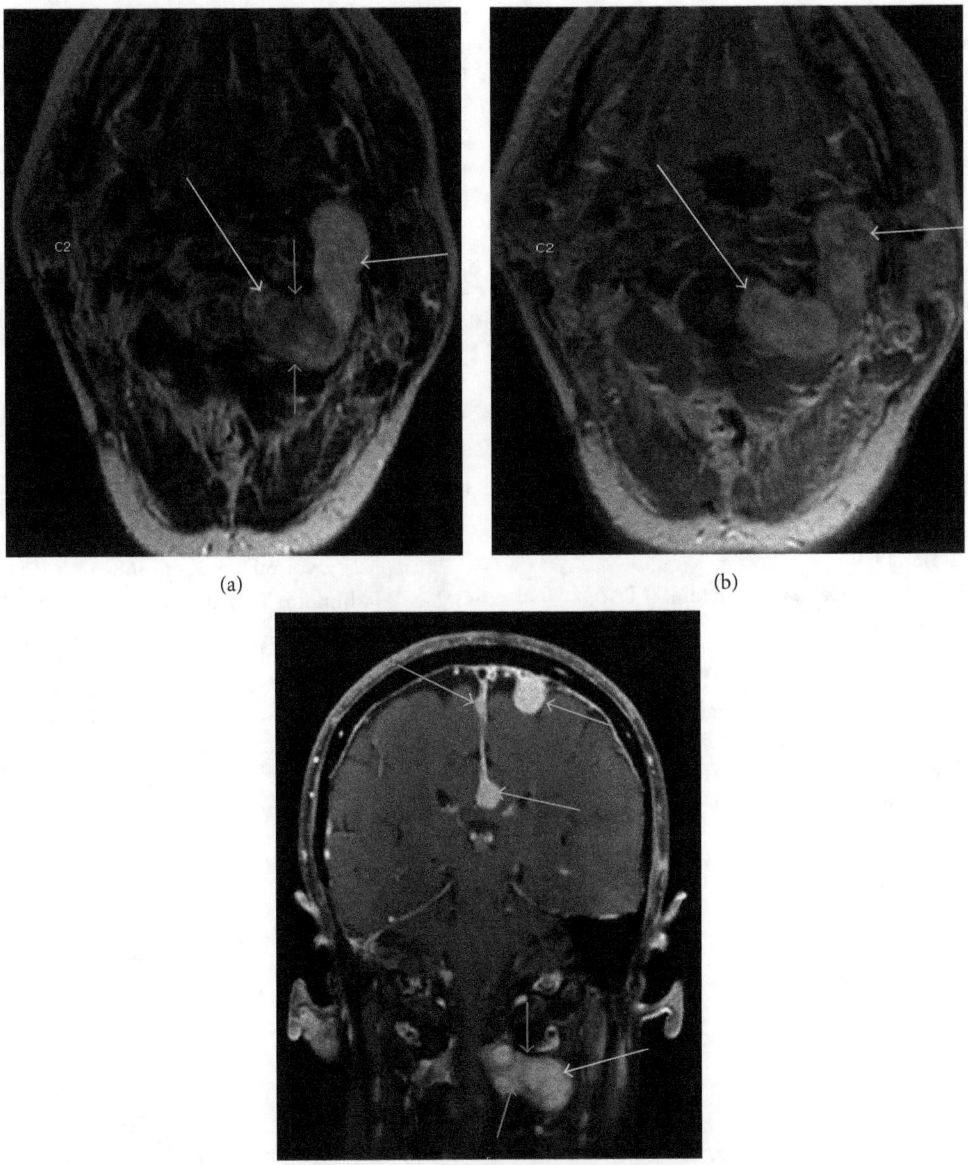

(a) (b) (c)

FIGURE 8: Axial T2WI (Figure 8(a)), axial postgadolinium (Figure 8(b)), and coronal postgadolinium (Figure 8(c)) demonstrate a well-defined extramedullary heterogeneously enhancing T2 hyperintense lobulated lesion representing a schwannoma (green arrow) extending along the left C2 nerve root in this patient with neurofibromatosis type 2 (NF2). This lesion causes effacement of left lateral thecal space at C1-C2 level and abuts the cervical spinal cord on the left, which is demonstrated on Figures 8(a) and 8(b). There is widening of left C1-C2 neural foramen (pink arrow) by this lesion. Additional multiple intracranial meningioma (blue arrows) are also identified on coronal postgadolinium image (Figure 8(c)) in this patient with NF2.

chondrosarcoma when aforementioned diagnostic imaging features are witnessed.

References

[1] W. Nussbeck, D. Neureiter, S. Söder, C. Inwards, and T. Aigner, "Mesenchymal chondrosarcoma: An immunohistochemical study of 10 cases examining prognostic significance of proliferative activity and cellular differentiation," *Pathology*, vol. 36, no. 3, pp. 230–233, 2004.

[2] H. Xu, M. Shao, H. Sun, and S. Li, "Primary mesenchymal chondrosarcoma of the kidney with synchronous implant and infiltrating urothelial carcinoma of the ureter," *Diagnostic Pathology*, vol. 7, no. 1, article no. 125, 2012.

[3] A. G. Huvos, G. Rosen, M. Dabska, and R. C. Marcove, "Mesenchymal chondrosarcoma. A clinicopathologic analysis of 35 patients with emphasis on treatment," *Cancer*, vol. 51, no. 7, pp. 1230–1237, 1983.

[4] Y. Nakashima, K. K. Unni, T. C. Shives, R. G. Swee, and D. C. Dahlin, "Mesenchymal chondrosarcoma of bone and soft tissue. A review of 111 cases," *Cancer*, vol. 57, no. 12, pp. 2444–2453, 1986.

[5] D. Borof, I. Kowalina, W. Wesołowski, W. Kloc, E. Iżycka-Świeszewska, and M. Derenda, "Primary spinal intradural mesenchymal chondrosarcoma with several local regrowths treated with osteoplastic laminotomies: a case report," *The Surgery Journal*, vol. 3, no. 3, 2017.

[6] P. Rao, R. R. Colen, J. M. Bruner, and J. M. Meis, "Extraskeletal myxoid chondrosarcoma presenting as an intradural spinal mass: Report of a rare clinical presentation with an emphasis on differential diagnostic considerations," *Rare Tumors*, vol. 6, no. 4, article no. 5586, pp. 150–153, 2014.

[7] K.-F. Huang, W.-C. Tzaan, and C.-Y. Lin, "Primary intraspinal mesenchymal chondrosarcoma: A case report and literature review," *Chang Gung Medical Journal*, vol. 26, no. 5, pp. 370–376, 2003.

[8] L. Lichtenstein and D. Bernstein, "Unusual benign and malignant chondroid tumors of bone. A survey of some mesenchymal cartilage tumors and malignant chondroblastic tumors, including a few multicentric ones, as well as many atypical benign chondroblastomas and chondromyxoid fibromas," *Cancer*, vol. 12, no. 6, pp. 1142–1157, 1959.

[9] A. H. Salvador, J. W. Beabout, and D. C. Dahlin, "Mesenchymal chondrosarcoma—observations on 30 new cases," *Cancer*, vol. 28, no. 3, pp. 605–615, 1971.

[10] L. G. Shapeero, D. Vanel, D. Couanet, G. Contesso, and L. V. Ackerman, "Extraskeletal mesenchymal chondrosarcoma," *Radiology*, vol. 186, no. 3, pp. 819–826, 1993.

[11] C. R. Wheeless, J. A. Nunley, and J. R. Urbaniak, "Chondrosarcoma," in *Wheeless' Textbook of Orthopaedics*, Duke University. Medical Center, 2016.

[12] I. R. Whittle, C. Smith, P. Navoo, and D. Collie, "Meningiomas," *The Lancet*, vol. 363, no. 9420, pp. 1535–1543, 2004.

[13] M. D. Murphey, W. S. Smith, S. E. Smith, M. J. Kransdorf, and H. T. Temple, "From the archives of the AFIP. Imaging of musculoskeletal neurogenic tumors: radiologic-pathologic correlation," *RadioGraphics*, vol. 19, no. 5, pp. 1253–1280, 1999.

[14] M. Pilavaki, D. Chourmouzi, A. Kiziridou, A. Skordalaki, T. Zarampoukas, and A. Drevelengas, "Imaging of peripheral nerve sheath tumors with pathologic correlation: pictorial review," *European Journal of Radiology*, vol. 52, no. 3, pp. 229–239, 2004.

[15] K. Thamburaj, V. V. Radhakrishnan, B. Thomas, S. Nair, and G. Menon, "Intratumoral microhemorrhages on T2*-weighted gradient-echo imaging helps differentiate vestibular schwannoma from meningioma," *American Journal of Neuroradiology*, vol. 29, no. 3, pp. 552–557, 2008.

[16] G.-S. Bae, S.-W. Choi, J.-Y. Youm, and S.-H. Kim, "Primary spinal dumbbell-shaped mesenchymal chondrosarcoma located intradurally and extradurally," *Journal of Korean Neurosurgical Society*, vol. 50, no. 5, pp. 468–471, 2011.

[17] N. Hashimoto, T. Ueda, S. Joyama et al., "Extraskeletal mesenchymal chondrosarcoma: An imaging review of ten new patients," *Skeletal Radiology*, vol. 34, no. 12, pp. 785–792, 2005.

[18] G. R. Harsh IV and C. B. Wilson, "Central nervous system mesenchymal chondrosarcoma. Case report," *Journal of Neurosurgery*, vol. 61, no. 2, pp. 375–381, 1984.

55

Occipital Hypometabolism on FDG PET/CT Scan in a Child with Hodgkin's Lymphoma

Inci Uslu Biner,[1] Ebru Tatci,[1] Ozlem Ozmen,[1] Atila Gokcek,[2] Haci Ahmet Demir,[3] and Nadide Basak Gulleroglu[4]

[1]*Department of Nuclear Medicine, Ataturk Chest Diseases and Thoracic Surgery Training and Research Hospital, Ankara, Turkey*
[2]*Department of Radiology, Ataturk Chest Diseases and Thoracic Surgery Training and Research Hospital, Ankara, Turkey*
[3]*Department of Pediatrics, Memorial Ankara Hospital, Ankara, Turkey*
[4]*Department of Radiology, Ankara Hematology Oncology Children's Training and Research Hospital, Ankara, Turkey*

Correspondence should be addressed to Inci Uslu Biner; inciuslu@yahoo.com

Academic Editor: Amit Agrawal

It is known that Fluorodeoxyglucose (FDG) Positron Emission/Computed Tomography (PET/CT) images may be helpful for evaluation of brain function in newborns. Here we described the fluorine-18 [18-F] FDG PET/CT imaging findings of encephalomalacia due to perinatal asphyxia in a child with refractory Hodgkin's Lymphoma (HL) who underwent PET/CT scan to stage the primary disease. Prominent hypometabolism was incidentally detected in the occipital regions bilaterally apart from the FDG uptakes in the malign lymphatic infiltrations. This case highlights the potential coexistence of a malignancy and a functional brain disorder.

1. Introduction

Encephalomalacia, also named as cerebral softening, is an area of focal brain damage that is most commonly seen in areas with insufficient blood supply. Cystic encephalomalacia is a softening of neurological tissue within a cystic cavity of the brain in various sizes and usually occurs prenatally during mid-fetal life secondary to a congenital infection (e.g., cytomegalovirus (CMV)) or occlusion of a major cerebral artery. It may also occur secondary to birth asphyxia [1–3].

Neonatal encephalopathy (NE) is a general term to define cerebral injury that can be caused by a variety of conditions. The most common cause of NE is hypoxia-ischemia, which is clinically named as hypoxic ischemic encephalopathy (HIE). It is a significant complication of neonatal-perinatal asphyxia that can cause some severe and permanent neuropsychological sequela or death [4]. HIE can occur secondary to several conditions including hypoglycemia [5, 6].

When the cause is an obstruction of blood flow, the temporal and parietal lobes are the most expected sites to be affected as cystic encephalomalacia [2, 3] while thinning of cerebral cortex predominantly in parietooccipital lobes is reported in several studies in hypoglycemic conditions [7].

In examining infants with suspected hypoxic ischemic brain injury, the main method is Magnetic Resonance Imaging (MRI). It is known that FDG PET/CT images may be helpful for evaluation of brain function in newborns. Here we described the metabolic imaging patterns of encephalomalacia due to perinatal asphyxia by MRI images in a child with refractory Hodgkin's Lymphoma (HL) who underwent PET/CT to stage the primary disease.

2. Case Report

A 3-year-old girl who was admitted to hospital with palpable masses in her neck and diagnosed as Hodgkin's Lymphoma (HL) was referred to our department for F-18 FDG PET/CT scan to stage the primary disease. She also had history of birth asphixia and congenital hypothyroidism with some clinical findings such as cerebral palsy, neurodevelopmental delay, seizures, and cortical blindness. She was suffering from seizures since she was three months old and started to

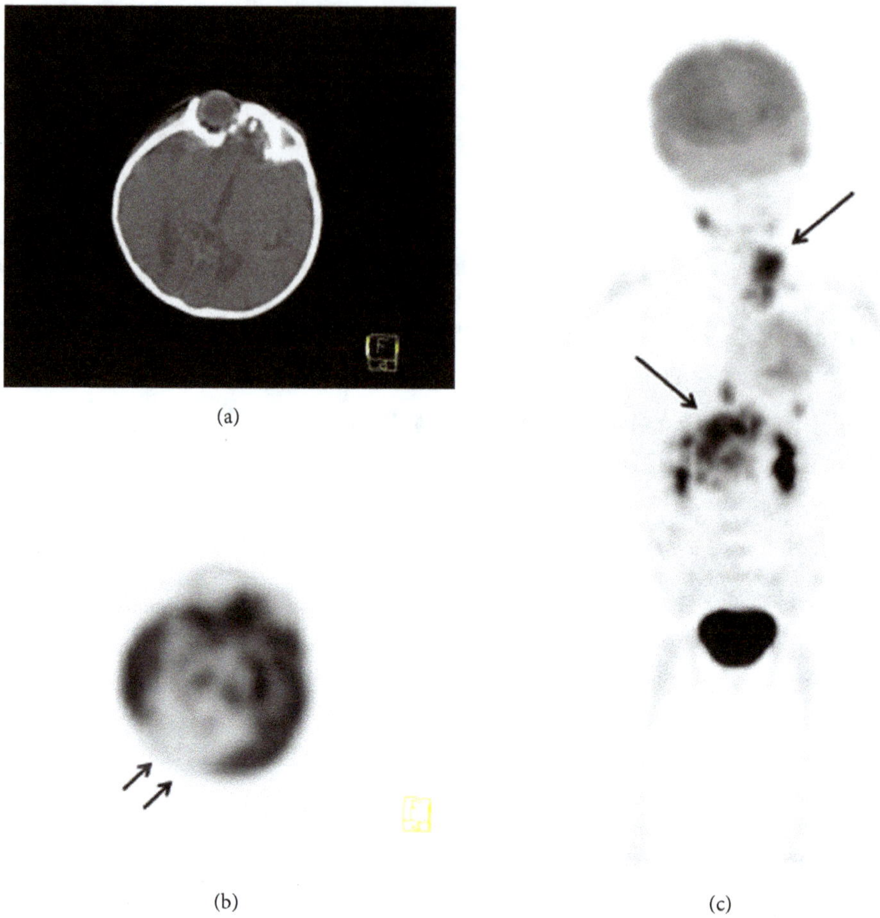

FIGURE 1: (a, b) In the cranial axial images of FDG PET/CT scan, hypometabolism in the occipital regions bilaterally was seen (arrows) and (c) maximum intensity projection (MIP) images of the staging PET/CT examination demonstrated focal increased FDG uptakes in the lymph nodes on the cervical and abdominal regions (long arrows).

take antiepileptics like Phenobarbital and Primidone. EEG was interpreted as showing epileptiform activity in the left temporoparietal region. Visual Evoked Potentials (VEP) showed abnormal visually evoked response (VER) with bilaterally affected nerves and deformed P1 waves. In the neurological examination, the deep tendon reflexes were normal if examined but mostly could not be examined since the child was agitated; the muscle tonus was increased in both upper and lower extremities without any pathological reflex. Additionally, she was microcephalic. She had not any seizure on the day of PET/CT scanning. She had not any history of brain operation and she and her parents had no history of any metabolic disorders and infections and that were retrospectively learned after evaluation of her PET/CT scan. Epstein Barr Virus sitology was negative. Also there is a history of consanguineous marriage of her parents. The glucose level was 40 mg/dL after birth but she did not have an episode of prominent and resistant hypoglycemia in the treatment period of lymphoma. The infant did not survive because of refractory HL. On cranial Computed Tomography (CT) images before the diagnosis of lymphoma, occupying mass lesion and hemorrhage were not seen in which volume loss and hypodensity were detected at the occipital region. FDG PET/CT images demonstrated prominent hypometabolism in the occipital regions bilaterally (Figures 1(a) and 1(b)) apart from the FDG uptakes in the malign lymphatic infiltrations in the cervical and abdominal regions (Figure 1(c)). On brain MRI, area of encephalomalacia was present in occipital region with surrounding gliosis. Both visual cortices were hyperintense on axial T2-weighted (a) series and in T2 and flair weighted series posterior parasagittal pattern of increased signal intensity in both occipital lobes (Figures 2(a) and 2(b)). On flair weighted series (Figure 2(b)), some subcortical cystic encephalomalacic changes in millimetric dimensions were seen and the thinning of the cerebral cortex also was noted in the occipital regions. MRI findings that were taken at different times (performed approximately interval of one year) were the same and not progressive. The diminished metabolic activity in PET/CT images was considered to be consistent with MRI findings and a part of encephalomalacia sequela. Informed consent was obtained from her parents prior to scanning.

3. Discussion

In our case, the findings of PET/CT and MRI were thought to be an encephalomalacia due to hypoglycemia and perinatal asphyxia because of the location and the corresponding

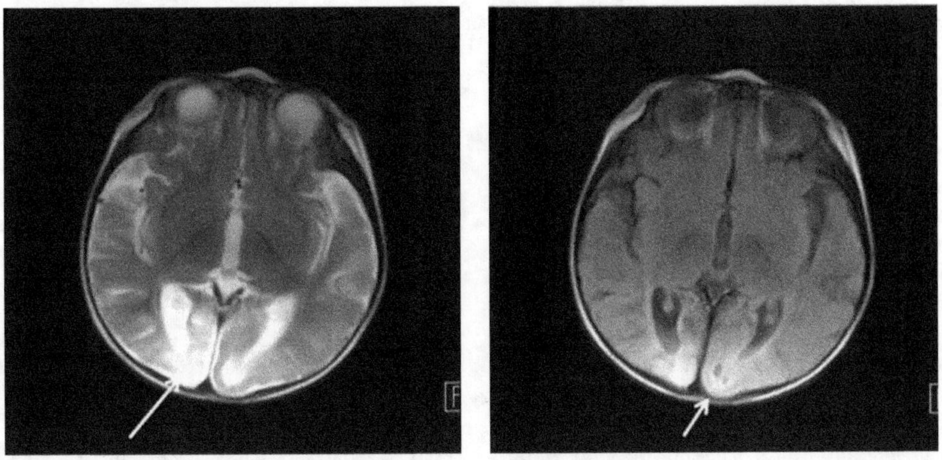

(a) (b)

Figure 2: On brain Magnetic Resonance (MR) images, both visual cortices were hyperintense (a) (long arrow) on T2-weighted and flair weighted (b) (arrow) series.

clinical symptoms, the presence of the same MRI findings that were taken at different times. Neonatal encephalopathy may result from a variety of conditions. When caused by hypoxic ischemic brain injury, it is called HIE. HIE is one of the most common causes of cerebral palsy and other severe neurological deficits in children and either atrophy or white matter demyelination may be seen [4]. The most sensitive and specific imaging technique for examining infants with suspected hypoxic ischemic brain injury is MRI [8]. FDG PET/CT may provide information about metabolic status of brain tissue and may be a complementary to other methods in the estimation of probable neurologic sequela in patients with HIE due to perinatal asphyxia. Studies in the literature revealed that rates of glucose utilization in the areas of cortical scarring were lower than the other regions of the brain in term newborns with hypoxic ischemic encephalopathy [9]. Occipital hypometabolism was a constant finding in follow-up PET/CT images that were performed for the evaluation of therapy response of lymphoma in this case.

HL is uncommon in children under 10 years of age and it is rarely seen in children under 5 years [10]. Since the HL was not expected to occur at this age group of children, it was also interesting that this infant had a diagnose of HL at an earlier age than expected and the lymphoma was refractory; the infant did not survive because of the lymphoma.

Inflammation of the brain nearly always is associated with white matter lymphoma in the brain and leads to demyelination. Brain biopsy has an importance in the differential diagnosis of primary central nervous system lymphoma (PCNSL) and inflammatory demyelination while any suspected contrast-enhanced white matter lesion was examined [11]. In MRI images of our case, inflammation findings like meningeal thickening and suppression of the brain sulcus secondary to edema were not seen and white matter myelination was found to be behind her age. Unfortunately, there was not any MRI scanning of this child performed after the diagnosis of lymphoma because of her convulsions and clinical status and her parent's demand. Therefore, any demyelination that might be caused by white matter lymphoma could not be evaluated and we could not have a chance to compare the pre and post diagnose MRI findings. However, demyelination secondary to lymphoma was not considered with priority by taking into account the previous MRI findings.

Hypoglycemia is a rare complication of Hodgkin's disease [12]. However, MRI of this child was performed previously because of the convulsions and the scan findings mentioned above were detected before the diagnosis of lymphoma. Additionally, any hypoglycemic episode was not seen in this child during the diagnosis and treatment period of the lymphoma. Therefore, the correlated clinical and imaging findings of this child are thought to be more coincidental rather than a paraneoplastic hypoglycemia sequel.

In conclusion, this is a presentation of coexistence of HL and a functional brain disorder in a child. The coexistence of development of lymphoma at an earlier age and the presence of perinatal asphyxia history is challenging and it may be discussed to search the probable trigger effect of hypoxic condition to the development of a following malignancy in early infantile period with further studies. Also, this case reminds us of the importance of incidental findings that can be detected in PET/CT scans.

Disclosure

Haci Ahmet Demir was formerly working at Ankara Hematology Oncology Children's Training and Research Hospital, Department of Pediatric Oncology, Ankara, Turkey.

References

[1] J. J. Volpe, *Neurology of the Newborn*, WB Saunders Company, Philadelphia, Pa, USA, 2008.

[2] K. M. Weidenheim, S. R. Bodhireddy, G. J. Nuovo, S. J. Nelson, and D. W. Dickson, "Multicystic encephalopathy: review of eight cases with etiologic considerations," *Journal of Neuropathology and Experimental Neurology*, vol. 54, no. 2, pp. 268–275, 1995.

[3] I. Ferrer and C. Navarro, "Multicystic encephalomalacia of infancy. Clinico-pathological report of 7 cases," *Journal of the Neurological Sciences*, vol. 38, no. 2, pp. 179–189, 1978.

[4] S. Shankaran, "Neonatal encephalopathy treatment with hypothermia," *Journal of Neurotrauma*, vol. 26, no. 3, pp. 437–443, 2009.

[5] P. Basu, S. Som, N. Choudhuri, and H. Das, "Contribution of the blood glucose level in perinatal asphyxia," *European Journal of Pediatrics*, vol. 168, no. 7, pp. 833–838, 2009.

[6] H. Kahraman, "Ischemic-hypoxic encephalopathy," *Turkiye Klinikleri Journal of Surgical Medical Sciences*, vol. 3, no. 37, pp. 49–54, 2007.

[7] J. A. Spar, J. D. Lewine, and W. W. Orrison Jr., "Neonatal hypoglycemia: CT and MR findings," *American Journal of Neuroradiology*, vol. 15, no. 8, pp. 1477–1478, 1994.

[8] E. Martin and A. J. Barkovic, "Magnetic resonanse imaging in perinatal asphixia Archives of Disease in Childhood," *Archives of Disease in Childhood—Fetal and Neonatal Edition*, vol. 72, no. 1, pp. 62–70, 1995.

[9] L. W. Doyle, C. Nahmias, G. Firnau, D. B. Kenyon, E. S. Garnett, and J. C. Sinclair, "Regional cerebral glucose metabolism of newborn infants measured by positron emission tomography," *Developmental Medicine and Child Neurology*, vol. 25, no. 2, pp. 143–151, 1983.

[10] J. F. Rico and C. K. Tebbi, "Hodgkin lymphoma in children: a review," *Austin Journal of Pediatrics*, vol. 1, no. 3, p. 1013, 2014.

[11] L. Husseini, A. Saleh, G. Reifenberger, H.-P. Hartung, and B. C. Kieseier, "Inflammatory demyelinating brain lesions heralding primary CNS lymphoma," *The Canadian Journal of Neurological Sciences*, vol. 39, no. 1, pp. 6–10, 2012.

[12] C. V. Soares-Welch, S. R. Zeldenrust, C. A. Conover, C. S. Grant, and F. J. Service, "Hodgkin's lymphoma manifesting with hypoglycemia," *Endocrine Practice*, vol. 9, no. 1, pp. 96–97, 2003.

Permissions

All chapters in this book were first published in CRR, by Hindawi Publishing Corporation; hereby published with permission under the Creative Commons Attribution License or equivalent. Every chapter published in this book has been scrutinized by our experts. Their significance has been extensively debated. The topics covered herein carry significant findings which will fuel the growth of the discipline. They may even be implemented as practical applications or may be referred to as a beginning point for another development.

The contributors of this book come from diverse backgrounds, making this book a truly international effort. This book will bring forth new frontiers with its revolutionizing research information and detailed analysis of the nascent developments around the world.

We would like to thank all the contributing authors for lending their expertise to make the book truly unique. They have played a crucial role in the development of this book. Without their invaluable contributions this book wouldn't have been possible. They have made vital efforts to compile up to date information on the varied aspects of this subject to make this book a valuable addition to the collection of many professionals and students.

This book was conceptualized with the vision of imparting up-to-date information and advanced data in this field. To ensure the same, a matchless editorial board was set up. Every individual on the board went through rigorous rounds of assessment to prove their worth. After which they invested a large part of their time researching and compiling the most relevant data for our readers.

The editorial board has been involved in producing this book since its inception. They have spent rigorous hours researching and exploring the diverse topics which have resulted in the successful publishing of this book. They have passed on their knowledge of decades through this book. To expedite this challenging task, the publisher supported the team at every step. A small team of assistant editors was also appointed to further simplify the editing procedure and attain best results for the readers.

Apart from the editorial board, the designing team has also invested a significant amount of their time in understanding the subject and creating the most relevant covers. They scrutinized every image to scout for the most suitable representation of the subject and create an appropriate cover for the book.

The publishing team has been an ardent support to the editorial, designing and production team. Their endless efforts to recruit the best for this project, has resulted in the accomplishment of this book. They are a veteran in the field of academics and their pool of knowledge is as vast as their experience in printing. Their expertise and guidance has proved useful at every step. Their uncompromising quality standards have made this book an exceptional effort. Their encouragement from time to time has been an inspiration for everyone.

The publisher and the editorial board hope that this book will prove to be a valuable piece of knowledge for researchers, students, practitioners and scholars across the globe.

List of Contributors

Serap Dogan, Serkan Senol, Hakan Imamoglu, Afra Ekinci and Mustafa Ozturk
Department of Radiology, Erciyes University Medical Faculty, Kayseri, Turkey

Ummuhan Abdulrezzak
Department of Nuclear Medicine, Erciyes University Medical Faculty, Kayseri, Turkey

Imdat Yuce
Department of Otorhinolaryngology, Erciyes University Medical Faculty, Kayseri, Turkey

Kei Shibuya, Yoshinori Koyama and Yoshito Tsushima
Department of Diagnostic and Interventional Radiology, Gunma University Hospital, 3-39-22 Showa-machi, Maebashi, Gunma 371-8511, Japan

Hiroki Tahara and Suguru Takeuchi
Department of Gastroenterology, Saiseikai Maebashi Hospital, 564-1 Kamishinden-machi, Maebashi, Gunma 371-0821, Japan

Ebru Ozan and Gokce Kaan Atac
Department of Radiology, Ufuk University School of Medicine, 06520 Ankara, Turkey

Egemen Akincioglu
Department of Pathology, Ufuk University School of Medicine, 06520 Ankara, Turkey

Mete Keskin and Kamil Gulpinar
Department of General Surgery, Ufuk University School of Medicine, 06520 Ankara, Turkey

Ahmed Fathala, Alaa Alduraibi and Moheieldin M. Abouzied
Department of Radiology, Division Nuclear Medicine Division and Cardiothoracic Radiology Division, King Faisal Specialist Hospital and Research Centre, MBC 28, Riyadh 11211, Saudi Arabia

Sharad M. Malvadkar, Madhuri S. Malvadkar, Shilpa V. Domkundwar and Shariq Mohd
Department of Radiodiagnosis, Grant Medical College and Sir JJ Group of Hospitals, Byculla, Mumbai 400008, India

Nicholas Beckmann and Susanna Spence
Department of Diagnostic and Interventional Imaging, Memorial Hermann, University of Texas Health Science Center, 6431 Fannin Street, No. 2.130B, Houston, TX 77030, USA

Elijah Burton
David Grant USAF Medical Center, Fairfield, CA, USA
Kristian Schafernak
University of Arizona College of Medicine, Phoenix, AZ, USA
Mayo Clinic College of Medicine, Phoenix, AZ, USA

Elaine Morgan and Jonathan Samet
Northwestern University Feinberg School of Medicine, Chicago, IL, USA

Ahmad Enshaei
Isfahan University of Medical Science, Kashani Hospital, Kashani Ave, Isfahan, Iran

Arash A. Boora
University of Queensland, St. Lucia, QLD, Australia

Diana Taheri
Department of Pathology, Isfahan Kidney Diseases Research Centre, Isfahan University of Medical Sciences, Isfahan, Iran

Zahra Changizi
Department of Internal Medicine, Saadi Hospital, Isfahan, Iran

Nahid Bahmani
Department of Radiology, Saadi Hospital, Isfahan, Iran

Kazuhiko Morikawa, Hirokazu Ashida, Yosuke Nozawa, Kenji Motohashi, Takao Igarashi and Hiroya Ojiri
Department of Radiology, The Jikei University School of Medicine, Tokyo, Japan

Yuji Kanaoka and Takao Ohki
Department of Vascular Surgery, The Jikei University School of Medicine, Tokyo, Japan

Moulion Tapouh Jean Roger
Yaounde University Hospital Center, Yaounde, Cameroon

Fokou Marcus
Department of Surgery, Yaounde General Hospital, Yaounde, Cameroon

Fongang Emmanuel
Radiology Department, Yaounde General Hospital, Yaounde, Cameroon

Juimo Alain Georges
Radiology Department, Yaounde General Hospital, Yaounde, Cameroon
Faculty of Medicine and Biomedical Sciences (FMBS), Yaounde, Cameroon

Moifo Boniface
Faculty of Medicine and Biomedical Sciences (FMBS), Yaounde, Cameroon
Radiology Department, Yaounde Gynaeco-Obstetric and Paediatric Hospital, Yaounde, Cameroon

Lama K. Agoda-Koussema
Department of Radiology, Lom´e Teaching Hospital, University of Lom´e, Lom´e, Togo

Nicoleta Modruz, AnthonyMichelot, Samer Naffa, Véronique Jeudy and Raymond Kaczmarek
Department of Radiology, Cornouaille Intercommunal Hospital, 29000 Quimper, France

Mazamaesso Tchaou
Department of Radiology, Lom´e Teaching Hospital, University of Lom´e, Lom´e, Togo
Department of Radiology, Cornouaille Intercommunal Hospital, 29000 Quimper, France

F. Chegai, A. U. Cavallo, M. Forcina, V. Giuricin, F. Castellani, L. Greco and G. Sergiacomi
Department of Diagnostic and Molecular Imaging, RadiationTherapy and Interventional Radiology, University Hospital Tor Vergata, Viale Oxford 81, 00133 Rome, Italy

M. Manuelli and T. M. Manzia
Organ Transplantation Unit, University Hospital Tor Vergata, Rome, Italy

Haji Mohammed Nazir, Akshiitha Ramesh Baabhu, Yuvaraj Muralidharan and Seena Cheppala Rajan
Saveetha Medical College and Hospital, Saveetha Nagar, Thandalam, Chennai, Tamil Nadu 602105, India

Darren Fitzpatrick
Department of Radiology, Mount Sinai Medical Center, 1 Gustave Levy Place, New York, NY 10029, USA

Catherine Petchprapa and Leon Rybak
Department of Radiology, NYU School of Medicine, 660 1st Avenue, 1st Floor, New York, NY 10016, USA

Quoc-Bao D. Nguyen, Avital Perry, Christopher S. Graffeo, Cody L. Nesvick, Aditya Raghunathan, Mark E. Jentoft, Brian P. O'Neill, Padraig P. Morris, Jonathan M. Morris and Jamie J. Van Gompe
Texas A&M Health Science Center College of Medicine, Temple, TX, USA

Avital Perry, Christopher S. Graffeo and Cody L. Nesvick
Department of Neurological Surgery, Mayo Clinic, Rochester, MN, USA

Aditya Raghunathan and Mark E. Jentoft
Department of Laboratory Medicine and Pathology, Mayo Clinic, Rochester, MN, USA
Brian P. O'Neill
Department of Neurology, Mayo Clinic, Rochester, MN, USA

Padraig P.Morris and Jonathan M.Morris
Department of Radiology, Mayo Clinic, Rochester, MN, USA

Jamie J. Van Gompel
Department of Neurological Surgery, Mayo Clinic, Rochester, MN, USA
Department of Otolaryngology-Head and Neck Surgery, Mayo Clinic, Rochester, MN, USA

Ilkay Çamlidağ, Mehmet Selim Nural and Murat Danaci
Department of Radiology, Ondokuz MayısUniversity, Kurupelit, 55139 Samsun, Turkey

Ilhan Karabiçak and Kağan Karabulut
Department of General Surgery, Ondokuz Mayıs University, Kurupelit, 55139 Samsun, Turkey

Connie Hapgood
Department of Radiology, Memorial University, St. John's, NL, Canada

Allison DeLong
Faculty of Medicine, Memorial University, St. John's, NL, Canada

Sharandran Chandra Mohan, Krishna Mohan Gummalla and Martin Weng Chin H'ng
Diagnostic Radiology Department, Tan Tock Seng Hospital, 11 Jalan Tan Tock Seng, Singapore 308433

Rohit Aiyer
Department of Psychiatry, Hofstra Northwell Health, Staten Island University Hospital, Staten Island, NY, USA

Janice Hwang
Department of Radiology, Hofstra NorthwellHealth, Staten Island University Hospital, Staten Island, NY, USA

Edward H. Yu
Department of Neurology, Hofstra Northwell Health, Staten Island University Hospital, Staten Island, NY, USA

Danilo Coco and Massimo Viola
Department of Surgery, Card. G. Panico Hospital of Tricase, 73039 Tricase, Italy

Sara Cecchini and Stefano Ricci
Department of Radiology, INRCA Hospital of Ancona, 60125 Ancona, Italy

Silvana Leanza and Roberto Campagnacci
Department of Surgery, C. Urbani Hospital of Jesi, 60035 Jesi, Italy

Danilo Coco
Madre Teresa of Calcutta Hospital, Schiavonia, Padova, Italy

Silvana Leanza
Carlo Urbani Hospital, Jesi, Ancona, Italy

Xin Cao
Medical College, Shandong University, Jinan, Shandong 250012, China

Qiang Fang
Medical College, Taishan Medical University, Tai'an, Shandong 271000, China

Hao Shi
Department of Medical Imaging, Qianfoshan Hospital Affiliated to Shandong University, Jinan, Shandong 250014, China

Deepak Vallabhaneni
Department of Internal Medicine, SUNY Upstate Medical University, Syracuse, NY, USA

Muhammad Atif Naveed
Department of Radiology, Shaukat Khanum Memorial Cancer Hospital, Lahore, Pakistan
Department of Radiology, SUNY Upstate Medical University, Syracuse, NY 13210, USA

Rajiv Mangla
Department of Radiology, SUNY Upstate Medical University, Syracuse, NY 13210, USA

Awss Zidan
Department of Neurology, SUNY Upstate Medical University, Syracuse, NY, USA

Rashi I. Mehta
Department of Radiology, SUNY Upstate Medical University, Syracuse, NY 13210, USA
Department of Radiology, West Virginia University, Morgantown, WV, USA

George Rahmani and Sarah Power
Department of Radiology, Beaumont Hospital, Dublin, Ireland

Tanner R. Henrie1
Tulane University School of Medicine, New Orleans, LA, USA

John G. Skedros
The University of Utah Department of Orthopaedic Surgery, Salt Lake City, UT, USA
Utah Orthopaedic Specialists, Salt Lake City, UT, USA
Intermountain Medical Center, Salt Lake City, UT, USA

H. Q. C. Lim, X. W. J. Lee and N. Mathias
Hairmyres Hospital, Glasgow G75 8RG, UK

Maxine Darke, Anil Dasyam, Matthew Then, Kavita Varma, Amir A. Borhani and Rakesh Varma
University of Pittsburgh Medical Center, 200 Lothrop Street, Pittsburgh, PA 15213, USA

Necdet Poyraz
Department of Radiology, Meram Faculty of Medicine, Necmettin Erbakan University, Konya 42080, Turkey

Soner DemirbaŞ, Celalettin Korkmaz and KürŞat Uzun
Department of Pulmonary Disease, Meram Faculty of Medicine, Necmettin Erbakan University, Konya 42080, Turkey

Rashid AL Umairi and Anastasia Oikonomou
Department of Medical Imaging, Sunnybrook Health Sciences Centre, University of Toronto, Toronto, ON, Canada

Danielle Blunt and Matthew Cheung
Department of Medicine, Sunnybrook Health Sciences Centre, University of Toronto, Toronto, ON, Canada

Wedad Hana
Department of Anatomic Pathology, Sunnybrook Health Sciences Centre, University of Toronto, ON, Canada

Hidayatullah Hamidi, Fazel Rahman Faizi, Najibullah Rasouly and Mer Mahmood Shah Hoshang
French Medical Institute for Children (FMIC), Kabul, Afghanistan

Joseph Tseng
Department of Medicine, University of California Irvine School of Medicine, 333 City BoulevardWest, Suite 400, Orange, CA 92868, USA
Michael Leshen
Creighton University School of Medicine, Phoenix Regional Campus, 350WThomas Road, Phoenix, AZ 85013, USA

Todd Chapman, Ryan Scott and Olga Kalinkin
Department of Radiology, St. Joseph's Hospital, 350WThomas Road, Phoenix, AZ 85013, USA

Sayf Al-Katib, Robert Colvin and Farnoosh Sokhandon
Department of Diagnostic Radiology and Molecular Imaging, Oakland University William Beaumont School of Medicine, Beaumont Health, Royal Oak, MI, USA

Katherine Chung
Geisinger Commonwealth School of Medicine, Scranton PA 18510, USA

Umar Tariq, Rabia M. Khan, Thomas P. Nickles and Joseph H. Lock Jr.
Department of Radiology, Geisinger Medical Center, Danville PA 17821, USA

Jama A. Mohamud
Department of Medical Imaging, Subei People's Hospital of Jiangsu Province, Medical College of Yangzhou University, Yangzhou, China

Jingtao Wu and Ye Jing
Department of Medical Imaging, Subei People's Hospital of Jiangsu Province, Yangzhou University, Yangzhou, China

Yu Wang
Department of Neurology, Subei People's Hospital of Jiangsu Province, Dalian Medical University, Dalian, Liaoning Province, China

Mihiri Wettasinghe and Kumari Pussepitiya
Department of Radiology, Teaching Hospital, Peradeniya, Sri Lanka

Bandula Samarasinghe
Department of Surgery, Faculty of Medicine, University of Peradeniya, Peradeniya, Sri Lanka

Nuwan Wickramasinghe
Department of Community Medicine, Faculty of Medicine and Allied Sciences, Rajarata University of Sri Lanka, Saliyapura, Sri Lanka

C. L. Fonseka and C. K. Bodinayake
University Medical Unit, Teaching Hospital Karapitiya, Galle, Sri Lanka
Department of Internal Medicine, Faculty of Medicine, University of Ruhuna, Sri Lanka

A. G. T. A. Kariyawasam, S. A. G. L. Singhapura, C. M. de Silva, T. E. Kanakkahewa and I. G. T. M. Senarathna
Department of Internal Medicine, Faculty of Medicine, University of Ruhuna, Sri Lanka

Joana Ruivo Rodrigues
Radiology Unit, Medical Imaging Department, Centro Hospitalar e Universit´ario de Coimbra, Coimbra, Portugal

Manuel João Brito
Pediatric Oncology Department, Hospital Pedi´atrico, Centro Hospitalar e Universit´ario de Coimbra, Coimbra, Portugal

Rui Pedro Faria Pais and Sílvia Carvalho,
Neuroradiology Unit, Medical Imaging Department, Centro Hospitalar e Universit´ario de Coimbra, Coimbra, Portugal

Edwige Kafando and Derek Ndangoh
Faculty of Medicine and Biomedical Sciences, University of Yaounde I, Yaounde, Cameroon

Boniface Moifo
Faculty of Medicine and Biomedical Sciences, University of Yaounde I, Yaounde, Cameroon
Department of Radiology, Yaounde Gynaeco-Obstetric and Pediatric Hospital, Yaounde, Cameroon

Faustin Mouafo Tambo
Faculty of Medicine and Biomedical Sciences, University of Yaounde I, Yaounde, Cameroon
Department of Pediatric Surgery, Yaounde Gynaeco-Obstetric and Pediatric Hospital, Yaounde, Cameroon

Evelyn Mah
Faculty of Medicine and Biomedical Sciences, University of Yaounde I, Yaounde, Cameroon
Department of Neonatology, Yaounde Gynaeco-Obstetric and Pediatric Hospital, Yaounde, Cameroon

Landry Mbouche
Department of Pediatric Surgery, Yaounde Gynaeco-Obstetric and Pediatric Hospital, Yaounde, Cameroon

Pierluca Torcia, Silvia Squarza, Paolo Rigamonti, Giovanni Damiani and Maurizio Cariati
ASST Santi Paolo and Carlo, San Carlo Borromeo Hospital, Department of Diagnostic Science, Radiology and Interventional Radiology Unit, Via Pio II 3, 20153 Milano, Italy

Umberto G. Rossi
ASST Santi Paolo and Carlo, San Carlo Borromeo Hospital, Department of Diagnostic Science, Radiology and Interventional Radiology Unit, Via Pio II 3, 20153 Milano, Italy
Department of Diagnostic Imaging, Interventional Radiology Unit, Galliera Hospital, Mura delle Cappuccine 14, 16128 Genova, Italy

Lorenzo Carlo Pescatori
Postgraduation School in Radiodiagnostics, Universit`a degli Studi di Milano, Via Festa del Perdono 7, 20122 Milano, Italy

Sanjay M. Khaladkar, Sushen Kumar Kondapavuluri, Anubhav Kamal, Raghav Kalra and Vigyat Kamal
Department of Radio-Diagnosis, Dr. D. Y. PatilMedical College, Pimpri, Pune 411018, India

Sanjay Khaladkar, Avadhesh Chauhan, Arijit Ghosh, Kunaal Jain and Surbhi Chauhan
Department of Radio-Diagnosis, Dr. D. Y. PatilMedical College and Research Center, Pimpri, Pune, India

Anagha R. Joshi, Saurabh Joshi, Kiran Kale, Rahul Jain and Jernail Singh Bava
Department of Radiology, Lokmanya Tilak Municipal Medical College and General Hospital, Sion West, Mumbai, Maharashtra 400022, India

Joseph R. Stein and Daniel A. Reidman
The Regional Medical Center, 3000 St. Matthews Road, Orangeburg, SC 29118, USA

Daniel Jeong, Kenneth L. Gage, Claudia G. Berman and Jaime L. Montilla-Soler
Department of Radiology, H. Lee Moffitt Cancer Center, Tampa, FL 33612, USA

Ibtisam Musallam Aljohani
Ministry of National Guard, Health Affairs, King Abdulaziz Medical City, Medical Imaging Department, Riyadh, Saudi Arabia

Khalefa Ali Alghofaily
College of Medicine, Medical Imaging Department, Al-Qassim University, Buraydah, Saudi Arabia

Sebastian R. McWilliams
Mallinckrodt Institute of Radiology, Washington University, St. Louis, MO, USA

Mnahi Bin Saeedan
King Faisal Specialist Hospital and Research Center, Department of Radiology, Riyadh 1121, Saudi Arabia

Filipa Vilaverde and Alcinda Reis
Servic¸o de Imagiologia, Centro Hospitalar de Entre o Douro e Vouga, Santa Maria da Feira, Portugal

Ana Rocha
Servicio de Radiolog´ıa, Hospital Povisa, Vigo, Spain

Francisco Rego Costa, Cátia Esteves and Lina Melão
Department of Radiology, São João Hospital, Alameda Professor Hernâni Monteiro, 4200-319 Porto, Portugal

Rachna Rath, Punyashlok Pati and Sonalisa Sahoo
Department of Oral and Maxillofacial Pathology, SCB Government Dental College and Hospital, Cuttack 753007, India

Sheetal Kaur
Department of Radio Diagnosis, Acharya Harihar Regional Cancer Centre, Cuttack 753007, India

Shadab Ali Baig
Department of Oral and Maxillofacial Surgery, SCB Government Dental College and Hospital, Cuttack 753007, India

Víctor Manuel Suárez-Vega, Carlos Sánchez Almaraz, Ana Isabel Bernardo and Ricardo Rodríguez-Díaz
Radiology Department, Hospital Infanta Elena, Valdemoro, 28342Madrid, Spain

Ana Díez Barrio and Leticia Martín Gil
Neurology Department, Hospital Infanta Elena, Valdemoro, 28342Madrid, Spain

Romeu Duarte Mesquita and Marta Sousa
Department of Radiology, Centro Hospitalar de Entre o Douro e Vouga, Santa Maria da Feira, Portugal

Carmen Trinidad
Department of Radiology, Hospital Povisa, Vigo, Spain

Eugénia Pinto
Department of Pathology, Centro Hospitalar de Lisboa Central, Lisboa, Portugal

Iosu Antón Badiola
Department of Pathology, Hospital Povisa, Vigo, Spain

Isabel Sollozo-Dupont, Héctor Alejandro Domínguez-Hernández, Cecilia Pavón-Hernández, Yolanda Villaseñor-Navarro and M. Patricia Pérez-Badillo
Department of Radiology and Imaging, Instituto Nacional de Cancerolog´ıa (INCan), Mexico City, Mexico

Robin Shaw-Dulin
Department of Surgical Oncology, Instituto Nacional de Cancerolog´ıa (INCan), Mexico City, Mexico

Victor Manuel Pérez-Sánchez, Alejandro Javier España-Ferrufino, Laura Marysol Álvarez-Guadarrama and Fany Iris Porras-Reyes
Department of Surgical Pathology, Instituto Nacional de Cancerolog´ıa (INCan), Mexico City, Mexico

V. Chandra, E. Wajswol, M. Shahid, A. Kumar and S. Contractor
Department of Radiology, Rutgers New Jersey Medical School, Newark, NJ, USA

Khalefa Ali Alghofaily
Radiology Department, Al Qassim University, Buraydah, Saudi Arabia

Musab Hamoud Almushayqih and Abdullah Abdulrahman Bin Salamah
King Saud University and King Khalid University Hospital, Riyadh, Saudi Arabia

Muhannad Faleh Alanazi
Radiology Department, Al Jouf University, Al Jawf, Saudi Arabia

Halldor Benediktsson
King Faisal Specialist Hospital and Research Centre, Riyadh, Saudi Arabia

Tomohiro Kikuchi, Hiroyuki Fujii, Akifumi Fujita and Hideharu Sugimoto
Department of Radiology, Jichi Medical University, School of Medicine, 3311-1 Yakushiji, Shimotsuke, Tochigi 329-0498, Japan

Tomoko Sugiyama
Department of Dentistry, Oral and Maxillofacial Surgery, Jichi Medical University, School of Medicine, 3311-1 Yakushiji, Shimotsuke, Tochigi 329-0498, Japan

Elizabeth Presutto, Sejal Patel and Sajeev Ezhapilli
Department of Radiology, SUNY Upstate Medical University, Room 3530, 750 East Adams Street, Syracuse, NY 13210, USA

Joseph Fullmer
Department of Pathology, SUNY Upstate Medical University, 750 East Adams Street, Syracuse, NY, USA

Inci Uslu Biner, Ebru Tatci and Ozlem Ozmen
Department of Nuclear Medicine, Ataturk Chest Diseases andThoracic Surgery Training and Research Hospital, Ankara, Turkey

Atila Gokcek
Department of Radiology, Ataturk Chest Diseases andThoracic Surgery Training and Research Hospital, Ankara, Turkey

Haci Ahmet Demir
Department of Pediatrics, Memorial Ankara Hospital, Ankara, Turkey

Nadide Basak Gulleroglu
Department of Radiology, Ankara Hematology Oncology Children's Training and Research Hospital, Ankara, Turkey

Index